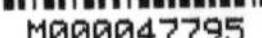

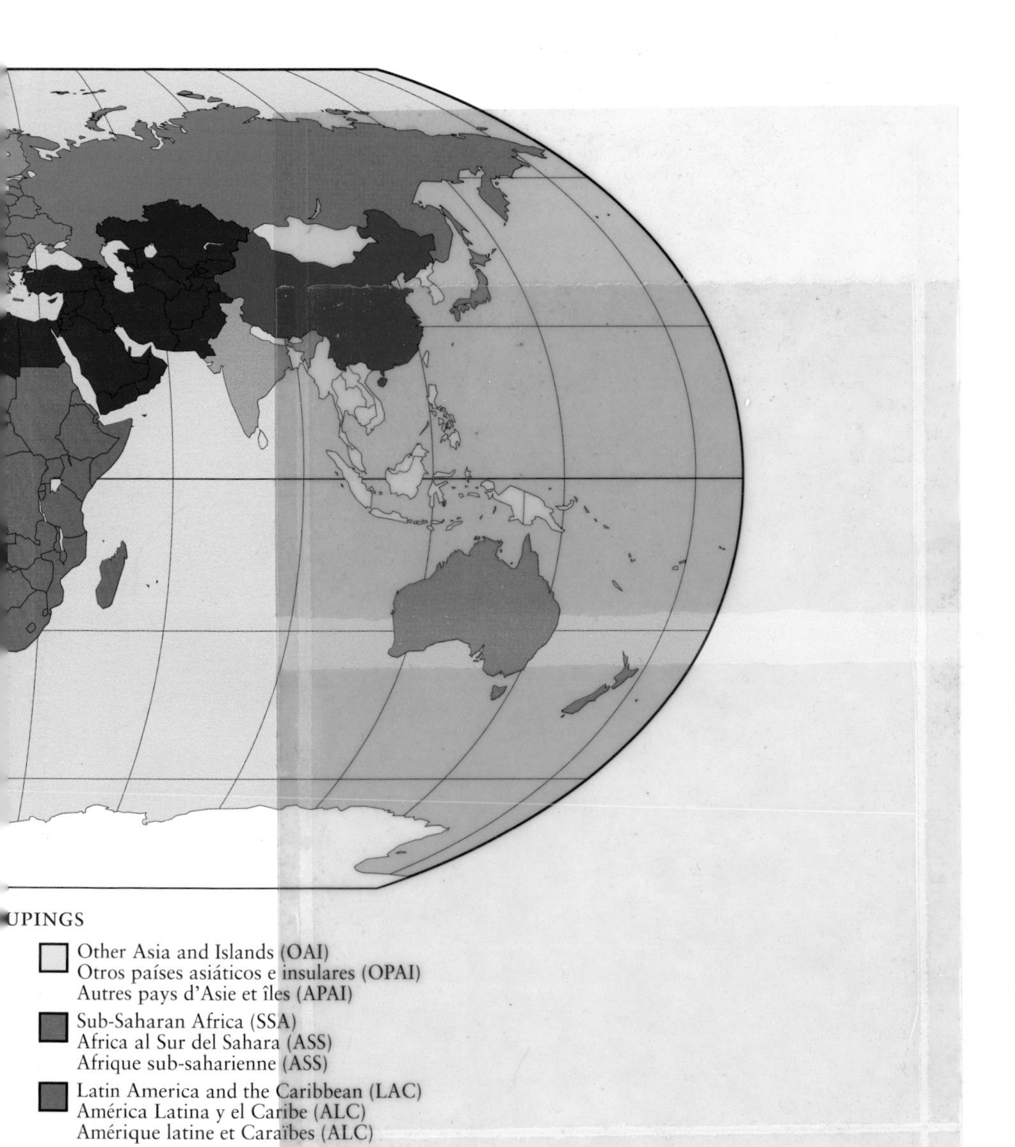

UPINGS

- Other Asia and Islands (OAI)
  Otros países asiáticos e insulares (OPAI)
  Autres pays d'Asie et îles (APAI)
- Sub-Saharan Africa (SSA)
  Africa al Sur del Sahara (ASS)
  Afrique sub-saharienne (ASS)
- Latin America and the Caribbean (LAC)
  América Latina y el Caribe (ALC)
  Amérique latine et Caraïbes (ALC)
- Middle Eastern Crescent (MEC)
  Arco del Oriente Medio (AOM)
  Croissant moyen-oriental (CMO)

GLOBAL BURDEN OF DISEASE AND INJURY SERIES
VOLUME III

HEALTH DIMENSIONS OF SEX AND REPRODUCTION

The global burden of sexually transmitted diseases, HIV, maternal conditions, perinatal disorders, and congenital anomalies

EDITED BY

Christopher J. L. Murray
Harvard University
Boston, MA, USA

Alan D. Lopez
World Health Organization
Geneva, Switzerland

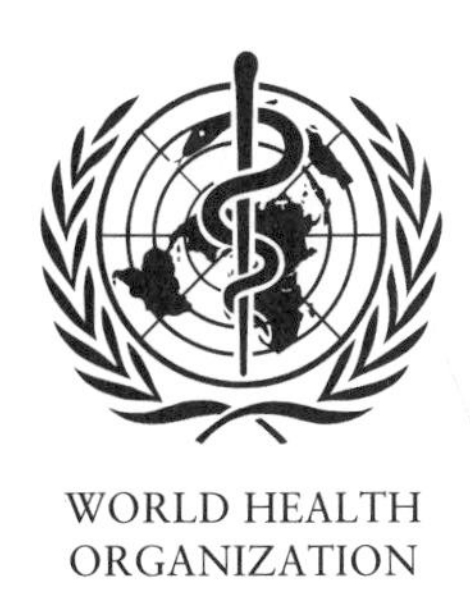
WORLD HEALTH ORGANIZATION

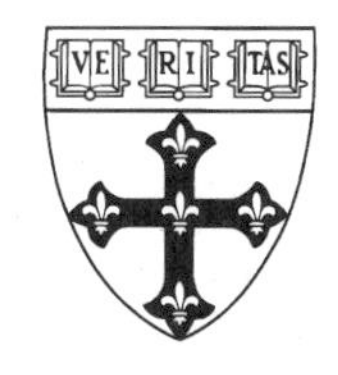

HARVARD SCHOOL OF PUBLIC HEALTH

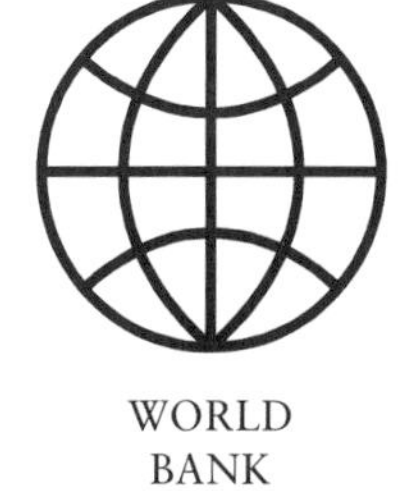
WORLD BANK

Published by The Harvard School of Public Health on behalf of
The World Health Organization and The World Bank
Distributed by Harvard University Press

Library of Congress Cataloging-in-Publication (CIP) Data

Health dimensions of sex and reproduction : the global burden of sexually transmitted diseases, HIV, maternal conditions, perinatal disorders, and congenital anomalies / edited by Christopher J. L. Murray and Alan D. Lopez.
580 p. 3 cm. -- (Global burden of disease and injury series ; v. 3)
Includes bibliographical references and index.
ISBN 0-674-38335-4
1. Pregnancy--Complications--Epidemiology.
2. Sexually transmitted diseases--Epidemiology.
3. HIV infections--Epidemiology. 4. Abnormalities, Human--Epidemiology. 5. Childbirth--Complications--Epidemiology. 6. World health--Statistics.
I. Murray, Christopher J. L. II. Lopez, Alan D.
III. Series.
RG106.3.H4 1998 98-30156
614.5' 9922--dc21 CIP

Printed in the United States of America.

Table of Contents

Foreword to The *Global Burden of Disease and Injury Series*

Ralph H. Henderson

The collection and use of timely and reliable health information in support of health policies and programmes have been actively promoted by the World Health Organization since its foundation. Valid health statistics are required at all levels of the health system, ranging from data for health services support at the local community level, through to national statistics and information used to monitor the effectiveness of national health strategies. Equally, regional and global data are required to monitor global epidemics and to continuously assess the effectiveness of global public health approaches to disease and injury prevention and control, as coordinated by WHO technical programmes. Despite the clear need for epidemiological data, reliable and comprehensive health statistics are not available in many Member States of WHO, and, indeed, in many countries the ascertainment of disease levels, patterns and trends is still very uncertain.

In recent years, monitoring systems, community-level research and disease registers have improved in both scope and coverage. Simultaneously, research on the epidemiological transition has increased our understanding of how the cause structure of mortality changes as overall mortality rates decline. As a consequence, estimates and projections of various epidemiological parameters, such as incidence, prevalence and mortality, can now be made at the global and regional level for many diseases and injuries. The Global Burden of Disease Study has now provided the public health community with a set of consistent estimates of disease and injury rates in 1990. The Study has also attempted to provide a comparative index of the burden of each disease or injury, namely the number of Disability-Adjusted Life Years (DALYs) lost as a result of either premature death or years lived with disability.

The findings published in the *Global Burden of Disease and Injury Series* provide a unique and comprehensive assessment of the health of populations as the world enters the third millennium. We also expect that the methods described in the various volumes in the series will stimulate

Member States to improve the functioning and usefulness of their own health information systems. Nonetheless, it must be borne in mind that the results from an undertaking as ambitious as the Global Burden of Disease Study can only be approximate. The reliability of the data for certain diseases, and for some regions, is extremely poor, with only scattered information available in some cases. To extrapolate from these sources to global estimates is clearly very hazardous, and could well result in errors of estimation. The methods that were used for some diseases (e.g. cancer) are not necessarily those applied by other scientists or institutions (e.g. the International Agency for Research on Cancer) and hence the results obtained may differ, sometimes considerably, from theirs. Moreover, the concept of the DALY as used in this Study is still under development, and further work is needed to assess the relevance of the social values that have been incorporated in the calculation of DALYs, as well as their applicability in different sociocultural settings. In this regard, WHO and its various partners are continuing their efforts to investigate burden-of-disease measurements and their use in health policy decision-making.

Dr Ralph H. Henderson is Assistant Director-General of the World Health Organization.

Foreword to The *Global Burden of Disease and Injury Series*

Dean T. Jamison

Rational evaluation of policies for health improvement requires four basic types of information: a detailed, reliable assessment of epidemiological conditions and the burden of disease; an inventory of the availability and disposition of resources for health (i.e. a system of what has become known as national health accounts); an assessment of the institutional and policy environment; and information on the cost-effectiveness of available technologies and strategies for health improvement. The *Global Burden of Disease and Injury Series* provides, on a global and regional level, a detailed and internally consistent approach to meeting the first of these information needs, that concerning epidemiological conditions and disease burden. It fully utilizes what information exists while, at the same time, pointing to great variation—across conditions and across countries—in data quality. In the *Global Burden of Disease and Injury Series*, Christopher Murray, Alan Lopez and literally scores of their collaborators from around the world present us with a *tour de force:* its (initial) 10 volumes summarize epidemiological knowledge about all major conditions and most risk factors; they generate assessments of numbers of deaths by cause that are consistent with the total numbers of deaths by age, sex and region provided by demographers; they provide methodologies for and assessments of aggregate disease burden that combine—into the Disability-Adjusted Life Year or DALY measure—burden from premature mortality with that from living with disability; and they use historical trends in main determinants to project mortality and disease burden forward to 2020. Publication of the *Global Burden of Disease and Injury Series* marks the transition to a new era of health outcome accounting—an era for which these volumes establish vastly higher standards for rigour, comprehensiveness and internal consistency. I firmly predict that by the turn of the century the official reporting of health outcomes in dozens of countries and globally will embody the approach and standards described in this series.

The *Global Burden of Disease and Injury Series* culminates an evolutionary process that began in the late 1980s. Close and effective collaboration between the World Bank and the World Health Organization initiated, supported and contributed substantively to that process.

Background

Work leading to the *Global Burden of Disease and Injury Series* proceeded in three distinct phases beginning in 1988. Intellectual antecedents go back much further (see Murray 1996, or Morrow and Bryant 1995); perhaps the most relevant are Ghana's systematic assessment of national health problems (Ghana Health Assessment Project Team 1981) and the introduction of the QALY (quality-adjusted life year)—see, for example Zeckhauser and Shepard (1976). My comments here focus on the three phases leading directly to the *Global Burden of Disease and Injury Series*.

Phase 1 constituted an input to a four-year long "Health Sector Priorities Review" initiated in 1988 by the World Bank; its purpose was to assess "...the significance to public health of individual diseases (or related clusters of diseases)...and what is now known about the cost and effectiveness of relevant interventions for their control" (Jamison et al. 1993, p. 3; that volume provides the results of the review). Dr Christopher Murray of Harvard University introduced the DALY as a common measure of effectiveness for the review to use across interventions dealing with diverse diseases, and Dr Alan Lopez of the World Health Organization prepared estimates of child death by cause that were consistent with death totals provided by demographers at the World Bank (Lopez 1993). At the same time, and in close coordination, a World Bank effort was preparing consistent estimates for adult (ages 15–59) mortality by cause for much of the developing world (Feachem et al. 1992). Ensuring this consistency was a major advance and is a precondition for systematic attempts to measure disease burden. (Estimates of numbers of deaths by cause that are not constrained to sum to a demographically-derived total seem inevitably to result in substantial overestimates of deaths due to each cause.) Phase I of this effort, then, introduced the DALY and established important consistency standards to guide estimation of numbers of deaths by cause.

Phase 2 constituted the first attempt to provide a comprehensive set of estimates not only of numbers of deaths by cause but also of total disease burden including burden from disability. This effort was commissioned as background for the World Bank's *World Development Report 1993: Investing in Health*; it was co-sponsored by the World Bank and the World Health Organization; and it was undertaken under the general guidance of a committee chaired by Dr JP Jardel (then Assistant Director-General of WHO). The actual work was conceptualized, managed and integrated by Drs Murray and Lopez and involved extensive efforts by a large number of individuals, most of whom were on the WHO staff. First publication of the estimates of 1990 disease burden appeared in Appendix B of *Investing in Health* (World Bank 1993); the World Health Organization subsequently published a volume containing a full account of the methods used and a somewhat revised and far more extensive presentation of the results (Murray and Lopez 1994).

Preparation and publication of the *Global Burden of Disease and Injury Series* constitutes Phase 3 of this sequence of efforts. As in the earlier phases, the *Global Burden of Disease and Injury Series* was undertaken to inform a policy analysis—in this case an assessment of priorities for health research and development in developing countries being guided by WHO's Ad Hoc Committee on Health Research Relating to Future Intervention Options. The Committee sought updated estimates of disease burden for 1990, projections to 2020 and an extension of the methods to allow assessment of burden attributable to selected risk factors (volume IX of the *Global Burden of Disease and Injury Series*). The committee's report (Ad Hoc Committee 1996) and the *Global Burden of Disease and Injury Series* appear as companion documents.

Chapters summarizing results from the *Global Burden of Disease and Injury Series* appear in volume I, *The Global Burden of Disease;* underlying epidemiological statistics for over 200 conditions appear in volume II, *Global Health Statistics*. The next six volumes of the *Series* provide, for the first time, chapters detailing the data on each condition or cluster of conditions. These condition-specific chapters were extremely difficult to prepare under the constraints of time, consistency and comprehensiveness imposed by Murray and Lopez. (As co-author of the chapter on intestinal helminthiases I am well aware of the difficulties involved!) Yet the results, individually and collectively, enrich greatly the summaries that were hitherto published. The selection of subjects for the individual volumes—reproductive health, infectious diseases, non-communicable diseases, neurological and psychiatric disorders, injury and malnutrition—will make individual volumes of value to specialist communities. Volume IX reports on the burden due to selected risk factors. The tenth and final volume for the initial series—additional volumes are in the planning stage—reports country-specific analyses (the first of which, for Mexico, had been published previously by Lozano et al. 1994), describes applications of the analyses and introduces alternative methodological approaches.

Will there be a fourth phase? I am sure there will. Reporting of the disease-specific and risk factor analysis in the *Global Burden of Disease and Injury Series* will provoke constructive and perhaps substantial criticism and improvements; country-specific assessments will multiply (over 20 are now under way) and they, too, will modify and enrich current estimates. Country and global estimates for times in the past will most likely be prepared; estimates of years of life lost for the Unites States in 1900 have already been made (Jamison 1995). Methodologies will be criticized and, I would predict, constructively revised. Unfinished elements of the agenda discussed in the next section will be completed. Phase 4, perhaps centred on the estimation of global and regional disease burden for 1995 and including a look at the past, will take us well beyond where we now are.

The Agenda

Disease burden (or numbers of deaths by cause) can be partitioned in three separate ways for different age, sex and regional groupings (Murray et al. 1994). One partition is by *risk factor*—genetic, behavioural, environmental and physiological. The second is by *disease*. The third is by consequence—*premature mortality* at different ages and different *types of disability* (e.g. sensory, cognitive functioning, pain, affective state, etc.).

Disaggregation by risk factor helps guide policy concerning primary and secondary prevention, including development of new preventive measures. Disaggregation by disease helps guide policy concerning cure, secondary prevention and palliation; and disaggregation by consequence helps guide policies for rehabilitation.

Work on the disease burden assessment agenda began with assessments of mortality and burden by disease; the *Global Burden of Disease and Injury Series* advances the agenda in that domain by revising and adding great detail on disease burden estimates. Additionally the *Global Burden of Disease and Injury Series* makes a major advance by assessing burden due to selected major risk factors (Volume IX); this extends usefulness of the work to the domain of prevention policy.

There remains, however, an important unfinished agenda. The disease burden associated with different types of disability remains to be assessed; perhaps part of the reason for neglect of rehabilitation in most discussion of health policy is the lack of even approximate information on burden due to disability or on the DALY gains per unit cost of rehabilitative intervention.

A related agenda item—relevant to planning for curative and, particularly, rehabilitative intervention—is to present disease burden estimates from a current prevalence perspective. The dominant perspective of work so far undertaken, including in the *Global Burden of Disease and Injury Series*, is that of adding up over time the burden that will result from all conditions incident in a given year (here 1990); this well serves the development of primary prevention policy and of treatment policy for diseases of short duration. The prevalence perspective complements the incidence one by assessing how much burden is being experienced during a particular year by chronic conditions or by disabilities; those conditions or disabilities will often have been generated some time in the past. From an incidence perspective, disability in this year from, say, an injury occurring a decade ago would generate DALY loss in the year of incidence; but to guide investment in rehabilitation we need to know how much disability exists today, i.e., we need a prevalence perspective. Murray and Lopez in *The Global Burden of Disease* and in *Global Health Statistics* provide the basic estimates of prevalence of different disabilities and first glimpses of the prevalence perspective.

A final major agenda item is to establish for each condition and in the aggregate how much of the potential current burden is in fact being averted by existing interventions and how much of the remaining burden persists because of lack of any intervention, lack of cost-effective interventions, or because of inefficiency of the system.

Uses of DALYs and Disease Burden Measurement

DALYs have six major uses to underpin health policy. Five of these relate to measurement of the burden of disease; the final one concerns judging the relative priority of interventions in terms of cost-effectiveness.

Assessing performance. A country-specific (or regional) assessment of the burden of disease provides a performance indicator that can be used over time to judge progress or across countries or regions to judge relative performance. These comparisons can be either quite aggregated (in terms of DALYs lost per thousand population) or finely disaggregated to allow focused assessment of where relative performance is good and where it is not. The *Global Burden of Disease and Injury Series* with its burden assessments for eight regions in 1990—and with the increasing number of country-specific assessments that it will report—will provide, I predict, the benchmark for all subsequent work. The most natural comparison is to the development of National Income and Product Accounts (NIPAs) by Simon Kuznets and others in the 1930s, which culminated in 1939 with a complete NIPA for the United Kingdom prepared by James Meade and Richard Stone at the request of the UK Treasury. NIPAs have, in the subsequent decades, transformed the empirical underpinnings of economic policy analysis. One of the leading proponents of major changes in NIPAs has put it this way:

> The national income and product accounts for the United States (NIPAs), and kindred accounts in other nations, have been among the major contributions to economic knowledge over the past half century....Several generations of economists and practitioners have now been able to tie theoretical constructs of income, output, investment, consumption, and savings to the actual numbers of these remarkable accounts with all their fine detail and soundly meshed interrelations. (Eisner 1989)

My own expectation is that this series will, over a decade or two, initiate a transformation of health policy analysis analogous to that initiated for economic policy by the introduction of NIPAs in the late 1930s. Today most health policy work concerns only cost, finance, process and access; burden of disease (and risk factor) assessments should soon allow full incorporation of performance measures in policy analysis.

Generating a forum for informed debate of values and priorities. The assessment of disease burden in a country-specific context in practice involves participation of a broad range of national disease specialists, epidemiologists and, often, policy makers. Debating the appropriate values for, say, disability weights or for years of life lost at different ages helps clarify values and objectives for national health policy. Discussing the inter-relations among diseases and their risk factors in the light of local conditions sharpens consideration of priorities. And the entire process brings technically informed participants to the table where policy is discussed. The preparation of a well-defined product generates a process with much value of its own.

Identifying national control priorities. Many countries now identify a relatively short list of interventions, the full implementation of which becomes an explicit priority for national political and administrative attention. Examples include interventions to control tuberculosis, poliomyelitis, HIV infection, smoking and specific micronutrient deficiencies. Because political attention and administrative capacity are in relatively fixed and short supply, the benefits from using those resources will be maximized if they are directed to interventions that are both cost-effective and aimed at problems associated with a high burden. Thus, national assessments of disease burden are instrumental for establishing this short list of control priorities.

Allocating training time for clinical and public health practitioners. Medical schools offer a fixed number of instructional hours; training programmes for other levels and types of practitioners are likewise limited. A major instrument for implementing policy priorities is to allocate this fixed time resource well—again that means allocation of time to training in interventions where disease burden is high and cost-effective interventions exist.

Allocating research and development resources. Whenever a fixed effort will have a benefit proportional not to the size of the effort but rather to the size of the problem being addressed, estimates of disease burden become essential for formulation of policy. This is the case with political attention and with time in the medical school curriculum; and it is likewise true for the allocation of research and development resources. Developing a vaccine for a broad range of viral pneumonias, for example, would have perhaps hundreds of times the impact of a vaccine against disease from Hanta virus infection. Thus information on disease or risk factor burden is one (of several) vital inputs to inform research and development resource allocation. Indeed, as previously noted, this series—with its disease burden assessments for 1990, its projections to 2020 and its initial assessment of burden due to risk factors—was commissioned to inform a WHO Committee charged with assessing health research and development priorities for developing countries (Ad Hoc Committee 1996).

The Committee sought not only to know the burden by condition, but also to partition the burden remaining for each condition into several distinct parts reflecting the importance of the reasons for the remaining disease burden. This division into four parts was undertaken for several conditions; a major agenda item for future analysis is to undertake such a partitioning systematically for all conditions so that there could be reasonably approximate answers to such questions as "How much of the remaining disease burden cannot be addressed without major biomedical advances?" or, "How much of the remaining disease burden could be averted by utilizing existing interventions more efficiently?" Arguably most of the spectacular gains in human health of the past century have resulted from advances in knowledge (although improvements in income and education have also played a role). If so, improving research and development policy in health may be more important than improving policy in health systems or finance; improved assessments and projections of disease burden will be critical to that undertaking.

Allocating resources across health interventions. Here disease burden assessment often plays a minor role; the task is to shift resources to interventions which, at the margin, will generate the greatest reduction in DALY loss. When there are major fixed costs in mounting an intervention—as is the case with political and managerial attention for national control priorities—burden estimates are indeed required to optimize resource allocation. But, typically, much progress can be made with only an understanding of how the DALYs gained from an intervention vary with the level of expenditure on it; such assessments are the stuff of cost-effectiveness analysis. The DALY as a common measure of effectiveness allows comparison of cost-effectiveness across interventions addressing all conditions; such an initial effort was undertaken for the World Bank's "Health Sector Priorities Review" (Jamison et al. 1993) in the late 1980s using a forerunner to the DALY utilized in this series.

* * *

The *Global Burden of Disease and Injury Series* contains the only available internally consistent, comprehensive and comparable assessments of causes of death, incidence and prevalence of disease and injury, measures and projections of disease burden, and measures of risk factor burden. In that sense the authors' contributions represent a landmark achievement and provide an invaluable resource for policy analysts and scholars. This effort dramatically raises the standard by which future reporting of health conditions will be judged. Yet, the very need for the ad hoc assessments that the volumes in this series report, points to important gaps in the international system for gathering, analysing and distributing policy-relevant data on the health of populations. Without information on how levels and trends in key indicators in their own countries compare with other countries, national decision-makers will lack benchmarks for judging performance. Likewise students of health systems will lack the empirical basis for forming outcome-based judgements on which policies work—and which do not. I hope, then, that one follow-on to the *Global*

Burden of Disease and Injury Series will be the institutionalization of continued efforts to generate and analyse internationally comparable data on health outcomes.

Dean T. Jamison is Professor of Public Health and of Education at the University of California, Los Angeles, and Economic Adviser to the Human Development Department of the World Bank. He recently served as Chairman of the World Health Organization's Ad Hoc Committee on Health Research Relating to Future Intervention Options.

References

Ad Hoc Committee on Health Research Relating to Future Intervention Options (1996) *Investing in health research and development*. World Health Organization. Geneva (Document TDR/Gen/96.1).

Eisner R (1989) *The total incomes system of accounts*. Chicago, University of Chicago Press.

Feachem RGA et al., eds. (1992) *The health of adults in the developing world*. New York, Oxford University Press for the World Bank.

Ghana Health Assessment Project Team (1981) A quantitative method of assessing the health impact of different diseases in less developed countries. *International journal of epidemiology*, 10: 73–80.

Goerdt A et al. (1996) Disability: definition and measurement issues. In: Murray CJL and Lopez AD, eds., *The global burden of disease: a comprehensive assessment of mortality and disability from diseases, injuries, and risk factors in 1990 and projected to 2020*. Cambridge, Harvard University Press.

Jamison DT et al., eds. (1993) *Disease control priorities in developing countries*. New York, Oxford University Press for the World Bank.

Jamison JC (1995) The mortal burden: disability adjusted life years lost to premature mortality in the United States in 1900. Economic history paper, MIT Department of Economics.

Lopez AD (1993) Causes of death in industrial and developing countries: estimates for 1985–1990. In: Jamison DT et al., eds. *Disease control priorities in developing countries*. New York, Oxford University Press for the World Bank, 35–50.

Lozano R et al. (1994) *El peso de la enfermedad en México: un doble reto*. [The national burden of disease in México: a double challenge.] Mexico, Mexican Health Foundation, (Documentos para el análisis y la convergencia, No. 3).

Morrow RH, Bryant JH (1995) Health policy approaches to measuring and valuing human life: conceptual and ethical issues. *American journal of public health*, 85(10): 1356–1360.

Murray CJL (1996) Rethinking DALYs. In: Murray CJL and Lopez AD, eds., *The global burden of disease: a comprehensive assessment of mortality and disability from diseases, injuries, and risk factors in 1990 and projected to 2020*. Cambridge, Harvard University Press.

Murray CJL and Lopez AD, eds. (1994) *Global comparative assessments in the health sector: disease burden, expenditures and intervention packages.* Geneva, World Health Organization.

Murray CJL, Lopez AD, Jamison DT (1994) The global burden of disease in 1990: summary results, sensitivity analysis and future directions. *Bulletin of the World Health Organization*, 72(3):495–509.

World Bank (1993) *World development report 1993: investing in health.* New York, Oxford University Press for the World Bank.

World Health Organization. *World health statistics annual*, various years. Geneva, WHO.

Zeckhauser R, Shepard D (1976) Where now for saving lives? *Law and contemporary problems*, 40:5–45.

Foreword

Adrienne Germain

This volume, like the Global Burden of Disease (GBD) study overall, makes pathbreaking contributions to our understanding of the magnitude of the health risks of sex and reproduction, widely lamented but little quantified until the debut of HIV/AIDS in the early 1980's and the promulgation of a global *Safe Motherhood Initiative* in 1987. The GBD emphasis on ill-health, not only mortality; its consideration of multiple aspects of reproductive health, not just complications due to pregnancy; and its disaggregation of data by age and sex, begin to expose the enormity of the physical health burden that women especially bear due to sex and reproduction. Further, the GBD methodology makes possible initial assessments of the magnitude of these health risks relative to others, and should strengthen the rationale for enhanced policy attention and resource allocation to them.

The volume focuses on selected, major elements of reproductive health, namely, sexually transmitted diseases, maternal risks, conditions arising during the perinatal period, congenital anomalies, HIV and unsafe sexual practices. Chapters 2–12 provide very useful reviews and analyses of existing data on these elements, and also point to severe short-comings in the database. Generation of data on these health issues, perhaps more than any other cluster of health risks, are deeply affected by societal norms, by gender inequalities, and by myths and taboos. Estimations of disability and illness due to sex and reproduction are further hampered by biological factors, e.g. half or more women who have sexually transmitted infections are not easily identified because they have no symptoms. These social and biological factors, as well as resource constraints, severely restrict collection of data on fundamental issues such as the incidence of STDs and the probability of developing complications if infected, gynecological disabilities, unsafe abortion, and low birth weight, among others.

Chapter 1, which reveals the dramatic extent to which quantification of risks is affected by changes in the definition of reproductive health, and

Chapter 13, which looks at unsafe sexual behaviour as a risk factor, effectively illuminate some of the limitations of current techniques which cannot assess and appropriately weight synergies among the various health dimensions of sex and reproduction; the significance of behavioural, socio-cultural, political and economic factors that determine disability and death, and/or obstruct effective intervention; and the relative values of specific interventions.

This volume will therefore be best used as a stimulus for further work to improve databases and estimation techniques; to refine basic analytic tools to take account of the socio-behavioral causes and consequences of health risks; and to enhance the utility, as well as understand the limits, of the GBD approach for policy making. Some of the major challenges for future work include measurement of not only the physical, but also the emotional and social, costs to the individual of events such as the millions of stillbirths that occur each year, obstetric fistulae, infertility, HPV infections and cervical cancer; female genital cutting, or sexual violence; quantification and weighting of the intergenerational effects of maternal conditions and services (e.g., one half of all infant deaths could be averted by prenatal, delivery and post-partum care); deaths and disabilities due to indirect maternal complications such as malaria or anaemia; and significant health dimensions of sex and reproduction not yet measured, including numerous gynaecological disabilities.

For example, a recent study of gynaecological morbidity in a district of India (Bhatia et al. 1997) suggests the kind of expansion needed in the conditions to be considered in future burden of disease estimates. The study (using clinical examination, laboratory tests, and self-reports) reveals a very high burden of reproductive tract infections, infections that would have been missed if only STDs had been assessed. The two most common conditions were bacterial vaginosis and mucopurulent cervicitis; approximately one-fourth of the women had clinical evidence of pelvic inflammatory disease, cervical ectopy, and fistula; 17 per cent suffered severe anaemia, and 12 per cent severe chronic energy deficiency. Only two other such community-based studies of overall gynaecological morbidity have been reported from developing countries.

In addition to the need to expand and improve the basic databases on which GBD analysis is based, the values and assumptions underlying the DALY methodology require further consideration. For example, the weights assigned to particular disabilities affect the estimation of disease. Similarly, it will be important as further work is done to develop methods to capture inequalities among individuals or subgroups of the population identified by income or other variables. An important challenge will be to refine the methodology and/or add complementary studies to describe and weight health dimensions of sex and reproduction. These include the impacts of cumulative insults to an individual's health over time (e.g. childhood malnutrition, sexually transmitted diseases and pregnancy in adolescence, botched abortion); the multiple impacts of a single health insult (e.g. the emotional and the physical impacts of domestic violence or of stillbirth and miscarriage); and the synergies among multiple sources of increased health risks (e.g. the interactions of malaria and pregnancy).

No one methodology is likely to capture the full complexity of such health problems.

The full benefit of future investments in burden of disease estimates will therefore only be realized with greater investment in complementary studies, such as the one in India, and additional measurement methods. Continuing refinement of the GBD/DALY methodology will also benefit from engagement of the broadest possible range of stakeholders in discussion about the weights assigned to various health states, the social and emotional dimensions of these health risks, and use of this methodology to assess policy and investment options.

Adrienne Germain is President of the International Women's Health Coalition.

References

Bhatia, JC et al. (1997) Levels and determinants of gynecological morbidity in a district of South India, *Studies in Family Planning*, 28(2):98–102.

Foreword

Tomris Türmen

Advocacy for health must be founded on fact not conviction. Health interventions must be based on evidence not habit and tradition. Knowing the burden of disease, and the specific composition of the burden in different places and for different groups of people, is essential for the formulation of health policy and for monitoring change. Yet gathering that essential knowledge, separating fact from opinion, identifying what is really happening as opposed to what people *say* is happening or what we *think* is happening, requires a constant effort of research, analysis and interpretation. In the area of reproductive health, bringing together the basic body of facts needed for advocacy and for the identification of interventions poses particular problems. Reproductive health concerns not merely reproduction but a range of issues related to human sexuality. These issues are different in men and women and change over a person's lifetime. Finding out about reproductive health means delving into intimate aspects of life which are everywhere bound by rules and regulations, traditions and taboo. It is often said that the three aspects of life most difficult to discuss openly are sex, birth and death: reproductive health must deal with all three.

Despite these difficulties, in recent years, monitoring and surveillance systems have improved in scope and coverage and community-based research has broadened the knowledge base in reproductive health. Only a decade ago, little was known about the extent of pregnancy-related mortality; today estimates are available for most countries. At the start of the HIV/AIDS pandemic, monitoring incidence and prevalence seemed an impossible challenge; today many countries have established the vital surveillance systems we need. At the same time, our knowledge about the burden of disease caused by other sexually transmitted diseases — gonorrhoea, syphilis, chlamydia — has increased dramatically. Slowly, the epidemiological data about cancers of the reproductive organs — cervix, breast, uterus, prostate — is beginning to accumulate. And we are starting to document the dimensions of ill-health resulting from harmful practices such as female genital mutilation. Yet there remain vast areas about which we are ignorant. The burden of disabilities resulting from pregnancy-related complications remains poorly documented and measured. We suspect that a huge toll of needless suffering is caused by reproductive tract infections but we do not yet have the means needed to measure them at the population level. We are gradually becoming aware of the importance of the mental as well as the physical ill-health and suffering associated with sexual abuse and violence but again, we are not yet in a position to quantify this burden. We remain unable to capture positive aspects of reproductive health. The contraceptive prevalence rate, for example, while easily measurable and long used to demonstrate improvements in reproductive health, is in reality a poor reflection of the benefits that accrue from avoiding unwanted fertility.

The concept of reproductive health, as defined by WHO and elaborated at the International Conference on Population and Development in Cairo in 1994, poses challenges particularly from a measurement perspective. This is because it cuts across the lines along which diseases have traditionally been classified — communicable and non-communicable diseases; infectious diseases versus those related to lifestyles and behaviours. Reproductive health deals with both diseases — cancers, HIV/AIDS, STDs — and with normal physiological processes — pregnancy and childbirth. The interventions to address the burden of reproductive ill-health must address not only the behaviours of pathogens and the clinical interventions needed to deal with them but also, and more critically, the behaviours of people in some of the most intimate aspects of their lives.

A more fundamental measurement problem is that in reproductive health as perhaps in no other aspect of health, people's own perceptions of health and disease and the value they put on different health states may differ from what the clinician diagnoses or the epidemiologist investigates. What can appear trivial from a clinical perspective may have profound consequences for the health and well-being of the individual. Good sexual and reproductive health is manifestly far more than just the absence of disease. Everywhere and throughout human history people and societies have placed great value on — and allocated effort and resources to — the ability to achieve sexual fulfilment and successful reproduction. Yet our ability to measure such positive health states remains limited.

Given our current limited measurement tools, we must, as Murray and Lopez observe, fall back on measures of mortality, morbidity and disability. This volume represents an important first step in bringing together what is currently known about deaths and disabilities related to sex and reproduction. It is particularly noteworthy because the DALY methodology permits us, for the first time, to count not only the deaths but also the immense burden of suffering among those who do not die. We have here a unique compilation and assessment of what is known about the burden of reproductive ill-health. At the same time, for those of us working in the area of reproductive health, this volume represents only a first important step. There must be a next time and we must do better next time to capture the full dimensions and complexity of reproductive health conditions. This means that we must find better ways of measuring deaths and disabilities; we must develop more sophisticated tools for analysing the multidimensional nature and complex aetiology of reproductive health conditions; we must develop innovative approaches for finding out about the impact of the burden on different groups of people.

The data assembled in this volume paint a sombre picture of premature death and disability, particularly among women on whom the bulk of the burden of sexual and reproductive ill-health falls. The importance of unsafe sex as a risk factor is now becoming apparent and with it the realization that public health interventions must address the full range of behavioural, social, cultural and economic factors that contribute to reproductive ill-health. The information assembled here will help us to take the next steps forward in identifying and implementing the needed interventions.

Tomris Türmen is Executive Director, Family and Reproductive Health, of the World Health Organization.

Preface

In this volume we have tried to provide detail on the epidemiology of the major diseases or conditions which are largely or exclusively related to reproductive health, irrespective of whether the outcome is related to the mother, to sexually-active adults in general, or to children. The structure of the book is arranged accordingly. Following our assessment of the approximate size of the disease burden arising from sex and reproduction, given in Chapter 1, Rowley and Berkley in Chapter 2 provide a comprehensive overview of the epidemiology of sexually transmitted diseases with information on the incidence and prevalence of the most common STDs and on numerous sequelae with often follow infection.

Chapters 3 to 7 by AbouZahr and colleagues focus on pregnancy-related outcomes and thus exclusively concern women in the reproductive ages. Following a consolidated analysis of maternal mortality worldwide in Chapter 3, the next five chapters deal with the epidemiology of major pregnancy-related risks, namely haemorrhage (Chapter 4), sepsis (Chapter 5); hypertensive disorders of pregnancy (Chapter 6), obstructed labour (Chapter 7) and unsafe abortion (Chapter 8).

Chapter 9 by Low-Beer and colleagues describes the global epidemiology of HIV infection in 1990. While HIV is not only caused by sexual contact, much of it is. We have therefore decided to include this chapter in the volume related to the public health aspects of sex and reproduction, although the chapter could equally well have appeared in Volume IV of this series on infectious diseases. This chapter provides an epidemiological assessment for 1990 when AIDS cases and deaths were primarily the result of the much lower HIV infection rates of the early 1980s compared to what was observed in the late 1980s and early 1990s. The comparatively low disease burden attributable to HIV infection in 1990 is therefore to some extent illusory; projections indicate that the HIV disease burden will rise dramatically into early next century.

In contrast to earlier chapters, where adult health is the primary concern, Chapters 10, 11 and 12 by Shibuya and Murray focus on the principal risks of pregnancy for the live-born fetus, namely low birth weight (Chapter 10), birth trauma and birth asphyxia (Chapter 11) and congenital anomalies (Chapter 12).

The final chapter of the book by Berkley (Chapter 13) does not address one or more specific outcomes related to sex and reproduction. Rather the chapter, for the first time to our knowledge, attempts to quantify the entire disease burden arising from unsafe sexual practices. The analysis is not a comparison of the disease burden related to sex with that which might be avoided if sex were avoided altogether — far from it! By listing and then quantifying the extensive range of disease and conditions associated with unsafe sex, unwanted pregnancy, contraception and sex-related risks such as cervical cancer, the author estimates that about 3 to 4 per cent of the global burden of disease and injury in 1990 was attributable to unsafe sexual practices as a risk factor. While there are substantial uncertainties surrounding the reliability of this estimate, it is nonetheless worth noting that this figure is comparable to other major risk factors such as tobacco, or diseases which are principal public health concerns, such as tuberculosis and measles.

In compiling these chapters into one volume we have attempted to provide a global overview of the probable dimensions of the public health burden of sex and reproduction in 1990. We realize that this overview has not addressed all the issues surrounding reproductive health; for example, the broader gender issues underlying reproductive health for women have been largely ignored in the calculation of disease burden. Nevertheless, the databases, assumptions and methods used to calculate the disease burden have been described. Future global assessments of the public health burden associated with sex and reproduction will hopefully benefit from a debate about their validity and efforts to improve on them.

CJLM
ADL

Acknowledgements

Many good and useful ideas remain just that, ideas, without the vision, perseverance, organization and dedication to bring them to fruition. The energy and drive to bring this book to completion have come from our editorial manager, Emmanuela Gakidou. Without her tireless efforts to obtain chapter submissions, critically review them for consistency with the computations based on the Global Burden of Disease Study and manage the entire production process, this book would still be a hope, not a reality. Her extraordinary contribution to the production of this book is very gratefully acknowledged.

We are also grateful to Carla AbouZahr and Jane Rowley for making extra efforts at short notice to complete several chapters.

We would like to thank the Eli Lilly Foundation for providing financial support for the editing of this book.

CJLM
ADL

Chapter 1

Quantifying the Health Risks of Sex and Reproduction: Implications of Alternative Definitions

Christopher JL Murray
Alan D Lopez

The Global Burden of Disease Study (GBD) is unique in the sense that, for the first time, estimates of mortality and disability have been prepared for 483 disabling sequelae of 107 diseases and injuries. Details of the methods and procedures used in the GBD have been published in *The Global Burden of Disease* (Murray and Lopez 1996a); *Global Health Statistics* contains detailed tabulations of epidemiological estimates for the various diseases, injuries and their sequelae, by sex, age and eight geographic regions (Murray and Lopez 1996b).

The goals of Volumes III through IX of the *Global Burden of Disease and Injury Series* are to: provide more detailed information in a series of chapters on each disease and risk factor included in the Study; review the state of empirical knowledge, describe the methods used to estimate incidence, duration, prevalence and mortality; and analyse these findings in a broader context. Because of the considerable interest in recent years in the health risks of sex and reproduction, we have chosen to cluster in this volume chapters on sexually transmitted diseases, maternal causes, conditions arising during the perinatal period, congenital anomalies, HIV and unsafe sexual practices. In doing so, the question arises as to what might reasonably be included as a health risk of sex and reproduction, and what is the relationship between the cluster of conditions that are so defined and the broader concept of reproductive health. As there are clearly many variants of what conditions should be included in the set of health risks of sex and reproduction, we have proposed in this chapter a variety of alternative definitions and have estimated premature mortality and disability according to these different conceptualizations of reproductive health.

What Is Reproductive Health?

During the 1980s, many groups working on population began shifting their emphasis from a focus on fertility reduction and contraception to the broader concept of women themselves, their reproductive rights and, ultimately, their reproductive health (Fathalla 1991, Ford Foundation 1991, Germain and Ordway 1989). This focus was widely acknowledged and supported at the International Conference on Population and Development held in Cairo in September 1994 (United Nations 1994). Given the increasing emphasis on the reproductive health movement (e.g. Benagiano 1996, Diczfalusy et al. 1994, Garcia-Moreno and Turmen 1995, Miller and Rosenfield 1996, Neilson et al. 1995), there has been considerable debate in the scientific community about the precise meaning of "reproductive health" and "reproductive health services."

The most widely recognized positive definition of health is that of the World Health Organization, namely that health is a state of complete physical, mental and social well-being and not merely the absence of disease or infirmity (World Health Organization 1996). Reproductive health has been defined as a state of complete physical, mental and social well-being in all matters relating to the reproductive system and to its functions and processes (World Health Organization 1994). According to the Cairo Conference report, this was further specified: "It implies that people are able to have a satisfying and safe sex life and that they have the capability to reproduce and the freedom to decide if, when and how often to do so. .... [It implies] the right of access to appropriate information and services. It also includes sexual health, the purpose of which is the enhancement of life and personal relations, and not merely counselling and care related to reproduction and sexually transmitted diseases." (United Nations 1994). Despite this statement, there remains considerable scope for ambiguity and interpretation as to what is and what is not reproductive health.

Notwithstanding the obvious appeal of such positive definitions, the fact remains that, given the current state of health measurement, most analyses must ultimately fall back on measures of mortality, morbidity and disability. Analyses of outcomes, determinants, resources and even intervention effectiveness in reproductive health require clear and unambiguous specificity to facilitate meaningful measurement. What conditions should be included in order to assess and monitor over time the health risks of reproduction? One has to decide, for example, whether to include all diseases of the reproductive organs, to include men and women, to include perinatal outcomes, or to restrict the focus to the reproductive age groups despite the fact that some conditions (e.g. cervical cancer) can manifest themselves several years after sexual contact. For example, Garcia-Moreno and Turmen (1995) include infertility, maternal morbidity and mortality, perinatal mortality, low birth weight, HIV, sexually transmitted diseases and female genital mutilation in their list of major reproductive concerns. Fathalla (1991) focuses his discussion of reproductive health on fertility, low birth weight, safe motherhood, infant and child survival, growth and development, sexually transmitted diseases, and AIDS.

The reproductive health programmes of the World Health Organization have defined reproductive health in terms of four guiding programme goals, namely, that people should be able to exercise their sexual and reproductive rights in order to:

- experience healthy sexual development and maturation and have the capacity for equitable and responsible and fulfilment;
- achieve their desired number of children safely and healthily, when and if they decide to have them;
- avoid illness, disease and disability related to sexuality and reproduction and receive appropriate care when needed; and
- be free from violence and other harmful practices related to sexuality and reproduction (World Health Organization 1997).

According to the World Health Organization, achieving these goals requires attention to nine reproductive health issues: sexual development, maturation and health with special reference to adolescents; fertility regulation; maternal health; perinatal health; unsafe abortion; infertility; endogenous and exogenous reproductive tract infections, including sexually transmitted diseases, HIV/AIDS, and cervical cancer; violence and its consequences for sexual and reproductive health; and female genital mutilation and other harmful practices such as inappropriate use of technologies. Clearly, different variants of reproductive health could have been defined based on some combination of these issues.

It is not our intention in this chapter to argue for a single, most appropriate definition of the concept "reproductive health". Rather, we provide a range of possible definitions and summary calculations of the disease burden estimated to occur in 1990 and 2000 from the health risks of sex and reproduction according to the following conceptualization of reproductive health. We do so, fully aware that these frameworks are undoubtedly incomplete or otherwise inadequate descriptions of the various issues surrounding reproductive health. We hope, however, that the variation in ill health suggested by these alternative definitions will provide a useful perspective on the approximate size of disease burden due to reproductive health.

Six Alternative Definitions of Reproductive Health

One obvious way to define the health risks of reproduction is to limit consideration to outcomes linked to the act of sex itself. Health risks directly attributable to sexual contact would include sexually transmitted diseases in people engaging in sex, as well as the health consequences of pregnancy. There is potential for ambiguity when this definition is applied to pathogens that are normally identified as sexually transmitted diseases, such as syphilis, where they afflict children. For example, congenital syphilis is due to unsafe sexual contact by the mother but not of the child. Where do we draw the "line"? In other words, how far should we follow the consequences of sexual contact? According to the classical definition of attributable risk, one should include all health events that would not otherwise occur in the absence of sexual contact (Rothman 1986). If there were no sexual contact there would of course be no children (excluding *in vitro* fertilization). Carrying this argument to its logical conclusion would suggest, for example, that ischaemic heart disease in a future 68 year old is "attributable" to the sexual contact of his or her parents. It is perhaps more meaningful to argue that we should assess the disease burden related to sex holding the number of children in the future constant.

Focussing on sexual contact as the paradigm for assessing health risks related to reproductive health, two operational definitions may be proposed. In *Option A: Consequences of Sex in Adults*, we use a narrow focus and include only the consequences linked to sex in those participating in the sexual contact. This would include sexually transmitted diseases in the sexually active population, maternal causes and the fraction of adult cancers, HIV and hepatitis B that is sexually transmitted — see Chapter 13 for a more detailed discussion. In *Option B: Consequences of Sex in Children and Adults*, we follow the consequences of sex one step further and include, in addition to everything in *Option A*, the burden of congenital anomalies and conditions arising during the perinatal period, the burden in age groups 0–4 and 5–14 from sexually transmitted diseases, and the fraction of cancers, HIV and hepatitis B that is sexually transmitted.

A third option is to conceptualize health risks of sex and reproduction in terms of anatomy, namely the reproductive organ systems of women and men. Such a definition would logically include diseases primarily afflicting these organ systems such as cancers of the breast, cervix, uterus, ovaries, prostate, penis and testes, disorders of pregnancy, and a number of sexually transmitted diseases and reproductive tract infections. Clearly, many other diseases involve the reproductive organ system, such as tuberculous salpingitis or mumps orchitis. Conversely, many of the diseases of the reproductive organs affect other organ systems. In practice, a definition of burden due to reproductive health risks needs to be restricted to a concise set of conditions. For the purposes of illustration, we have therefore chosen to include in *Option C: Conditions of the Reproductive Organ System* all sexually transmitted diseases, maternal conditions, and the reproductive cancers.

Another approach to defining reproductive health is to focus on categories of health services that are commonly regarded as reproductive health services. In most countries, the cluster of services that would be labelled reproductive health services would include family planning services, antenatal and postnatal care, labour and delivery services, and most child health services (Ford Foundation 1991). To reflect this conception, we have defined *Option D: Conditions Managed Through Reproductive Health Services* to include all causes of burden in children aged 0–4 years

Table 1 Estimated deaths due to health risks of reproduction (in thousands), according to alternative definitions of reproductive health, by region, 1990

Burden of Reproductive Health Defined as:

	Consequences of sex in adults	Consequences of sex in children and adults	Conditions of the reproductive organ system	Conditions managed through reproductive health services	Burden in the reproductive age group (15-44 years)	Conditions predominantly afflicting the reproductive age group (15-44 years)
EME	53	139	311	106	427	106
FSE	32	95	102	116	343	58
IND	200	1 077	294	3 365	1 161	216
CHN	68	450	104	1 100	1 090	251
OAI	105	540	187	1 668	799	139
SSA	368	1 057	370	4 216	1 489	498
LAC	65	315	119	728	532	148
MEC	65	549	95	1 912	584	87
WORLD	*956*	*4 223*	*1 583*	*13 211*	*6 425*	*1 503*

Table 2 Percentage of deaths from all causes due to the health risks of reproduction, according to alternative definitions of reproductive health, by region, 1990

EME	0.7	2.0	4.4	1.5	6.0	1.5
FSE	0.8	2.5	2.7	3.1	9.1	1.5
IND	2.1	11.5	3.1	35.9	12.4	2.3
CHN	0.8	5.1	1.2	12.4	12.3	2.8
OAI	1.9	9.8	3.4	30.1	14.4	2.5
SSA	4.5	12.9	4.5	51.4	18.2	6.1
LAC	2.2	10.5	4.0	24.2	17.7	4.9
MEC	1.4	12.1	2.1	42.0	12.8	1.9
WORLD	*1.9*	*8.4*	*3.1*	*26.2*	*12.7*	*3.0*

Table 3 Percentage of deaths due to the health risks of reproduction which occur in females, according to alternative definitions of reproductive health, by region, 1990

EME	43.1	43.5	69.5	43.4	29.6	17.7
FSE	70.5	51.2	84.3	43.3	24.8	16.0
IND	90.2	57.9	86.0	52.4	48.8	76.3
CHN	80.6	56.2	91.0	54.1	42.6	56.8
OAI	90.7	53.4	81.0	46.0	42.9	57.5
SSA	81.0	60.6	80.1	48.6	45.8	55.7
LAC	73.1	49.4	77.6	44.7	39.7	27.2
MEC	92.2	54.0	87.3	50.0	43.9	62.7
WORLD	*81.7*	*56.1*	*80.4*	*49.6*	*42.6*	*52.4*

Table 4 DALYs due to the health risks of reproduction (in thousands), according to alternative definitions of reproductive health, by region, 1990

Burden of Reproductive Health Defined as:

	Consequences of sex in adults	Consequences of sex in children and adults	Conditions of the reproductive organ system	Conditions managed through reproductive health services	Burden in the reproductive age group (15-44 years)	Conditions predominantly afflicting the reproductive age group (15-44 years)
EME	1 810	5 738	3 521	6 205	37 763	20 101
FSE	1 308	4 047	2 098	6 039	23 944	9 297
IND	12 014	47 980	14 620	136 717	70 571	26 725
CHN	3 239	19 781	3 790	53 547	77 529	31 905
OAI	7 270	25 137	9 386	70 689	55 843	22 981
SSA	17 455	46 101	16 825	164 321	76 637	31 334
LAC	3 591	13 905	4 052	31 720	38 584	18 212
MEC	4 253	23 576	4 949	79 379	38 273	14 025
WORLD	*50 940*	*186 264*	*59 242*	*548 616*	*419 144*	*174 580*

Table 5 Percentage of DALYs from all causes due to the health risks of reproduction, according to alternative definitions of reproductive health, by region, 1990

EME	1.8	5.8	3.6	6.3	38.2	20.3
FSE	2.1	6.5	3.4	9.7	38.5	14.9
IND	4.2	16.7	5.1	47.5	24.5	9.3
CHN	1.6	9.5	1.8	25.7	37.2	15.3
OAI	4.1	14.1	5.3	39.8	31.4	12.9
SSA	5.9	15.6	5.7	55.6	26.0	10.6
LAC	3.7	14.1	4.1	32.3	39.3	18.5
MEC	2.8	15.6	3.3	52.6	25.4	9.3
WORLD	*3.7*	*13.5*	*4.3*	*39.8*	*30.4*	*12.7*

Table 6 Percentage of DALYs from all causes due to the health risks of reproduction which occur in females, according to alternative definitions of reproductive health, by region, 1990

EME	57.2	48.9	81.9	47.6	41.6	42.2
FSE	86.0	57.2	91.2	49.0	37.8	44.7
IND	90.2	60.7	86.5	53.6	54.3	69.5
CHN	93.2	58.4	95.9	54.4	48.1	58.5
OAI	89.7	58.3	83.7	48.3	49.3	59.9
SSA	83.4	62.7	84.9	49.8	48.6	61.3
LAC	80.5	53.8	88.0	47.3	45.6	43.0
MEC	96.3	57.6	93.0	51.2	50.2	62.3
WORLD	*86.5*	*59.3*	*86.7*	*51.0*	*48.2*	*57.0*

as well as all maternal conditions. We wish to emphasize that this is but one arbitrary definition linked to a service delivery construct; many others, perhaps more restrictive, are possible.

An alternative approach to defining the health risks of reproduction could be based on the concept of the reproductive age group. *Option E: Burden of the Reproductive Age Group (15–44 years)* is defined to include all causes of premature mortality and disability in the age group 15–44 years. Such an all-inclusive construct would address the concerns expressed that many of the hazards for reproductively health are not traditional reproductive causes (Katz et al. 1995). Thus in the quantification of *Option E*, we have included all sources of disease and injury burden in both men and women.

A slightly more restrictive definition can be developed by identifying those causes of premature mortality and disability that are more common during the reproductive ages (taken here to be 15–44 years) than at other stages of the life cycle. In order to do so, *Option F: Health Problems Predominantly Affecting the Reproductive Age Group* includes all causes of disease and injury for which the age-specific DALY rates at ages 15–44 is more than 1.5 times higher than the crude DALY rate for all age groups. The list of conditions meeting this criterion in males includes the sexually transmitted diseases, HIV, Chagas disease, unipolar major depression, bipolar affective disorder, schizophrenia, alcohol dependence, multiple sclerosis, drug dependence, obsessive-compulsive disorder, panic disorder, self-inflicted injuries, and violence. In women, the list is similar with the inclusion of maternal causes and the exclusion of violence.

RESULTS

Tables 1–6 summarize the estimated burden of disease and injury in 1990 arising from the health risks of sex and reproduction as defined by the various options defined above. Projections of the burden of reproductive health according to these six definitions are also summarized in Tables 7–12 based on the GBD baseline projection (Murray and Lopez 1996a). Separate tabulations have been provided for each of the six options. For both 1990 and 2000, estimates are presented for deaths (absolute numbers (Tables 1 and 7) and proportionate mortality (Tables 2 and 8)) and DALYs (numbers (Tables 4 and 10), per cent of total (Tables 5 and 11)), for each of the six operational definitions of reproductive health risks (A through F), and for each region. In addition, the percentage of the estimated attributable burden which occurs in females is given in Tables 3 and 6 for the year 1990 and Tables 9 and 12 for 2000.

The results provide an interesting perspective of how the quantification of these health risks is affected by changes in the definition of what constitutes "reproductive health." From the tables, it is clear that the six options can be effectively clustered into three groups on the basis of the estimated number of deaths and DALYs, their sex ratio and their regional distribution.

Mortality

Conceptually, the most restrictive definitions of reproductive health risks are *Option A: Consequences of Sex in Adults* and *Option C: Conditions of the Reproductive Organ System* which are estimated to have accounted for 1 million and 1.6 million deaths respectively in 1990. Nonetheless, even *Option A*, the most restrictive of all, still implies that hazards of sex and reproduction cause more than two times as many deaths as did maternal conditions alone, often thought of as an indirect measure of reproductive health. More than one-third of the 1990 deaths under this option occurred in Sub-Saharan Africa, and a further 21 per cent in India. If the reproductive organ system (*Option C*) is used to define attributable deaths, the proportion contributed by Sub-Saharan Africa declines to 23 per cent, but rises dramatically in EME (about 20 per cent of the total), reflecting the importance of breast, prostate, ovarian and uterine cancers in EME. By the year 2000, deaths from *Options A* are projected to increase to 1.4 million largely because of the HIV epidemic, while deaths from *Option C* are expected to be comparable (1.5 million).

The majority of deaths in 1990 measured under *Option C* occurred in females (70–91 per cent, depending on the region) as was the case under *Option A*, with the notable exception of EME due to the larger role of HIV. This sex pattern undoubtedly reflects the higher incidence of total diseases of the reproductive system in women, the consequences of which are exacerbated in poorer populations. Globally, 82 per cent of deaths under *Option A* and 80 per cent under *Option C* in 1990 were deaths among women, although some attenuation of this excess female mortality is expected by 2000, with the proportion female falling to 61 per cent and 72 per cent for *Options A and C*, respectively.

The six alternative definitions vary vastly in the proportion of all-cause mortality they ascribe to reproductive health risks. Thus in 1990, the percentage of all deaths which might be attributed to reproductive health risks ranged from 2 to 13 per cent for what might be termed the more restrictive options, but rose to 26 per cent if one were to choose *Option D: Conditions Managed Through Reproductive Health Services*. The lowest proportionate mortality can be ascribed to *Option A: Consequences of Sex in Adults*, *Option C: Conditions of the Reproductive Organ System*, and *Option F: Conditions Predominantly Afflicting the Reproductive Age Group*, each suggesting that reproductive health risks accounted for about 2–4 per cent of all deaths in 1990. Little change in this proportion at the global level is foreseen for the year 2000.

Important regional variations in the range of proportionate mortality are evident in Table 2. For example, omitting *Option D*, reproductive health-related deaths contributed between 5 and 18 per cent of all deaths in Sub-Saharan Africa in 1990, substantially higher than the global aver-

Table 7 Projected deaths due to the health risks of reproduction, GBD baseline projection for 2000, according to alternative definitions of reproductive health, by region

Burden of Reproductive Health Defined as:

	Consequences of sex in adults	Consequences of sex in children and adults	Conditions of the reproductive organ system	Conditions managed through Reproductive health services	Burden in the reproductive age group (15-44 years)	Conditions predominantly afflicting the reproductive age group (15-44 years)
EME	92	161	341	85	435	129
FSE	34	84	113	90	321	52
IND	305	948	237	2 152	1 319	272
CHN	61	303	112	669	1 051	126
OAI	167	492	180	1 163	886	152
SSA	536	1 328	318	4 265	1 891	530
LAC	135	330	140	546	653	214
MEC	57	508	84	1 739	642	72
WORLD	*1 382*	*4 148*	*1 525*	*10 710*	*7 200*	*1 547*

Table 8 Percentage of deaths from all causes due to the health risks of reproduction, GBD baseline projection for 2000, for alternative definitions of reproductive health, by region

EME	1.2	2.0	4.3	1.1	5.5	1.6
FSE	0.7	1.8	2.4	1.9	6.9	1.1
IND	3.2	10.0	2.5	22.7	13.9	2.9
CHN	0.6	2.9	1.1	6.5	10.2	1.2
OAI	2.9	8.4	3.1	19.8	15.1	2.6
SSA	5.8	14.4	3.5	46.3	20.5	5.8
LAC	3.8	9.3	4.0	15.4	18.5	6.1
MEC	1.1	10.0	1.6	34.1	12.6	1.4
WORLD	2.5	7.4	2.7	*19.1*	*12.8*	2.8

Table 9 Percentage of deaths due to the health risks of reproduction which occur in females, GBD baseline projection for 2000, for alternative definitions of reproductive health, by region

EME	30.5	36.2	67.1	43.3	27.9	1.7
FSE	65.8	51.6	79.3	43.2	24.0	5.5
IND	61.1	53.6	84.7	50.8	42.6	40.0
CHN	70.8	55.0	88.2	51.8	38.0	4.1
OAI	66.5	51.4	80.2	44.9	38.1	22.9
SSA	66.9	55.9	72.9	46.3	42.0	25.6
LAC	43.5	43.3	75.3	43.9	33.1	5.7
MEC	78.0	51.4	84.1	48.5	39.1	29.5
WORLD	*61.8*	*52.5*	*76.7*	*47.6*	*38.3*	*20.9*

Table 10 Projected DALYs due to the health risks of reproduction (in thousands), GBD baseline projection for 2000, according to alternative definitions of reproductive health, by region

Burden of Reproductive Health Defined as:

	Consequences of sex in adults	Consequences of sex in children and adults	Conditions of the reproductive organ system	Conditions managed through reproductive health services	Burden in the reproductive age group (15-44 years)	Conditions predominantly afflicting the reproductive age group (15-44 years)
EME	2 363	5 578	3 336	4 942	35 546	20 037
FSE	1 005	3 314	1 807	4 756	22 523	8 655
IND	11 762	38 692	9 093	89 280	74 340	26 146
CHN	1 499	13 152	2 266	34 206	70 763	30 497
OAI	7 051	20 891	6 677	50 025	59 637	24 642
SSA	19 415	51 984	12 497	166 043	90 920	34 357
LAC	4 638	13 203	3 363	24 476	44 175	22 285
MEC	3 000	21 624	3 541	72 836	42 534	13 849
WORLD	*50 496*	*168 228*	*42 579*	*446 564*	*440 438*	*180 469*

Table 11 Percentage of DALYs from all causes due to the health risks of reproduction, GBD baseline projection for 2000, according to alternative definitions of reproductive health, by region

EME	2.4	5.5	3.3	4.9	35.4	19.9
FSE	1.5	5.1	2.8	7.3	34.5	13.3
IND	4.7	15.5	3.6	35.7	29.7	10.5
CHN	0.7	6.5	1.1	17.0	35.2	15.2
OAI	4.3	12.7	4.1	30.5	36.4	15.0
SSA	6.1	16.3	3.9	52.1	28.5	10.8
LAC	4.5	12.9	3.3	24.0	43.3	21.8
MEC	1.9	13.9	2.3	46.9	27.4	8.9
WORLD	*3.7*	*12.4*	*3.1*	*32.9*	*32.5*	*13.3*

Table 12 Percentage of DALYs due to the health risks of reproduction which occur in females, GBD baseline projection for 2000, according to alternative definitions of reproductive health, by region

EME	36.5	41.6	78.7	46.6	27.9	1.7
FSE	80.6	55.1	88.1	47.8	24.0	5.5
IND	68.2	55.8	84.3	51.7	42.6	40.0
CHN	81.6	54.4	91.2	51.7	38.0	4.1
OAI	73.1	54.8	81.9	47.0	38.1	22.9
SSA	71.9	57.5	79.9	47.3	42.0	25.6
LAC	52.3	47.3	86.1	46.1	33.1	5.7
MEC	89.5	54.2	90.6	49.4	39.1	29.5
WORLD	*69.5*	*54.8*	*83.4*	*48.7*	*38.3*	*20.9*

Table 13 Percentage of DALYs due to the health risks of reproduction that are attributed to maternal causes, GBD baseline projection for 2000, according to alternative definitions of reproductive health, by region

Burden of Reproductive Health Defined as:

	Consequences of sex in adults	Consequences of sex in children and adults	Conditions of the reproductive organ system	Conditions managed through reproductive health services	Burden in the reproductive age group (15-44 years)	Conditions predominantly afflicting the reproductive age group (15-44 years)
EME	18.2	5.7	9.4	5.3	0.9	1.6
FSE	43.2	14.0	27.0	9.4	2.4	6.1
IND	61.7	15.4	50.7	5.4	10.5	27.7
CHN	80.9	13.2	69.1	4.9	3.4	8.2
OAI	55.6	16.1	43.0	5.7	7.2	17.6
SSA	54.5	20.6	56.5	5.8	12.4	30.4
LAC	47.4	12.2	42.0	5.4	4.4	9.4
MEC	85.7	15.5	73.7	4.6	9.5	26.0
WORLD	*58.6*	*16.0*	*50.3*	*5.4*	*7.1*	*17.1*

age. Under *Option D*, more than half of all deaths in Sub-Saharan Africa would be attributed to hazards of sex and reproduction. Typically, the proportionate mortality from reproductive ill-health is significantly lower in low mortality regions such as EME, FSE and China.

No matter which option is used to define reproductive hazards, mortality from them is significantly higher in Sub-Saharan Africa and India. The share of reproductive ill-health deaths which occur in Sub-Saharan Africa varied from about one-quarter (*Options B, C, D, E and F*) to 39 per cent (*Option A*). In India, the contribution to global mortality was more stable across options — about 19–26 per cent, but markedly lower (14 per cent) for the definition encompassing the increased risk ratio (*Option F*).

Somewhat surprisingly, the proportion of global reproductive health-related deaths that occur in EME and FSE does not remain uniformly low across the six definitions. While the contribution of these two regions is typically around 1–7 per cent, it increases to 20 per cent for EME when reproductive health is defined as *Option C: Conditions of the Reproductive Organ System*. This highlights the importance of the reproductive organ cancers, especially breast and prostate, as causes of death in high-income regions.

The second cluster of definitions is the pair comprising *Option B: Consequences of sex in Children and Adults*, and *Option F: Conditions Predominantly Afflicting the Reproductive Age Group*. The inclusion of the perinatal and congenital causes under *Option B* is largely responsible

Figure 1 Components of reproductive ill-health burden by cause for options A, B and C (global deaths and DALYs)

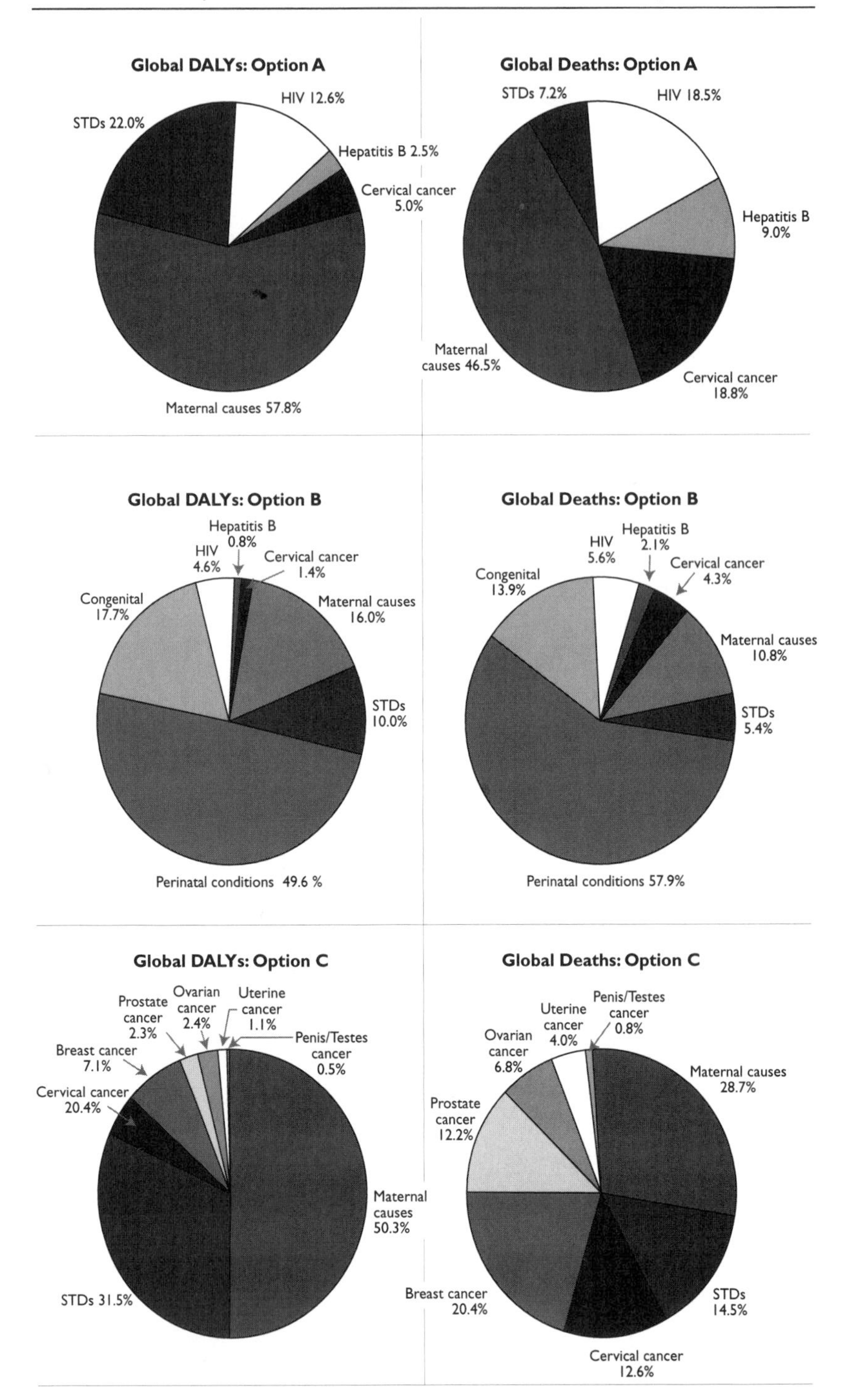

for the three-fold difference in mortality (4.2 million deaths in 1990) compared with *Option F* (1.5 million), and indeed with *Option A* (1 million). Each of these two options shows a similar sex ratio of deaths, with just over half of all so-defined reproductive risk deaths occurring among women.

The last cluster of definitions, *Option D: Conditions Managed Through Reproductive Health Services* and *Option E: Burden of the Reproductive Age Group (15–44 years)* are much more inclusive and as a consequence they define a less coherent collection of causes. Because *Option D* includes all causes of death in children aged 0–4 years, the total number of deaths attributed to the risks of reproduction is 13.2 million, or 26.2 per cent of global mortality. *Option E* includes all causes of burden in the population of reproductive age, resulting in an estimated 6.4 million deaths or 12.7 per cent of global mortality.

Figure 1 illustrates the composition of reproductive ill-health burden by cause for *Options A, B* and *C* in terms of global reproductive deaths and DALYs. In *Option A: Consequences of Sex in Adults* which is a narrow definition, both deaths and DALYs are dominated by maternal causes. In terms of deaths, cervical cancer due to human papilloma virus is the next most important component but in terms of DALYs, STDs are the next largest. Using the definition in *Option C: Consequences of Sex in Children and Adults* which is also relatively narrow, maternal causes and STDs make up over 80 per cent of the estimated global DALYs from reproductive health but in terms of mortality reproductive organ system cancers account for over half of the global burden. Because *Option B: Consequences of sex in Children and Adults* includes perinatal and congenital causes which are major contributors to overall disease burden, these two childhood causes dominate the cause composition. Childhood causes account for the vast majority of the burden of reproductive ill health calculated according to *Option D* while there is a wide variety of causes that contribute to the burden in *Options E* and *F*.

DALYs

The pattern of DALYs from reproductive ill-health is substantially different than deaths because of the young age of many of the deaths associated with reproductive ill-health and the large component of Years Lived with Disability (YLDs) from many of these conditions. For example, the share of all DALYs attributable to reproductive risks as defined by *Option E: Burden of the Reproductive Age Group (15–44 years)* and *Option F: Conditions Predominantly Afflicting the Reproductive Age Group* is two to four times higher than that suggested by deaths alone (see Tables 2 and 5). Measuring the burden of reproductive ill-health in terms of DALYs also increases the comparative importance of *Option E* compared to *Option D: Conditions Managed Through Reproductive Health Services*. In terms of mortality, the disease burden suggested by *Option E* is about half that of *Option D*; when disability is included as well, the disease burden of *Option E* increases to about 80 per cent of the *Option D*.

The tendency for much of the disease burden from reproductive ill-health to arise in Sub-Saharan Africa and India is not nearly so evident when DALYs are compared rather than deaths. Indeed, under *Options E* and *F*, these two regions together account for only about one-third of the global burden arising from reproductive ill-health, not very much higher than the proportionate contribution from other developing regions.

It is interesting to note that when DALYs are considered, the estimated amount of total disease burden attributable to reproductive health is similar for *Options B and F* (about 13 per cent), despite the very different conceptualizations of these two definitions. This was not the case for deaths where proportionate mortality from *Option B* (8.4 per cent) was three times that of *F* (3 per cent). The use of DALYs also leads to a substantially higher proportion of the reproductive disease burden in females, compared with what is suggested from deaths alone. This is particularly evident for the low mortality regions LAC, FSE and EME, because of the disabilities associated with maternal causes and STDs.

As mentioned earlier, reproductive health is often equated with complications related to pregnancy whereas the disease burden due to the hazards of sex and reproduction is in reality much greater. This is illustrated by the data presented in Table 13 which shows the percentage of all DALYs attributable to the health risks of sex and reproduction that are accounted for by the cluster of maternal conditions. Maternal conditions range from accounting for over half of the reproductive health burden for *Option A* and *Option C*, to around one-sixth of the burden for *Option B* and *Option F* to less than 10 per cent of the burden for *Option C* and *Option E*.

Figure 2 Global DALYs due to health risks of reproduction

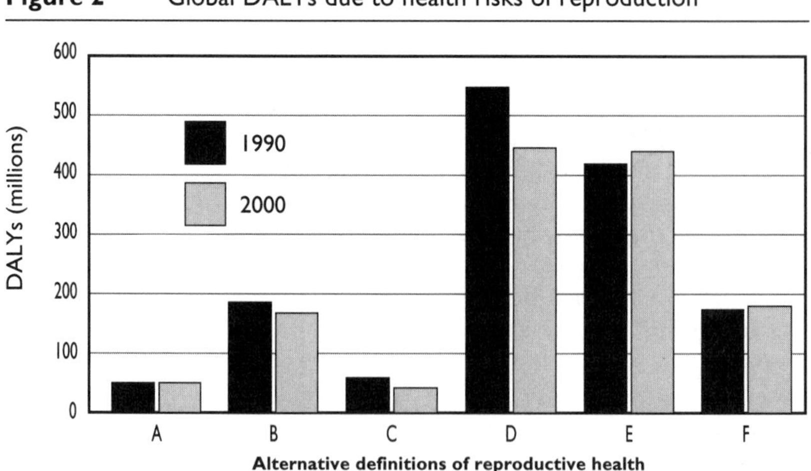

Changes in Reproductive Health DALYs 1990–2000

Figure 2 illustrates the expected changes in the burden of reproductive ill-health between 1990 and 2000, according to the six definitions. This heterogeneity reiterates the need for a clear specification of what is meant by reproductive health when discussing epidemiological patterns and trends. For example, under *Option A: Consequences of Sex in Adults*, the change in DALYs between 1990 and 2000 is minor, declining slightly in some regions (FSE, China), and rising marginally elsewhere. Modest declines are expected according to *Option B: Consequences of sex in Children and Adults* and *Option C: Conditions of the Reproductive Organ System*. Given the major contribution of child mortality to *Option D: Conditions Managed Through Reproductive Health Services* which is declining substantially, the burden of reproductive health according to this definition will drop by 19 per cent. Conversely, both definitions related to the reproductive age group (*Option E* and *Option F*) imply that the burden of reproductive health risks will rise over the decade.

Discussion

Political debates on the scope of reproductive health and the associated boundaries defining the health risks of reproduction will undoubtedly continue. The analyses presented in this chapter clearly indicate, however, that the proposed definitions of reproductive health can lead to enormous differences in the magnitude of premature mortality and disability from the health risks of reproduction. Even the direction of the trends in the burden of reproductive ill-health depend critically on the definition used. It is not our intention to argue for one or and other of the definitions presented in this chapter. Rather, we hope that this exercise in quantification will contribute to a more informed debate on the scope and nature of reproductive health. Progress in epidemiological surveillance and assessment will be severely hampered until a consensus on the definition of reproductive health and the boundaries defining the health risks of reproduction is attained.

The six definitions proposed here range from focussed, restrictive definitions such as *Option A: Consequences of Sex in Adults* and *Option C: Conditions of the Reproductive Organ System* to more inclusive but also more diffuse definitions such as *Option B: Consequences of sex in Children and Adults* and *Option F: Conditions Predominantly Afflicting the Reproductive Age Group*, to definitions that are so inclusive that there is little relationship to problems commonly associated with sex and reproduction such as *Option D: Conditions Managed Through Reproductive Health Services* and *Option E: Burden of the Reproductive Age Group (15–44 years)*. In the case of *Option D,* inclusion of all childhood causes of premature mortality and disability completely swamps the contribution of health events related to sex and reproduction in adult women. Likewise, *Option E* gives little focus to the health problems that are generally associated with the domain of reproductive health. This chapter clearly demonstrates that the magnitude of specific health problems must be considered when drawing the boundaries that define the health risks of sex and reproduction.

Despite the heterogeneity of patterns that emerge using different definitions, we can draw several substantive conclusions on the cause composition of reproductive ill-health. In all of the definitions, a significant component of the burden is due to premature mortality and disability in males – ranging from 14 per cent in *Option A* to over half in *Option E*. Little of the literature on reproductive health has focussed on male reproductive ill-health. In the narrower definitions such as *Option A* and *Option C*, it is clear that maternal causes and STDs are extremely important components of reproductive ill-health. Comparison of the deaths and DALYs attributable to the health risks of sex and reproduction clearly indicates that there is disproportionately large component of burden due to disability and to the young average age of death from these causes. Research and intervention studies on reproductive health will need to pay particular attention to disabling outcomes from these causes.

What is clear from this analysis is that the burden of reproductive health hazards is large and of major public health concern, irrespective of what definition is used. Ten-year projections over the period 1990–2000 also suggest that this disease burden is unlikely to diminish rapidly. With a proportionate contribution to overall disease burden of 5–15 per cent even by the most restrictive definitions, the improvement of reproductive health conditions, especially in developing countries will remain a public health priority for the foreseeable future.

References

Benagiano G (1996) Reproductive health as an essential human right. Advances in Contraception 12(4):243–50.

Diczfalusy E et al. (1994) Reproductive health: towards a brighter future. World Health Forum 15(1):1–8.

Fathalla MF (1991) Reproductive health: a global overview. Annals of the New York Academy of Science 626:1.

Ford Foundation (1991) Reproductive health: a strategy for the 1990s. New York: Ford Foundation.

Garcia-Moreno C, Turmen T (1995) International perspectives on women's reproductive health. Science 269:790–792.

Germain A, Ordway J (1989) Population control and women's health: balancing the scales. International Women's Health Coalition and the Overseas Development Council, New York.

Katz ME et al. (1995) Mortality rates among 15 to 44-year-old women in Boston: looking beyond reproductive status. American Journal of Public Health 85(8):1135–8.

Murray CJL and Lopez AD, eds. (1996a) *The global burden of disease: a comprehensive asessment of mortality and disability from diseases, injuries, and risk factors in 1990 and projected into 2020.* Cambridge, Harvard University Press.

Murray CJL and Lopez AD (1996b) *Global health statistics: a compendium of incidence, prevalence and mortality estimates for over 200 conditions.* Cambridge, Harvard University Press.

Miller K, Rosenfield A (1996) Population and women's reproductive health: an international perspective. Annual Review of Public Health 17:359–82.

Neilson JP, Molyneux DH, Peel KR (1995) Reproductive health in developing countries: a new initiative. British Journal of Obstetrics and Gynecology 102(5):353–4.

Rothman KJ (1986) *Modern epidemiology.* Boston: Little Brown and Company.

United Nations (1994) Report of the International Conference on Population and Development. United Nations: New York.

World Health Organization (1996) *Constitution of the World Health Organization. Basic documents (41st edition).* Geneva.

World Health Organization (1994) *Health, Population and Development: WHO position paper for the International Conference on Population and Development,* WHO/FHE/94, Geneva.

World Health Organization (1997) *Proposed programme budget for 1998–1999, Division of Reproductive Health,* WHO/FRH/RHT/97.5, Geneva.

Chapter 2

Sexually Transmitted Diseases

Jane Rowley
Seth Berkley

Introduction

Sexually transmitted diseases (STDs) are found throughout the world and are recognized as an important public health problem. Their health and social consequences, however, are much greater for women than for men, especially women in the reproductive age groups and their offspring, reflecting a variety of biological, economic and social factors. In addition, STDs and their complications are found more often in resource poor settings.

Increased recognition of the range of sexually transmitted infections and their sequelae through the use of new diagnostic methods has made the field of STDs one of the more dynamic areas of medicine in recent years. Over 40 bacterial, viral, and parasitic diseases have been identified that can be transmitted sexually (see Table 1). Unraveling the relationships between a STD and its complications, however, is a complex exercise and involves examining correlations among conditions with varying definitions, imprecise diagnoses, different microbial organisms, and temporal lags. In addition, there are few data on the relative frequencies of different complications or on their duration in those untreated.

The diagnosis and management of STDs is complicated by the lack of rapid and inexpensive diagnostic tests for most STDs. As a result, health care workers usually diagnose infections based on their symptoms. However, many STDs, particularly in women, are asymptomatic or minimally symptomatic with non-specific symptoms. In addition, current methods for diagnosing a number of STDs in women require a pelvic examination. This in turn requires a private setting, good light source, appropriate training, sterile speculums, and cultural acceptance. These characteristics mean that in many parts of the world only a fraction of infected individuals are treated.

Complications in females result primarily from the migration of STD pathogens upwards from the lower reproductive tract. This can lead to

Table 1 The most important sexually transmitted pathogens and the diseases they cause

Pathogens	*Disease or syndrome*
Bacterial agents	
Neisseria gonorrhoeae	Urethritis, epididymitis, proctititis, bartholinitis, cervicitis, endometritis, salpingitis and related sequelae (infertility, ectopic pregnancy), perihepatitis; complications of pregnancy (e.g., chorioamnionitis, premature rupture of membranes, premature delivery, postpartum endometritis); conjunctivitis; disseminated gonococcal infection (DGI)
Chlamydia trachomatis	Same as *N. gonorrhoeae*, except for DGI. Also trachoma, lymphogranuloma venereum, Reiter's syndrome, infant pneumonia
Treponema pallidum	Syphilis
Haemophilus ducreyi	Chancroid
Mycoplamsa hominis	Postpartum fever, salpingitis
Ureaplasma urealyticum	Urethritis, low birth weight, chorioamnionitis
Gardnerella vagnialis, etc.*	Bacterial vaginosis
Calymmatobacterium granulomatis	Donovanosis
Shigella species, *Campylobacter* spp.	Shigellosis, campylobacteriosis (sexually transmitted among homosexual men)
Group B ß-hemolytic streptococcus	Neonatal sepsis, neonatal meningitis
Viral agents	
Herpes simplex virus	Primary and recurrent genital herpes, asceptic meningitis, neonatal herpes with associated mortality or neurological sequelae. Spontaneous abortion and premature delivery
Hepatitis A virus	Acute hepatitis A (sexually transmitted among homosexual men)
Hepatitis B virus	Acute, chronic, and fulminant hepatis B, with associated immune complex phenomena and sequelae including cirrhosis and hepatocellular carcinoma
Cytomegalovirus	Congenital infection: gross birth defects and infant mortality, cognitive impairment (e.g., mental retardation, sensorineural deafness), heterophile-negative infectious mononucleosis, protean manifestations in the immunosupressed host
Human papilloma virus	Condyloma acuminata, laryngeal papilloma in infants, squamous epithelial neoplasias of the cervix, anus, vagina, vulva, and penis
Molluscum contagiosum virus	Genital molluscum contagiosum
Human immunodeficiency virus	AIDS and related conditions
HTLV-1	T-cell leukemia/lymphoma, tropical spastic paraperesis

Table 1 (continued)

Pathogens	*Disease or syndrome*
Protozoan agents	
Trichomonas vaginalis	Vaginitis, urethritis, balanitis
Entamoeba histolytica	Amebiasis (sexually transmitted among homosexual men)
Giardia lamblia	Giardiasis (sexually transmitted among homosexual men)
Fungal agents	
Candida albicans	Vulvovaginitis, balanitis, balanoposthitis
Ectoparasites	
Phthirus pubis	Pubic lice infestation
Sarcoptis scabies	Scabies

* Vaginal bacteria associated with bacterial vaginosis include *G. vaginalis, Mobiluncus* spp. (*M. curtisii, M. mulieris*), *Bacteroides* spp. (e.g. *B. bivius, B. disiens*, black pigmented species), *Mycoplasma hominis, Ureaplasma urealyticum*.

Source: Piot and Holmes 1990

pelvic inflammatory disease (inflammation of the uterus, fallopian tubes, ovaries, or other pelvic structures), chronic pelvic pain, tubo-ovarian abscesses, ectopic pregnancies and infertility. In pregnant women untreated STDs can also result in fetal wastage, stillbirths, low birth weight, eye damage, lung damage, and congenital abnormalities. In adult males infection spreads from the urethra to the epididymis and may cause urethral stricture and infertility. In both adult males and females untreated syphilis can lead to cardiovascular and neurological disease. Many STDs also facilitate the transmission of HIV and are associated with particular types of cancer.

Data on the incidence of STDs and their complications are limited and substantially underestimate the burden of these diseases. This is particularly true in regions with limited access to health facilities for the diagnosis and treatment of STDs, and where there is a social stigma attached to STDs. In most countries, the data that are available are of uncertain quality and are not representative of the general population. Studies have primarily been carried out in "convenient" population groups, such as those attending STD or antenatal care (ANC) clinics, and often have a small sample size. In addition, the use of different diagnostic methods further complicates the interpretation and comparison of results.

It is estimated that in 1990 there were over 160 million new cases of the three "classic" bacterial STDs—gonorrhoea, chlamydia and syphilis in adults between the ages of 15 and 49. These three STDs, however, represent only a fraction of the new STD cases each year. STDs, including HIV (but not hepatitis B or human papilloma virus (HPV)), are estimated globally to account for 33.3 million DALYs and in the worst affected region, Sub-Saharan Africa, they account for 15.6 million DALYs—5.3 per cent of the total burden: 15.6 per cent of the burden in females between the ages of 15 and 44 and 6.8 per cent in males in the same age group.

The direct and indirect costs in the United States of just one STD, chlamydia, were estimated to be US$ 2.4 billion in 1990—more than 70 per cent of which was attributable to the complications and sequelae (Washington et al. 1987). STDs also place a major burden on the health care system. For example, in Africa it is estimated that STDs account for 2.5 to 15 per cent of all adult outpatient diagnoses (Piot and Holmes 1990) and in the United States women with pelvic inflammatory disease (PID) make over 2.5 million outpatient visits for PID each year and account for 275,000 hospital admissions.

Effective and accessible STD treatment and prevention programmes are key to reducing the global burden associated with STDs. Improved access to STD treatment, information and education campaigns designed to change sexual behaviour patterns, condom promotion, and contact tracing all have important roles to play in reducing the spread of STDs, the incidence of complications and sequelae, the development of drug resistance, and HIV transmission. STD treatment programmes also provide an opportunity to target behavioural change activities at those individuals at greatest risk of transmitting or acquiring STDs or HIV.

The focus of this chapter is on the three "classic" sexually transmitted bacterial diseases—gonorrhoea, chlamydia, and syphilis. HIV (human immunodeficiency virus) and HPV (human papilloma virus), which is closely linked with cervical cancer, the most common cancer in women in many parts of the world, two viral diseases that can be transmitted sexually and are associated with a high disease burden are discussed in detail in Chapters 9 and 13 of this volume.

Natural History of STDs

STDs are part of the wider spectrum of reproductive tract infections which include: endogenous infections caused by an overgrowth of organisms normally found in the reproductive tract of healthy women; sexually transmitted infections such as non-specific bacterial vaginosis and moniliasis (candidiasis); and iatrogenic infections associated with medical instrumentation related to different procedures such as induced abortion.

STDs infect the reproductive tract as their primary site with transmission primarily occuring during sexual intercourse or from mother to child during pregnancy or childbirth. As a result, the groups at greatest risk of infection are sexually active individuals and infants born to infected mothers. Many STDs, however, can also be transmitted through other routes. The relative importance of the various transmission routes reflects the biology of the pathogen and behavioural and environmental factors. For example, Hepatitis B and Cytomegalovirus (CMV) are frequently acquired in childhood through non-sexual routes in populations with low hygiene standards or poor living conditions. *Trichomonas vaginalis* can also be transmitted non sexually—in a study of girls under the age of 10 in Nigeria *T. vaginalis* was the most common cause of vaginitis. Contaminated bed clothing, sharing of underwear and towels with older household members, and digitogenital contamination from infected adults were believed to be the most important ways of transmission (Osoba and Alausa 1974)

STDs share a number of biological, medical and behavioural characteristics that distinguish them from other infectious diseases and have implications for the design and implementation of prevention programmes (Aral and Holmes 1991, Wasserheit 1989).

Biological

- STD micro-organisms can only survive outside the human host for short periods of time (minutes to hours) and as a result direct contact (e.g., genital mucosal contact) is required for efficient transmission.
- Most STD micro-organisms are uniquely adapted to humans and have no non-human reservoirs.
- STD micro-organisms have elaborate pathogenic mechanisms that permit persistence or reinfection in the face of an immune response.
- The genetic structure of most STD agents varies widely.

Medical

- STDs may be asymptomatic or minimally symptomatic, especially in females.
- No vaccines have been approved for a STD except for sexually transmitted hepatitis B.

Behavioural

- A subset of individuals with high rates of sexual partner change play an important role in transmission and in maintaining infection in a population. Individuals with high rates of sexual partner change include prostitutes and, in some areas, truck drivers, members of the military, and migrant workers. These individuals are frequently difficult to reach with prevention programmes especially when their activities are illegal.
- Women are not only more likely than men to be asymptomatic and to develop complications and pathological sequelae but are also (1) less likely to be treated when they have symptoms and (2) more likely to continue having sex while symptomatic as their symptoms often manifest in the less well innerverated cervix, and hence are less painful during intercourse.
- Individuals who are asymptomatic or minimally symptomatic may spread their infection without realizing it.

- The social stigma of infection often makes patients reluctant to admit they have a problem or to name their sexual contacts hence allowing individuals who are not aware of their infection to transmit it to others, and also leaving themselves open to reinfection.

Boxes 1 to 3 briefly review the natural history of gonorrhoea, chlamydia, and syphilis while Table 2 provides information on the natural history of some of the other important sexually transmitted pathogens.

Epidemiology of Sexually Transmitted Diseases

Epidemiological data show that the prevalence and incidence of the various STDs vary widely between countries and within a country. Differences in the epidemiological patterns of STDs reflect differences in the characteristics of each microorganism (e.g. duration of infectivity, transmissibility) and other biological, behavioural, medical, social and economic factors (see Table 3). Multiple infections within an individual are also frequent, as is reinfection either from the original source or secondary sources if these partners have not been adequately treated.

In general, the prevalence of detected STDs, tends to be higher in men, in urban residents, in unmarried persons, and in young adults. Highest rates of infection occur in the 15–44 year old age group—over 90 per cent of infections have been documented in this age group. For most STDs infections in females occur at an earlier age than in males. This relates to patterns of sexual mixing as well as to relative rates of transmission from males to females and vice versa—for many STDs the probability of transmission is higher from males to females than from females to males.

A number of epidemological studies have looked at risk factors for acquiring STDs through sexual intercourse. Factors identified include: large number of sexual partners; marital status; sexual intercourse with a commercial sex worker; history of STDs; urban residence; age; and gender. In males circumcision status has also been identified as a risk factor for genital ulcers—uncircumcised males have a greater susceptibility probably as a result of the frequent cracks and tears that occur in the foreskin. In females the use of oral contraceptives has been found to predispose users to candidiasis and thereby increasing the risk of attachment for *C trachomatis*. The data, however, also suggest that oral contraceptives may decrease the risk of upper tract infections by making the cervical mucus plug less penetrable to organisms (Stamm and Holmes 1990).

At the population level the rate of spread of a STD depends upon the average number of new cases generated by each infected person which is often described in terms of the basic or case reproduction ratio (R_0). The basic reproduction ratio for a STD is determined by the efficiency of transmission (β), the effective mean rate of sexual partner change (c), and the average duration of infectiousness (D).

Table 2 Natural history of selected STDs.

Disease & Pathogen	*First Symptoms*	*Incubation Period*	*Natural History/Sequlae*	*Transmissibility*
Chancroid — *Haemophilus ducreyi*	*Females:* Painful, irregularly shaped ulcers at entrance to vagina and around anus. May cause pain on urination or defecation, rectal bleeding, pain on intercourse, or vaginal discharge. May have no symptoms. *Males:* Painful, irregularly shaped ulcers on penis or tenderness in groin.	Usually 3 to 7 days, up to10 days.	Ulcers disappear without treatment usually in about a months but may last to 12 weeks. Causes inguinal buboes in up to one-half of cases. Lesions are difficult to distinguish from ulcers caused by syphilis or genital herpes.	*Sexual:* Acquired through vaginal or anal intercourse. People are infectious as long as they have ulcers. *Mother to child:* No transmission from mother to fetus or during delivery.
Trichomaniasis — *Trichomaniasis vaginalis*	*Females:* Green or yellow, abundant, frothy vagnial discharge with foul odour, itching, pain on urination, pain on intercourse. *Males:* Usually without symptoms but may involve urethral discharge, pain on urination, or itching.	3 to 28 days	*Females:* Without treatment initial symptoms may persist for years. Symptoms worsen during or after menses. No complications or sequelae in most cases. *Males:* Most cases resolve spontaneously. Sequelae include urethritis, prostatitis and infertility. *Infants:* May contribute to pregnancy complications, especially premature delivery and low birth weight.	*Sexual:* Up to 85% of the female sexual partners of infected men are infected. 30% to 40% of male partners of infected women are infected. *Mother to infant:* About 5% of girls born to infected women are infected during birth.
Donovanosis (Granuloma inguinale) — *C. granulomatis*	Nodules below the skin that break through to form a beefy lesion. In women lesions usually form on the labia and in men on the prepuce or glans of the penis. Women may have no symptoms.	8 to 80 days	Without treatment, may erode genitalia or block urethra.	Not available.

Table 2 (continued)

Disease & Pathogen	*First Symptoms*	*Incubation Period*	*Natural History/ Sequlae*	*Transmissibility*
Herpes — Herpes simplex virus (HSV types 1 and 2)	*Females:* First episode: Painful blisterlike lesions in and around vagina, around anus, or on thighs. Pain may be more severe than in men. May cause painful urination or vaginal discharge. As many as 70% may have no symptoms. Symptoms last about 2 to 3 weeks. *Males:* First episode: Painful penile lesions. May cause urethral discharge or pain on urination. Same systemic symptoms as in women.	1 to 26 days; average 6 to 7 days	In both men and women primary infection can affect central nervous system, causing stiff neck, headache, fever, malaise and abnormal sensitivity to light. Can lead to cervicitis in women and proctitis in both sexes. Half of those infected have recurrences. Compared with first episode, recurrent episodes involve smaller and fewer lesions and systemic symptoms are less common. Pain, numbness, or tingling in buttocks, legs, or hips may precede outbreak. *Infants:* Women who develop a first episode of genital herpes during pregnancy may be at higher risk for premature delivery. Half of infants who become infected die or suffer serious brain damage.	*Sexual:* In a study of 144 couples with one infected partner followed for a median of 344 days, 17% of women and 4% of men became infected. HSV can be transmitted while person is without symptoms. *Mother to infant:* If mother has first episode, 20% to 50% of infants are infected at birth; during recurrent episode, 3% to 5%. Most transmission occurs while mother has no symptoms.

Source: Based on Lande 1993 (Table 1) and Donovan 1993 (Figures 3 & 4).

Table 3 Factors affecting the spread of STDs in a population

Biological
- duration of infection
- presence of other STDs
- infectivity of particular strain of the pathogen
- age and presence of cervical erosion
- immunologic status
- circumcision status

Behavioural
- rates of sexual partner change
- type of sexual intercourse (anal, oral, vaginal)
- use of condoms and other contraceptives
- patterns of sexual contact ("who mixes with whom")

Medical
- access to health care facilities
- access to laboratory facilities
- availability of appropriate treatment

Social and economic
- migration patterns
- ease of travel
- level of education
- religion
- civil unrest
- position of women in society

$$R_0 = \beta c D$$

The higher the value of R_0 the greater the potential for the of spread of a STD (Anderson and May 1991, Brunham and Plummer 1990).

a. Efficiency of transmission (β)

The efficiency of transmission depends upon the infectiousness of the pathogen, the infectivity of the infected individual, the susceptibility of the host, and the type of sexual act (vaginal, anal, or oral). The infectivity of an individual is also related to the size of the microbial inoculum and is generally highest during early infection and when lesions or exudate are present. Condom use or microbial agents both reduce an individual's infectivity by reducing the size of the inoculum.

Various biological factors increase the risk that a susceptible individual will acquire an STD after exposure. For example, infection with another STD may increase the probability of acquiring infection. Cervical ectopy has also been shown to increase susceptibility to chlamydial infection and perhaps to gonorrhoea. Since cervical ectopy decreases with advancing age and increases with oral contraceptive use very young women and oral contraceptive users may be particularly susceptible to infection.

Box 1 Natural history of gonorrhoea

Description	A bacterial infection of the cervix, urethra, rectum or throat acquired through vaginal, anal or oral sex. The bacteria responsible for the disease, *Neisseria gonorrhoeae,* is a fastidious non-motile, small gram-negative diplococcus that has complex growth requirements and only infects humans.
First symptoms	*Females:* Vaginal discharge, dysuria (pain on urination), menstrual abnormalities, spotting after sexual intercourse, and/or lower abdominal pain. Up to 30% of women are asymptomatic. *Males:* Urethral discharge and/or pain on urination. Approximately 95% of infected males develop symptoms, usually within 2 to 5 days of infection. *Female and Males:* Anal gonorrhoea is usually asymptomatic although 10-20% may have symptomatic proctitis. Gonococcal pharyngitis tends to be asymptomatic although in a small percentage of persons, sore throat may be present.
Incubation period	1 to 14 days. Most symptoms develop within 2 to 5 days.
Natural history & sequelae	*Females:* Cervicitis, urethritis, and bartholinitis. Untreated infections may ascend and result in PID and its associated complications including infertility, ectopic pregnancy, chronic pelvic pain, tubo-ovarian abscesses. *Males:* In untreated males infection may lead to urethritis, epididymitis, stricture, and prostatitis. *Female and Males:* Untreated infection may spread to the blood stream and infect the joints, heart valves and the brain, although this is unusual. *Infants:* Clinical outcomes of neonatal infection are ophthalmia neonatorum and the systemic complications of gonococcemia (e.g. meningitis and septic arthritis). Maternal infection may also be detrimental to pregnancy outcome.
Transmissibility	*General:* Humans are infected through intimate mucosa-to-mucosa contact and the most common routes of transmission are vaginal, anal or oral sex. Transmission through other routes, however, has been documented. *Sexual intercourse:* Transmission from females to males is less efficient than from males to females. Studies have documented that 50-90% of females acquire infection from an infected male after one exposure (Platt et al. 1983) while 20% of males are infected after one exposure and 60-80% after 4 exposures (Holmes et al. 1970). *Mother to infant:* In the absence of eye prophylaxis 30 to 40 % of infants exposed during birth will develop gonococcal ophthalmia neonatorum (Laga et al. 1986, Galega et al. 1984, also see de Schryver and Meheus 1990). The use of tetracycline or silver nitrate reduces the risk to less than 6% (Laga et al. 1988).
Treatment	Infection can be cured with antibiotics but owing to the development of antibiotic resistance it is important that treatment is based upon the antibiotic resistance patterns in the local area. As patients may be co-infected with *C. trachomatis* dual therapy is often prescribed.

Box 2	Natural history of chlamydia
Description	A bacterial infection acquired chiefly through vaginal or anal intercourse, although it can also be transmitted through oral sex. The bacteria responsible for the disease, *Chlamydia trachomatis,* is an obligate intracellular parasite and requires live tissue culture for laboratory growth. There are two biovars that infect humans: lymphogranuloma venereum (LGV) and trachoma. The former causes an STD found predominantly in the tropics and results in lymph node infections while the latter causes ocular and genital infections.
First symptoms	*Females:* Vaginal discharge, pain on urination, spotting after sexual intercourse, lower abdominal pain and/or pain during intercourse. The clinical spectrum is similar to gonorrhoea but, in general, with less inflammation. Approximately 25-30% of women develop symptoms which are usually non-specific. *Males:* Urethral discharge, pain on urination, and/or swelling or pain in the testicles. Symptoms are similar to gonorrhoea although less purulent. Approximately 70-80% of males develop symptoms. *Female and Males:* Symptomatic rectal infections may occur and are similar to rectal gonococcal infections. Ocular infections may also occur as a result of inoculation of the eye with infected genital secretions. Symptoms include redness and discharge from the eye.
Incubation period	7 to 21 days before symptoms appear (if present).
Natural history & sequelae	*Females:* Can cause cervicitis, urethritis, and bartholinitis. If untreated up to 30% of infections may ascend into the uterus, fallopian tubes, ovaries or peritoneum, causing PID (salpingitis and endometritis) which in turn may lead to ectopic pregnancy, infertility, and chronic pelvic pain. Often the first symptom of chlamydia infection is the pain of PID. *Males:* Can cause urethritis and epididymitis. If untreated may lead to infertility. *Infants:* Clinical outcomes of neonatal infection are ophthalmia neonatorum and pneumonia. In pregnant women may also cause premature rupture of membranes and preterm delivery.
Transmissibility	*Sexual intercourse:* Chlamydia appears to be less contagious than gonorrhoea. In a study of individuals with dual infection (gonorrhoea and chlamydia) 45% of women and 30% of men whose sexual partners had chlamydia were infected. Partners were infected with chlamydia 1/3 to 2/3 as frequently as with gonorrhoea (Lycke et al. 1980). Actual transmission, however, may be higher than this when assessed using more sensitive diagnostic methods (e.g. PCR, LCR). *Mother to infant:* 60-70% of infants exposed during birth develop respiratory, lung or eye infections. Epidemiological data suggest that infants generally become infected via delivery through an infected cervix as infection after Cesarean sections are rare.
Treatment	Infection can be cured with tetracyclines, however, prolonged therapy is required raising issues of compliance. There is also evidence suggesting that some chlamydial organisms may survive after the currently recommended therapy although the clinical significance of this has not been determined. Single oral dose therapy with newer antibiotics such as azithromycin is also possible but currently expensive. As patients mey be co-infected with *N. gonorrhoeae* dual therapy is often prescribed.

Box 3	Natural history of syphilis
Description	A bacterial infection caused by the spirochete *Treponema pallidum*. The bacteria can spread throughout the body and is usually transmitted sexually. *T. pallidum* is a member of the Treponema family which includes two other spirochetes that are pathogenic in man: *T. pertenue* (yaws) and *T. carateum* (pinta). So far no antigenic or chemical differences has been found between the various pathogenic treponemas and hence differentiation is only possible by clinical means.
First symptoms	*Adults:* Small painless sore (chancre) on vulva, cervix, penis, nose, mouth, or anus. Multiple lesions may occur and atypical presentations are common. Without therapy, the chancres heal within 3-6 weeks. In males chancres usually occur on the external genitalia. In females chancres frequently occur internally and hence primary infections are less likely to be identified in women.
Incubation period	10 to 90 days post infection (average 21 days).
Natural history & sequelae	*Adults:* Symptoms of secondary syphilis appear 2 to 8 weeks after the primary lesion develop. Secondary syphilis is usually marked by a rash that may cover the entire body or only a few areas. Other symptoms include: malaise, fever, general lymph-node enlargement, hepatitis, arthritis, and/or hearing loss. Symptoms resolve after several weeks or months even when left untreated. About 30% of untreated individuals go on to develop late syphilis where they may experience symptomatic destruction of the central nervous and cardiovascular systems or develop large soft lesions in other organs (gummas). *Infants:* Most children with congenital syphilis are apparently normal at birth - clinical features usually appear between 2 and 8 weeks of age and may be quite variable (Hira and Hira, 1987). If untreated infants may suffer damage to the heart, brain or eyes.
Transmissibility	*General:* The most common way to acquire syphilis is through vaginal, anal or oral sex with someone who has an active infection. It can also be spread by nonsexual contact between sores produced by the disease and broken skin of another individual. *Sexual intercourse:* The probability of transmission from males to females and from females to males appears to be similar. 30-60% of partners become infected after a single exposure to someone with infectious lesions. The secondary stage is also highly infectious, however, syphilis is rarely transmitted more than 2 years after acquisition. *Mother to child:* Syphilis can pass through the placenta as early as the ninth week of pregnancy and in two thirds or more of pregnancies results in spontaneous abortion, stillbirth or neonatal death. Women with untreated syphilis may be infectious to fetus for many years although the proportion of affected fetuses appears to decrease with duration of maternal infection (Brunham et al. 1990).
Treatment	Syphilis is easily treated with penicillin. In late syphilis and in patients suspected of having neurosyphilis higher doses may be required. Damage done to body organs cannot be reversed.

b. Effective mean rate of sexual partner change (c)
The extent of spread of an STD depends upon: the average number of sexual partnerships formed per unit of time by infected individuals; heterogeneity in rates of sexual partner change; patterns of sexual contact (i.e. who mixes with whom); and the type of contraceptives used and when they are used. In general, those individuals with high rates of sexual partner change (often referred to as the "core") contribute disproportionately to STD transmission. The contribution of this group, however, varies greatly. For example, in Africa and Asia up to 80 per cent of male STD patients named commercial sex workers, a key component of the "core", as their source of infection, while in Europe and North America this figure is less then 20 per cent (Piot and Holmes 1990).

The main source of quantitative data on sexual behaviour patterns is the former WHO Global Programme on AIDS supported sexual behaviour surveys (Carael 1995).

In all of the surveys males reported a higher number of sexual partners than women. Age differences between regular partners were between three and five years in most societies. Large age differences were associated with high levels of polygamy or of multiple partnerships. Urban-rural disparities in proportions sexually active were less pronounced than expected and there was a strong correlation between behaviour in rural and urban areas. An additional independent predictor of sexual activity among youths was education—among males secondary schooling was associated with a substantial increase in risk behaviour, while among females primary schooling was associated with an increase in risk behaviour.

WHO studies also documented large differences between countries in a number of areas including:

- the percentage of men and women reporting non-regular sex (defined as sex with a person who is not a spouse and has lasted less than one year) and commercial sex (sex that involved the exchange of money, gift or favours) in the last 12 months;
- the number of non-marital partners reported by men and women;
- the age at first intercourse;
- levels of premarital sexual activity and rates of partner change among persons aged 15 to 19 years;
- the age at which men and women first marry or enter a stable partnership.

Data from studies carried out in Guinea Bissau and Cote d'Ivoire provide additional information on the age distribution of sexual activity. In Guinea Bissau (Hogsborg and Aaby 1992) the highest mean number of sexual partners was reported by men between the ages of 20 and 29. In Cote d'Ivoire in men the highest mean number of sexual partners was in the age group 25–29 and in women in the age group 15–19 (Carael, personal communication). Women in the Cote d'Ivoire study also reported much lower mean number of sexual partners per year than men.

c. Duration of infectiousness (D)
The average duration of infectiousness depends upon the pathogen as well as the quality, accessibility, and use of health services. Early diagnosis and treatment shortens the average length of time infected individuals are infectious and hence reduces both the rate of spread of the infection as well as the probability of developing complications and sequelae.

Diagnosing infection

The clinical presentation of the initial symptoms of STDs are limited in nature, and each presentation can be caused by a variety of organisms. For example, genital ulcers are commonly associated with syphilis as well as chancroid and herpes simplex, and urethritis and cervicitis with both gonorrhoea and chlamydia. Vaginitis may also be caused by gonorrhoea or chlamydia but is more commonly caused by trichomonas or candida. Without the help of diagnostic tests it is therefore difficult to make a definitive diagnosis. Rapid and easily administered diagnostic tests that are both sensitive and specific however are not available for most STDs. Box 4 provides a brief summary of the diagnostic tests currently available for each of the STDs.

Where diagnostic tests are not available the WHO recommends following a syndromic approach where diagnosis is based upon the presence of vaginal or urethral discharge and lower abdominal pain, and strict treatment protocols are then followed. Syndromic diagnosis may result in over treatment or in inappropriate treatment. For example, a male who presents with urethritis may be presumptively treated for both gonorrhoea and chlamydia even though the individual may have been suffering from one or neither of these infections. In general, syndromic diagnosis is more useful for males than for females as many infected women do not generate symptoms or develop non-specific symptoms—in Zaire a simple hierarchical algorithm based only on symptoms had a sensitivity of 48 per cent and a specificity of 75 per cent in pregnant women (Vuylsteke et al. 1993).

Definition and Measurement

The quantity and quality of data on the prevalence and incidence of STDs vary widely by country and disease. The two main sources of information are national surveillance systems and epidemiological surveys. Broadly, surveillance systems provide information on the number of people diagnosed with a particular infection or complication, while epidemiological surveys provide data on the levels of infection in a particular population group.

Box 4 Diagnostic tests

Gonorrhoea: Culture is the gold standard for diagnosis of infection with *N. gonorrhoeae* and when performed by experienced technicians it has a sensitivity of 90-95% and specificity of 100%. However, culture is complicated to perform and time consuming; cultures must be incubated at a high temperature in a humid and CO_2 enriched atmosphere, and read after 18-20 hours, and, if negative, again after 48 hours. Positive specimens can then be confirmed by sugar degradation or antibody testing. In symptomatic individuals gonorrhoea can also be diagnosed by direct microscopy of a gram stained specimen from the urethra of males or the cervix of females. Gram stains are estimated to be over 90% sensitive and 95% specific in males, but even with careful sampling of the cervix only 40 to 60% sensitive in females. Other approaches include immunoassays (estimated to have a sensitivity of 83-100% for males and 73-100% for females and a specificity of 96-100% for males and 88-100% for females (Mårdh and Danielsson, 1990)), direct immunofluorescence, PCR (polymerase chain reaction amplification of DNA sequences), and LCR (ligase chain reaction). PCR and/or LCR will probably replace culture as the gold standard as they are more sensitive than culture. But at present they require expensive equipment and trained personnel and without a major technological breakthrough will remain out of reach for widespread use in developing countries for the foreseeable future.

Chlamydia: Tissue culture is the reference technique for diagnosis of *C. trachomatis* infection. However, tissue culture is slow and technically difficult, and is beyond the capacity of many laboratories. Even in good laboratories, sensitivity may only be as high as 70-80%. In the 1980s and 90's a number of new non-culture tests were developed which are significantly easier to perform (see Table B4.1). PCR or LCR, will almost certainly replace tissue culture as the gold standard and with the finding that LCR assays are highly effective for the detection of *C. trachomatis* infection in urine from both men and women with or without signs or symptoms of genitourinary tract infection (Lee et al. 1995) they are likely to become more widely used for diagnostic purposes.

Table B4.1: Sensitivity (in per cent) of different diagnostic assays for chlamydia

Assay	Sensitivity
Direct Florescent Antibody (DFA)	60-90
Enzyme Immunoassay for Antigen (EIA)	70-90
Solid Phase Rapid EIA	70-90
Nucleic Acid Hybridization	78-96
Polymerase Chain Reaction (PCR)	95-100
Ligase Chain Reaction (LCR)	95-100
Leukocyte Esterase Test	40-70

Source: Quinn TC et al. 1994

SURVEILLANCE SYSTEMS

In countries with good reporting systems the number of reported cases is a good proxy for the total number of infections for a disease with very definite symptoms. STDs, however, are often asymptomatic and when there are symptoms these are often not specific. As a result, many infected individuals do not present at health centers and, even when they do, they may not be correctly diagnosed or treated.

Box 4 (continued)

Syphilis: Treponemes can be detected using dark field microscopes at the site of entry during primary infections and from humid lesions in the secondary stage. This technique, however, can only be done in specialized facilities as it requires considerable experience and a suitable microscope. As a result, most diagnoses are done using serologic tests. There are two types of serologic tests: nonspecific nontreponemal reagin tests and specific treponemal tests. Neither, however, can differentiate between the different pathogenic treponemes (e.g. yaws). Nontreponemal tests such as RPR (rapid plasma reagin) and VDRL detect the antibody that reacts with a component of treponemas, and are inexpensive, easy to use, and do not require sophisticated laboratory equipment. False positives, however, may occur in any condition accompanied by a strong immunologic response or in pregnancy. Treponemal tests such as FTA-ABS (fluorescent treponemal-antibody absorption) and MHA-TP (microhaemaglutination antibody) are more expensive and remain positive for life, and hence are not able to differentiate between recent and older infections. As a result, treponemal tests are usually used to confirm a reactive nontreponemal test. Table B4.2 compares the sensitivity of three different tests during the different stages of syphilis. Syphilis ELISA tests capable of distinguishing IgM antibody and hence of indicating recent infection, are currently being tested in developed country settings. If these tests prove practical for widespread use they could radically alter the screening of populations for syphilis worldwide.

Table B4.2 Sensitivity (in per cent) of serologic tests for syphilis in untreated infected individuals by stage of disease

		Stage of Disease			
Type of test		Primary	Secondary	Latent	Late (tertiary)
Nontreponemal	VDRL	59-87	100	73-91	37-94
Treponemal	FTA-ABS	86-100	99-100	96-99	96-100
	MHA-TP	64-87	96-100	96-100	94-100

Source: Jaffe and Musher 1990

In some countries reporting is mandatory for certain STDs while in others it is voluntary. Sources of information include reports from office-based medical practices, other health care facilities, commercial and reference laboratories, or research projects. A recent survey of the national surveillance systems in Europe found that the completeness of reporting for mandatory notification systems for STDs ranged from over 90 per cent to less than 10 per cent (European Center for the Epidemiological Monitoring of AIDS 1992).

Even high quality report-based STD surveillance systems tend to underestimate substantially the total number of new cases since for many STDs a substantial proportion of infected individuals do not develop symptoms. Other circumstances in which cases may not be detected by the system include:

- individuals with symptoms not seeking treatment from the formal medical system but rather self-treating or seeking treatment from pharmacists or traditional practitioners or doing nothing; and;
- information not being reported to the national body.

Data from these systems, however, have an important role in informing the design, implementation and evaluation of STD treatment and prevention programmes. Ideally, every country would have an active surveillance system where reports of disease occurrence are continually being solicited.

In general, specialty STD clinics tend to be the most reliable at reporting, other government facilities less good and private practitioners the least reliable. Some countries collect data from commercial and reference laboratories to ensure more complete reporting rather than relying on practitioners. This simplifies the surveillance system by reducing the number of organizations reporting data and also reduces any effect the social stigma of STDs may have on doctors' reporting patterns. However, for those diseases where laboratory procedures are simple and can be done in a doctors' office, for example syphilis, data from commercial and reference laboratories substantially underestimate the number of diagnosed cases.

The ICD codes for STDs are listed in Tables 4 and 5 respectively. Substantial revisions were made to the classification scheme prior to the publication of ICD 10 and the number of codes relating to STDs more than doubled.

The most comprehensive and reliable reporting systems for STDs are in the EME region. Throughout the region there has been a marked reduction in the number of reported cases of STDs. In the United States reported cases declined by just under 40 per cent between 1975 and 1990, and in Sweden an aggressive campaign of STD treatment, reporting, screening and case finding led to a dramatic reduction in all types of STDs. However, this decline in incidence has been inconsistent both between and within countries. In the US, for example, despite the overall decline in reported cases, an increase in the incidence of STDs has been documented in some impoverished urban communities, and racial differences have widened.

While the number of reported cases has fallen in EME there have been dramatic increases in other parts of the world. Chinese epidemiologists, however, estimate that the actual number of cases is in excess of 1.5 million.

Epidemiological surveys

A large number of epidemiological surveys have been conducted that provide data on the point or period prevalence of one or more STDs. Only a handful of these surveys however provide information on the incidence of infection, as incidence studies are significantly more complicated and expensive to conduct.

The majority of studies have been conducted among STD clinic attendees and female commercial sex workers in urban areas. These studies are of limited usefulness in understanding the epidemiology and prevalence of a particular STD at the population level. Community based surveys and studies conducted in groups such as pregnant women, women attending

Table 4 ICD 8 and 9 codes for STDs

Syphilis and other venereal diseases (090-099)	
090	Congenital syphilis
091	Early syphilis, symptomatic
092	Early syphilis, latent
093	Cardiovascular syphilis
094	Syphilis of central nervous system
095	Other forms of late syphilis, with symptoms
096	Late syphilis, latent
097	Other syphilis and not specified
098	Gonococcal infections
099	Other venereal diseases

Table 5 ICD 10 codes for STDs

Infections with a predominantly sexual mode of transmission (A50-A64)	
A50	Congenital syphilis
A51	Early syphilis
A52	Late syphilis
A53	Other and unspecified syphilis
A54	Gonococcal infection
A55	Chlamydial lymphogranuloma
A56	Other sexually transmitted chlamydial diseases
A57	Chancroid
A58	Granuloma inguinale
A59	Trichomaniasis
A60	Anogenital herpesviral [herpes simplex] infections
A63	Other predominantly sexually transmitted diseases, not elsewhere classified
A64	Unspecified sexually transmitted diseases
Other categories	
B20-24	Human immunodeficiency virus [HIV] disease
N34.1	Nonspecific and nongonococcal urethritis
M02.3	Reiter's disease
P39.1	Chlamydial neonatal conjunctivitis
P23.1	Chlamydial neonatal pneumonia
B08.1	Molluscum contagiosum
D26.0	Papilloma of cervix

Table 6 Sources of bias in commonly studied population groups

Population group	*Source of bias*
Pregnant women attending antenatal clinics	• younger than the general female population • must have been sexually active in the recent past • only includes women who make use of health care facilities (in low income developing countries not all women have access to health care facilities; those that do are, in general, better off, better educated, and live closer to the facilities). • infertile women are excluded
Family planning clinic attendees	• more likely to be married, better educated, and wealthier
Blood donors	• representativeness depends upon the type of blood transfusion service and who gives blood (e.g. voluntary/ paid/ family members)
STD clinic attendees	• only individuals who seek treatment are included
Commercial sex workers	• only individuals identified as commercial sex workers are included

family planning clinics, and blood donors often provide more helpful information (see Table 6 for a discussion of the sources of bias with these groups).

Other pertinent factors when interpreting study results are sample size, the duration of time over which specimens were collected, and the sensitivity and specificity of the particular diagnostic approach used depends upon the type of test, the skill of the laboratory technicians involved, and the methods used to collect and transport specimens. For example, PCR/ LCR technologies can detect much lower levels of infection in an individual than direct microscopy, while some serum antibody tests remain positive for life or cross react with antibodies produced in response to other species.

The remainder of this section provides a brief summary of data for gonorrhoea, chlamydia and syphilis in the eight GBD regions. The regional summaries are based on data collected by the former WHO Global Programme on AIDS and The Rockefeller Foundation as part of an exercise to estimate the annual incidence of different STDs and focus on "low-risk" populations (World Health Organization 1995). For other reviews of STD prevalence data see DeSchryer and Meheus 1990, and Stanecki 1995.

The amount of data available varies considerably by region and by disease. In addition, the distribution of studies within a region or within a particular country not necessarily correlate with the population distribution. For example, in the MEC region only one prevalence study was identified in Pakistan (obstetric and gynaecology patients), one study in Egypt (patients with schistosomiasis), and no studies in Iran. Together these three countries account for over 40 per cent of the region's population. In addition, the studies are biased towards women and urban areas. Very few studies have been conducted in "low risk" men, and the studies from rural areas are frequently based in district level clinics that act a referral centres or in convenient locations (i.e., close to transportation routes), factors that are likely to bias results towards higher levels of infection). In general, prevalence rates for STDs are higher in developing countries than in developed countries and are more common in Africa than in Asia or Latin America. Within countries the prevalence is generally higher in urban areas than in rural areas. Differences reflect a number of factors including behavioural, medical, and social and economic factors, study design, type of diagnostic test used and experience of the laboratory technicians.

Established Market Economies (EME)

Data on the prevalence of chlamydia from various studies conducted in women living in EME are summarized in Figure 1. The graph shows the marked range in documented prevalence rates (also see Table 7). Estimates of the ratio of the prevalence of chlamydia to gonorrhoea in women seeking abortions also vary considerably, ranging from 11:1 to 44:1 in studies where data have been collected on both (see Table 7). In the United States it is estimated that the prevalence of chlamydia in asymptomatic adult females and males is between 3 and 5 per cent; in pregnant women between 5 and 7 per cent; in sexually active young men attending adolescent clinics between 13 and 15 per cent; and in STD clinic attendees (both males and females) between 10 and 20 per cent (Quinn and Cates 1992).

All of the EME have taken active steps to reduce the prevalence of syphilis. As a result the prevalence is low throughout the region. For example, in pregnant women in the Netherlands, Spain and Switzerland in the late 1980s recorded prevalences were 0.15 per cent, 0.15 per cent, and 0.53 per cent respectively, and in French blood donors 0.01 per cent (Bindels et al. 1991, Moreno et al. 1992, Ministère des Affaires Sociales 1991, Zimmerman 1993).

A large general population based screening programme in Manitoba, Canada is one of the few new studies providing data on the incidence of infection (Jolly et al. 1995). The authors estimated that there were 3.7 cases of chlamydia for every case of gonorrhoea. Reinfection was estimated to account for 15 per cent of all chlamydia cases and 13 per cent of all gonorrhoea cases. Some 27 per cent of the identified cases of chlamydia were in males and 73 per cent in females, with the highest incidence in the 15–24 age group (females 3 256 per 100 000 and males 1 081 per 100 000).

Formerly Socialist Economies of Europe (FSE)

No prevalence data were identified for syphilis or gonorrhoea in low risk populations in FSE. Three studies of chlamydia in pregnant women were identified. In Czechoslovakia a prevalence of 28.0 was recorded in 276

Figure 1 Established Market Economies: Prevalence of chlamydia in pregnant women, women attending family planning clinics and abortion seekers

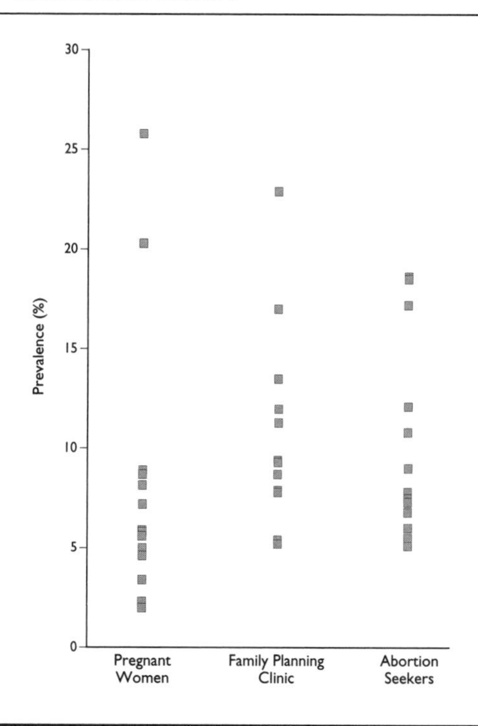

Table 7 Established Market Economies: Prevalence of infection in women seeking abortions

Country	*Year*	*Prevalence (%)* *Gonorrhoea*	*Chlamydia*	*Sample size*	*Diagnostic method*	*Reference*
Belgium	1985*	0.6	12.0	170	Culture	Avnts and Piot 1985
Denmark	1992*	0.7	7.9	428		Sorensen et al. 1992
Denmark	1989*	0.6	7.8	335	Culture	Prien-Larsen and Kjer 1989
Netherlands	1988	0.4	9.4	560	Culture	Thewessen et al. 1990
Norway	1991	0.5	5.4	2110		Skjeldestad and Jerve 1992
UK	1992*	0.2	8.7	1784		Cohn and Stewart 1992
USA	1996*	0.9	9.3	210	Culture	Amortegul et al. 1986

*year of publication

women in 1989–90 (smear test) (Cislakova et al. 1992) while data presented at a European Society of Chlamydial Research meeting documented a prevalence of 3.1 per cent in Russia in 1988 and 3.0 per cent in Romania (Country files, Office of HIV, AIDS and STDs, WHO).

India (IND)

Data on the prevalence of gonorrhoea in low risk populations in India are limited and no studies were identified providing information on the prevalence of chlamydia. In Jaipur the prevalence of gonorrhoea in 250 women attending antenatal clinics in 1992 was 1.6 per cent and in 519 male transport and industrial workers 2.1 per cent (Country files, Office of HIV, AIDS and STDs, WHO). Similar figures were recorded in women attending gynaecology clinics in Chandigarh (2.0 per cent; n=271) (Dhall et al. 1990), while in a community based study of rural women in 1986 the prevalence was 0.3 per cent (n=650) (Bang et al. 1989).

Table 8 records the prevalence of syphilis from studies conducted in pregnant woman, primary health care (PHC) attendees, and male workers. The study of PHC attendees in rural Tamil Nadu documented a slightly higher prevalence in males (3.6 per cent) than in females (3.3 per cent) (Kantharaj et al. 1993). Data from blood donors in Madras (both sexes) show a decline in the prevalence of syphilis between 1987 and 1989—the

Table 8 India: Prevalence of syphilis in selected low risk population groups

Location		*Year*	*Prevalence (%)*	*Sample size*	*Diagnostic method*	*Reference*
A. Pregnant women and ANC clinic attendees						
Bombay		1988-89	5	10 181		Hira 1991
Delhi		1988*	1	9 380	VDRL	Health Information India 1988**
Jaipur		1992	1.6	250	VDRL	WHO country file
Madras		1992	1.7	750		Kantharaj et al. 1993
B. Primary health care attendees						
Rural Tamil Nadu	Female	1992	3.3	300		Kantharaj et al. 1993
Rural Tamil Nadu	Male	1992	3.6	300		Kantharaj et al. 1993
C. Male workers						
Jaipur	Transport & industrial workers	1992	4.2/4.4	519	TPHA/VDRL+	WHO country file
Madras	Industrial workers	1992	0.8	250		Kantharaj et al. 1993
Madras	Transport workers	1992	4.4	250		Kantharaj et al. 1993

*year of publication

**studies cited in Luthra et al. 1992

percentage of blood donors with a reactive VDRL test fell from 8.4 to 3.9 per cent and the number with a reactive test greater than 8 dilutions fell from 2.4 to 1.2 per cent (Bhargava 1993)

China (CHN)

Prevalence data from China are limited. Two studies were identified providing data on the prevalence of gonorrhoea in women at low risk of infection. The first study conducted in 300 women of childbearing age in 1988 recorded a prevalence of 1.0 per cent (Dong 1991), while a 1990 study of 1 000 pregnant women recorded a prevalence of 0.5 per cent (Fan and Dong 1991). Both studies used a smear test to detect infection and were conducted in Beijing.

A study by Gao et al. (1995) of 269 pregnant women attending a gynaecology clinic in Beijing recorded a prevalence of chlamydia 23.7 per cent using DFA staining. This figure is substantially higher than the 1.0 per cent reported by Hodgson et al. (1988) in 100 women attending family planning or gynaecology clinics in Hangzhou using a DFA test.

Other Asia and Islands (OAI)

Data on the prevalence of gonorrhoea and chlamydia are limited, and are disproportionately from small countries (see Table 9). Figure 2 summarizes data on the prevalence of syphilis in pregnant women and in blood donors. Within countries where more than one data set is available for pregnant women there is considerable variation. For example, in Vietnam

Table 9 Other Asia and Islands: Prevalence of infection in pregnant women and women attending ANC clinics

Country	*Location*	*Year*	*Prevalence (%)*		*Sample size*	*Diagnostic method*	*Reference*
			Gonorrhoea	*Chlamydia*			
Fiji	Suva - Fijians	1985-86	3.1	50.0	257		Gyanseshwar et al. 1987
Fiji	Suva - Indians	1985-86	1.1	38.0	183		Gyanseshwar et al. 1987
New Caledonia		1988-89		19.0	400	culture	Morillon M et al. 1992
Papua New Guinea	Port Moresby General Hospital	1991		17.7	181	DFA	Klufio 1992
Singapore		1987	0.8				WHO country file
Sri Lanka		1992		30.0			WHO country file
Sri Lanka		1992	0.5			culture	WHO country file
Taiwan	Taipei	1986-87		7.8	514	DFA	Yang et al. 1988
Thailand	Bangcock	1988		24.0	126	culture	Niamsanti et al. 1988
Vanuatu			11.0	20.0	200		WHO country file

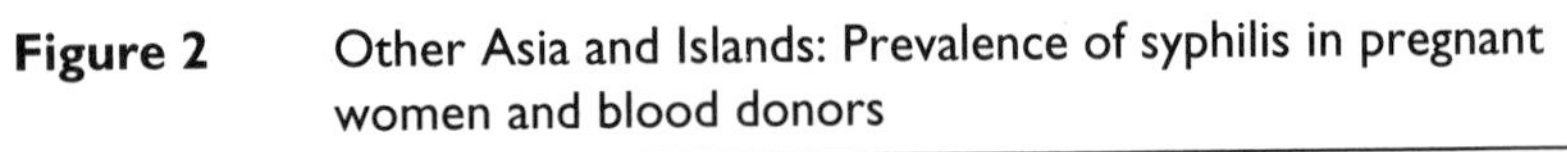

Figure 2 Other Asia and Islands: Prevalence of syphilis in pregnant women and blood donors

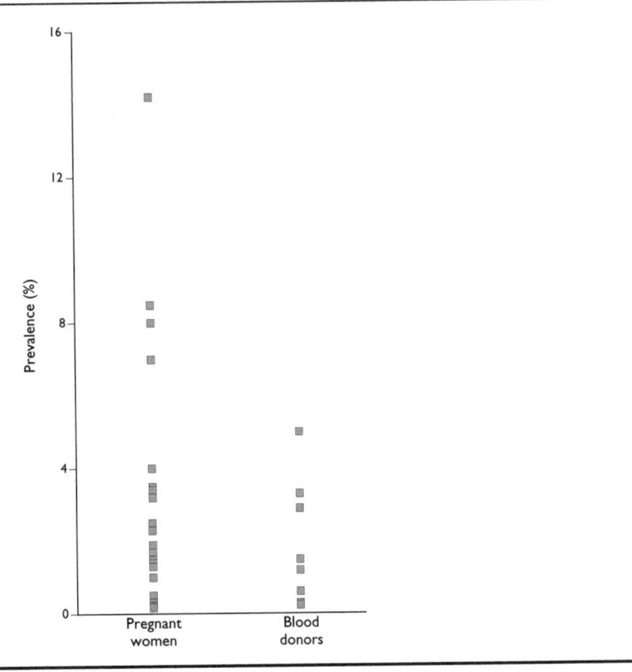

estimates for the early 1990s range from 0.3 per cent to 4.0 per cent (Country Files, Office of HIV, AIDS and STDs, WHO).

Sub-Saharan Africa (SSA)

More epidemiological studies have been conducted on STDs in Africa than in any other region of the world, despite the weak public health infrastructure and health care delivery system. This reflects both a historical interest in STDs in the region and, more recently, the rapid spread of HIV. Figure 3 summarizes the studies conducted in pregnant women by disease and geographical area (rural, urban, unknown). For both syphilis and chlamydia the median and average prevalences were higher in rural areas than in urban areas, while for gonorrhoea they were broadly similar. Studies, however, that provide data on both rural and urban prevalences for syphilis show higher prevalences in urban areas than in rural areas, e.g. in Gabon (19.1 per cent in urban and 13.3 per cent in rural areas) (Schrijvers et al. 1989).

Studies in the region that provide data on the prevalence of all three STDs show no common pattern in the relationship between the STDs (see Table 10). Data on levels of STD infection in men at low risk of infection are limited, and the number of studies providing data for both males and females even fewer (see Table 11). In most of the studies, the prevalence

Figure 3 Sub-Saharan Africa: Prevalence in pregnant women by geographical area

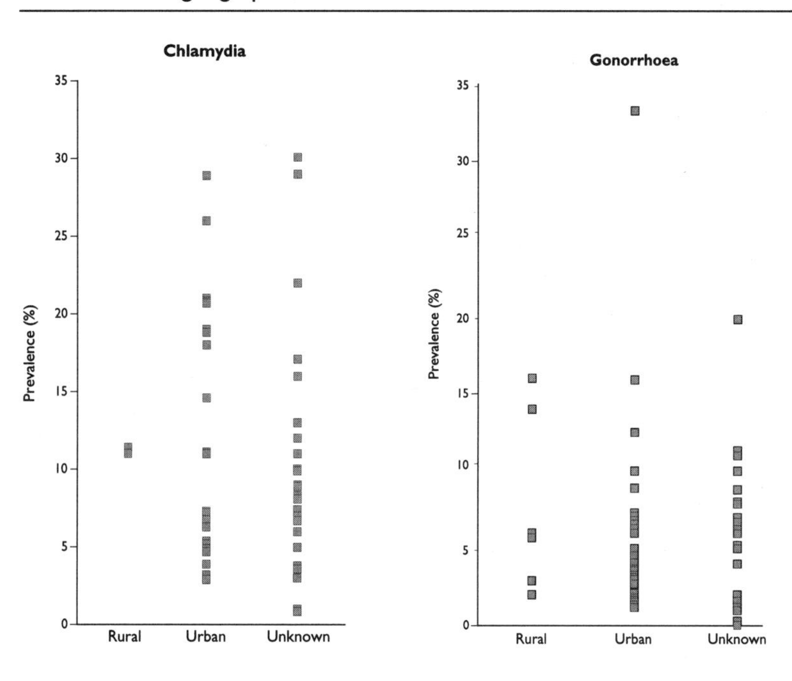

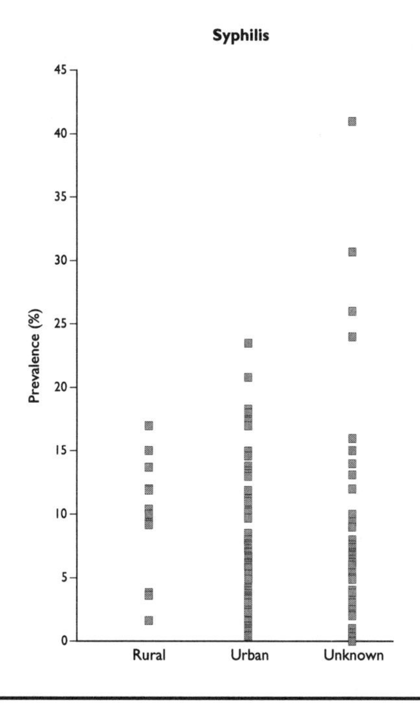

Table 10 Sub-Saharan Africa: Prevalence of STDs among pregnant women and women attending antenatal clinics

Country	*Location*	*Year of study*	*Gonorrhoea*	*Chlamydia*	*Syphilis*	*Sample Size*	*Diagnostic Method*	*References*
Burkina Faso		1991	1.0	5.0	2.0	288	smear & serology	AIDSTECH 1993
Cote d'Ivoire	Abidjan	1992*	3.7	2.9	0.7	500	RPR, TPHA	Diallo et al. 1992
Malawi	Liomba	1990*	4.6	2.9	11.2	648	RPR, FTA confirmation	Chipangwi et al. 1990
Niger	Niamey	1993*	1.5	1.5	4.0	400	RPR, TPHA	Hassane et al. 1993
Senegal	national	1989-93	1.1	7.4	4.0	900		Samb et al. 1993
South Africa	rural Natal	late 80's	6.0	11.0	12.0		Non T + Trep	O'Farrell et al. 1989
South Africa	Durban	1991	4.1	4.7	7.6	170	RPR, TPHA	Dietrick et al. 1992
Tanzania	Mwanza	1992*	3.1	6.7	6.2	100	RPR, TPHA	Mayaud et al. 1992
Tanzania	Mwanza	1992-93	2.1	6.3	10.3	1000	RPR, TPHA	Todd et al. 1993
Uganda	Kampala	1991	1.0	7.2	10.2			Nsubuga et al. 1992
Zaire	Kinshasa	1990	1.5	5.4	1.0	1160	Culture; EIA; RPR TPHA	Vuylsteke et al. 1993

*year of publication

Table 11 Sub-Saharan Africa: Prevalence of syphilis by gender

Country	*Location*	*Population group*	*Year of study*	*Female (%)*	*Male (%)*	*Diagnostic Method*	*References*
Burundi	Central region	rural	1986	10.2	5.9	TPHA	Lalla et al. 1990
Central African Republic	Bangui	general	1987	12.4	13.3	TPHA	Georges-Courbot et al. 1989
Gabon	Franceville	general	1988	7.4	8.6	RPR/TPHA	Schrijvers et al. 1989
Somalia		general	1987	22.5	24.0	TPHA	
Sudan		general	1989	27.5	35.2	VDRL/RPR	Genitourin 1990
Tanzania	Mwanza region	roadside	1990-91	13.2	12.3	TPHA	Mosha et al. 1993
				21.7	22.4	TPHA&RPR	
Tanzania	Mwanza region	rural	1990-91	7.9	7.0	TPHA	Mosha et al. 1993
				13.5	13.1	TPHA&RPR	
Tanzania	Mwanza region	urban	1990-91	12.4	9.3	TPHA	Mosha et al. 1993
				20.5	15.9	TPHA&RPR	
Uganda	Northern area	rural	1986	42	26.3	TPHA	Mosha et al. 1993

in the two sexes was similar—although in Burundi and Uganda found that the prevalence was markedly higher in women.

Latin America and the Caribbean (LAC)

The prevalence of gonorrhoea and chlamydia in pregnant women from studies conducted in 7 LAC countries are recorded in Table 12.

Figure 4 summarizes data on the prevalence of syphilis in pregnant women and in blood donors. Two studies in Brazil also provide information on males at low risk of infection—municipal civil servants (0 per cent), and policemen (0.7 per cent) (Faundes and Tanaka 1992).

Middle Eastern Crescent (MEC)

Data on the prevalence of gonorrhoea and chlamydia in pregnant women in 4 MEC countries are presentd in Table 13. Only one of the studies provides data on the prevalence of chlamydia, a study by Genc et al. (1993) in Turkey, where none of the 190 women studied had evidence of chlamydia (culture based test).

The only large scale surveys in the region are for syphilis. In studies conducted in pregnant women or women attending ob/gyn clinics in Turkey, Tunisia, and Saudi Arabia the reported prevalence was under 1 per cent (Akan et al. 1987; Ben Salem et al. 1993; Hossain 1986). In blood donors, however, the prevalence was 2.0 per cent in Morocco (n=116 904) (Country Files Office of HIV, AIDS and STDs, WHO) and 3.0 per cent in Saudi Arabia (n=1 263) (Hossain 1986).

Methods and review of empirical databases

Regional estimates of disease burden were calculated for each of the three diseases by estimating annual incidence rates and the burden of disease per incident infection. This section describes the methods used to estimate

Table 12 Latin America and the Caribbean: Prevalence of infection in pregnant women

Country or Region	*Year*	*Prevalence (%) Gonorrhoea*	*Chlamydia*	*Sample size*	*Diagnostic method*	*Reference*
Eastern Caribbean	1993		13.0	160		AIDSTECH 1993
El Salvador	1989		44.0	129	EIA & DFA	Posada et al. 1992
Guatemala	1992	1.0	5.0	301		AIDSTECH 1993
Ecuador	1989*		1.6	61		Narvaez et al. 1989
Nicaragua	1993*	1.0	4.0	636		Espinoza et al. 1993

*year of publication

Figure 6 Latin America and the Caribbean: Prevalence of syphilis in low risk populations

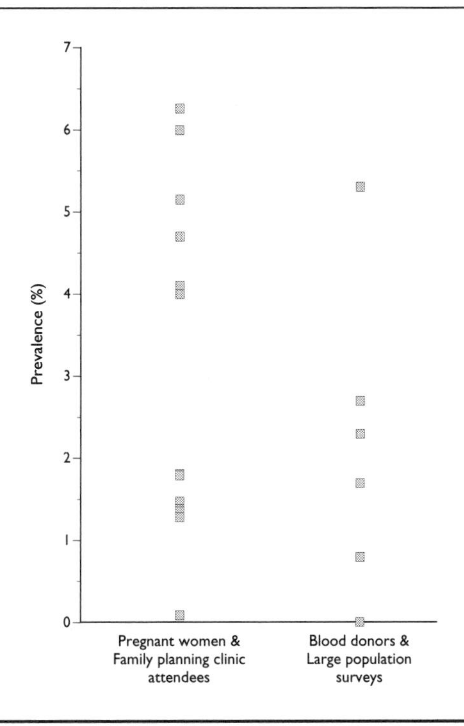

Table 13 Middle Eastern Crescent: Prevalence of infection in pregnant women

Country	*Year*	*Chlamydia Prevalence (%)*	*Sample size*	*Diagnostic method*	*Reference*
Israel		7.8/23.1	281		Tadmor OP et al. 1993
Saudi Arabia	1989	9	106	EIA	Bakir TMF et al. 1989
Tunisia	1991	2.9	1030	serum	Ben Salem N et al. 1993
Turkey		12.2	220	IgG and/ or IgM	Akan E et al. 1987
Turkey	1987-88	1.6	63	EIA-IgG>19	Yildiz A et al. 1990
Turkey	1992	1.1	190	ct:culture; gc: EIA & gram staining	Genc M et al. 1993

these values, reviews the available literature, and presents the values used in the analysis.

INCIDENCE OF INFECTION

Data on the incidence of STDs are limited and vary widely. Even in countries with good disease surveillance systems many STDs are not reported because they are asymptomatic or are treated outside the formal health care sector. As a result, incidence estimates were based on regional prevalence estimates adjusted for the average period an individual is infected for and continues to give a positive response on a diagnostic test.

a. Age group 15 –44 years

The relationship used to estimate the annual incidence rate among individuals of sex *k* living in region *r* in age group 15–44, *I(k,r)* was:

$$I(k,r) = \frac{P(k,r)}{(1 - P(k,r))} * \frac{1}{D(k,r)}$$

where:

P(k,r) is the prevalence of infection among individuals of sex *k* living in region *r*

D(k,r) is the average duration of infection among individuals of sex *k* living in region *r*. This approach provides useful approximate estimates of incidence rates, but does not allow for changes in prevalence or population size through time, nor for age-relation variation in the duration or incidence of infection within the 15–44 age group.

Estimating the prevalence of infection P(k,r)

An extensive review of the medical literature using computer searches and, personal contacts was carried out by the Office of STD of the former WHO Global Programme on AIDS and the Health Sciences Division of The Rockefeller Foundation (Stanecki et al. 1995, World Health Organization 1995). Information collated include: population sampled (age, sex, geographical location, type of population (e.g., blood donors, STD clinic attendees, commercial sex workers, students)), date samples collected, and study design (sampling procedure, size of sample, time period over which samples were collected, and diagnostic methods).

The subset of studies in the database that met specified criteria (see Table 14) formed the basis of the regional estimates after adjusting for the nature of the populations sampled, the diagnostic tests used, and regional population distributions. Different adjustment factors were used in the 8 regions and for the 3 diseases reflecting our subjective views of the quantity and quality of data available. For those regions where only a small number of studies were available the excluded studies were also looked at in detail. When no data were available, estimates were based on the prevalence of other STDs and the prevalence in surrounding regions. Table

Table 14 Criteria for study inclusion

1. Population sampled	Studies conducted in low risk populations such as pregnant women, women attending family planning clinics, and blood donors.
2. Date samples collected	Specimens collected in 1985 or later. For those studies where no information was provided on when specimens were collected the data of publication was used.
3. Sample size	Sample size was at least 50. Studies where no information on sample size was provided were also included.

Table 15 Estimated prevalence (%) of infection in the age group 15-44 by region, 1990

Region	*Gonorrhoea*		*Chlamydia*		*Syphilis*	
	Males	*Females*	*Males*	*Females*	*Males*	*Females*
EME	0.11	0.28	0.92	3.02	0.06	0.06
FSE	0.31	0.50	1.57	3.41	0.07	0.07
IND	1.19	1.57	4.31	5.66	1.75	2.17
CHN	0.04	0.05	0.15	0.20	0.002	0.003
OAI	1.12	1.48	3.85	5.06	1.40	1.75
SSA	2.19	3.10	5.32	7.77	3.47	4.31
LAC	0.70	1.19	2.72	4.46	0.64	0.79
MEC	0.23	0.40	1.38	1.84	0.48	0.60

15 shows the estimated prevalence of infection in the age group 15–44 by sex for each of the eight regions in 1990.

Estimating the duration of infection D(k,r)

The average duration of infection depends upon a number of factors including: the proportion of infected individuals who develop symptoms; the probability that symptomatic individuals are treated; the probability asymptomatic individuals are treated; the average length of time between infection and treatment; the appropriateness of the treatment; and the length of time it takes to develop an antibody response and duration of this response (which may relate to previous exposure).

Gonorrhoea and chlamydia

The relationship used to estimate $D(k,r)$, the average duration of infection with gonorrhoea and chlamydia was:

$$D(k,r) = M(k,r)\,[VS(k,r)\,TS(k,r) + (1-VS(k,r))\,US(k,r)] + (1-M(k,r))[\,VA(k,r)TA(k,r) + (1-VA(k,r))UA(k,r)]$$

where:

M(k,r) is the probability that individuals of sex *k* in region *r* are symptomatic,

VS(k,r) is the probability that symptomatic individuals of sex *k* in region *r* are treated,

TS(k,r) is the average duration of infection for symptomatic individuals of sex *k* in region *r* who are treated,

US(k,r) is the average duration of infection for untreated symptomatic individuals of sex *k* in region *r*,

VA(k,r) is the probability asymptomatic individuals of sex *k* in region *r* are treated,

TA(k,r) is the average duration of infection for asymptomatic individuals of sex *k* in region *r* who are treated, and

UA(k,r) is the average duration of infection for untreated asymptomatic individuals of sex *k* in region *r*

Data from clinical and laboratory studies suggest that approximately 95 per cent of males with gonorrhoea and 75 to 80 per cent of males with chlamydia develop symptoms. The proportion of women developing symptoms is much smaller—approximately 50 per cent of women infected with gonorrhoea and 25 to 30 per cent with chlamydia develop symptoms. In the analysis we assumed that the proportion of individuals who developed symptoms was the same in all regions. Infection with gonorrhoea was assumed to lead to symptoms in 95 per cent of infected males and 50 per cent of infected females. The corresponding figures for chlamydia were estimated to be 80 per cent and 25 per cent, respectively.

Information on the duration of infection in the absence of treatment for both chlamydia and gonorrhoea is limited. Apart from a study of women with chlamydial infection conducted in the late 1970's where 50 per cent of untreated women remained culture positive when tested 15 months apart (McCormack et al. 1979), the only data available are from the pre-antibiotic era and are difficult to interpret owing to the diagnostic approaches used. Table 16 provides the values used in this exercise. These values are based on the figures used in other modelling exercises (e.g., Brunham and Plummer 1990) and were assumed to be the same for men and for women.

Table 16 Average duration of infection with gonorrhoea and chlamydia (in years) for treated and untreated individuals

	Untreated	*Treated*	
		symptomatic	*asymptomatic*
Gonorrhoea	0.5	0.06 (3 weeks)	0.25
Chlamydia	1.25	0.08 (4 weeks)	0.625

Source: Brunham and Plummer 1990

Data on the proportion of infected individuals who receive treatment are also limited. Treatment levels vary by disease sex, socioeconomic characteristics, geographical location, attitude toward STDs, and, in general, are biased towards symptomatic males and certain age groups. In rural India Bang et al. (1989) found that only a negligible proportion of women with symptoms or signs of reproductive tract disorder had sought or received treatment while in rural Nigeria less then 3 per cent of adolescent females had sought treatment (Brabin et al. 1995). For those who present, the length of time prior to presentation varies considerably. Table 17 sumarizes the results from a study of 380 patients with STDs presenting for treatment at health care centers in Kenya. Over 27 per cent of the patients had already sought treatment elsewhere without relief of symptoms before coming to the clinic. For individuals who do not develop symptoms the proportion treated is even lower—although some may receive treatment through screening programmes, partner notification schemes, or inadvertently when receiving treatment for another health problem.

To estimate the probability that symptomatic individuals are treated, *VS(k,r)*, the eight regions were assigned to one of three levels of health care based on an estimate of the relative quality and accessibility of health care for STDs:

- Level A: high level of care and easy access—most people are diagnosed using accurate tests and treated appropriately.
- Level B: mix of services with some high quality services serving urban areas and wealthier clients.
- Level C: most services of low quality

Table 17 Per cent of patients reporting different lengths of time between developing symptoms and attending a health centre in Kenya, by presenting complaints

	Duration of symptoms (days)					
Parenting complaint	**1-3**	**4-7**	**8-14**	**15-30**	**31-60**	**60+**
Vaginal discharge (n=120)	16.7	32.5	19.2	11.7	6.7	13.3
Lower abdominal or back pain in women (n=88)	25.0	25.0	23.9	12.5	4.5	9.1
Urethral discharge (n=104)	31.7	44.2	10.6	10.6	1.0	1.9
Genital ulcers or sores (n=121)	15.7	35.5	24.8	6.6	6.6	10.7
Men (n=66)	19.7	30.3	25.8	12.1	3.0	9.1
Women (n=55)	10.9	41.8	23.6	0.0	10.9	12.7
All complaints (n=377)	22.3	35.8	18.8	9.8	4.5	8.8
Men (n=187)	28.9	39.0	16.6	9.1	1.6	4.8
Women (n=190)	15.8	32.6	21.2	10.5	7.4	12.6

Source: Moses et al. 1994

Table 18 records how the regions were allocated to the different levels of health care, Table 19 the probability that a symptomatic individual is treated in each level and Table 20 the calculated average duration of infection for men and women in each region, $D(k,r)$. It should be noted, that within each region services vary considerably; however, in this analysis we have focused on the regional rather than the national level. For both diseases the proportion of symptomatic and asymptomatic individuals treated was assumed to be the same, but to be lower for women than men. The proportion of asymptomatic individuals treated as a result of screening programmes, partner tracing, or inadvertent correct therapy when being treated for other health problems was set at $1/10^{th}$ of the value assigned to symptomatics.

Syphilis

For syphilis a similar procedure was followed taking into account for each stage of infection (primary, secondary, latent, tertiary) the probability that infected individuals develop symptoms, the likelihood that symptomatic or asymptomatic individuals are treated, and the average length of time spent in each stage in the absence of treatment or when treated. Ninety per cent of individuals with primary syphilis were assumed to develop symptoms, while 60 per cent of individuals with secondary syphilis and none of those in the latent stage were assumed to be symptomatic. The probability of moving from one stage to the next in the absence of treatment was assumed to be independent of the development of symptoms—

Table 18 Assignment of regions to the three levels of care.

Level A	*Level B*	*Level C*
EME	FSE	SSA
	China	OAI
	LAC	India
	MEC	

Source: Authors' estimates

Table 19 Estimated proportion of individuals with gonorrhoea or chlamydia treated, by level of health care

	Level of Health Care		
Sex	**A**	**B**	**C**
Males	0.9	0.65	0.35
Females	0.85	0.55	0.25

Source: Authors' estimates

all untreated individuals with primary syphilis were assumed to progress to secondary syphilis and then into the latent stage. Thirty per cent of those in the latent phase were assumed to develop tertiary syphilis.

The estimated probabilities that individuals with syphilis are treated for each of the three levels of health care are given in Table 21. The probability of treatment was assumed to depend on the stage of syphilis and to be independent of sex. It was also assumed that a high proportion of individuals in the long latent period are treated even though they are asymptomatic primarily as a result of active screening programmes. In the absence of treatment it was assumed that the average duration of primary syphilis was four weeks, secondary syphilis three months and latent syphilis three years. Individuals who developed tertiary syphilis or who were not treated at all were assumed, on average, to remain positive for 10 years. The estimated duration of infection by level of health care is shown in Table 20.

b. Other age groups

Most prevalence and incidence data are from studies conducted among individuals between the ages of 15 and 44. Very few studies have been conducted outside this age range.

Table 20 Estimated average duration of infection for adults (years)

		Level of Health Care		
Disease	**Sex**	**A**	**B**	**C**
Gonorrhoea	Males	0.12	0.23	0.35
	Females	0.30	0.37	0.44
Chlamydia	Males	0.39	0.63	0.92
	Females	0.91	1.03	1.15
Syphilis	Both	0.48	1.28	2.63

Source: Authors' estimates

Table 21 Estimated proportion of individuals with syphilis who are treated, by level of health care and stage of infection

		Level of Health Care		
Stage		**A**	**B**	**C**
primary	symptomatic	0.85	0.6	0.35
	asymptomatic	0.00	0.00	0.00
secondary	symptomatic	0.85	0.60	0.35
	asymptomatic	0.00	0.00	0.00
latent		0.95	0.85	0.75

Source: Authors' estimates

As a first approximation, the incidence rates in the age groups 5–14, 45–59 and 60+ were assumed to be directly proportional to the incidence in the age group 15–44 and to be the same for all three diseases, for all eight regions and for both sexes. The ratio of the incidence in the 5–14 age group to the 15–44 age groups were 0.1 and 0.025. No transmission was assumed to occur in the age group 0–4.

All three diseases can be transmitted from an infected mother to her child during pregnancy or at birth with the likelihood of transmission depending on a number of factors including the length of time the other mother has been infected, the delivery method, and the likelihood of being treated when pregnant. Incidence rates for the age group 0–1 were not explicitly calculated—rather estimates of the incidence of the different complication rates were calculated.

In order to estimate the global burden of disease from STDs it was necessary to estimate the age individuals acquire infection. For the purpose of this exercise it was assumed that the average age of infection was the same for all three diseases, but that women acquire infection at an earlier age than males.

Epidemiological data on mortality were used to derive a first set of regional mortality estimates. The estimates, however, when combined with mortality estimates proposed by the authors for other diseases and injuries in the Global Burden of Disease Study, usually exceeded the level of overall mortality estimated by various demographic methods. In order to not exceed this upper bound for mortality within each age-sex and broad-cause group, an algorithm was applied by the editors to reduce mortality estimates for specific conditions. The algorithm has been described in more detail in *The Global Burden of Disease* (Murray and Lopez 1996).

Burden of disease per incident infection

Unravelling the relationships between an STD and its consequences is a complex exercise and involves exploring correlations among conditions with varying definitions, imprecise diagnoses, different microbial organisms, and temporal lags. This section describes the methods used to estimate the burden of disease per incident infection and examines the relationships between infection with the etiologic agents causing gonorrhoea, chlamydia and syphilis and the probability of developing different complications and sequelae. The focus is on the major complications from a health perspective—not all possible complications and sequelae are included.

The literature on the potential complications and sequelae following infection with *N. gonorrhoea, C. trachomatis* and *T. pallidum* in developed and developing countries was reviewed. Based on this review a set of probability maps was drawn for each disease illustrating the relationship between infection and the major complications and sequelae from a health perspective (see Figures 5–9). In reality, the relationships are much more complex than recorded in the maps. Each infection has many other complications that have not been included in the analysis e.g., disseminated gonococcal infection. Box 5 describes the approach used for females with gonorrhoea.

The probability of developing different complications in the presence and absence of treatment and the duration and level of disability were estimated for each disease. The values assigned to the probabilities were based on the literature review and supplemented by personal communications with STD experts.

Most research has been carried out in developed countries reflecting in part the technical difficulties involved in performing these studies—sophisticated equipment (e.g., laparoscope), laboratories and pathology services are required. How generalizable these data are to other regions of the world is unknown—although it is very probable that the consequences of these infections will be as likely, if not more likely, in areas where treatment is inadequate or delayed. For many of the relationships there were no data available and for others the data are limited and not necessarily generalizable. Box 5 describes the approach used for females with chlamydia infection. For some outcomes (e.g., mortality related to low birth weight and prematurity) differences in access to health care facilities were also taken into account.

A. Gonorrhoea and Chlamydia

Adult females

1. Initial infection

Approximately 50 per cent of women infected with *N. gonorrhoeae* and 25 to 30 per cent of women infected with *C. trachomatis* develop non-specific signs of infection although these are generally mild and usually do not interfere with daily activities. Symptoms for the two infections are similar but tend to be less severe for chlamydia than gonorrhoea and include increased vaginal discharge, dysuria, inter-menstrual uterine bleeding, and menorrhagia, and usually develop within 10 days of infection (Hook and Handsfield 1990, Platt et al. 1983).

Parameter Values: 50 per cent of women infected with *N. gonorrhoeae* and 25 per cent of women infected with *C. trachomatis* were assumed to develop symptoms within two weeks of infection. In the absence of treatment symptoms were assumed to last three weeks and to result in low level disability (level I). Treatment was assumed to halve the duration of symptoms (see Table 22). The probability of being treated is recorded in Table 23 for women with symptoms. The probability asymptomatic women are treated was set at 1/10th of the value for symptomatic women.

2. Pelvic Inflammatory Disease (PID)

Infection with *N. gonnorrhoeae* and *C. trachomatis* can lead to pelvic inflammatory disease (PID), a syndrome that results from infection of the upper genital tract and most commonly manifests itself as endometritis (infection of the lining of the uterus) or salpingitis (infection of the fallo-

Box 5 Estimating the burden of disease for women with gonorrhoea living in a region with Level B health care services

Initial infection

- 50 % develop symptomatic initial infection
- For those with symptomatic initial infection: 55% are treated
- For those with asymptomatic initial infection: 5% are treated
- If symptomatic and treated: average duration of symptoms is 1.5 weeks with a disability weight of I
- If symptomatic and not treated: average duration of symptoms is 1.3 weeks with a disability weight of I
- If symptomatic or asymptomatic and treated: 0% chance of developing PID
- If symptomatic or asymptomatic and not treated: 20% chance of developing PID

For those women who develop PID

- 80% develop symptomatic PID and average duration of symptoms is 2 weeks with a disability weight of I
- 60% of women who develop PID are treated
- If PID is treated:
  - 0% chance of developing recurrent symptomatic PID
  - 3% chance of developing tubo-ovarian abscess
  - 3% chance of being infertile
  - 2% chance of having an ectopic pregnancy
  - 4% chance of developing chronic pelvic pain
- If PID is untreated:
  - 30% chance of developing recurrent symptomatic PID if initially had symptoms
  - 15% chance of developing tubo-ovarian abscess
  - 15% chance of being infertile
  - 10% chance of having an ectopic pregnancy
  - 20% chance of developing chronic pelvic pain

For those women who develop recurrent symptomatic PID

- average duration of symptoms is 2 weeks with a disability weight of II

For those women who develop tubo-ovarian abscesses

- average duration of symptoms is 4 weeks with a disability weight of III
- 18% chance of dying

For those women who have an ectopic pregnancy

- average duration of symptoms is 4 weeks with a disability weight of III
- 16.5% chance of dying
- 20% chance of becoming infertile

For those women who develop chronic pelvic pain

- average duration of symptoms is 4 years with a disability weight of II

Table 22 Gonorrhoea and chlamydia: Average duration and level of disability associated with major complications and sequelae (excluding infertility)

	Duration of symptoms		*Level of Disability*
Females			
Symptomatic cervical infection	not treated:	3 weeks	I
	treated:	1.5 weeks	I
Symptomatic PID	not treated:	2.6 weeks*	I (chlamydia); II (gonorrhoea)
	treated:	1 week	I (chlamydia); II (gonorrhoea)
Ectopic pregnancy	4 weeks		III
Tubo-ovarian abscess	4 weeks		III
Chronic pelvic pain	3 years		III
Males			
Symptomatic Urethritis	not treated:	3 weeks	II
	treated:	1.5 weeks	II
Stricture	not treated:	5 years	II
	treated:	6 months	II
Epididymitis	not treated:	5 weeks	II
	treated:	2 weeks	II

* includes disability associated with recurrent symptomatic PID (30% of women with initial symptoms who are not treated are assumed to have recurrent bouts and each bout to result in 2 weeks disability at level II).

Source: Authors' estimates

Table 23 Gonorrhoea and chlamydia: Probability symptomatic individuals are treated.

	Level of Health Care		
	A	**B**	**C**
Females			
Cervical infection	0.85	0.55	0.25
PID	0.9	0.6	0.3
Males			
Urethritis	0.9	0.65	0.35
Stricture	1.0	0.8	0.6
Epididymitis	1.0	0.8	0.4

Source: Authors' estimates

pian tubes). Other manifestations include parametritis, oophoritis, pelvic peritonitis, and pelvic abscesses. From the clinical point of view PID is often difficult to diagnose without the use of use of sophisticated and expensive diagnostic techniques (laparoscopy) as a substantial proportion of cases are only mildly or non-specifically symptomatic.

The onset of a substantial proportion of PID occurs following abortion or the insertion of an intrauterine contraceptive device which suggests that the risk of PID is enhanced by instrumentation (Cates and Stone 1992, Washington et al. 1991). Invasive procedures are thought to increase the risk of developing PID by altering the cervicovaginal environment, disrupting protective mucus, altering the normally protective vaginal flora, or by passively carrying lower genital tract organisms into the upper genital tract. Data also suggest that the incidence of acute PID is higher in women who are about to start their menstrual cycle and have cervicitis from *N. gonorrhoeae* or *C. trachomatis* and in younger women (see review by Washington et al. 1991). Cigarette smoking has also been implicated as a risk factor (Scholes et al. 1992). Oral contraceptives, on the other hand, appear to decrease the risk of developing symptomatic PID despite their known risk to increase susceptibility to chlamydia infection (Wolner Hanssen et al. 1990, Washington et al. 1991).

Acute PID—gonorrhoea: In industrialized countries it is estimated that 10 to 20 per cent of women with untreated cervical gonorrhoea infection go on to develop symptoms of acute PID (Eschenbach et al. 1975, Holmes et al. 1980, Weström 1980). Women with acute PID due to gonococcal infection usually present with various combinations of lower abdominal pain, pain with sexual intercourse, abnormal menses, intermenstrual bleeding, or other complaints compatible with intra-abdominal infection (Hook and Handsfield 1990). Symptoms usually appear within 1 to 2 menstrual cycles and often occur following the end of menses.

Acute PID—chlamydia: In industrialized countries it is estimated that 8 to 30 per cent of women with cervical chlamydial infection will develop clinically apparent salpingitis if not treated with appropriate antibiotics (Moore and Cates 1990, Weström and Mårdh 1990). The 8 per cent figures comes from a Swedish study and represents the proportion of women with untreated chlamydial infections who progressed to overt salpingitis (Weström et al. 1981). The higher figure comes from a study of women treated for gonorrhoeal infection whose subsequent culture showed simultaneous infection with cervical chlamydia—30 per cent developed signs of upper genital tract infection during the 7-day follow up interval (Stamm et al. 1984).

Silent (asymptomatic) PID: The proportion of women infected with cervical gonorrhoea or chlamydia who develop silent PID is unknown although acute cases probably represent only a small percentage of the total cases of endometrial and tubal infections. In the United States it is estimated that asymptomatic PID is 3 to 5 times more common than the number of clinically diagnosed cases. These estimates are based on studies that use laparoscopy or endometrial biopsy studies to detect PID in women who present with evidence of lower genital tract infection but no signs and symptoms of PID, and from studies conducted in women with ectopic pregnancies or who have tubal damage and are infertile and show serologic evidence of chlamydial or gonococcal infection but have no history of clinical salpingitis (Jones et al. 1982, Rosenfeld et al. 1983, Washington et al. 1991).

Recurrent PID: Data also suggest that up to one third of women who have had an episode of acute PID suffer from repeated bouts (Weström 1988, Weström and Mårdh 1990). Recurrent PID occurs for a number of reasons including: inadequate treatment, failure to examine and treat sex partners resulting in reinfection, unchanged sexual behavioural patterns, and post-infection damage to normal tubal clearance patterns (Meheus 1992).

Parameter Values: The proportion of symptomatic and asymptomatic individuals who develop PID in the absence of treatment was assumed to be the same (20 per cent of women infected with *N. gonorrhoeae* and 40 per cent of women infected with *C. trachomatis*). Treatment was assumed to reduce the probability of developing symptoms to 1/10th of their value in the absence of treatment. The probability that PID is symptomatic was assumed to be 80 per cent for women infected with *N. gonorrhoeae* and 50 per cent for women infected with *C. trachomatis*. Table 23 records the probability that symptomatic PID is treated and Table 22 the average duration and level of disability associated with symptomatic PID. The probability asymptomatic infected females are was set at 1/10th of the value for symptomatic women.

3. Complications and sequelae of PID

The majority of women with acute PID recover completely even without treatment. Some, however, are left with post-infection damage to different structures of the reproductive system such as ectopic pregnancy, infertility, chronic pelvic pain and tubo-ovarian abscesses. Treatment reduces the likelihood of developing complications if irreversible scarring and distortion of the fallopian tubes have not already occurred.

Chronic pelvic pain: Chronic pelvic pain is estimated to develop in 15 to 18 per cent of women after an upper reproductive tract infection and is often associated with infertility. The probability of developing chronic pelvic pain also appears to be positively correlated with the number of episodes of PID. The pain may wax and wain but is often so severe as to interfere with daily activities (Weström 1975).

Ectopic pregnancy: PID by permanently scarring and narrowing the fallopian tubes increases the risk that a pregnancy will be ectopic. Comprehensive reviews of retrospective studies estimate that after one or more episodes of PID the risk of an ectopic pregnancy is increased 7 to 10 fold when compared to women who have never had PID (Weström and Mårdh 1990). In the Lund cohort study 7 per cent of first pregnancies in women with acute salpingitis were ectopic (n = 544) while in the control population ectopic pregnancies occurred in less than 1 per cent of women. Studies from the EME suggest that more than 50 per cent of ectopic pregnancies can be attributed to previous PID (Weström et al. 1981).

In some cases ectopic pregnancies may heal spontaneously. In others, maternal mortality can result from sudden and severe internal bleeding when the out of place pregnancy ruptures the fallopian tube. Repeat ectopic pregnancies almost certainly increase the risk of maternal mortality. In the developing world, studies have estimated that ectopic pregnancies account for between 1 and 15 per cent of all maternal deaths (Meheus 1992), although these may underestimate the true attributable risk as the studies were primarily done in areas with reasonable access to health facilities.

Infertility: Laparoscopic investigations of infertile women show evidence of tubal occlusion and/or past PID in a large proportion of cases. Bilateral tubal occlusion was estimated to be the cause of 49 per cent of female infertility in Africa, 14 per cent in Asia, 15 per cent in Latin America, and 11 per cent in developed countries (Moore and Cates 1990). Investigators from around the world have documented that tubal occlusion is strongly associated with the presence of chlamydial antibody (measuring lifetime exposure). When these studies are combined, 70 per cent of women with tubal infertility had antibodies to chlamydia vs. 26 per cent of control women. The majority of these (39–81 per cent, median 63 per cent) had no history of symptoms or signs of PID (Moore and Cates 1990).

The cohort studies from Lund, Sweden provide the best evidence for the link between salpingitis and infertility. Seventeen per cent of the women with laparoscopically documented acute salpingitis subsequently became infertile from tubal occlusion. In the control population of women with similar pelvic symptoms but non-inflamed fallopian tubes there were no cases of infertility. The proportion that became infertile varied with the number of episodes of PID (increasing from 11 per cent after one episode to 54 per cent after 3 or more episodes) and with the severity of tubal inflammation (Weström and Mårdh 1990).

There is some evidence to suggest that infection with chlamydia may carry a worse fertility prognosis than infection with other organisms despite its mild clinical signs. Women who delayed seeking care for PID symptoms had a threefold worse fertility prognosis if the salpingitis was associated to chlamydial infection than to gonococcal infection. Chlamydia appears to cause more severe subclinical tubal inflammation and ultimately tubal damage than other agents (Moore and Cates 1990, Weström and Mårdh 1990). Work on laboratory animals illustrates the potential mechanisms behind PID-induced tubal damage. After a single inoculation of chlamydia in the ovarian tubes of monkeys there is negligible or no damage. Serial inoculations, however, cause alterations in the tubal mucosa, intratubular adhesion, and distal obstruction. This may represent an immune-mediated destruction or exacerbation of chronic infection.

Figure 5 Consequences of gonorrhoeal and chlamydial infection in females in the absence of treatment

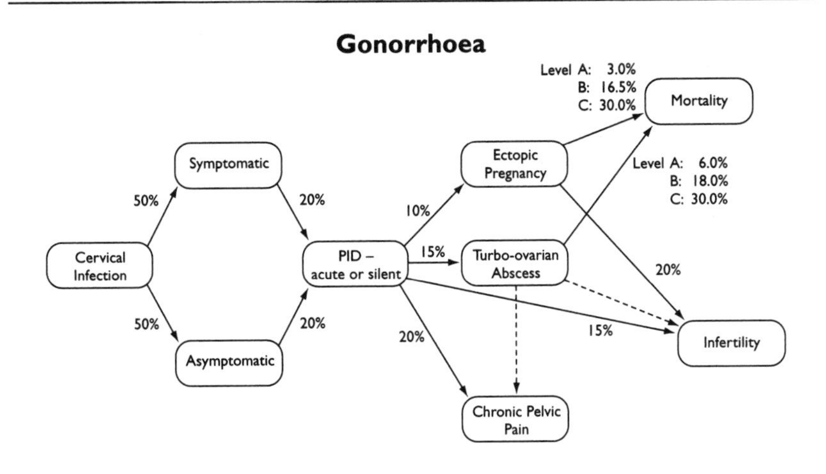

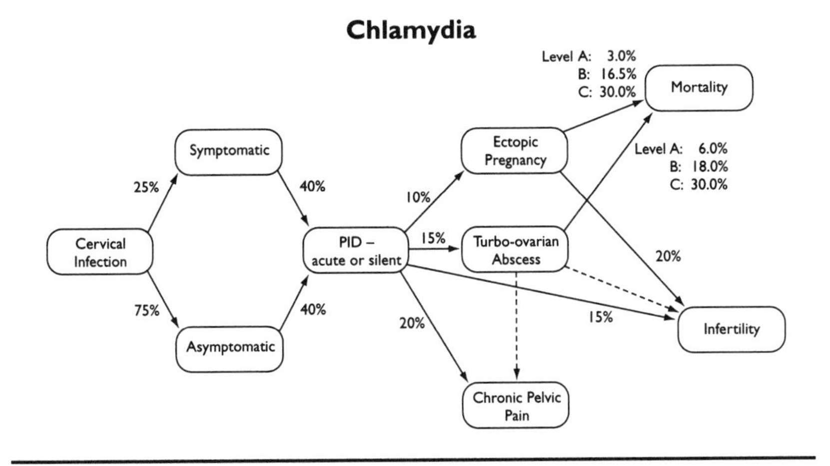

In the pre-antibiotic era the rates of pregnancy after acute PID in women who were followed and attempted to become pregnant ranged from 25 to 45 per cent. After the advent of chemotherapy the rates increased to between 70 and 80 per cent. In the Lund study treatment of PID with a variety of different antibiotic regimens had no impact on infertility, a more recent study, however, found that a ten day delay in start of therapy increased the risk of infertility 3.5 fold (Hillis et al. 1993) suggesting that the rapid start of therapy may help prevent the development of infertility.

Tubo-ovarian abscesses: The most common cause of mortality from PID is rupture of tubo-ovarian abscesses with generalized peritonitis. In such cases the mortality rate is around 6 to 8 per cent in EME countries

Table 24 Gonorrhoea and chlamydia: Average time between acquiring infection and developing a particular complication

	Average time (years)
Females	
Acute PID	0.167 (2months)
Recurrent PID	0.5
Ectopic pregnancy	3
Tubo-ovarian abscess	3
Chronic pelvic pain	1
Infertility — PID	1
Infertility — ectopic pregnancy	3
Mortality — ectopic pregnancy	3
Males	
Epididymitis	0.167 (2 months)
Stricture	0.167 (2months)
Infertility — epididymitis	2

Source: Authors' estimates

(Weström and Mårdh 1990). In developing countries the mortality is probably much higher.

Recurrent PID: Data suggest that up to 1/3 of women who have had an episode of acute PID suffer from repeated bouts. Recurrent PID ocurs for a number of reasons including: inadequate treatment and post-infection damage to normal tubal clearance patterns.

Parameter Values: The values assigned to the proportion of symptomatic and asymptomatic individuals who develop complications and sequelae from PID in the absence of treatment are shown in Figure 5. Treatment was assumed to reduce the probability of developing recurrent PID to zero and the other complications by 80 per cent. Figure 5 also records the value assigned to the probability of becoming infertile or dying. Table 22 records the average duration and level of disability associated with the different complications and Table 24 the average time between developing infection and a particular complication. In addition, 30 per cent of women who developed PID but were not treated were assumed to have recurrent episodes. These were assumed to last the same length of time as initial cases and to have the same level of disability.

Adult males

1. Urethritis

Symptoms and signs of gonococcal and chlamydial urethritis are similar and it is difficult to make an absolute distinction on clinical grounds. Both may cause urethral discharge, dysuria, or urethral itching. Discharges are more profuse and usually purulent in men with gonorrhoea while they are generally mucoid in men with non-gonocccocal urethritis.

Gonococcal urethrititis: Symptoms usually develop between 2 and 6 days after exposure and while most cases are symptomatic a small percentage of males may carry the organism and be asymptomatic or minimally symptomatic (perhaps up to 5 per cent of males have no or minimal symptoms) (Bowie 1990). The severity of symptoms is partly determined by the pathogenicity of the infecting strain of *N. gonorrhoeae* (Hook and Handsfield 1990). Gonococcal urethritis is a self-limiting disease and without treatment the usual course is spontaneous resolution over a period of several weeks, with over 95 per cent of untreated patients becoming asymptomatic within 6 months (Pelouze 1941).

Non-gonoccocal urethritis: C. trachomatis is one of the two most common causes of what is referred to as non-gonococcal urethritis. It is estimated that in heterosexual men living in North America and Europe 30 to 50 per cent of NGU is due to infection with *C. trachomatis* and 10 to 40 per cent with ureaplasma urealyticum (Bowie 1990). NGU has similar symptoms to gonococcal urethritis, although in general, they are less severe and have a longer incubation time. NGU usually develops between 1 to 4 weeks after infection with the time of acquisition peaking around 2 to 3 weeks. As many as 25 per cent of men identified with urethral infection, however, have no symptoms or signs of infection (Stamm et al. 1984, Stamm and Cole 1986). NGU is a self limiting disease and even without therapy the physical consequences to the individual are slight. If untreated symptoms may wax and wane for weeks to months.

Parameter Values: 95 per cent of men infected with *N. gonorrhoeae* and 80 per cent of men infected with *C. trachomatis* were assumed to develop symptoms (see Figure 6). Table 23 records the vaslues assigned to the proportion of symptomatic people treated and Table 22 the average duration and level of disabilityfor treated and untreated urethritis.

2. Complications and sequelae of urethritis

Complications following gonococcal urethritis or NGU include epididymitis, stricture, acute or chronic prostatis, posterior urethritis, seminal vesiculitis, infections of Cowper's and Tyson's glands, and infrequently disseminated with arthritis and synovitis. Since the introduction of antibiotics these complications have become rare in many countries although they still occur in parts of the developing world (Hook and Handsfield 1990).

Stricture: Mild to severe urethral stricture is the most important complication and may occur after untreated or late treated urethritis in up to 3 per cent of men (Bewes 1973, Osegbe and Amaku 1981).

Epididymitis: Epididymitis was a frequent complication of infection with *N. gonorrhoeae* in the pre-antimicrobial era. Pelouze (1941) reported that epididymitis occurred in 10 to 30 per cent of cases of gonorrhoeal urethritis. The use of antimicrobials has substantially reduced the incidence of epididymitis and it is now estimated that acute and chronic epididymitis occur in 1–2 per cent of cases of urethritis in developed countries (Bowie

Figure 6 Consequences of gonorrhoeal and chlamydial infection in males in the absence of treatment

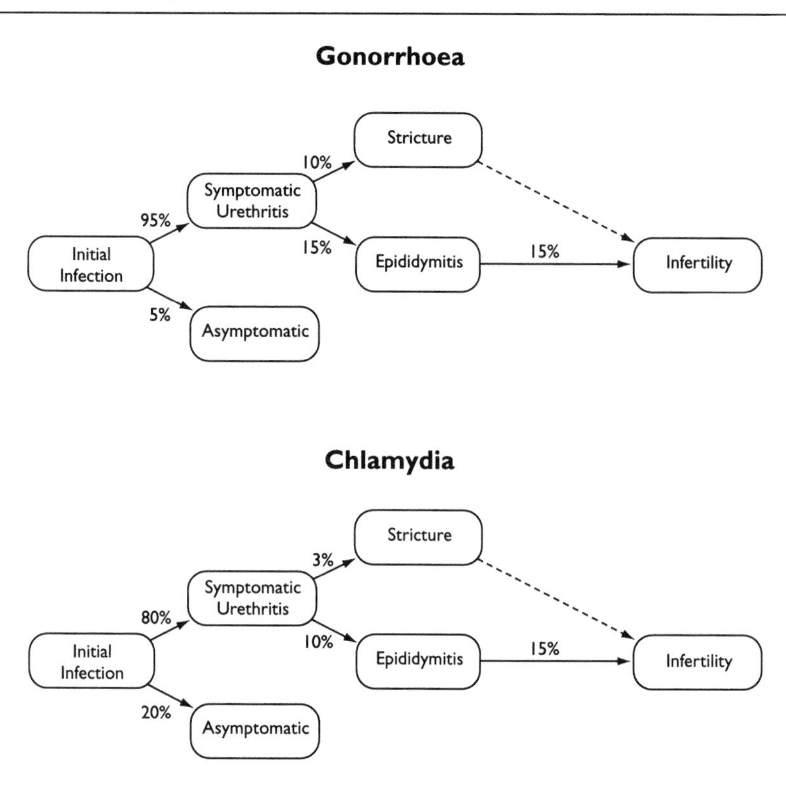

1990). In areas where urethritis often goes untreated epididymitis is still likely to be a leading cause of male infertility. Acute inflammation and damage may also lead to decreased fertility even in the absence of occlusion of the epididimis.

Prostatis: In the pre-antimicrobial era prostatis was a frequent (20–40 per cent) complication of gonococcal urethritis (Colleen and Mårdh 1990). Gonococcal prostatis can lead to septicemia, prostatic abscess, and fistula to the rectum, urethra, and perineal surface and, in the absence of antibiotics mortality from these complications approached 30 per cent.

Parameter values: The values assigned to the proportion of individuals who develop complications and sequelae in the absence of treatment are shown in Figure 6. Treatment was assumed to reduce the probability of developing complications to 1/10th of their value in the absence of treatment. Figure 6 also records the probability that epididymitis will result in infertility in the absence of treatment. If treated the probability of becoming infertile was assumed to be 0. Tables 22 and 24 record the average duration and level of disability associated with the different complications and the average time between developing infection and a particular complication.

Pregnancy outcome and infants

Maternal infection with gonorrhoea or chlamydia can be detrimental to pregnancy outcome and the health of her newborn infant. The most common clinical outcomes among neonates born to mothers with gonorrhoea are ophthalmia neonatorum and the systemic complications of gonococcemia. Other local forms include vaginitis, rhinitis, anorectal infection, urethritis, scalp abscesses, and neonatal sepsis. In infants born to mothers with chlamydia the most common clinical outcomes are opthalmia neonatorum and pneumonia.

1. Pregnancy outcome

Gonorrhoea: A review paper by Gutman and Wilfert (1990) documented that the outcomes for infants born to infected mothers were significantly worse than for infants born to uninfected mothers—rates of premature delivery ranged from 13 to 67 per cent, perinatal death from 2 to 11 per cent, and perinatal distress from 5 to 10 per cent. The effects of gonococcal infection on early pregnancy are less well studied but early infection may also cause septic abortion (Brunham et al. 1990).

Chlamydia: The role of *Chlamydia trachomatis* infection in prematurity and perinatal mortality is still under investigation. Studies of birth weights and gestational ages of infants with chlamydia infection have given conflicting results (see review in Brunham et al. 1990). It is also not clear if *C. trachomatis* infection can cause abortion. *C. psittaci* infection, however, is an important cause of abortion in lower mammals (Page and Smith 1974) and a study of first-trimester spontaneous abortions by Schachter (1967) isolated chlamydia from 4 of 22 abortions.

Parameter Values: The values assigned to the proportion of births ending in fetal wastage, low birth weight or premature delivery are recorded in Figure 7 for an untreated infected mother. In mothers who were treated it was assumed that infection had no affect on pregnancy outcome. Table 25 records the values assigned to the average duration and level of disability associated with low birth weight/premature deliver. Low birth weight/prematurity was also assumed to result in an increase in mortality (see Figure 7) with the mortality rate depending upon the level of health care.

2. Opthalmia neonatorum

Ophthalmia neonatorum is a purulent conjunctivitis in infants less than 30 days. Infection is acquired during delivery through the infected birth canal. Occasionally the disease is transmitted to infants delivered by cesarean section after prolonged rupture of the membranes (Thompson et al. 1974). Gonorrhoea ophthalmia neonatorum (GCON) tends to appear earlier and to be more severe than chlamydial infection although the symp-

Table 25 Gonorrhoea and chlamydia in infants born to untreated infected mothers: Average duration and level of disability from major complications and sequelae in the absense of treatment.

	Duration	*Level of disability*
Low Birth Weight/premature	6 months	II
Pneumonia (chlamydial infection only)	6 months	II
Opthalmia neonatorum	2 weeks	III
Mild corneal ulceration	2 weeks	II
Severe corneal ulceration	lifelong	III

Source: Authors' estimates

toms are not sufficiently distinctive to lead to an etiologic diagnosis from clinical signs alone.

Gonorrhoea: GCON begins between 1 and 13 days from birth and is mostly bilateral and purulent with the conjunctivae and eyelids swollen with edema and hyperemia. If untreated the ulcerations can lead to perforation of the eyeball with loss of vision. Corneal scarring from new blood vessels invading the cornea may also develop. GCON is associated with keratitis in 10–20 per cent of cases and it is estimated that 1 to 6 per cent of affected infants who are not treated will have permanently damaged vision (Fransen et al. 1986).

Two prospective studies in Kenya and Cameroon looked at the probability infants born to infected mothers develop GCON. In the Kenyan study 28 out of 67 babies born to infected mothers developed GCON in the absence of prophylaxis (transmission rate of 42 per cent) (Laga et al. 1986) while in Cameroon 14 out of 40 babies were infected (transmission rate of 30 per cent). In the Kenyan study it was also found that the transmission rate in mothers infected with both *N. gonorroheae* and *C. trachomatis* was significantly higher (68 per cent versus 31 per cent) (Laga et al. 1986).

The introduction of prophylaxis at birth drastically reduces the incidence of GCON. A large controlled study in Kenya by Laga showed a 93 per cent reduction in incidence when tetracycline ointment was used and an 83 per cent reduction for silver nitrate (Laga et al. 1988). Treatment once symptoms have developed also substantially reduces the probability of developing more permanent damage.

Chlamydia: Estimates of the probability of an infant developing conjunctivitis range from 18 to 50 per cent in the absence of prophylaxis (Harrison and Alexander 1990). Prophylaxis at birth does not appear to be as effective at preventing development of chlamydial ophthalmia neonatorum as GCON. It is estimated that 15 to 25 per cent of infants exposed who receive prophylaxis develop conjunctivitis (Bell et al. 1987,

Figure 7 Consequences of gonorrhoeal and chlamydial infection for infants born to untreated infected women

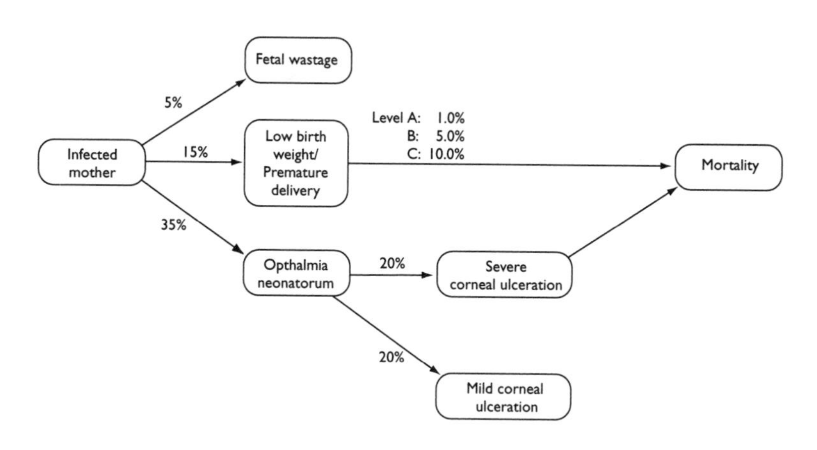

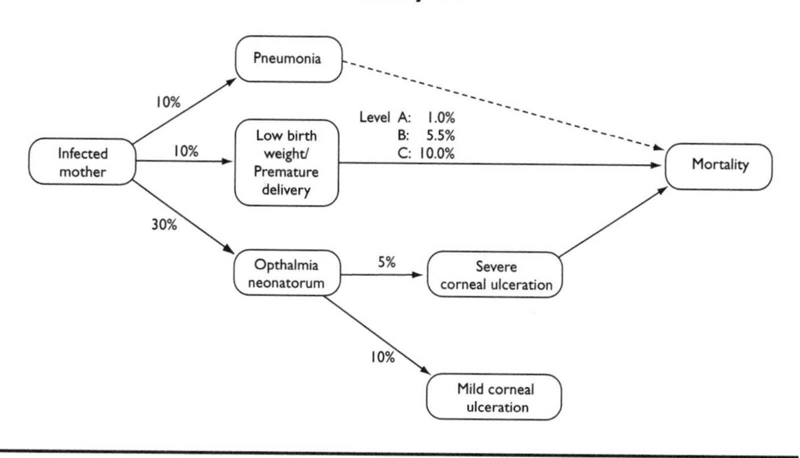

Hammerschlag et al. 1989, Preece et al. 1989); in a large controlled trial in Kenya prophylaxis resulted in a 77 per cent reduction in evidence of chlamydia ophthalmia with tetracycline prophylaxis and a 68 per cent reduction with silver nitrate (Laga et al. 1988). Once symptoms have developed, treatment substantially reduces the probability of developing more permanent damage.

Parameter Values: The probability of developing opthalmia neonatorum in infants born to untreated mothers and who did not receive prophylaxis is recorded in Figure 7. Twenty per cent of untreated infants were assumed to develop severe corneal ulceration and 20 per cent mild cor-

Table 26 Gonorrhoea and chlamydia in infants born to untreated infected mothers: Probability infants receive prophylaxis against opthalmia neonatorum or are treated.

	Level of Health Care		
	A	B	C
Prophylaxis	0.9	0.5	0.1
Treatment	1.0	0.8	0.5

Source: Authors' estimates

neal ulceration (see Figure 7). Maternal treatment and prophylaxis were assumed to reduce the probability of developing opthalmia neonatorum to 0. Table 28 records the estimated duration and level of disability and Table 26 the probability infants receive prophylaxis or are treated for opthalmia neonatorum.

3. Infant pneumonitis

It is not clear how infants acquire chlamydial pneumonitis nor has the pathology been thoroughly elucidated. Prospective studies of mothers infected with chlamydia have recorded attack rates for pneumonia of between 12 and 22 per cent in their infants (Harrison and Alexander 1990). Untreated pneumonia may last for several months and may predispose infants to respiratory problems in later life (Brasfield et al. 1987).

Parameter Values: The probability of developing pneumonia in infants born to untreated mothers is presented in Figure 7, which also records the probability of dying from pneumonia for the three levels of health care. Table 25 records the values assigned to the estimated duration and level of disability.

B. SYPHILIS

Syphilis can affect most organs and as a result was known as the "great imitator". The principal morbidity and mortality from syphilis results from the variable occurrence of later manifestations in untreated patients of systemic illnesses in the skin, bones, central nervous system, or viscera, particularly the heart and great vessels. The use of penicillin has considerably changed the course of infection as treating early syphilis almost always prevents the development of late complications. Present understanding of the course of untreated syphilis is based primarily on the large prospective studies of patients conducted in Oslo between 1890 and 1910, in Tuskegee during the 1930s, and on a review of all autopsies conducted at Yale University School of Medicine from 1917 to 1941 (See Sparling 1990 for a review of these studies).

Adults

1. Primary and secondary syphilis

Untreated infection typically results in a primary lesion, which develops 10 to 90 days post exposure (average 3 weeks). The lesion is usually single and painless, and left untreated heals in a few weeks. Within a few weeks or months of exposure a variable systemic illness develops (described as secondary syphilis). Symptoms may include low grade fever, malaise, sore throat, headache, adenopathy, cutaneous or mucosal rash, alopecia, and mild hepatitis. In a number of individuals these symptoms may be very mild (see Thin 1990).

Parameter Values: It was assumed that 90 per cent of infected individuals develop symptoms and in the absence of treatment all symptomatic and asymptomatic individuals develop secondary syphilis (see Figure 8). 60 per cent of people with secondary syphilis were assumed to develop symptoms (see Table 27). Table 27 also records the average duration and level of disability associated with each sequelae as well as the average time between acquiring infection and developing symptoms.

Tertiary syphilis

Approximately one third of patients with untreated syphilis will progress to the tertiary phase. Tertiary complications include:

Gummas: Cutaneous and osseous manifestations that develop 2 to 40 years post exposure, and usually respond well to specific therapy although untreated can lead to destruction of soft tissues or bone. Gummas of critical organs (heart, brain, liver) can be fatal (see Kampmeier 1990).

Cardiovascular: Cardiovascular syphilis involves the heart and main vessels leading from it and is not usually recognized until 10 to 30 years after initial infection. Manifestations include aortitis, aortic incompetence, aortic aneurysm, coronary ostitis, and angina pectoris (see Healy 1990).

Neurologic: Neurological complications include: inflammation of the arteries leading to the brain resulting in a stroke (occurs 5 –12 years post infection), general paresis, a combination of dementia and other neurological changes (occurs 15–20 years post infection), and tabes dorsalis which involves the spinal cord and results in loss of sensation especially in the legs (occurs 20–25 years post infection) (see Swartz 1990).

A follow-up study of the Oslo cohort 50 years after the start of the original study found that 28 per cent of the patients followed up had developed late complications whilst 72 per cent had survived to old age without obvious ill effects (Gjestland 1955). These figures, however, probably underestimate the proportion of individuals who developed tertiary syphilis as only a minority of those who died were autopsied. Both the

Figure 8 Consequences of syphilis in the absence of treatment in adults.

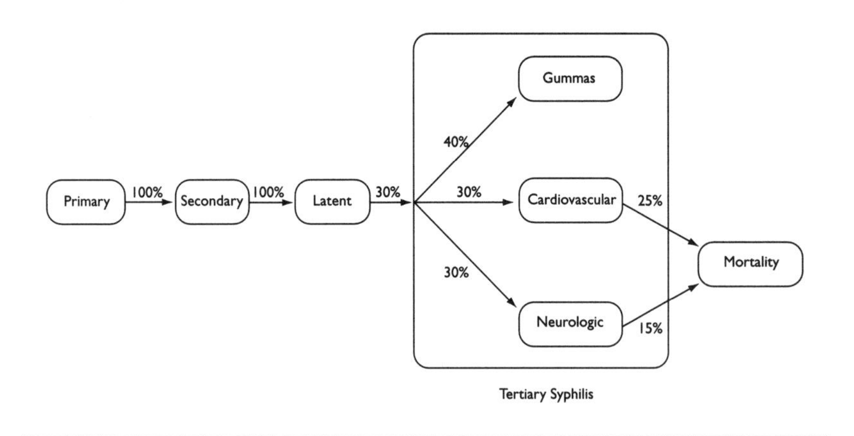

Table 27 Syphilis in adults: Probability of developing symptoms and their duration and level of disability.

Symptoms	*Probability of developing symptoms*	*Average duration of symptoms*	*Average time between infection and developing symptoms (years)*	*Level of disability*
Primary	0.9	treated: 2 weeks not treated: 3 weeks	0	II II
Secondary	0.6	treated: 3 weeks not treated: 6 weeks	0.1667 (2 months)	II II
Latent	0.3	- -		
Tertiary—Gummas	1.0	2 years	10	II
Tertiary —Cardiovascular	0.5	10 years	10	III
Tertiary —Neurologic	1.0	10 years	10	III

Source: Authors' estimates

Tuskegee study and the Rosahn study also demonstrated increased mortality and indicate that 15 to 40 per cent of untreated patients develop recognizable late complications.

Parameter Values: It was assumed that 30 per cent of individuals with latent syphilis in the absence of treatment develop symptoms and that 40 per cent of these will develop gummas, 30 per cent cardiovascular problems, and 30 per cent neurosyphilis (see Figure 8). All individuals who developed gummas or neurologic syphilis were assumed to be symptomatic and 50 per cent of those with cardiovascular syphilis. Table 27 records the average duration and level of disability associated with each of the sequelae as well as the average time between acquiring infection and developing symptoms. Mortality from tertiary syphilis was assumed to occur on average 15 years after acquiring infection. Treatment was assumed to have no impact on the duration or level of disability.

Infants

Syphilis in a pregnant woman can result in a number of different complications in the absence of treatment. Data from a study of pregnancy outcome in syphilitic women in Zambia documented that almost 58 per cent of syphilitic pregnancies had some adverse outcome, namely abortion (14.8 per cent), stillbirth (7 per cent) preterm/premature (12.2 per cent), low birth weight (21.3 per cent), and congenital syphilis (2.2 per cent) (Hira et al. 1990). By comparison 10 per cent of nonsyphilitic pregnancies had adverse outcomes.

Pregnancy outcome: A study conducted in England in 1917 and another study in Philadelphia in 1951 on the effect of untreated syphilis on pregnancy outcomes found that approximately one-third of pregnancies yielded a non syphilitic infant (Shulz et al. 1992). The Philadelphia study also highlighted relationship between the stage of maternal infection and pregnancy outcome. Prematurity, perinatal death, and congenital syphilis were all found to be directly related to the stage of maternal syphilis during pregnancy.

Congenital infection: Congenital syphilis is a serious condition that is often disfiguring and debilitating if not fatal. The pattern of histopathology seen in congenital syphilis depends on gestational age at the time of infection. Traditionally congenital syphilis is divided into two clinical syndromes:

early: features typically appear within the first 2 years of life

late: features occur later than 2 years—most often at puberty

In the Oslo study of untreated syphilis (1891–1910) 26 per cent of babies born to syphilitic mothers remained free of disease or recovered spontaneously, 25 per cent were seropositive but remained clinically unaffected, and 49 per cent displayed manifest disease (see Schlz et al. 1990). Treatment of pregnant women with penicillin, however, is 98 per cent effective in preventing congenital infection (Ingraham 1950, Platou 1949). Approximately 80 per cent of children ultimately diagnosed as having congenital syphilis pass through the early stage undetected and without specific treatment (Kauffman et al. 1977). Inadvertent partial treatment (i.e. treatment for other infections) appears to modify the expression of disease so that the classic syndromes of late congenital infection are now rare.

Parameter values: The probability of a child developing each complication was assumed to depend on how long his or her mother had been

Figure 9 Consequences of syphilis in infants born to untreated mothers with primary of secondary syphilis.

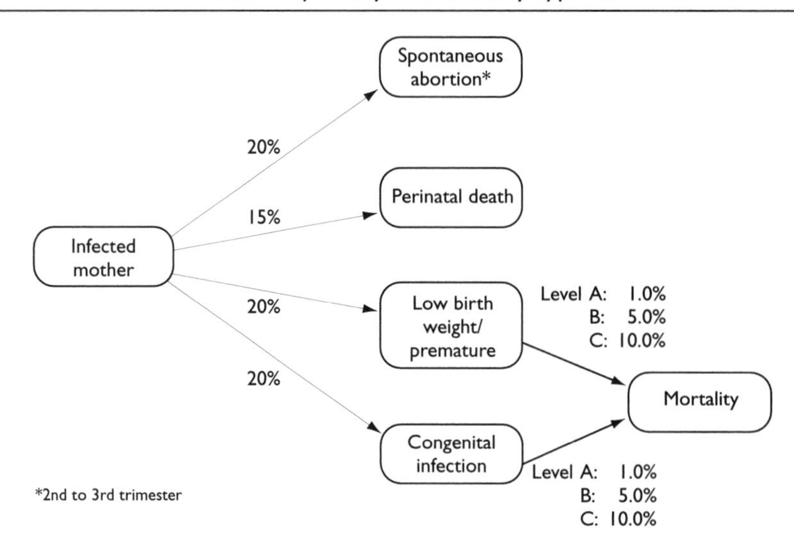

infected. The probability of developing a particular complication was assumed to be the same for women with primary and secondary syphilis, and half this value for women with latent syphilis (see Figure 11). Transmission from women with tertiary syphilis was assumed not to take place. The average duration of low birth weight/premature delivery was assumed to be six months at disability level II and for congenital syphilis three years at disability level III. Figure 9 also presents the values assigned to the mortality rate from low birth weight/premature delivery and congenital infection by level of health care.

Results

This section describes the results presented in the Global Burden of Disease. It should be noted that these figures do not include all of the complications and sequelae related to the three STDs highlighted in the previous section. In order to avoid double counting deaths and disability, the following complications were allocated to other sections:

1. ectopic pregnancies (allocated to maternal conditions)
2. neonatal pneumonia (allocated to lower respiratory infections)
3. low birth weight (allocated to perinatal conditions)
4. infertility (allocated to maternal conditions)

In addition, spontaneous abortions were excluded from the GBD estimates.

Like many other conditions STDs assume a much greater public health significance when, in addition to mortality, their prevalence and common disabling sequelae are taken into account. In terms of mortality, the three STDs (as defined above) collectively accounted for 230 000 deaths or 0.4 per cent of global deaths in 1990. In terms of DALYs, STDs were estimated to have resulted in 18.6 million DALYs lost in 1990 or about 1.5 per cent of the global burden of all diseases and injuries. Roughly two-thirds of DALYs due to STDs arise from the disabling sequelae of these infections and one-third from the premature mortality they cause (see Tables 28 to 31). These figures are, however, underestimates of the true burden of STDs as not only have a number of their consequences been allocated to other conditions, but there are a large number of STDs which have not been included, most notably HIV (which is the subject of Chapter 9, in this volume).

Syphilis accounts for almost 90 per cent of STD deaths, or some 200 000 deaths in 1990. Almost 80 per cent of these cases were congenital syphilis. The other STD related deaths (about 30 000) were in women between the ages of 15 and 45 and were related to complications and sequelae following infection with chlamydia or gonorrhoea.

Even with the restricted GBD definition of STDs, regional priorities for prevention and treatment are clear (see Tables 28 to 31). Virtually all of the deaths and DALYs from STDs occurred in developing regions with Sub-Saharan Africa accounting for roughly one-third of the entire STD burden, and India accounting for another one-third. The differential impact on women is also clear. In all regions of the world mortality and DALYs lost from STDs are greater in women than in men. Globally mortality from STDs in females in 1990 was 20 per cent fold greater than in males (126 146 deaths for females and 104 768 for males). In terms of DALYs, the excess female burden was even greater, being twice that of males (12.44 million DALYs versus 6.25 million).

For males, among whom chlamydia and gonorrhoea cause very few deaths, premature death from syphilis (largely at ages 0–4 years) accounted for about one-half of the entire STD burden. The remainder was attributable to disabilities arising primarily from gonorrhoeal infections, and to a lesser extent chlamydia and syphilis. In comparison, among females, 70 per cent of the STD disease burden in 1990 was estimated to result from the non-fatal consequences of infection, mostly chlamydia (which accounted for two-thirds of the DALYs lost).

Almost all of the deaths and DALYs lost from STDs occur in two broad age groups: 0–4 years, where the effects of maternal-fetal transmission predominate, and during the reproductive ages, defined here as the age group 15–44 years. In the 0–4 age group mortality and DALYs lost from STDs are similar for males and females. In the reproductive age classes the balance changes. In 1990 the mortality rate in women was 92 times greater than in men (6.42 per 100 000 versus 0.07 per 100 000) and the number of DALYs lost was 3.8 times greater (713.13 per 100 000 versus 189.05).

Table 28a Epidemiological estimates for sexually transmitted diseases, 1990, males.

Age group (years)	*Deaths* Number ('000s)	*Deaths* Rate per100 000	*YLLs* Number ('000s)	*YLLs* Rate per100 000	*YLDs* Number ('000s)	*YLDs* Rate per100 000	*DALYs* Number ('000s)	*DALYs* Rate per100 000
	Established Market Economies							
0-4	0.02	0.07	0.65	2.48	0.09	0.35	0.75	2.83
5-14	0.00	0.00	0.08	0.14	0.12	0.23	0.20	0.37
15-44	0.03	0.02	0.92	0.50	21.85	11.87	22.77	12.37
45-59	0.04	0.06	0.57	0.86	0.28	0.42	0.85	1.28
60+	0.14	0.24	0.64	1.05	0.08	0.13	0.72	1.19
All Ages	*0.24*	*0.06*	*2.86*	*0.73*	*22.42*	*5.74*	*25.28*	*6.48*
	Formerly Socialist Economies of Europe							
0-4	0.01	0.06	0.28	2.05	4.99	36.28	5.27	38.33
5-14	0.00	0.01	0.12	0.43	0.68	2.49	0.80	2.92
15-44	0.09	0.11	2.30	3.02	42.03	55.10	44.33	58.12
45-59	0.07	0.27	1.06	3.92	0.44	1.62	1.50	5.55
60+	0.04	0.20	0.33	1.57	0.11	0.55	0.44	2.12
All Ages	*0.21*	*0.13*	*4.09*	*2.47*	*48.26*	*29.19*	*52.34*	*31.66*
	India							
0-4	21.85	36.55	729.08	1,219.43	282.43	472.38	1 011.51	1 691.80
5-14	0.00	0.03	0.00	0.00	12.74	12.52	12.74	12.52
15-44	0.83	0.42	23.54	11.74	780.03	388.99	803.57	400.73
45-59	1.02	2.15	15.25	32.06	3.84	8.08	19.09	40.14
60+	4.86	16.33	23.42	78.69	0.79	2.65	24.21	81.34
All Ages	*28.57*	*6.50*	*791.30*	*180.09*	*1 079.83*	*245.75*	*1 871.13*	*425.84*
	China							
0-4	0.03	0.05	0.96	1.59	1.50	2.49	2.46	4.08
5-14	0.00	0.00	0.11	0.11	0.15	0.16	0.26	0.27
15-44	0.05	0.02	1.36	0.44	17.19	5.61	18.55	6.06
45-59	0.05	0.07	0.79	1.08	0.10	0.14	0.89	1.22
60+	0.20	0.42	0.94	1.92	0.02	0.04	0.96	1.97
All Ages	*0.34*	*0.06*	*4.15*	*0.71*	*18.97*	*3.24*	*23.12*	*3.95*
	Other Asia and Islands							
0-4	17.11	39.10	577.74	1 320.15	200.24	457.55	777.98	1 777.71
5-14	0.00	0.00	0.00	0.00	9.57	11.39	9.57	11.39
15-44	0.46	0.29	12.90	8.02	568.16	353.28	581.06	361.30
45-59	0.66	1.94	9.87	28.91	2.48	7.25	12.34	36.16
60+	3.25	16.06	15.35	75.97	0.48	2.39	15.84	78.36
All Ages	*21.48*	*6.26*	*615.86*	*179.57*	*780.93*	*227.70*	*1 396.79*	*407.27*
	Sub-Saharan Africa							
0-4	33.01	69.51	1 121.56	2 361.97	365.40	769.52	1 486.96	3 131.49
5-14	0.00	0.00	0.00	0.00	14.60	20.79	14.60	20.79
15-44	0.67	0.64	18.71	18.03	686.54	661.64	705.25	679.66
45-59	1.08	5.33	16.31	80.33	2.88	14.17	19.19	94.50
60+	5.22	49.68	26.07	248.05	0.49	4.70	26.56	252.75
All Ages	*39.98*	*15.84*	*1 182.65*	*468.70*	*1 069.91*	*424.03*	*2 252.56*	*892.73*

Table 28a continued

Age group (years)	Deaths Number ('000s)	Deaths Rate per100 000	YLLs Number ('000s)	YLLs Rate per100 000	YLDs Number ('000s)	YLDs Rate per100 000	DALYs Number ('000s)	DALYs Rate per100 000
	Latin America and the Caribbean							
0-4	5.17	18.00	174.23	606.64	23.89	83.17	198.12	689.80
5-14	0.00	0.00	0.00	0.00	1.74	3.33	1.74	3.33
15-44	0.09	0.09	2.56	2.46	124.09	118.99	126.66	121.45
45-59	0.13	0.57	1.88	8.45	0.67	3.01	2.55	11.46
60+	0.60	4.23	2.79	19.60	0.14	0.98	2.93	20.58
All Ages	*5.99*	*2.70*	*181.46*	*81.88*	*150.52*	*67.92*	*331.99*	*149.81*
	Middle Eastern Crescent							
0-4	6.32	15.35	213.58	518.88	12.89	31.31	226.46	550.19
5-14	0.00	0.00	0.00	0.00	0.95	1.45	0.95	1.45
15-44	0.06	0.05	1.71	1.50	59.14	51.93	60.85	53.43
45-59	0.10	0.46	1.53	6.85	0.30	1.36	1.83	8.21
60+	0.48	3.54	2.25	16.50	0.06	0.45	2.31	16.94
All Ages	*6.97*	*2.72*	*219.07*	*85.45*	*73.34*	*28.61*	*292.42*	*114.05*
	Developed Regions							
0-4	0.03	0.07	0.94	2.33	5.08	12.67	6.02	15.00
5-14	0.01	0.01	0.20	0.24	0.80	0.99	1.00	1.24
15-44	0.12	0.05	3.22	1.24	63.88	24.54	67.10	25.78
45-59	0.11	0.12	1.63	1.75	0.72	0.77	2.34	2.52
60+	0.19	0.23	0.97	1.19	0.20	0.24	1.16	1.43
All Ages	*0.45*	*0.08*	*6.95*	*1.25*	*70.68*	*12.72*	*77.63*	*13.97*
	Developing Regions							
0-4	83.49	33.07	2 817.15	1 115.97	886.34	351.11	3 703.49	1 467.08
5-14	0.00	0.00	0.11	0.02	39.76	8.89	39.87	8.92
15-44	2.16	0.23	60.79	6.48	2 235.15	238.43	2 295.94	244.92
45-59	3.05	1.01	45.63	15.14	10.27	3.41	55.90	18.55
60+	14.62	10.06	70.82	48.72	1.99	1.37	72.81	50.09
All Ages	*103.32*	*5.51*	*2 994.50*	*159.60*	*3 173.50*	*169.14*	*6 168.00*	*328.74*
	World							
0-4	83.52	25.99	2 818.08	877.08	891.42	277.44	3 709.51	1 154.52
5-14	0.01	0.00	0.31	0.06	40.56	7.36	40.87	7.41
15-44	2.28	0.18	64.01	5.12	2 299.03	183.93	2 363.04	189.05
45-59	3.16	1.01	47.26	15.13	10.98	3.52	58.24	18.64
60+	14.80	6.76	71.79	32.80	2.18	1.00	73.97	33.80
All Ages	*103.77*	*3.91*	*3 001.45*	*113.10*	*3 244.18*	*122.25*	*6 245.63*	*235.36*

Table 28b Epidemiological Estimates for sexually transmitted diseases, 1990, females.

Age group (years)	*Deaths* Number ('000s)	*Deaths* Rate per100 000	*YLLs* Number ('000s)	*YLLs* Rate per100 000	*YLDs* Number ('000s)	*YLDs* Rate per100 000	*DALYs* Number ('000s)	*DALYs* Rate per100 000
	Established Market Economies							
0-4	0.04	0.00	0.41	1.64	0.09	0.35	0.50	1.99
5-14	0.10	0.03	0.08	0.15	2.55	5.04	2.63	5.19
15-44	0.01	0.10	1.34	0.75	369.87	206.40	371.21	207.15
45-59	0.00	0.37	0.72	1.06	1.74	2.56	2.45	3.62
60+	0.01	0.62	1.48	1.74	0.60	0.71	2.07	2.45
All Ages	*0.17*	*0.21*	*4.02*	*0.99*	*374.84*	*92.03*	*378.86*	*93.02*
	Formerly Socialist Economies of Europe							
0-4	0.04	0.00	0.21	1.58	5.12	38.95	5.32	40.52
5-14	0.01	0.03	0.00	0.00	4.19	15.84	4.19	15.84
15-44	0.01	0.10	1.06	1.41	316.49	422.21	317.54	423.62
45-59	0.00	0.37	0.60	2.01	1.08	3.60	1.68	5.61
60+	0.01	0.62	0.33	0.91	0.43	1.19	0.76	2.09
All Ages	*0.06*	*0.21*	*2.20*	*0.91*	*327.30*	*134.84*	*329.50*	*135.74*
	India							
0-4	1.30	0.00	795.45	1 403.42	270.09	476.53	1 065.54	1 879.96
5-14	3.56	0.03	8.00	8.40	43.20	45.35	51.20	53.75
15-44	23.35	0.10	273.34	149.17	2 247.49	1 226.51	2 520.83	1 375.68
45-59	0.21	0.37	21.51	46.75	5.31	11.55	26.82	58.29
60+	4.60	0.62	29.31	101.33	1.07	3.69	30.38	105.02
All Ages	*33.02*	*0.21*	*1 127.61*	*274.95*	*2 567.16*	*625.96*	*3 694.77*	*900.91*
	China							
0-4	0.06	0.00	0.60	1.04	1.61	2.78	2.21	3.82
5-14	0.15	0.03	0.13	0.14	0.91	1.00	1.03	1.14
15-44	0.02	0.10	3.42	1.20	75.66	26.63	79.07	27.83
45-59	0.00	0.37	0.34	0.53	0.14	0.22	0.48	0.75
60+	0.06	0.62	0.68	1.31	0.04	0.07	0.71	1.38
All Ages	*0.28*	*0.21*	*5.16*	*0.94*	*78.35*	*14.28*	*83.51*	*15.23*
	Other Asia and Islands							
0-4	0.85	0.00	410.55	977.78	200.31	477.05	610.85	1 454.83
5-14	2.39	0.03	5.08	6.33	32.57	40.60	37.65	46.93
15-44	12.02	0.10	178.72	111.97	1 748.72	1 095.61	1 927.44	1 207.58
45-59	0.14	0.37	15.41	43.90	3.57	10.18	18.98	54.08
60+	2.66	0.62	18.67	82.40	0.73	3.23	19.40	85.63
All Ages	*18.06*	*0.21*	*628.43*	*185.07*	*1 985.89*	*584.83*	*2 614.32*	*769.90*
	Sub-Saharan Africa							
0-4	1.37	0.00	1 069.07	2 273.16	390.25	829.79	1 459.32	3 102.95
5-14	3.85	0.03	8.15	11.67	50.27	72.00	58.42	83.67
15-44	31.24	0.10	270.78	254.84	2 080.13	1 957.64	2 350.91	2 212.48
45-59	0.22	0.37	26.45	119.57	4.23	19.13	30.68	138.70
60+	4.84	0.62	38.20	300.11	0.59	4.62	38.79	304.73
All Ages	*41.52*	*0.21*	*1 412.65*	*547.64*	*2 525.46*	*979.04*	*3 938.11*	*1 526.68*

Table 28b continued

Age group (years)	Deaths Number ('000s)	Deaths Rate per100 000	YLLs Number ('000s)	YLLs Rate per100 000	YLDs Number ('000s)	YLDs Rate per100 000	DALYs Number ('000s)	DALYs Rate per100 000
	Latin America and the Caribbean							
0-4	0.16	0.00	144.61	522.50	23.94	86.51	168.55	609.01
5-14	0.44	0.03	0.55	1.09	12.14	23.93	12.69	25.02
15-44	4.28	0.10	30.92	29.71	668.02	641.80	698.94	671.51
45-59	0.01	0.37	2.76	11.82	1.31	5.61	4.07	17.42
60+	0.51	0.62	3.61	21.48	0.29	1.75	3.91	23.23
All Ages	*5.41*	*0.21*	*182.45*	*81.93*	*705.71*	*316.91*	*888.16*	*398.84*
	Middle Eastern Crescent							
0-4	0.13	0.00	205.28	516.63	12.78	32.15	218.05	548.78
5-14	0.35	0.03	0.27	0.44	5.81	9.37	6.08	9.81
15-44	6.04	0.10	9.96	9.29	271.92	253.63	281.88	262.92
45-59	0.01	0.37	2.02	9.06	0.53	2.37	2.55	11.43
60+	0.16	0.62	2.75	17.82	0.12	0.75	2.87	18.57
All Ages	*6.70*	*0.21*	*220.28*	*89.30*	*291.15*	*118.02*	*511.43*	*207.32*
	Developed Regions							
0-4	0.08	0.20	0.62	1.62	5.20	13.62	5.82	15.24
5-14	0.11	0.14	0.08	0.10	6.74	8.74	6.81	8.84
15-44	0.02	0.01	2.40	0.94	686.35	270.05	688.75	270.99
45-59	0.00	0.00	1.32	1.35	2.82	2.88	4.14	4.23
60+	0.02	0.02	1.81	1.49	1.03	0.85	2.83	2.34
All Ages	*0.23*	*0.03*	*6.22*	*0.96*	*702.14*	*108.01*	*708.36*	*108.97*
	Developing Regions							
0-4	3.87	1.43	2 625.55	968.65	898.98	331.66	3 524.53	1 300.31
5-14	10.75	2.40	22.18	4.95	144.89	32.31	167.07	37.26
15-44	76.95	8.15	767.14	81.22	7 091.92	750.88	7 859.06	832.10
45-59	0.59	0.28	68.48	32.11	15.09	7.08	83.57	39.19
60+	12.84	8.66	93.23	62.88	2.83	1.91	96.06	64.79
All Ages	*104.99*	*5.18*	*3 576.58*	*176.58*	*8 153.72*	*402.55*	*11 730.30*	*579.13*
	World							
0-4	3.94	1.28	2 626.17	849.20	904.18	292.38	3 530.35	1 141.57
5-14	10.86	2.07	22.26	4.24	151.63	28.85	173.89	33.09
15-44	76.96	6.42	769.54	64.20	7 778.28	648.92	8 547.82	713.13
45-59	0.59	0.19	69.80	22.44	17.91	5.76	87.71	28.20
60+	12.86	4.78	95.04	35.30	3.86	1.43	98.89	36.73
All Ages	*105.21*	*4.03*	*3 582.80*	*137.08*	*8 855.86*	*338.82*	*12 438.66*	*475.90*

Table 29a Epidemiological estimates for gonorrhoea, 1990, males.

Age group (years)	*Deaths*		*YLLs*		*YLDs*		*DALYs*	
	Number ('000s)	Rate per100 000	Number ('000s)	Rate per100 000	Number ('000s)	Rate per100 000	Number ('000s)	Rate per100 000
	Established Market Economies							
0-4	0.00	0.00	0.00	0.00	0.00	0.00	0.00	0.00
5-14	0.00	0.00	0.00	0.00	0.04	0.08	0.04	0.08
15-44	0.00	0.00	0.00	0.00	7.56	4.11	7.56	4.11
45-59	0.00	0.00	0.00	0.00	0.09	0.14	0.09	0.14
60+	0.00	0.00	0.01	0.02	0.03	0.05	0.04	0.07
All Ages	*0.00*	*0.00*	*0.01*	*0.00*	*7.72*	*1.98*	*7.73*	*1.98*
	Formerly Socialist Economies of Europe							
0-4	0.00	0.00	0.00	0.00	3.01	21.88	3.01	21.88
5-14	0.00	0.00	0.00	0.00	0.22	0.80	0.22	0.80
15-44	0.00	0.00	0.00	0.00	22.54	29.55	22.54	29.55
45-59	0.00	0.00	0.02	0.06	0.19	0.71	0.21	0.77
60+	0.00	0.00	0.00	0.00	0.05	0.23	0.05	0.23
All Ages	*0.00*	*0.00*	*0.02*	*0.01*	*26.01*	*15.73*	*26.02*	*15.74*
	India							
0-4	0.00	0.00	0.00	0.00	208.91	349.41	208.91	349.41
5-14	0.00	0.00	0.00	0.00	6.83	6.72	6.83	6.72
15-44	0.00	0.00	0.00	0.00	438.42	218.64	438.42	218.64
45-59	0.00	0.00	0.00	0.00	1.99	4.19	1.99	4.19
60+	0.00	0.00	0.00	0.00	0.41	1.38	0.41	1.38
All Ages	*0.00*	*0.00*	*0.00*	*0.00*	*656.57*	*149.42*	*656.57*	*149.42*
	China							
0-4	0.00	0.00	0.00	0.00	1.18	1.95	1.18	1.95
5-14	0.00	0.00	0.00	0.00	0.09	0.09	0.09	0.09
15-44	0.00	0.00	0.00	0.00	10.48	3.42	10.48	3.42
45-59	0.00	0.00	0.00	0.00	0.06	0.08	0.06	0.08
60+	0.00	0.00	0.00	0.00	0.01	0.03	0.01	0.03
All Ages	*0.00*	*0.00*	*0.00*	*0.00*	*11.82*	*2.02*	*11.82*	*2.02*
	Other Asia and Islands							
0-4	0.00	0.00	0.00	0.00	150.58	344.07	150.58	344.07
5-14	0.00	0.00	0.00	0.00	5.32	6.33	5.32	6.33
15-44	0.00	0.00	0.00	0.00	331.21	205.95	331.21	205.95
45-59	0.00	0.00	0.00	0.00	1.35	3.95	1.35	3.95
60+	0.00	0.00	0.00	0.00	0.26	1.31	0.26	1.31
All Ages	*0.00*	*0.00*	*0.00*	*0.00*	*488.72*	*142.50*	*488.72*	*142.50*
	Sub-Saharan Africa							
0-4	0.00	0.00	0.00	0.00	287.27	604.98	287.27	604.98
5-14	0.00	0.00	0.00	0.00	8.82	12.55	8.82	12.55
15-44	0.00	0.00	0.00	0.00	423.91	408.53	423.91	408.53
45-59	0.00	0.00	0.00	0.00	1.59	7.85	1.59	7.85
60+	0.00	0.00	0.00	0.00	0.27	2.61	0.27	2.61
All Ages	*0.00*	*0.00*	*0.00*	*0.00*	*721.87*	*286.09*	*721.87*	*286.09*

Table 29a continued

Age group (years)	*Deaths* Number ('000s)	Rate per 100 000	*YLLs* Number ('000s)	Rate per 100 000	*YLDs* Number ('000s)	Rate per 100 000	*DALYs* Number ('000s)	Rate per 100 000
	Latin America and the Caribbean							
0-4	0.00	0.00	0.00	0.00	16.89	58.82	16.89	58.82
5-14	0.00	0.00	0.00	0.00	0.92	1.77	0.92	1.77
15-44	0.00	0.00	0.00	0.00	68.42	65.60	68.42	65.60
45-59	0.00	0.00	0.00	0.00	0.35	1.57	0.35	1.57
60+	0.00	0.00	0.00	0.00	0.07	0.51	0.07	0.51
All Ages	*0.00*	*0.00*	*0.00*	*0.00*	*86.66*	*39.10*	*86.66*	*39.10*
	Middle Eastern Crescent							
0-4	0.00	0.00	0.00	0.00	8.09	19.66	8.09	19.66
5-14	0.00	0.00	0.00	0.00	0.38	0.59	0.38	0.59
15-44	0.00	0.00	0.00	0.00	24.80	21.78	24.80	21.78
45-59	0.00	0.00	0.00	0.00	0.12	0.52	0.12	0.52
60+	0.00	0.00	0.00	0.00	0.02	0.17	0.02	0.17
All Ages	*0.00*	*0.00*	*0.00*	*0.00*	*33.42*	*13.03*	*33.42*	*13.03*
	Developed Regions							
0-4	0.00	0.00	0.00	0.00	3.01	7.50	3.01	7.50
5-14	0.00	0.00	0.00	0.00	0.26	0.32	0.26	0.32
15-44	0.00	0.00	0.00	0.00	30.10	11.56	30.10	11.56
45-59	0.00	0.00	0.02	0.02	0.28	0.31	0.30	0.32
60+	0.00	0.00	0.01	0.02	0.08	0.09	0.09	0.11
All Ages	*0.00*	*0.00*	*0.03*	*0.01*	*33.73*	*6.07*	*33.76*	*6.07*
	Developing Regions							
0-4	0.00	0.00	0.00	0.00	672.91	266.56	672.91	266.56
5-14	0.00	0.00	0.00	0.00	22.37	5.00	22.37	5.00
15-44	0.00	0.00	0.00	0.00	1 297.24	138.38	1 297.24	138.38
45-59	0.00	0.00	0.00	0.00	5.47	1.81	5.47	1.81
60+	0.00	0.00	0.00	0.00	1.06	0.73	1.06	0.73
All Ages	*0.00*	*0.00*	*0.00*	*0.00*	*1 999.05*	*106.54*	*1 999.05*	*106.54*
	World							
0-4	0.00	0.00	0.00	0.00	675.93	210.37	675.93	210.37
5-14	0.00	0.00	0.00	0.00	22.63	4.11	22.63	4.11
15-44	0.00	0.00	0.00	0.00	1 327.34	106.19	1 327.34	106.19
45-59	0.00	0.00	0.02	0.00	5.75	1.84	5.77	1.85
60+	0.00	0.00	0.01	0.01	1.14	0.52	1.15	0.53
All Ages	*0.00*	*0.00*	*0.03*	*0.00*	*2 032.78*	*76.60*	*2 032.81*	*76.60*

Table 29b Epidemiological estimates for gonorrhoea, 1990, females.

Age group (years)	Deaths Number ('000s)	Deaths Rate per 100 000	YLLs Number ('000s)	YLLs Rate per 100 000	YLDs Number ('000s)	YLDs Rate per 100 000	DALYs Number ('000s)	DALYs Rate per 100 000
	Established Market Economies							
0-4	0.00	0.00	0.00	0.00	0.00	0.00	0.00	0.00
5-14	0.00	0.00	0.04	0.08	0.38	0.74	0.41	0.82
15-44	0.00	0.00	0.06	0.03	35.89	20.03	35.94	20.06
45-59	0.00	0.00	0.00	0.00	0.12	0.18	0.12	0.18
60+	0.00	0.00	0.00	0.00	0.05	0.05	0.05	0.06
All Ages	*0.00*	*0.00*	*0.10*	*0.02*	*36.43*	*8.94*	*36.53*	*8.97*
	Formerly Socialist Economies of Europe							
0-4	0.00	0.01	0.04	0.32	3.12	23.73	3.16	24.05
5-14	0.00	0.00	0.00	0.00	0.62	2.33	0.62	2.33
15-44	0.01	0.01	0.20	0.26	46.49	62.02	46.68	62.28
45-59	0.01	0.02	0.10	0.35	0.15	0.51	0.26	0.86
60+	0.01	0.03	0.07	0.18	0.06	0.16	0.12	0.34
All Ages	*0.03*	*0.01*	*0.41*	*0.17*	*50.43*	*20.78*	*50.84*	*20.94*
	India							
0-4	0.00	0.00	0.00	0.00	199.80	352.51	199.80	352.51
5-14	0.07	0.07	2.66	2.79	10.37	10.89	13.03	13.68
15-44	2.81	1.53	82.46	45.00	526.17	287.14	608.63	332.14
45-59	0.07	0.15	1.10	2.40	1.03	2.23	2.13	4.62
60+	0.00	0.00	0.00	0.00	0.20	0.70	0.20	0.70
All Ages	*2.95*	*0.72*	*86.22*	*21.02*	*737.57*	*179.84*	*823.78*	*200.87*
	China							
0-4	0.00	0.00	0.00	0.00	1.16	2.00	1.16	2.00
5-14	0.00	0.03	0.02	0.02	0.20	0.22	0.22	0.25
15-44	0.03	0.01	0.90	0.32	16.85	5.93	17.76	6.25
45-59	0.00	0.00	0.01	0.02	0.03	0.05	0.04	0.07
60+	0.00	0.00	0.00	0.00	0.01	0.02	0.01	0.02
All Ages	*0.03*	*0.01*	*0.93*	*0.17*	*18.26*	*3.33*	*19.19*	*3.50*
	Other Asia and Islands							
0-4	0.00	0.00	0.00	0.00	150.78	359.11	150.78	359.11
5-14	0.05	0.06	1.75	2.18	8.17	10.18	9.92	12.36
15-44	1.95	1.22	56.36	35.31	428.80	268.65	485.16	303.96
45-59	0.06	0.16	0.91	2.58	0.73	2.09	1.64	4.68
60+	0.00	0.00	0.00	0.00	0.15	0.66	0.15	0.66
All Ages	*2.06*	*0.61*	*59.01*	*17.38*	*588.64*	*173.35*	*647.65*	*190.73*
	Sub-Saharan Africa							
0-4	0.00	0.00	0.00	0.00	307.77	654.41	307.77	654.41
5-14	0.09	0.13	3.38	4.83	15.42	22.09	18.80	26.92
15-44	3.32	3.13	99.46	93.61	618.53	582.11	718.00	675.72
45-59	0.12	0.53	1.83	8.29	0.99	4.49	2.83	12.79
60+	0.00	0.00	0.00	0.00	0.18	1.42	0.18	1.42
All Ages	*3.53*	*1.37*	*104.67*	*40.58*	*942.90*	*365.53*	*1,047.57*	*406.11*

Table 29b continued

Age group (years)	*Deaths*		*YLLs*		*YLDs*		*DALYs*	
	Number ('000s)	Rate per100 000	Number ('000s)	Rate per100 000	Number ('000s)	Rate per100 000	Number ('000s)	Rate per100 000
	Latin America and the Caribbean							
0-4	0.00	0.00	0.00	0.00	16.98	61.35	16.98	61.35
5-14	0.00	0.01	0.18	0.35	2.86	5.64	3.04	5.99
15-44	0.30	0.29	8.71	8.36	155.85	149.73	164.56	158.10
45-59	0.01	0.03	0.11	0.45	0.28	1.22	0.39	1.67
60+	0.00	0.00	0.00	0.00	0.06	0.38	0.06	0.38
All Ages	*0.31*	*0.14*	*8.99*	*4.04*	*176.04*	*79.05*	*185.03*	*83.09*
	Middle Eastern Crescent							
0-4	0.00	0.00	0.00	0.00	8.05	20.25	8.05	20.25
5-14	0.00	0.00	0.08	0.12	1.18	1.90	1.25	2.02
15-44	0.08	0.07	2.21	2.06	53.99	50.36	56.20	52.42
45-59	0.00	0.01	0.04	0.16	0.09	0.41	0.13	0.57
60+	0.00	0.00	0.00	0.00	0.02	0.13	0.02	0.13
All Ages	*0.08*	*0.03*	*2.32*	*0.94*	*63.32*	*25.67*	*511.00*	*207.15*
	Developed Regions							
0-4	0.00	0.00	0.04	0.11	3.12	8.16	3.16	8.27
5-14	0.00	0.00	0.04	0.05	0.99	1.29	1.03	1.34
15-44	0.01	0.00	0.26	0.10	82.37	32.41	82.63	32.51
45-59	0.01	0.01	0.10	0.11	0.27	0.28	0.38	0.39
60+	0.01	0.01	0.07	0.06	0.10	0.08	0.17	0.14
All Ages	*0.03*	*0.00*	*0.51*	*0.08*	*86.86*	*13.36*	*87.37*	*13.44*
	Developing Regions							
0-4	0.00	0.00	0.00	0.00	684.54	252.55	684.54	252.55
5-14	0.21	0.05	8.05	1.80	38.20	8.52	46.26	10.31
15-44	8.49	0.90	250.10	26.48	1 800.19	190.60	2 050.29	217.08
45-59	0.26	0.12	4.00	1.87	3.16	1.48	7.16	3.36
60+	0.00	0.00	0.00	0.00	0.62	0.42	0.62	0.42
All Ages	*8.96*	*0.44*	*262.15*	*12.94*	*2 526.72*	*124.75*	*2 788.87*	*137.69*
	World							
0-4	0.00	0.00	0.04	0.01	687.66	222.36	687.70	222.37
5-14	0.22	0.04	8.09	1.54	39.20	7.46	47.29	9.00
15-44	8.50	0.71	250.35	20.89	1 882.57	157.06	2 132.92	177.94
45-59	0.26	0.08	4.10	1.32	3.43	1.10	7.53	2.42
60+	0.01	0.00	0.07	0.03	0.73	0.27	0.80	0.30
All Ages	*8.99*	*0.34*	*262.66*	*10.05*	*2 613.58*	*99.99*	*2 876.24*	*110.04*

Table 30a Epidemiological estimates for chlamydia, 1990, males.

Age group (years)	Deaths Number ('000s)	Deaths Rate per 100 000	YLLs Number ('000s)	YLLs Rate per 100 000	YLDs Number ('000s)	YLDs Rate per 100 000	DALYs Number ('000s)	DALYs Rate per 100 000
	Established Market Economies							
0-4	0.00	0.00	0.00	0.00	0.00	0.00	0.00	0.00
5-14	0.00	0.00	0.00	0.00	0.07	0.14	0.07	0.14
15-44	0.00	0.00	0.00	0.00	13.30	7.23	13.30	7.23
45-59	0.00	0.00	0.00	0.00	0.17	0.25	0.17	0.25
60+	0.00	0.00	0.00	0.00	0.05	0.08	0.05	0.08
All Ages	*0.00*	*0.00*	*0.00*	*0.00*	*13.59*	*3.48*	*13.59*	*3.48*
	Formerly Socialist Economies of Europe							
0-4	0.00	0.00	0.00	0.00	1.87	13.61	1.87	13.61
5-14	0.00	0.00	0.00	0.00	0.19	0.70	0.19	0.70
15-44	0.00	0.00	0.00	0.00	17.40	22.82	17.40	22.82
45-59	0.00	0.00	0.00	0.00	0.15	0.55	0.15	0.55
60+	0.00	0.00	0.00	0.00	0.04	0.18	0.04	0.18
All Ages	*0.00*	*0.00*	*0.00*	*0.00*	*19.65*	*11.89*	*19.65*	*11.89*
	India							
0-4	0.00	0.00	0.00	0.00	66.56	111.32	66.56	111.32
5-14	0.00	0.00	0.00	0.00	4.64	4.56	4.64	4.56
15-44	0.00	0.00	0.00	0.00	238.81	119.09	238.81	119.09
45-59	0.00	0.00	0.00	0.00	0.97	2.04	0.97	2.04
60+	0.00	0.00	0.00	0.00	0.20	0.67	0.20	0.67
All Ages	*0.00*	*0.00*	*0.00*	*0.00*	*311.17*	*70.82*	*311.17*	*70.82*
	China							
0-4	0.00	0.00	0.00	0.00	0.32	0.52	0.32	0.52
5-14	0.00	0.00	0.00	0.00	0.06	0.07	0.06	0.07
15-44	0.00	0.00	0.00	0.00	6.52	2.13	6.52	2.13
45-59	0.00	0.00	0.00	0.00	0.04	0.05	0.04	0.05
60+	0.00	0.00	0.00	0.00	0.01	0.02	0.01	0.02
All Ages	*0.00*	*0.00*	*0.00*	*0.00*	*6.95*	*1.19*	*6.95*	*1.19*
	Other Asia and Islands							
0-4	0.00	0.00	0.00	0.00	45.46	103.87	45.46	103.87
5-14	0.00	0.00	0.00	0.00	3.42	4.07	3.42	4.07
15-44	0.00	0.00	0.00	0.00	170.58	106.07	170.58	106.07
45-59	0.00	0.00	0.00	0.00	0.62	1.81	0.62	1.81
60+	0.00	0.00	0.00	0.00	0.12	0.60	0.12	0.60
All Ages	*0.00*	*0.00*	*0.00*	*0.00*	*220.20*	*64.20*	*220.20*	*64.20*
	Sub-Saharan Africa							
0-4	0.00	0.00	0.00	0.00	65.21	137.34	65.21	137.34
5-14	0.00	0.00	0.00	0.00	4.01	5.70	4.01	5.70
15-44	0.00	0.00	0.00	0.00	154.48	148.88	154.48	148.88
45-59	0.00	0.00	0.00	0.00	0.52	2.56	0.52	2.56
60+	0.00	0.00	0.00	0.00	0.09	0.85	0.09	0.85
All Ages	*0.00*	*0.00*	*0.00*	*0.00*	*224.31*	*88.90*	*224.31*	*88.90*

Table 30a continued

Age group (years)	Deaths Number ('000s)	Deaths Rate per100 000	YLLs Number ('000s)	YLLs Rate per100 000	YLDs Number ('000s)	YLDs Rate per100 000	DALYs Number ('000s)	DALYs Rate per100 000
	Latin America and the Caribbean							
0-4	0.00	0.00	0.00	0.00	5.63	19.59	5.63	19.59
5-14	0.00	0.00	0.00	0.00	0.65	1.24	0.65	1.24
15-44	0.00	0.00	0.00	0.00	41.96	40.23	41.96	40.23
45-59	0.00	0.00	0.00	0.00	0.21	0.96	0.21	0.96
60+	0.00	0.00	0.00	0.00	0.04	0.31	0.04	0.31
All Ages	*0.00*	*0.00*	*0.00*	*0.00*	*48.49*	*21.88*	*48.49*	*21.88*
	Middle Eastern Crescent							
0-4	0.00	0.00	0.00	0.00	3.24	7.88	3.24	7.88
5-14	0.00	0.00	0.00	0.00	0.41	0.63	0.41	0.63
15-44	0.00	0.00	0.00	0.00	23.10	20.28	23.10	20.28
45-59	0.00	0.00	0.00	0.00	0.11	0.48	0.11	0.48
60+	0.00	0.00	0.00	0.00	0.02	0.16	0.02	0.16
All Ages	*0.00*	*0.00*	*0.00*	*0.00*	*26.89*	*10.49*	*26.89*	*10.49*
	Developed Regions							
0-4	0.00	0.00	0.00	0.00	1.87	4.66	1.87	4.66
5-14	0.00	0.00	0.00	0.00	0.27	0.33	0.27	0.33
15-44	0.00	0.00	0.00	0.00	30.70	11.79	30.70	11.79
45-59	0.00	0.00	0.00	0.00	0.31	0.34	0.31	0.34
60+	0.00	0.00	0.00	0.00	0.09	0.11	0.09	0.11
All Ages	*0.00*	*0.00*	*0.00*	*0.00*	*33.24*	*5.98*	*33.24*	*5.98*
	Developing Regions							
0-4	0.00	0.00	0.00	0.00	186.42	73.85	186.42	73.85
5-14	0.00	0.00	0.00	0.00	13.19	2.95	13.19	2.95
15-44	0.00	0.00	0.00	0.00	635.46	67.79	635.46	67.79
45-59	0.00	0.00	0.00	0.00	2.47	0.82	2.47	0.82
60+	0.00	0.00	0.00	0.00	0.49	0.33	0.49	0.33
All Ages	*0.00*	*0.00*	*0.00*	*0.00*	*838.01*	*44.66*	*838.01*	*44.66*
	World							
0-4	0.00	0.00	0.00	0.00	188.29	58.60	188.29	58.60
5-14	0.00	0.00	0.00	0.00	13.45	2.44	13.45	2.44
15-44	0.00	0.00	0.00	0.00	666.16	53.30	666.16	53.30
45-59	0.00	0.00	0.00	0.00	2.78	0.89	2.78	0.89
60+	0.00	0.00	0.00	0.00	0.57	0.26	0.57	0.26
All Ages	*0.00*	*0.00*	*0.00*	*0.00*	*871.25*	*32.83*	*871.25*	*32.83*

Table 30b Epidemiological estimates for chlamydia, 1990, females.

Age group (years)	*Deaths* Number ('000s)	Rate per100 000	*YLLs* Number ('000s)	Rate per100 000	*YLDs* Number ('000s)	Rate per100 000	*DALYs* Number ('000s)	Rate per100 000
	Established Market Economies							
0-4	0.00	0.00	0.00	0.00	0.00	0.00	0.00	0.00
5-14	0.01	0.01	0.26	0.52	3.52	6.95	3.79	7.47
15-44	0.01	0.01	0.40	0.23	329.99	184.15	330.40	184.37
45-59	0.00	0.00	0.00	0.00	0.99	1.46	0.99	1.46
60+	0.00	0.00	0.00	0.00	0.37	0.44	0.37	0.44
All Ages	*0.02*	*0.01*	*0.67*	*0.16*	*334.88*	*82.22*	*335.55*	*82.38*
	Formerly Socialist Economies of Europe							
0-4	0.00	0.03	0.14	1.10	1.94	14.76	2.08	15.86
5-14	0.00	0.00	0.00	0.00	3.56	13.47	3.56	13.47
15-44	0.03	0.03	0.69	0.92	268.20	357.79	268.89	358.71
45-59	0.02	0.08	0.37	1.22	0.86	2.87	1.23	4.09
60+	0.00	0.00	0.00	0.00	0.32	0.89	0.32	0.89
All Ages	*0.05*	*0.02*	*1.20*	*0.49*	*274.88*	*113.24*	*276.08*	*113.73*
	India							
0-4	0.00	0.00	0.00	0.00	63.67	112.33	63.67	112.33
5-14	0.14	0.15	5.35	5.61	31.34	32.90	36.69	38.51
15-44	5.65	3.09	165.98	90.58	1 603.71	875.19	1 769.69	965.76
45-59	0.14	0.31	2.22	4.82	3.22	7.01	5.44	11.83
60+	0.00	0.00	0.00	0.00	0.65	2.24	0.65	2.24
All Ages	*5.94*	*1.45*	*173.54*	*42.32*	*1 702.59*	*415.15*	*1 876.13*	*457.47*
	China							
0-4	0.00	0.00	0.00	0.00	0.44	0.76	0.44	0.76
5-14	0.00	0.00	0.05	0.06	0.70	0.78	0.75	0.83
15-44	0.07	0.03	2.15	0.76	58.62	20.63	60.77	21.39
45-59	0.00	0.00	0.03	0.04	0.11	0.16	0.13	0.21
60+	0.00	0.00	0.00	0.00	0.03	0.05	0.03	0.05
All Ages	*0.08*	*0.01*	*2.22*	*0.41*	*59.90*	*10.92*	*62.12*	*11.33*
	Other Asia and Islands							
0-4	0.00	0.00	0.00	0.00	45.51	108.40	45.51	108.40
5-14	0.09	0.11	3.33	4.16	23.40	29.17	26.73	33.32
15-44	3.73	2.34	107.56	67.39	1 237.98	775.62	1 345.55	843.02
45-59	0.11	0.31	1.73	4.93	2.19	6.23	3.92	11.16
60+	0.00	0.00	0.00	0.00	0.45	1.98	0.45	1.98
All Ages	*3.93*	*1.16*	*112.63*	*33.17*	*1 309.53*	*385.65*	*1 422.16*	*418.81*
	Sub-Saharan Africa							
0-4	0.00	0.00	0.00	0.00	69.85	148.51	69.85	148.51
5-14	0.13	0.18	4.77	6.84	32.64	46.75	37.42	53.59
15-44	4.70	4.43	140.70	132.42	1 323.74	1 245.79	1 464.44	1 378.21
45-59	0.17	0.75	2.59	11.73	2.20	9.95	4.79	21.68
60+	0.00	0.00	0.00	0.00	0.41	3.19	0.41	3.19
All Ages	*4.99*	*1.94*	*148.07*	*57.40*	*1 428.84*	*553.92*	*1 576.91*	*611.32*

Table 30b continued

Age group (years)	Deaths Number ('000s)	Deaths Rate per100 000	YLLs Number ('000s)	YLLs Rate per100 000	YLDs Number ('000s)	YLDs Rate per100 000	DALYs Number ('000s)	DALYs Rate per100 000
	Latin America and the Caribbean							
0-4	0.00	0.00	0.00	0.00	5.65	20.43	5.65	20.43
5-14	0.01	0.02	0.38	0.74	9.08	17.90	9.46	18.64
15-44	0.64	0.61	18.52	17.79	495.17	475.73	513.68	493.52
45-59	0.01	0.06	0.22	0.96	0.89	3.80	1.11	4.76
60+	0.00	0.00	0.00	0.00	0.20	1.19	0.20	1.19
All Ages	*0.66*	*0.30*	*19.11*	*8.58*	*510.99*	*229.47*	*530.11*	*238.05*
	Middle Eastern Crescent							
0-4	0.00	0.01	0.00	0.00	3.23	8.13	3.23	8.13
5-14	0.01	0.01	0.19	0.31	4.45	7.18	4.65	7.49
15-44	0.19	0.18	5.64	5.26	204.65	190.89	210.29	196.15
45-59	0.01	0.03	0.09	0.42	0.34	1.52	0.43	1.93
60+	0.00	0.00	0.00	0.00	0.07	0.48	0.07	0.48
All Ages	*0.20*	*0.08*	*5.93*	*2.40*	*212.75*	*86.24*	*511.00*	*207.15*
	Developed Regions							
0-4	0.00	0.01	0.14	0.38	1.94	5.07	2.08	5.45
5-14	0.01	0.01	0.26	0.34	7.08	9.18	7.35	9.53
15-44	0.04	0.02	1.09	0.43	598.19	235.36	599.28	235.79
45-59	0.02	0.02	0.37	0.38	1.85	1.89	2.22	2.27
60+	0.00	0.00	0.00	0.00	0.70	0.57	0.70	0.57
All Ages	*0.08*	*0.01*	*1.87*	*0.29*	*609.76*	*93.80*	*611.62*	*94.09*
	Developing Regions							
0-4	0.00	0.00	0.00	0.00	188.35	69.49	188.35	69.49
5-14	0.37	0.08	14.08	3.14	101.61	22.66	115.69	25.80
15-44	14.99	1.59	440.54	46.64	4 923.87	521.33	5 364.42	567.97
45-59	0.44	0.21	6.89	3.23	8.94	4.19	15.83	7.42
60+	0.00	0.00	0.00	0.00	1.80	1.22	1.80	1.22
All Ages	*15.80*	*0.78*	*461.51*	*22.78*	*5 224.58*	*257.94*	*5 686.09*	*280.73*
	World							
0-4	0.00	0.00	0.14	0.05	190.29	61.53	190.43	61.58
5-14	0.38	0.07	14.34	2.73	108.70	20.68	123.03	23.41
15-44	15.03	1.25	441.64	36.84	5 522.07	460.69	5 963.70	497.54
45-59	0.46	0.15	7.25	2.33	10.79	3.47	18.05	5.80
60+	0.00	0.00	0.00	0.00	2.50	0.93	2.50	0.93
All Ages	*15.88*	*0.61*	*463.37*	*17.73*	*5 834.34*	*223.22*	*6 297.71*	*240.95*

Table 31a Epidemiological estimates for syphilis, 1990, males.

Age group (years)	*Deaths* Number ('000s)	Rate per 100 000	*YLLs* Number ('000s)	Rate per 100 000	*YLDs* Number ('000s)	Rate per 100 000	*DALYs* Number ('000s)	Rate per 100 000
	Established Market Economies							
0-4	0.02	0.07	0.65	2.48	0.09	0.35	0.75	2.83
5-14	0.00	0.00	0.08	0.14	0.01	0.01	0.08	0.16
15-44	0.03	0.02	0.90	0.49	0.98	0.53	1.88	1.02
45-59	0.04	0.05	0.52	0.79	0.01	0.02	0.54	0.81
60+	0.14	0.23	0.61	1.00	0.00	0.01	0.61	1.01
All Ages	*0.24*	*0.06*	*2.76*	*0.71*	*1.09*	*0.28*	*3.86*	*0.99*
	Formerly Socialist Economies of Europe							
0-4	0.00	0.02	0.11	0.77	0.05	0.39	0.16	1.16
5-14	0.00	0.00	0.04	0.14	0.01	0.04	0.05	0.18
15-44	0.01	0.01	0.20	0.26	1.16	1.53	1.36	1.78
45-59	0.01	0.05	0.22	0.81	0.01	0.05	0.23	0.86
60+	0.02	0.08	0.13	0.60	0.00	0.02	0.13	0.61
All Ages	*0.04*	*0.03*	*0.68*	*0.41*	*1.25*	*0.75*	*1.93*	*1.17*
	India							
0-4	21.85	36.55	729.08	1 219.43	6.96	11.64	736.04	1 231.07
5-14	0.00	0.00	0.00	0.00	1.27	1.24	1.27	1.24
15-44	0.83	0.42	23.54	11.74	102.80	51.27	126.34	63.01
45-59	1.02	2.15	15.25	32.06	0.88	1.85	16.13	33.91
60+	4.86	16.33	23.42	78.69	0.18	0.60	23.60	79.29
All Ages	*28.57*	*6.50*	*791.30*	*180.09*	*112.08*	*25.51*	*903.38*	*205.59*
	China							
0-4	0.03	0.05	0.96	1.59	0.01	0.01	0.97	1.60
5-14	0.00	0.00	0.11	0.11	0.00	0.00	0.11	0.12
15-44	0.05	0.02	1.36	0.44	0.19	0.06	1.55	0.50
45-59	0.05	0.07	0.79	1.08	0.00	0.00	0.79	1.09
60+	0.20	0.42	0.94	1.92	0.00	0.00	0.94	1.92
All Ages	*0.34*	*0.06*	*4.15*	*0.71*	*0.20*	*0.03*	*4.35*	*0.74*
	Other Asia and Islands							
0-4	17.11	39.10	577.74	1 320.15	4.20	9.61	581.94	1 329.76
5-14	0.00	0.00	0.00	0.00	0.84	1.00	0.84	1.00
15-44	0.46	0.29	12.90	8.02	66.36	41.26	79.27	49.29
45-59	0.66	1.94	9.87	28.91	0.51	1.49	10.37	30.39
60+	3.25	16.06	15.35	75.97	0.10	0.48	15.45	76.46
All Ages	*21.48*	*6.26*	*615.86*	*179.57*	*72.01*	*21.00*	*687.87*	*200.57*
	Sub-Saharan Africa							
0-4	33.01	69.51	1 121.56	2 361.97	12.92	27.20	1 134.47	2 389.17
5-14	0.00	0.00	0.00	0.00	1.78	2.53	1.78	2.53
15-44	0.67	0.64	18.71	18.03	108.15	104.22	126.85	122.25
45-59	1.08	5.33	16.31	80.33	0.76	3.76	17.08	84.09
60+	5.22	49.68	26.07	248.05	0.13	1.23	26.19	249.28
All Ages	*39.98*	*15.84*	*1 182.65*	*468.70*	*123.73*	*49.04*	*1 306.38*	*517.74*

Table 31a continued

Age group (years)	*Deaths*		*YLLs*		*YLDs*		*DALYs*	
	Number ('000s)	Rate per100 000	Number ('000s)	Rate per100 000	Number ('000s)	Rate per100 000	Number ('000s)	Rate per100 000
	Latin America and the Caribbean							
0-4	5.17	18.00	174.23	606.64	1.37	4.76	175.60	611.39
5-14	0.00	0.00	0.00	0.00	0.16	0.32	0.16	0.32
15-44	0.09	0.09	2.56	2.46	13.72	13.16	16.28	15.61
45-59	0.13	0.57	1.88	8.45	0.11	0.47	1.98	8.92
60+	0.60	4.23	2.79	19.60	0.02	0.15	2.81	19.75
All Ages	*5.99*	*2.70*	*181.46*	*81.88*	*15.38*	*6.94*	*196.84*	*88.82*
	Middle Eastern Crescent							
0-4	6.32	15.35	213.58	518.88	1.55	3.78	215.13	522.66
5-14	0.00	0.00	0.00	0.00	0.15	0.24	0.15	0.24
15-44	0.06	0.05	1.71	1.50	11.23	9.86	12.95	11.37
45-59	0.10	0.46	1.53	6.85	0.08	0.35	1.61	7.21
60+	0.48	3.54	2.25	16.50	0.02	0.11	2.27	16.61
All Ages	*6.97*	*2.72*	*219.07*	*85.45*	*13.04*	*5.08*	*232.11*	*90.53*
	Developed Regions							
0-4	0.03	0.06	0.76	1.89	0.15	0.36	0.91	2.26
5-14	0.00	0.00	0.12	0.14	0.02	0.02	0.13	0.17
15-44	0.04	0.02	1.10	0.42	2.14	0.82	3.24	1.24
45-59	0.05	0.05	0.74	0.80	0.03	0.03	0.77	0.83
60+	0.15	0.19	0.73	0.90	0.01	0.01	0.74	0.91
All Ages	*0.27*	*0.05*	*3.45*	*0.62*	*2.34*	*0.42*	*5.79*	*1.04*
	Developing Regions							
0-4	83.49	33.07	2 817.15	1 115.97	27.01	10.70	2 844.16	1 126.67
5-14	0.00	0.00	0.11	0.02	4.21	0.94	4.32	0.97
15-44	2.16	0.23	60.79	6.48	302.45	32.26	363.24	38.75
45-59	3.05	1.01	45.63	15.14	2.33	0.77	47.96	15.92
60+	14.62	10.06	70.82	48.72	0.44	0.30	71.27	49.03
All Ages	*103.32*	*5.51*	*2 994.50*	*159.60*	*336.44*	*17.93*	*3 330.94*	*177.53*
	World							
0-4	83.51	25.99	2 817.91	877.02	27.16	8.45	2 845.06	885.47
5-14	0.01	0.00	0.23	0.04	4.22	0.77	4.45	0.81
15-44	2.20	0.18	61.89	4.95	304.59	24.37	366.48	29.32
45-59	3.10	0.99	46.37	14.84	2.36	0.76	48.73	15.60
60+	14.77	6.75	71.56	32.70	0.45	0.21	72.01	32.90
All Ages	*103.59*	*3.90*	*2 997.95*	*112.97*	*338.78*	*12.77*	*3 336.73*	*125.74*

Table 31b Epidemiological estimates for syphilis, 1990, females.

Age group (years)	Deaths Number ('000s)	Deaths Rate per 100 000	YLLs Number ('000s)	YLLs Rate per 100 000	YLDs Number ('000s)	YLDs Rate per 100 000	DALYs Number ('000s)	DALYs Rate per 100 000
	Established Market Economies							
0-4	0.01	0.05	0.41	1.64	0.09	0.35	0.50	1.99
5-14	0.00	0.00	0.04	0.08	0.01	0.01	0.04	0.09
15-44	0.01	0.01	0.25	0.14	0.96	0.53	1.21	0.67
45-59	0.01	0.02	0.20	0.30	0.01	0.02	0.22	0.32
60+	0.10	0.1	0.41	0.48	0.00	0.01	0.41	0.49
All Ages	*0.13*	*0.03*	*1.31*	*0.32*	*1.07*	*0.26*	*2.38*	*0.58*
	Formerly Socialist Economies of Europe							
0-4	0.00	0.00	0.00	0.00	0.05	0.39	0.05	0.39
5-14	0.00	0.00	0.00	0.00	0.01	0.04	0.01	0.04
15-44	0.00	0.00	0.08	0.10	1.12	1.50	1.20	1.60
45-59	0.01	0.02	0.08	0.26	0.02	0.05	0.10	0.32
60+	0.00	0.00	0.00	0.00	0.01	0.02	0.01	0.02
All Ages	*0.01*	*0.00*	*0.16*	*0.06*	*1.21*	*0.50*	*1.36*	*0.56*
	India							
0-4	23.35	41.19	795.45	1 403.42	6.63	11.70	802.08	1 415.12
5-14	0.00	0.00	0.00	0.00	1.49	1.56	1.49	1.56
15-44	0.87	0.47	24.91	13.59	117.61	64.18	142.52	77.78
45-59	1.16	2.53	18.19	39.53	1.06	2.31	19.25	41.84
60+	5.56	19.24	29.31	101.33	0.21	0.74	29.52	102.07
All Ages	*30.94*	*7.54*	*867.85*	*211.61*	*127.00*	*30.97*	*994.85*	*242.58*
	China							
0-4	0.02	0.03	0.60	1.04	0.01	0.01	0.61	1.06
5-14	0.00	0.00	0.05	0.06	0.00	0.00	0.06	0.06
15-44	0.01	0.00	0.37	0.13	0.18	0.06	0.55	0.19
45-59	0.02	0.03	0.30	0.47	0.00	0.00	0.31	0.48
60+	0.14	0.28	0.68	1.31	0.00	0.00	0.68	1.31
All Ages	*0.20*	*0.04*	*2.01*	*0.37*	*0.19*	*0.04*	*2.20*	*0.40*
	Other Asia and Islands							
0-4	12.02	28.62	410.55	977.78	4.01	9.54	414.56	987.32
5-14	0.00	0.00	0.00	0.00	1.00	1.25	1.00	1.25
15-44	0.52	0.33	14.80	9.27	81.93	51.33	96.73	60.61
45-59	0.82	2.32	12.77	36.39	0.65	1.85	13.42	38.24
60+	3.68	16.25	18.67	82.40	0.13	0.59	18.81	82.99
All Ages	*17.04*	*5.02*	*456.79*	*134.52*	*87.73*	*25.83*	*544.51*	*160.35*
	Sub-Saharan Africa							
0-4	31.24	66.42	1 069.07	2 273.16	12.63	26.86	1 081.70	2 300.02
5-14	0.00	0.00	0.00	0.00	2.20	3.15	2.20	3.15
15-44	1.07	1.01	30.62	28.81	137.86	129.74	168.47	158.55
45-59	1.40	6.34	22.02	99.55	1.04	4.69	23.05	104.23
60+	6.77	53.17	38.20	300.11	0.00	0.01	38.20	300.12
All Ages	*40.48*	*15.69*	*1 159.90*	*449.66*	*153.73*	*59.60*	*1 313.63*	*509.25*

Table 31b continued

Age group (years)	Deaths		YLLs		YLDs		DALYs	
	Number ('000s)	Rate per100 000	Number ('000s)	Rate per100 000	Number ('000s)	Rate per100 000	Number ('000s)	Rate per100 000
	Latin America and the Caribbean							
0-4	4.28	15.48	144.61	522.50	1.31	4.73	145.92	527.23
5-14	0.00	0.00	0.00	0.00	0.20	0.39	0.20	0.39
15-44	0.13	0.13	3.70	3.55	17.00	16.33	20.70	19.89
45-59	0.16	0.67	2.43	10.41	0.14	0.59	2.57	11.00
60+	0.75	4.43	3.61	21.48	0.03	0.18	3.65	21.67
All Ages	*5.32*	*2.39*	*154.35*	*69.31*	*18.67*	*8.39*	*173.03*	*77.70*
	Middle Eastern Crescent							
0-4	6.04	15.21	205.28	516.63	1.50	3.78	206.78	520.40
5-14	0.00	0.00	0.00	0.00	0.18	0.30	0.18	0.30
15-44	0.07	0.07	2.11	1.97	13.27	12.38	15.39	14.35
45-59	0.12	0.54	1.89	8.48	0.10	0.45	1.99	8.92
60+	0.55	3.56	2.75	17.82	0.02	0.14	2.78	17.97
All Ages	*6.79*	*2.75*	*212.03*	*85.95*	*15.08*	*6.11*	*511.00*	*207.15*
	Developed Regions							
0-4	0.01	0.03	0.41	1.08	0.14	0.36	0.55	1.44
5-14	0.00	0.00	0.04	0.05	0.02	0.02	0.05	0.07
15-44	0.01	0.00	0.33	0.13	2.08	0.82	2.41	0.95
45-59	0.02	0.02	0.28	0.29	0.03	0.03	0.31	0.32
60+	0.10	0.08	0.41	0.34	0.01	0.01	0.42	0.34
All Ages	*0.14*	*0.02*	*1.46*	*0.23*	*2.28*	*0.35*	*3.74*	*0.58*
	Developing Regions							
0-4	76.95	28.39	2 625.55	968.65	26.09	9.62	2 651.64	978.27
5-14	0.00	0.00	0.05	0.01	5.08	1.13	5.13	1.14
15-44	2.68	0.28	76.50	8.10	367.85	38.95	444.35	47.05
45-59	3.68	1.73	57.60	27.01	2.99	1.40	60.58	28.41
60+	17.45	11.77	93.23	62.88	0.40	0.27	93.63	63.16
All Ages	*100.76*	*4.97*	*2 852.93*	*140.85*	*402.41*	*19.87*	*3 255.34*	*160.72*
	World							
0-4	76.96	24.89	2 625.96	849.13	26.23	8.48	2 652.19	857.61
5-14	0.00	0.00	0.09	0.02	5.09	0.97	5.18	0.99
15-44	2.69	0.22	76.82	6.41	369.94	30.86	446.76	37.27
45-59	3.70	1.19	57.88	18.61	3.02	0.97	60.90	19.58
60+	17.55	6.52	93.64	34.78	0.41	0.15	94.05	34.93
All Ages	*100.90*	*3.86*	*2 854.39*	*109.21*	*404.68*	*15.48*	*3 259.08*	*124.69*

Much of the excess female disease burden at ages 15–44 is from chlamydia and, to a lesser extent, gonorrhoea. Globally, chlamydia accounted for 70 per cent of DALYs due to STDs among women of reproductive age in 1990 and gonorrhoea accounted for another 25 per cent (see Tables 29 and 30). However, in males, unlike females, gonorrhoea accounts for a greater proportion of the disease burden than chlamydia. In 1990 gonorrhoea accounted for 56 per cent of DALYs due to STDs among men whereas chlamydia accounted for 28 per cent. While syphilis is only a relatively minor (5–15 per cent) cause of the STD burden in both sexes at ages 15–44, it is the major cause at ages 0–4 (primarily through congenital syphilis). Roughly three-quarters of all DALYs lost from STDs in the 0–4 age class are due to syphilis (100 per cent in the case of EME).

Other Considerations in Calculating Disease Burden

This section summarizes the burden associated with some of the complications and sequelae associated with gonorrhoea, chlamydia and syphilis that were excluded from the STD component of the Global Burden of Disease Study. We also briefly discuss the burden associated with other STDs and review some of the assumptions behind our estimates.

Additional Disease Burden Associated with Gonorrhoea, Chlamydia and Syphilis

In order to avoid double counting deaths and disability, ectopic pregnancies, neonatal pneumonia, low birth weight, and infertility were not included in the global STD estimates. Together these complications were estimated to have accounted for an additional 184 000 deaths and 5.8 million DALYs lost in 1990 . These figures highlight the importance of these conditions. Including them in the STD estimates would have increased global mortality from STDs in 1990 to 414 000 deaths and the number of lost DALYs to 24.4 million. In addition, there are a number of other potential complications associated with these STDs that were not included as they have a low incidence (e.g., gonococcal arthritis and meningitis).

Other Sexually Transmitted Infections

Over forty bacteriae, viral and parasitic diseases have been identified that can be transmitted sexually (see Table 1). Three of these were described in this chapter—and another three are the subject of other chapters in the *Global Burden of Disease and Injury Series* (HIV, Human Papilloma Virus, Hepatitis). Expanding the definition of STDs to include HIV (sexual transmission and mother to child), and the sexually transmitted components of HPV and Hepatitis B would increase the total global disease burden caused by STDs in 1990 by more than 450 000 deaths and 12 million DALYs.

In addition there are a number of other STDs such as chancroid, herpes simplex, lymphogranuloma venereum, and trichomoniasis which are linked to adverse health outcomes, enhancing HIV transmission, and premature delivery. As more data become available on the relationships between STDs and the development of complications, the scope of the diseases included in future estimates of the global burden of disease associated with STDs is likely to increase.

ASSUMPTIONS MADE IN ESTIMATING THE DISEASE BURDEN

Incidence of Infection

The incidence of infection was assumed to depend upon the prevalence of infection and the average duration of infection in each region, both of which are uncertain. This approach provides useful approximate estimates of incidence rates, but does not allow for changes in prevalence or population size over time, nor for age-related variation in the incidence or duration of infection. Unfortunately, the data are insufficient to permit a more detailed analysis that allows for these factors.

Prevalence of infection: Regional prevalence estimates were based on a comprehensive survey of the available information. Presenting the information at the regional level, however, conceals the many sub-epidemics both within the region and within countries. In addition, the prevalence figures, while based on a comprehensive survey of the available information, are limited by the quantity and quality of data available from the different regions (for example, in North Africa and the Middle East we were only able to identify a small number of studies that met the inclusion criteria). Collating and interpreting data from different studies is also complicated by the variety of different methods used to diagnose infection.

Duration of infection: Duration of infection was assumed to depend upon the particular pathogen, the health seeking behaviour of the population, and access to health care. Information on all three of these factors is very limited and, as a result, there is considerable uncertainty regarding regional estimates of duration of infection for males and females. For example, the spread of strains of gonorrhoea resistant to one or more antibiotics is making treatment more difficult and expensive, and in many areas alternative drugs are not available. In addition, in the absence of routine antimicrobial testing, even when drugs are available it may turn out that inappropriate drugs are being prescribed. In our estimates of treatment rates, no specific adjustment was made to take antibiotic resistance into account. In areas where this is prevalent, our estimates of successful treatment may be too high.

Development of Complications and Sequelae

Complications and sequelae were identified for each infection and values assigned to the different parameters based on a review of the literature and discussions with experts. For many of the parameters little or no information was available and we had to make a number of assumptions. We also had to make a number of other assumptions on how different factors affected the development of complications, four of which are described below.

Infection with more than one organism: STDs (including HIV) tend to cluster in the same individuals. For example, in some STD clinics in the Established Market Economies over 50 per cent of individuals with gonorrhoea are co-infected with chlamydia, and in Nairobi, Kenya 36 per cent of commercial sex workers were found to be infected with 2 or more STDs (D'Costa et al. 1985). In the analysis coexisting infections were treated as two single infections as, at present, it is not known how infection with more than one organism affects the probability of developing complications beyond potentially delaying correct treatment.

Repeat infections: Many infections occur in individuals who have been infected before. For example, a large scale screening programmeme in Manitoba, Canada found that reinfection accounted for 15 per cent of all chlamydia cases and 13 per cent of gonorrhoea cases (Jolly et al. 1995) and in Wisconsin, United States 30 per cent of young women diagnosed with chlamydia had a recurrent chlamydia infection within two years (Hillis et al. 1994). How repeat infections affect the development of complications is not clear, although in the case of PID, women who have had two cases of PID are more than twice as likely to develop an ectopic pregnancy (Westrom and Mardh 1990). On the other hand there is also evidence to suggest that commercial sex workers who are continually exposed to infections develop partial immunity such that their symptoms become quite mild. In this analysis repeat infections were treated as two primary infections with similar probabilities of developing complications. Treating repeat infections as two primary infections will overestimate disability in some cases (e.g. women who are infertile cannot become infertile again) and underestimate it in others.

Age at infection: The genital tract changes with age, with repercussions for the development of complications and sequelae. For example, data from a study in Sweden suggests that women younger than 25 years who develop gonococcal or chlamydial PID have significantly better infertility prognosis than those who develop these infections at an older age (Westrom et al. 1992). However, other data on how the probabilities of developing complications and their serverity vary with age are limited. As a result, in the analysis the probability of developing complications was assumed to be independent of age.

Relationship between severity of symptoms and final outcome: A proportion of individuals who become infected, especially women, are asymptomatic or minimally symptomatic. Whilst we know that asymptomatic women do develop complications, it is not clear whether in the absence of treatment they are more or less likely than symptomatic individuals to develop complications. In the analysis we assumed that the probability of developing complications from gonorrhoea and chlamydia was the same for asymptomatic and symptomatic women. For men, however, it was assumed that those who were asymptomatic did not develop complications.

STDs as a Risk Factor for Other Diseases

Infection with a STD can lead to the development of a variety of different complications and sequelae. They can also influence the natural history and transmission of other diseases, including HIV, and cause problems following the introduction of interuterine devices (IUDs).

STDs and HIV

Quantitative data on the interaction between HIV and STDs are limited because of methodological problems in designing and interpreting such studies (see Mertens et al. 1990; Berkley 1991 for reviews of the issues surrounding the design of these studies). Infection with an STD may be a marker for high-risk sexual behaviour rather than a causal link in HIV transmission and, as a result, studies investigating the relationship between STDs and HIV have to control for sexual activity. The analysis is further complicated by the fact that HIV affects the natural history of other STDs making it difficult to interpret studies without documented data on the order of acquiring infection.

HIV is thought to alter the natural history and response to therapy for a number of STDs, including chancroid, syphilis, genital HSV, and HPV (see Table 32). For example, single dose treatment for chancroid was six times less likely to succeed in HIV positive individuals than in HIV negative individuals (Cameron et al. 1988). With syphilis, rapid progression from early syphilis to central nervous system involvement has been documented after an interval of months in HIV infected individuals as opposed to years in those without HIV infection, and skin lesions and VDRL antibody levels in HIV-infected patients with secondary syphilis respond more slowly to conventional penicillin therapy (Musher et al. 1990). This suggests that HIV may increase the period of infectivity as well as increasing the likelihood of diagnosis of symptomatic disease, and hence could accentuate the syphilis epidemic as well as change reporting of the disease.

Table 32 Possible impact of HIV infection on the presentation, natural history, diagnosis and therapy of other STDs

	Clinical Presentation	*Natural History*	*Performance of Standardized Laboratory Tests*	*Response to Standard Therapy*
Chancroid	(?) Multicentric, extragenital lesions; systemic symptoms; less lymphadenitis	(?) Larger, more persistent lesions	(#) Altered accuracy of culture or serology for H. ducreyi	(++) Increased risk of treatment failure with single dose regimes
Syphilis	(?) Atypical presentations	(+) More persistent primary lesions (?) Accelerated progression to CNS or tertiary disease (+) Seroreversion in advancing HIV disease	(?) Delayed or persistently negative serologies (?) Abnormally high titers	(+) Increased risk of treatment failure with single dose bicillin for secondary syphilis
Herpes	(?) Atypical sites, multicentric disease	(?) Increased frequency of recurrences (?) Increased size and duration of lesions (#) Increased incidence of disseminated disease	(#) Altered accuracy of culture or serology for HSV	(+) Increased incidence of acyclovir resistence
Genital Warts/ HPV Infection	(?) Multicentric disease, larger lesions (+) Increased frequency of infection with multiple HPV types	(+) Increased incidence of recurrences (++) Increased incidence of progression to dysplasia or neoplasia	(+) Increased HPV viral load (++) Increased HPV detection with advancing HPV disease	(++) Decreased responsiveness to topical, laser, or surgical therapy
Gonorrhoea	(#) Atypical presentations	(+) Increased incidence of gonoccocal PID (?) Increased incidence of disseminated gonococcal infection	(#) Altered accuracy of culture for N. gonorrhoea	(+) Increased incidence of PPNG (#) Increased incidence of treatment failure
Chlamydia and Trichomaniasis	No published data currently support or refute associations in any of the four categories			

Source: Wasserheit 1991

Key:
(++) = Likely (supported by multiple studies in humans which include a comparison group);
(+) = Probable (supported by a single study in animals or humans which includes a comparison group);
(?) = Possible (supported by anecdotal information or case reports);
(#) = Unknown (supported by no published data)

HIV infection has also been found to change the immunologic response to STD infection (Spence and Abrutyn 1987).

It has been postulated that infection with a STD (ulcerative or non-ulcerative) enhances sexual transmission of HIV by increasing susceptibility and/or infectivity. Disruption of the normal epithelial barrier (e.g. as a result of genital ulcers) or microscopic discontinuity in cervical or vaginal mucosa (e.g. as a result of gonococcal or chlamydial cervicitis or trichomonas vaginitis) is thought to influence susceptibility by providing a means of entry for the virus and/or infectivity by enhancing viral shedding. It has also been postulated that STDs which result in genital inflammation may facilitate HIV transmission by increasing the recruitment of HIV-target cells in the genital tract, such as lymphocytes and macrophages. In addition, HIV has been isolated directly from the base of ulcers in men and women.

Studies conducted in the United States and Africa have documented increased rates of seroconversion to HIV among high-risk individuals with genital ulcers from chancroid, syphilis, and herpes (see Table 33). For example, a study of commercial sex workers in Zaire found that the incidence of genital ulcer disease was 3 times higher among those with HIV infection than in those who were HIV negative independent of sexual behaviour. Data on non-ulcerative STDs are more limited but also support an association (see Wasserheit 1992).

Recent data from a study of HIV positive men in Malawi documented that in men with urethritis HIV RNA concentrations in seminal fluid were eight times higher than in men without urethritis, but that after appropriate antimicrobial therapy there was a significant decline in HIV RNA levels (Cohen et al. 1997). Similar data exist for cervicitis in women although these are not as definitive (Mostad and Kreiss 1996). There is also evidence to suggest that HIV viral replication is enhanced by infection with an STD; co-cultures of HIV and chlamydia showed increased rates of viral replication (Cohen 1997).

STDs and IUDs

IUDs are one of the most common contraceptive methods used in the world, and when inserted in a woman with a lower or upper tract reproductive tract infection can lead to the development of serious complications. As a result, it is recommended that women should be screened for gonorrhoea and chlamydia before insertion of an IUD. However, without inexpensive, simple and reliable tests for these conditions this is a recommendation that cannot be implemented in many parts of the world.

Burden and Intervention

STD and HIV prevention programmes have played an important role in reducing the incidence of STDs and their complications by encouraging people to modify their behaviour and adopt safer sex practices (e.g. in-

Table 33 Summary of studies of the relationship between STDs and HIV

	Prospective or nested case- control studies	*Cross-sectional case-control studies*
Gonorrhoea		
Number of studies	4	6
Number detecting significant association	2	3
Risk estimate - median (range)		
Women	3.5 [Lab]	5.6 (3.8-8.9) [Lab]
Heterosexual men	NA	NS [Hx]
Homosexual men	1.5 [Hx]	
Chlamydial infection		
Number of studies	2	2
Number detecting significant association	2	0
Risk estimate — median (range)		
Women	4.5 (3.2-5.7) [Lab]	NS [Lab]
Heterosexual men	NA	NA
Homosexual men	NA	NA
Syphilis		
Number of studies	2	9
Number detecting significant association	2	7
Risk estimate — median (range)		
Women	NA	1.8 [Hx]; 4.0 (2.5-5.4) [Lab]
Heterosexual men	NA	2.0 [Hx]; 6.0 (3.3-8.7) [Lab]
Homosexual men	1.5 [Hx]; 2.2 [Lab]	3.0 [Hx]; 8.4 (2.0-9.9) [Lab]
Genital Ulcers		
Number of studies	3	7
Number detecting significant association	2	4
Risk estimate — median (range)		
Women	3.7 [Px]	3.3 [Px]
Heterosexual men	4.7 [Px]	2.4 [Hx]; 13.2 (8.2-18.2) [Px]
Homosexual men	NA	NA

Key: NA = not available; NS = not significant; Hx = by history; Px = by physical examination; Lab = by laboratory studies

Source: Wasserheit 1991

crease use of condoms or virucides, limit the number of sexual partners, postpone initiation of sexual intercourse, choose partners at low risk of infection, and seek early treatment for STDs), and by ensuring that appropriate treatment is widely available. The challenge today is to increase access to, and improve the quality of these programmes in the most cost-effective manner, and, to ensure that they are sustainable.

STD prevention programmes have an important role to play in improving public health by:

- reducing the secondary spread of infection
- reducing the incidence of complications and sequelae in the infected individual
- reducing the incidence of complications and sequelae in infants born to infected individuals
- reducing the probability of acquiring or transmitting other STDs, including HIV

In countries or regions where STD prevention has been a public health priority, a marked decline in STDs has been seen. For example:

- in Sweden, a programme including free STD diagnosis and treatment, partner notification, sex education in schools, general population messages and condom promotion led to an almost 15-fold reduction in the incidence of gonorrhoea and a halving of the incidence of chlamydia over a fifteen year period.
- in the United States, a trial programme of chlamydia screening in 150 family planning clinics reported a decrease in the prevalence of chlamydia from 11 per cent to 5 per cent from 1988–1993.
- in Zambia, the creation of a national STD programme which included increasing the number of STD clinics from 2 to 54 and training clinicians and health educators led to a three-fold reduction in STD cases being seen at the national referral centre.

It is, however, difficult to project what levels of infection would have been without these programmes and hence to assess their cost-effectiveness.

Some of the characteristics of an effective STD control programme are highlighted in Table 34. Ensuring early and effective treatment is a key component as this reduces both the probability that an individual will develop complications and sequelae and the likelihood the individual will pass on infection to other people. However, the lack of rapid and inexpensive diagnostics and the high proportion of people who are asymptomatic make the identification of infected individuals difficult. At present, even with a well functioning laboratory, the inherent limitations in the current generation of tests frequently mean a delay of 24–48 hours for diagnosis which, especially for people who have travelled long distances, is too long to wait. To circumvent this problem the WHO has been promoting syndromic diagnosis where treatment decisions are based on a clinical flow chart which includes symptoms, clinical signs and risk assessment and, where practicable, simple and quick laboratory tests.

Targeting prevention activities at those at high risk, especially in the early stages of an epidemic, can play a crucial role in limiting its spread. Targeting strategies include: outreach activities to high risk groups; partner notification (identification and treatment of both the infector and

Table 34 Components of an effective STD control programme

- A structure to support STD services in primary health centers and referral clinics
- A reliable drug supply
- Epidemiological surveillance to identify the most prevalent STDs and to track the effectiveness of various antibiotics
- Primary health care providers who "think STDs," watch for their signs, counsel those at risk of STDs, and treat or refer those who are infected
- Training suited to each practitioner's role in STD services
- Condoms, readily and cheaply available and heavily promoted to the public. In addition, women urgently need more effective barrier methods that they can control
- Counseling to help STD patients understand their illnesses, take medication correctly and completely, and prevent future infections. Women often need special help to protect themselves
- Mass-media communication to alert people to STDs, encourage them to seek treatment, promote condoms, and support mutual monogamy
- Methods of notifying the sexual partners of STD patients so that they, too, can be treated

infectee); and re-screening of treated cases after several months to check for reinfection. Targeted programmes, however, face two constraints: those targeted may be, or feel, stigmatized; and those not targeted may react with a false sense of security. Furthermore, it may be difficult to define those at high risk—and denial may make self assessment impossible.

Treatment of pregnant women who are infected reduces the probability of transmission to infants. It is therefore important that high quality prenatal care is available to all women and that it includes STDs diagnosis and treatment. Ensuring that infants receive appropriate care is also important.

A study of STD treatment conducted in Mwanza, Tanzania suggests that improved STD case management can also play an important role in reducing the efficiency of HIV transmission. Over a 2 year period the rate of HIV seroconversion in the villages that had received health education and improved syndromic STD treatment was 42 per cent lower than in the control villages; in the intervention villages 48 of 4149 (1.2 per cent) seroconverted while in the control villages 82 of 4 400 (1.9 per cent) seroconverted (Grosskurth et al. 1995). However, the only STD differences that could be measured were a decrease in symptomatic male urethritis and in active syphilis.

A more aggressive approach has been tried in a mass treatment project in Rakai, Uganda. This study has documented a reduction in syphilis, chlamydia, trichomoniasis and bacterial vaginosis following mass antimicrobial treatment of the population. HIV data, however, will not be available until late 1998. If this study also shows reductions in HIV seroconversion it will reconfirm the important role that the treatment and prevention of STDs has to play in reducing the spread of HIV.

In some countries governments have also introduced policies directly related to reducing the spread of STDs. These include the regulation or prohibition of prostitution and mandatory partner notification by provider referral. The effectiveness of these policies, however, is not known.

Discussion

This chapter has provided details on the approach used to estimate the global and regional burden of disease associated with gonorrhoea, chlamydia and syphilis, three important STDs from a public health perspective. Generating the estimates involved two steps: (1) estimating the global prevalence and incidence of STDs; and (2) assessing the probability of developing different sequelae in infected individuals and the level of disability associated with each complication. As far as we are aware this is the first systematic attempt to estimate the global burden of disease from STDs, and despite the many methodological limitations we hope that this work will encourage others to generate new and better estimates.

In the Global Burden of Disease Study, STDs were estimated to account for 230 000 deaths and 18.7 million DALYs in 1990, or 0.5 per cent of global deaths and 1.5 per cent of the global burden of disease. However, these figures are based on only three STDs (gonorrhoea, syphilis and chlamydia), and include only a subset of their complications. If we were to expand the definition of STDs to include other complications associated with gonorrhoea, chlamydia and syphilis allocated to other conditions, this would increase the number of deaths in 1990 to 414 000 and the number of DALYs lost to 30.6 million, or 1 per cent of global deaths and 2.5 per cent of the global burden of disease (see Box 6).

A number of other infections can also be transmitted sexually, and three of them form the basis of other chapters in the *Global Burden of Disease and Injury Series*. Including the sexually transmitted components of HIV, HPV and Hepatitis B would increase the number of deaths in 1990 to 680 000 and the number of DALYs lost to 30 million, or 1.3 per cent of global deaths and 2.2 per cent of the global burden of disease.

These estimates refer to all age groups. If attention is confined to the reproductive age class (defined here as ages 15 to 44) STDs account for an even larger proportion of the global burden of disease. Using the GBD definition STDs in 1990 accounted for 4.2 per cent of DALYs lost in women and 1.1 per cent of DALYs lost in men at these ages. Expanding the definition of STDs to include HIV, HPV and hepatitis B increases the STD burden to 3.5 per cent of total disease burden in males and 6.3 per cent in females.

Geographically, the burden from STDs is greatest in the developing world and, in particular, in Sub-Saharan Africa where in 1990 STDs (based on the restricted GBD definition) accounted for 6.3 per cent of DALYs lost in women in the reproductive age group and 1.8 per cent of DALYs lost in men of the same age.

Box 6 Sequelae from gonorrhoea, chlamydia and syphilis, and other STDs not included in the GBD estimates of the burden of STDs

Ectopic pregnancies: Ectopic pregnancies resulting from a previous infection with chlamydia or gonorrhoea were estimated to have accounted for 28 000 deaths and 0.8 million DALYs in women of reproductive age in 1990. The majority of deaths and DALYs were due to chlamydial infection. Chlamydia was estimated to have accounted for 71 per cent of the deaths; three regions, SSA, IND and OAI, accounted for over 90 per cent of these deaths.

Neonatal pneumonia: Neonatal pneumonia, or chlamydial pneumonitis, was estimated to have accounted for 42 000 deaths and 1.4 million DALYs in 1990. Again, SSA, IND and OAI, accounted for over 90 per cent of these deaths.

Low birth weight: Low birth weight caused by maternal infection with gonorrhoea, chlamydia or syphilis was estimated to account for 114 000 deaths and 3.7 million DALYs in 1990. Of these deaths, gonorrhoea accounted for 42 per cent, chlamydia for 37 per cent, and syphilis for 21 per cent. The vast majority of these deaths and DALYs were in SSA, IND and OAI.

Infertility: Infertility was estimated to have resulted in 6 million DALYs in 1990. As for the other sequelae, the majority of DALYs were accounted for by SSA, IND and OAI.

HIV: HIV can be transmitted through blood, vertically from mother to child, and sexually. Globally more than 90 per cent of HIV is transmitted sexually (see Chapter 9 in this volume). The sexually transmitted proportion of HIV was estimated to account for 236 000 deaths and 8.5 million DALYs in 1990 in adults and another 52 300 deaths and 1.8 million DALYs in children born to infected mothers (see Chapters 9 and 13 in this volume).

Human Papilloma Virus (HPV): Particular serovars of HPV are associated with the development of cervical cancer. Sexual transmission of HPV was estimated to account for 180 000 deaths and 2.6 million DALYs in 1990 (see Chapter 13 in this volume).

Hepatitis B: Hepatitis B has been linked to the development of liver cancer. Sexual transmission of hepatitis B was estimated to have accounted for 90 000 deaths and 1.4 million DALYs in 1990 (see Chapter 13 in this volume).

These figures highlight the considerable contribution sexually transmitted infections make to the global disease burden, especially for women of reproductive age in developing countries. In these regions the STD DALY rate for women between ages 15 and 44 was more than 10 times greater than in the developed regions (see Table 28). These estimates, however, do not take into account the serious social and economic consequences that they may have for the affected individual and his or her family. For example, becoming infertile may lead to anxiety and depression in the infertile woman and, in some parts of the world, she may be abandoned or divorced with serious consequences for her survival.

Developing the framework for the GBD STD estimates highlighted how little information was available on the incidence of STDs and on the probability of developing complications if infected. To improve future estimates there is a need for more studies to provide information on: the prevalence of infection by age and sex in low risk populations over time; access to and use of appropriate treatment; the link between infection and the development of different complications; and the role played by different factors (e.g. genetic, environmental, and cultural) in the development of complications.

Reducing the global burden of disease associated with STDs will require a concerted effort by national health services, international and bilateral agencies, non-governmental organizations, the private sector, and academic and research institutions. There is also a need for improved diagnostic tools (i.e. tools that are rapid, non-invasive, easy to use, inexpensive, and that can detect infections in both symptomatic and asymptomatic individuals), treatment regimens (ideally a one dose drug that treats multiple infections) and prevention technologies, together with operational research directed at ensuring that STD prevention programmes use their resources efficiently and equitably. Investing today in STD prevention and treatment programmes and in developing new diagnostic, treatment and preventive methods should have a substantial impact on reducing the global burden of disease from STDs, including HIV, in the future.

ACKNOWLEDGEMENTS

The authors would like to acknowledge the following people who have contributed to this chapter of assisted in the reviewing sections of it: Drs Antonio Gerbase, Richard Rothenberg, Amy Pollack, Judith Wasserheit, Julius Schacter, Thomas Quinn, Peter Piot and Stephen Morse. We would also like to thank Stefani Janicki and Jacqueline Kellachan for their unflagging assistance and patience.

REFERENCES

AIDSTECH (1993) AIDSTECH final report. Durham, North Carolina: AIDSTECH.

Akan E et al. (1987) Determination of anti-chlamydial serum IgG and IgM levels in women and their mature infants born in term. *Journal of the Turkish Microbiology Association* 17:205–12.

Amortegul AJ et al. (1986) Prevalence of Chlamydia trachomatis and other microorganisms in women seeking abortions in Pittsburgh, Pennsylvania, United States of America. *Genitourinary Medicine* 62:88–92.

Anderson RM, May RM (1991) *Infectious diseases of humans: Dynamics and control.* Oxford: Oxford University Press.

Aral SO, Holmes KK (1991) Sexually transmitted diseases in the AIDS era. *Scientific American* 264:62–9.

Avonts D, Piot P (1985) Genital infections in women undergoing therapeutic abortion. *European Journal of Obstetrics, Gynaecology, & Reproductive Biology* 20:53–9.

Bakir TM et al. (1989) Enzyme immunoassay in the diagnosis of Chlamydia trachomatis infections in diverse patient groups. *Journal of Hygiene, Epidemiology, Microbiology & Immunology* 33:189–97.

Bang RA et al. (1989) High prevalence of gynaecological diseases in rural Indian women. *Lancet* 1:85–8.

Bell TA et al. (1987) Comparison of ophthalmic silver nitrate solution and erythromycin ointment for prevention of natally acquired Chlamydia trachomatis. *Sexually Transmitted Diseases* 14:195–200.

Ben Salem N et al. (1993) STD/HIV seroprevalence among women attending an antenatal clinic in Tunis. *Presented at the 9th International Conference on AIDS.*

Berkely SF (1991) Public health significance of STDs for HIV infection in Africa. In: Chen LC, Sepúlveda J and Segal SJ. *AIDS and women's reproductive health,* Plenum Press, New York.

Bewes PC (1973) Urethral stricture. *Tropical Doctor* 3:77–81.

Bhargava NC (1993) Sexually transmitted diseases in India. *Presented at STD Medical Orientation Workshop, Jaipur.*

Bindels PJ et al. (1991) [Benefit of the serological screening programme for syphilis in pregnant women in Amsterdam in the period 1985–1989]. [Dutch]. *Nederlands Tijdschrift voor Geneeskunde* 135:1319–22.

Bowie WR (1990) Urethritis in males. In: Holmes KK et al., eds. *Sexually transmitted diseases.* 2nd ed. New York: McGraw-Hill, Inc.

Brabin L et al. (1995) Reproductive tract infections and abortion among adolescent girls in rural Nigeria. *Lancet* 345:300–4.

Brasfield DM et al. (1987) Infant pneumonitis associated with cytomegalovirus, chlamydia, pneumocystis, and ureaplasma: follow-up. *Pediatrics* 79:76–83.

Brunham RC et al. (1990) Sexually transmitted diseases in pregnancy. In: Holmes KK et al. editors. *Sexually transmitted diseases.* 2nd ed. New York: McGraw-Hill, Inc.

Brunham RC, Plummer FA (1990) A general model of sexually transmitted disease epidemiology and its implications for control. *Medical Clinics of North America* 74:1339–52.

Cameron DN et al. (1988) Prediction of HIV infection by treatment failure for chncroid, a genital ulcer disease. IV International Conference on AIDS, Stockholm, Sweden.

Carael M. (1995) Sexual behaviour. In: Cleland J, Ferry B, eds. *AIDS in the developing world.* London: Taylor & Francis.

Cates Jr W, Stone KM (1992) Family planning: the responsibility to prevent both pregnancy and reproductive tract infections. In: Germain A et al., eds. *Reproductive tract infections: global impact and priorities for women's reproductive health.* New York: Plenum Press.

Chiphangwi J et al. (1990) Risk factors for HIV-1 infection in pregnant women in Malawi. *Presented at the VIth International Conference on AIDS.*

Cislakova L et al. (1992) [Detection of Chlamydia trachomatis in clinical material 1989–1990]. [Slovak]. *Ceskoslovenska Epidemiologie, Mikrobiologie, Imunologie* 41:240–4.

Cohen M (1997) Biology of HIV transmission: STD amplifications in vitro and in vivo. Abstracts of the 35th meeting of the Infectious Disease Society of America, San Francisco, California.

Cohen M et al. (1997) Treatment of urethritis reduces the concentration of HIV-1 in semen: implications for prevention of transmission of HIV-1. *Lancet,* 349:1868

Cohn M, Stewart P (1992) Prevalence of potential pathogens in cervical canal before termination of pregnancy. *British Medical Journal* 304:1479

Colleen S, Mårdh P (1990) Prostatitis. In: Holmes KK et al., eds. *Sexually transmitted diseases.* 2nd ed. New York: McGraw-Hill, Inc.

de Lalla F et al. (1990) HIV, HBV, delta-agent and Treponema pallidum infections in two rural African areas. *Transactions of the Royal Society of Tropical Medicine & Hygiene* 84:144–7.

De Schryver A, Meheus A (1990) Epidemiology of sexually transmitted diseases: the global picture. *Bulletin of the World Health Organization* 68:639–54.

Dhall K et al. (1990) Incidence of gonococcal infection and its clinicopathological correlation in patients attending gynaecological outpatient department. *Journal of Obstetric Gynaecology India* 40:410–3.

Diallo MO, et al. (1992) Sexually transmitted diseases and HIV-1/HIV-2 infections among pregnant women attending an antental clinic in Abidjan, Cote d'Ivoire. *Presented at the VIIth International Conference on AIDS in Africa.*

Dietrich M et al. (1992) Urogenital tract infections in pregnancy at King Edward VIII Hospital, Durban, South Africa. *Genitourinary Medicine* 68:39–41.

Dong Y (1991) Female simple gonorrhoea. *Journal of Practical Obstretrics and Gynaecology* 7:172–4.

Donovan, P (1993) *Testing Positive.* New York: The Alan Guttmacher Institute.

Eschenbach DA et al. (1975) Polymicrobial etiology of acute pelvic inflammatory disease. *New England Journal of Medicine* 293:166–71.

Espinoza F et al. (1993) STD in Nicaragua: population rate estimates and health seeking behaviour. *Presented at the 9th International Conference on AIDS.*

Fan SL, Dong Y (1991) Screening report for STD in 1000 pregnant women. *Beijing Medical Journal* 13:76.

Faundes A, Tanaka AC (1992) Reproductive tract infections in Brazil: solutions in a difficult economic climate. In: Germain A et al., eds. *Reproductive tract infections: global impact and priorities for women's reproductive health.* New York: Plenum Press.

Fransen L et al. (1986) Ophthalmia neonatorum in Nairobi, Kenya: the roles of Neisseria gonorrhoeae and Chlamydia trachomatis. *Journal of Infectious Diseases* 153:862–9.

Galega FP et al. (1984) Gonococcal ophthalmia neonatorum: the case for prophylaxis in tropical Africa. *Bulletin of the World Health Organization* 62:95–8.

Gao ZY, Li YL, Chai DF (1995) [Investigation of cervical Chlamydia trachomatis infection in gynecologic outpatients]. [Chinese]. *Chung-Hua Liu Hsing Ping Hsueh Tsa Chih Chinese Journal of Epidemiology* 16:211–2.

Genc M et al. (1993) Screening for Chlamydia trachomatis and Neisseria gonorrhoeae in pregnant Turkish women. *European Journal of Clinical Microbiology & Infectious Diseases* 12:395–6.

Georges-Courbot MC et al. (1989) Seroprevalence of HIV-I is much higher in young women than men in Central Africa. *Genitourinary Medicine* 65:131–2.

Ghana Health Assessment Project (1981) A quantitative method of assessing the health impact of different diseases in less developed countries. *International Journal of Epidemiology* 10:73–80.

Gjestland T (1955) The Oslo study of untreated syphilis: an epidemiologic investigation of the natural course of syphilitic infection based on a restudy of the Boeck-Bruusgaard material. *Acta Dermato-Venereologica* 35:1.

Grosskurth H et al. (1995) Impact of improved treatment of sexually transmitted diseases on HIV infection in rural Tanzania: randomized controlled trial. *Lancet* 346:530–6.

Gutman LT, Wilfert CM (1990) Gonococcal diseases in infants and children. In: Holmes KK et al., eds. *Sexually transmitted diseases.* 2nd ed. New York: McGraw-Hill.

Gyaneshwar R et al. (1987) The prevalence of sexually transmitted disease agents in pregnant women in Suva. *Australian and New Zealand Journal of Obstetrics & Gynaecology* 27:213–5.

Hammerschlag MR et al. (1989) Efficacy of neonatal ocular prophylaxis for the prevention of chlamydial and gonococcal conjunctivitis. *New England Journal of Medicine* 320:769–72.

Harrison HR, Alexander ER (1990) Chlamydial infections in infants and children. In: Holmes KK et al., eds. *Sexually transmitted diseases.* 2nd ed. New York: McGraw-Hill, Inc.

Hassane A et al. (1993) Estimation rapide de prevalence des MST/VIH a Niamey, Niger. *Presented at the VIIIth International Conference on AIDS in Africa.*

Healey BP (1990) Cardiovascular syphilis. In: Holmes KK et al., eds. *Sexually transmitted diseases.* 2nd ed. New York: McGraw-Hill, Inc.

Health Information India (1988) Central Bureau of Health Intelligence, Director General of Health Services, Ministry of Health and Family Welfare. New Delhi: Government of India.

Hillis SD et. al. (1994) Risk factors for recurrent Chlamydia trachomatis infections in women. *American Journal Obstetrics and Gynaecology* 170:801–6.

Hillis SD et al. (1993) Delayed care of pelvic inflammatory disease as a risk factor for impaired fertility. *American Journal of Obstetrics and Gynaecology* 168:1503–9.

Hira SK (1991) Guidelines for prevention of adverse outcomes of pregnancy due to syphilis. World Health Organization. Geneva, Switzerland.

Hira SK, Hira RS (1987) Congenital syphilis. In: Osoba AO. *Sexually transmitted diseases in the tropics.* London: Balliere'sTindall.

Hira SK et al. (1990) Syphilis intervention in pregnancy: Zambian demonstration project. *Genitourinary Medicine* 66:159–64.

Hodgson JE et al. (1988) Chlamydial infection in a Chinese gynecologic outpatient clinic. *Obstetrics & Gynaecology* 71:96–100.

Hogsborg M, Aaby P (1992) Sexual relations, use of condoms and perceptions of AIDS in an urban area of Guinea-Bissau with a high prevalence of HIV-2. In Dyson T, ed. *Sexual behaviour and networking: anthropological and socio-cultural studies on the transmission of HIV*. Liege: International Union for the Scientific Study of Population.

Holmes KK et al. (1970) An estimate of the risk of men acquiring gonorrhoea by sexual contact with infected females. *American Journal of Epidemiology* 91:170–4.

Hook EW, Handsfield HH (1990) Sexually transmitted diseases. In: Holmes KK et al., eds. 2nd ed. New York: McGraw-Hill, Inc.

Hossain A (1986) Serological tests for syphilis in Saudi Arabia. *Genitourinary Medicine* 62:293–7.

Ingraham NR. (1951) The value of penicillin alone in the prevention and treatment of congenital syphilis. *Acta Dermato-Venereologica* 31:60.

Ismail SO et al. (1990) Syphilis, gonorrhoea and genital chlamydial infection in a Somali village. *Genitourinary Medicine* 66:70–5.

Jaffe HW, Musher DM (1990) Management of the reactive syphilis serology. In: Holmes KK et al., eds. *Sexually transmitted diseases*. 2nd ed. New York: McGraw-Hill.

Jolly AM et al. (1995) Risk factors for infection in women undergoing testing for Chlamydia trachomatis and Neisseria gonorrhoeae in Manitoba, Canada. *Sexually Transmitted Diseases* 22:289–95.

Jones RB et al. (1982) Correlation between serum antichlamydial antibodies and tubal factor as a cause of infertility. *Fertility & Sterility* 38:553–8.

Kampmeier RH (1990) Late benign syphilis. In: Holmes KK et al., eds. *Sexually transmitted diseases*. 2nd ed. New York: McGraw-Hill, Inc.

Kantharaj K et al. (1993) STD baseline survey in Madras and Tamil Nadu. *Presented at the IXth International Conference on AIDS/ IVth STD World Congress*.

Kaufman RE et al. (1977) Questionnaire survey of reported early congenital syphilis: problems in diagnosis, prevention, and treatment. *Sexually Transmitted Diseases* 4:135–9.

Kiviat N et al. (1990) Anal human papillomavirus infection among human immunodeficiency virus-seropositive and -seronegative men. *Journal of Infectious Diseases* 162:358–61.

Klufio CA et al. (1992) Endocervical Chlamydia trachomatis infection in pregnancy: direct test and clinico-sociodemographic survey of pregnant patients at the Port Moresby General Hospital antenatal clinic to determine prevalence and risk markers. *Australian & New Zealand Journal of Obstetrics & Gynaecology* 32:43–6.

Laga M et al. (1986) Epidemiology of ophthalmia neonatorum in Kenya. *Lancet* 2:1145–9.

Laga M et al. (1988) Prophylaxis of gonococcal and chlamydial ophthalmia neonatorum. A comparison of silver nitrate and tetracycline. *New England Journal of Medicine* 318:653–7.

Lande R (1993) Controlling sexually transmitted diseases. *Population Reports—Series L: Issues in World Health* :1–31.

Lee HH et al. (1995) Diagnosis of Chlamydia trachomatis genitourinary infection in women by ligase chain reaction assay of urine [see comments]. *Lancet* 345:213–6.

Luthra UK et al. (1992) Reproductive tract infections in India: the need for comprehensive reproductive health policy and programmes. In: Germain A et al., eds. *Reproductive tract infections: global impact and priorites for women's reproductive health.* New York: Plenum Press.

Lycke E et al. (1980) The risk of transmission of genital Chlamydia trachomatis infection is less than that of genital Neisseria gonorrhoeae infection. *Sexually Transmitted Diseases* 7:6–10.

Malele B et al. (1990) Genital ulcer disease (GUD) among HIV(+) and HIV(-) prostitutes in Kinshasa: prevalence, incidence and etiology. *Presented at the 5th International Conference on AIDS in Africa.*

Mårdh P, Danielsson D (1990) Neisseria gonorrhoeae. In: Holmes KK et al., eds. *Sexually transmitted diseases.* 2nd ed. New York: McGraw-Hill, Inc.

Mayaud P et al. (1992) Risk score approach in the diagnosis of sexually transmitted diseases in an antenatal population in Mwanza, NW Tanzania. *Presented at the VIIth International Conference on AIDS in Africa.*

Mayer KH et al. (1990) Sexually transmitted diseases and genital tract inflammation among US heterosexuals at increased risk for HIV infection. *Presented at the 30th ICAAC.*

McCormack WM et al. (1979) Fifteen-month follow-up study of women infected with Chlamydia trachomatis. *New England Journal of Medicine* 300:123–5.

Meheus A (1992) Women's health: importance of reproductive tract infections, pelvic inflammatory disease and cervical cancer. In: Germain A et al., eds. *Reproductive tract infections: global impact and priorities for women's reproductive health.* New York: Plenum Press.

Ministry of Social Affairs and Assimilation, France (1991) Weekly Epidemiological Bulletin. 14. Director General of Health, France. [Ministere des Affaires Sociales et de l'Integration. Bulletin epidemiogique hebdomadaire. 14. Direction generale de la Sante, Republique Francaise.]

Moore DE, Cates WJ (1990) Sexually transmitted diseases and infertility. In: Holmes KK et al., eds. *Sexually transmitted diseases.* 2nd ed. New York: McGraw-Hill.

Moreno R et al. (1992) [Prevalence of human immunodeficiency virus infection, hepatitis B virus and syphilis in full term pregnancy]. [Spanish]. *Medicina Clinica* 98:768–70.

Morillon M et al. (1992) [Genital infections with Chlamydia trachomatis in pregnant women in New Caledonia]. [French]. *Bulletin de la Societe de Pathologie Exotique* 85:121–4.

Moses S et al. (1994) Health care-seeking behaviour related to the transmission of sexually transmitted diseases in Kenya [see comments]. *American Journal of Public Health* 84:1947–51.

Mosha F et al. (1993) A population-based study of syphilis and sexually transmitted disease syndromes in north-western Tanzania. 1. Prevalence and incidence. *Genitourinary Medicine* 69:415–20.

Mostad SB, Kreiss JK. (1996) Shedding of HIV-1 in the genital tract. *AIDS* 10:1305–1315

Murray CJL and Lopez AD, eds. (1996) *The global burden of disease: a comprehensive assesment of mortality and disability from diseases, injuries, and risk factors in 1990 and projected to 2020.* Cambridge, Harvard University Press.

Musher DM et al. (1990) Effect of human immunodeficiency virus (HIV) infection on the course of syphilis and on the response to treatment. [Review] [129 refs]. *Annals of Internal Medicine* 113:872–81.

Narvaez M et al. (1989) [Prevalence of Chlamydia trachomatis and Neisseria gonorrhoeae in 3 groups of Ecuadorian women with different sexual behaviours]. [Spanish]. *Boletin de la Oficina Sanitaria Panamericana* 107:220–5.

Niamsanit S et al. (1988) Prevalence of Chlamydia trachomatis among women attending an antenatal clinic in Bangkok. *Southeast Asian Journal of Tropical Medicine & Public Health* 19:609–13.

Nsubuga P et al. (1992) Reported sexual behaviour and sexually transmitted infection prevalence among women attending a prenatal clinic in Kampala, Uganda. *Presented at the VIIth International Conference on AIDS.*

O'Farrell N et al. (1989) Sexually transmitted pathogens in pregnant women in a rural South African community. *Genitourinary Medicine* 65:276–80.

Osegbe DN and Amaku EO (1981) Gonococcal strictures in young patients. *Urology* 18:37–41.

Osoba AO and Alausa KO (1974) *Nigerian Journal of Pediatrics* 1:26

Over M and Piot P (1993) HIV infection and sexually transmitted diseases. In: Jamison DT et al., eds. *Disease control priorities in developing countries.* New York: Oxford University Press.

Page LA, Smith PC (1974) Placentitis and abortion in cattle inoculated with chlamydiae isolated from aborted human placental tissue. *Proceedings of the Society for Experimental Biology and Medicine* 146:269–75.

Pelouze PS; (1941) Gonorrhoea in the male and female. Philadelphia: W.B. Saunders.

Piot P and Holmes KK (1990) Sexually transmitted diseases. In: Warren KS, Mahmoud AAF eds. *Tropical and geographical medicine.* 2nd ed. New York: McGraw-Hill, Inc.

Platou RV (1949) Treatment of congenital syphilis with penicillin. *Advanced Pediatrics* 4:39.

Platt R et al. (1983) Risk of acquiring gonorrhoea and prevalence of abnormal adnexal findings among women recently exposed to gonorrhoea. *Journal of the American Medical Association* 250:3205–9.

Posada AB et al. (1992) Prevalence of urogenital Chlamydia trachomatis infection in El Salvador. I. Infection during pregnancy and perinatal transmission. *International Journal of STD and AIDS* 3:33–7.

Preece PM et al. (1989) Chlamydia trachomatis infection in infants: a prospective study. *Archives of Disease in Childhood* 64:525–9.

Prien-Larsen JC, Kjer JJ (1989) [Prevalence of positive gonococcal and chlamydial findings in women applying for termination of pregnancy. A screening evaluation]. [Danish]. *Ugeskrift for Laeger* 151:1671–2.

Quinn TC, Cates Jr W (1992) Epidemiology of sexually transmitted diseases in the 1990s. In: Quinn TC, eds. *Sexually transmitted diseases.* New York: Raven Press Ltd.

Quinn TC et al. (1988) Human immunodeficiency virus infection among patients attending clinics for sexually transmitted diseases. *New England Journal of Medicine* 318:197–203.

Rosahn PD (1947) Autopsy studies in syphilis. *Journal of Venereal Disease Information (US Public Health Service, Venereal Disease Division)* supplement no 21.

Rosenfeld DL et al. (1983) Unsuspected chronic pelvic inflammatory disease in the infertile female. *Fertility & Sterility* 39:44–8.

Samb ND, et al. (1993) Prevention et traitement des MST dans le cadre du programme national de lutte contre les MST et le SIDA au Senegal. *Presented at the VIIIth International Conference on AIDS in Africa.*

Schachter J (1967) Isolation of Bedoniae from human arthritis and abortion tissue. *American Journal of Ophtalmology* 63:1082.

Scholes D et al. (1992) Current cigarette smoking and risk of acute pelvic inflammatory disease. *American Journal of Public Health* 82:1352–5.

Schrijvers D et al. (1989) Transmission of syphilis between sexual partners in Gabon. *Genitourinary Medicine* 65:84–5.

Schulz KF et al. (1990) Congenital syphilis. In: Holmes KK et al., eds. *Sexually transmitted diseases.* 2nd ed. New York: McGraw-Hill, Inc.

Schulz KF et al. (1992) Maternal health and child survival: opportunities to protect both women and children from the adverse consequences of reproductive tract infections. In: Germain A et al., eds. *Reproductive tract infections: global impact and priorities for women's reproductive health.* New York: Plenum Press.

Skjeldestad FE, Jerve F (1992) [Chlamydia trachomatis and Neisseria gonorrhoeae among women seeking abortion in Norway. Results from a nationwide study]. [Norwegian]. *Tidsskrift for Den Norske Laegeforening* 112:2082–4.

Sorensen JL et al. (1992) [Presence of genital Chlamydia trachomatis in abortion seekers—correlates with young age and nulliparity but not with previous genital infection]. [Danish]. *Ugeskrift for Laeger* 154:3053–6.

Sparling PF (1990) Natural history of syphilis. In: Holmes KK et al., eds. *Sexually transmitted diseases.* 2nd ed. New York: McGraw-Hill, Inc.

Spence MR, Abrutyn E (1987) Syphilis and infection with the human immunodeficiency virus. *Annals of Internal Medicine* 107:587.

Stamm WE, Cole B (1986) Asymptomatic Chlamydia trachomatis urethritis in men. *Sexually Transmitted Diseases* 13:163–5.

Stamm WE, Holmes KK (1990) Chlamydia trachomatis infections of the adult. In: Holmes KK et al., eds. *Sexually transmitted diseases.* 2nd ed. New York: McGraw-Hill, Inc.

Stamm WE et al. (1984) Chlamydia trachomatis urethral infections in men. Prevalence, risk factors, and clinical manifestations. *Annals of Internal Medicine* 100:47–51.

Stanecki KA et al. (1995) *Sexually transmitted diseases in sub-Saharan Africa and associated interactions with HIV.* Washington, DC, IPC Staff Paper 75.

Swartz MN (1990) Neurosyphilis. In: Holmes KK et al., eds. *Sexually transmitted diseases.* 2nd ed. New York: McGraw-Hill, Inc.

Tadmor OP et al. (1993) Pregnancy outcome in serologically indicated active Chlamydia trachomatis infection. *Israel Journal of Medical Sciences* 29:280–4.

Thewessen EA et al. (1990) Screening for cervical Chlamydia trachomatis infections in two Dutch populations. *Genitourinary Medicine* 66:361–6.

Thin RN (1990) Early syphilis in the adult. In: Holmes KK et al., eds. *Sexually transmitted diseases.* 2nd ed. New York: McGraw-Hill, Inc.

Thompson TR et al. (1974) Gonococcal ophthalmia neonatorum. Relationship of time of infection to relevant control measures. *Journal of the American Medical Association* 228:186–8.

Todd J et al. (1993) An examination of risk factors associated with STD/RTI infections among women attending rural ante-natal clinics. *Presented at the VIIIth International Conference on AIDS in Africa.*

Vuylsteke B et al. (1993) Clinical algorithms for the screening of women for gonococcal and chlamydial infection: evaluation of pregnant women and prostitutes in Zaire. *Clinical Infectious Diseases* 17:82–8.

Washington AE et al. (1987) Chlamydia trachomatis infections in the United States. What are they costing us? *Journal of the American Medical Association* 257:2070–2.

Washington AE et al. (1991) Assessing risk for pelvic inflammatory disease and its sequelae [see comments]. [Review] [77 refs]. *Journal of the American Medical Association* 266:2581–6.

Wasserheit JN. (1989) The significance and scope of reproductive tract infections among Third World women. [Review] [149 refs]. *Supplement to International Journal of Gynaecology & Obstetrics* 3:145–68.

Wasserheit JN. (1991) Epidemiological synergy: interrelationships between HIV infection and other STDs. In: Chen LC et al., eds. *AIDS and women's reproductive health.* New York: Plenum Press.

Weström L (1975) Effect of acute pelvic inflammatory disease on fertility. *American Journal of Obstetrics & Gynaecology* 121:707–13.

Weström L (1980) Incidence, prevalence, and trends of acute pelvic inflammatory disease and its consequences in industrialized countries. *American Journal of Obstetrics & Gynaecology* 138:880–92.

Weström L (1988) Decrease in incidence of women treated in hospital for acute salpingitis in Sweden. *Genitourinary Medicine* 64:59–63.

Weström L, Mårdh P (1990) Acute pelvic inflammatory disease (PID). In: Holmes KK et al., eds. *Sexually transmitted diseases.* 2nd ed. New York: McGraw-Hill.

Weström L et al. (1981) Incidence, trends, and risks of ectopic pregnancy in a population of women. *British Medical Journal.* 282:15–8.

Weström L et al. (1992) Pelvic inflammatory disease and fertility: a cohort study of 1, 844 women with laparoscopically verified disease and 657 control women with normal laproscopic results. *Sexually Transmitted Diseases*,19:185–92.

Wolff H, Anderson DJ (1988) Male genital tract inflammation associated with increased numbers of potential human immunodeficiency virus host cells in semen. *Andrologia* 20:404–10.

Wolner-Hansen P et al. (1990) Atypical pelvic inflammatory disease: subacute, chronic, or subclinical infection in women. In: Holmes KK et al., eds. *Sexually transmitted diseases.* 2nd ed. New York: McGraw-Hill, Inc.

World Health Organization/Global Programme on AIDS (1995) Global prevalence and incidence of selected curable sexually transmitted diseases: Overview and Estimates. WHO/GPA/STD 95.1

Yang YS et al. (1988) Chlamydia trachomatis infection in pregnant women. *Taiwan I Hsueh Hui Tsa Chih—Journal of the Formosan Medical Association* 87:1177–81.

Yildiz A et al. (1990) Prevalence of Chlamydia trachomatis infection in the Turkish female population. *Gynecologic & Obstetric Investigation* 29:282–4.

Zimmermann R (1993) [Syphilis screening in pregnancy]. [German]. *Geburtshilfe und Frauenheilkunde* 53:677–80.

Chapter 3

Maternal Mortality Overview

Carla AbouZahr[1]

Introduction

One of the reasons why maternal mortality was a neglected problem for so long was inadequate information. Countries with the highest levels of mortality seldom have good reporting of vital events such as births and deaths. And even countries with relatively complete vital registration (generally defined as covering some 90 per cent of the population) may have less than adequate attribution of causes of death. This is important because in order to decide whether the death of a women is a maternal death or not it is essential to know both the timing of the death in relation to the pregnancy status of the woman and the cause of death. Because this information is generally not readily available in developing countries, few have reliable national estimates of maternal mortality.

In the mid-1980s a number of community surveys, many of which were supported by the World Health Organization, brought to light the enormity of the problem of maternal mortality and the high risks women in developing countries undergo as a result of becoming pregnant. These studies set the stage for the first estimates of the magnitude of the health problem due to complications of pregnancy and childbirth. However, all such efforts focused exclusively on the calculation of numbers of deaths. It is important to stress that at that stage, no attempt was made to calculate the burden of disability and morbidity because of the dearth of information on the subject.

Intuitively, one would expect the definition of maternal death to be a simple matter. Childbirth is a memorable event and death in childbirth even more so. In practice, however, matters are not that clear. Childbirth is an event in a process comprising the nine months pregnancy period, as well as the puerperium which extends some time beyond the birth itself. If the definition of a maternal death is to include all pregnancy-related deaths it must include those that occur before childbirth (such as abortion, ectopic pregnancy), those taking place during childbirth (such as intrapartum haemorrhage or ruptured uterus) as well as deaths taking place some time after the event of childbirth (such as sepsis). Moreover, not all maternal deaths are directly due to conditions resulting solely from pregnancy. Some are caused by pre-existing conditions aggravated by pregnancy (such as cardiovascular disease or hepatitis).

The World Health Organization has estimated that 10–15 per cent of all pregnancies that end in a live birth develop life-threatening complications which require rapid and skilled intervention if the woman is to survive without lifelong disabilities (World Health Organization 1994). An additional proportion of pregnancies will result in complications that are not life-threatening but which may nevertheless compromise the health of the mother. The dimensions of this proportion of less serious complications are difficult to estimate. However, a study in the United Sates found that hospitalization for pregnancy complications is far more common than is widely appreciated. For every 100 hospitalizations involving a pregnancy or birth there were 22.2 hospitalizations for non-delivery complications (14.6 prenatal complications, 7.6 pregnancy loss complications) (Franks et al. 1992). Furthermore, a number of readmissions occurred during the postpartum period, yielding an average annual rate of 8.1 readmissions per 1000 deliveries (Piper 1992). Thus, nearly one in four pregnancies required hospitalization for conditions not directly related to the delivery. It is inappropriate to generalize from a single study in an industrialized country with a highly medicalized approach to pregnancy and childbirth (some would argue over-medicalized). Nonetheless, the figures are striking given the relatively good nutritional and health status of most women in the United States. In developing countries the proportion of pregnant women needing medical care could be even higher, given the generally poor health and nutritional status of women and the prevalence of communicable diseases. If the needed help is not available those with the severest complications will die and countless others who survive will suffer from permanently impaired health and from a variety of disabilities.

The sequelae of untreated pregnancy complications are both short and long term. Postpartum and post abortion infections, common in developing countries, can lead to pelvic inflammatory disease (PID) which, in addition to causing chronic pain and discomfort, can result in permanent infertility. Repeated and lengthy labours lead to uterine prolapse, which, depending on the degree of severity, may cause incontinence, permanent discomfort and pain. Poorly managed obstructed labour can cause uterine rupture, or obstetric fistulae (an unnatural opening between the vagina and bladder or rectum). This is without doubt the most debilitating and distressing condition of all. Leaking urine and/or faeces cause a permanent odour and painful skin rashes. Women suffering from this condition become social outcasts.

While organic illness accounts for most of the complications reported in pregnancy, childbirth and the puerperium, psychiatric illnesses also occur. Psychiatric illnesses may take one of several forms, which include neurotic reaction, states of confusion, affective disorders and schizophrenia. Usually such disorders become manifest within the first week following childbirth. Infections, including puerperal sepsis, can trigger psychiatric disturbance that can be severe, leading to infanticide and suicide (Kendell et al. 1989).

Early attempts to estimate maternal mortality

Past attempts at measuring the burden related to pregnancy and childbirth have focused exclusively on measures of mortality. Given the dearth of reliable national data, WHO adopted a strategy based on an intensive search of all published and unpublished information on maternal mortality, its compilation in the form of bibliographic and indicator databases, and the development of modelling approaches in order to formulate estimates of maternal mortality in countries lacking reliable data.

The first attempts at global and regional estimates of the scale of the problem were developed by WHO by building a statistical model of the maternal mortality ratio (MMR) based on widely available predictor variables. The relationship between MMR and the predictor variables was estimated on the basis of a set of countries with reliable estimates of maternal mortality, and the model was then used to predict maternal mortality in countries without good national estimates.

A number of predictor variables were explored, including demographic measures (infant mortality, female life expectancy at birth and at age 15 years, total fertility rate) and measures of health service access and utilization (coverage of prenatal care, percentage of live births with a trained attendant). The variable most closely correlated with maternal mortality turned out to be female life expectancy at birth which was, in the end, the only variable retained in the model. To avoid problems with negative predicted values, the dependent variable used in these models was the logarithm of the maternal mortality ratio.

A major problem with this approach was that most of the data used in the estimation model were derived from vital registration data, which are, with a few notable exceptions, available only for industrialised countries. This was particularly true of the first attempt in 1986. By 1991, when the same approach was used to update the figures, more data had become available for developing countries as a result of the development and use of community-based methodologies for calculating maternal mortality, such as the Reproductive Age Mortality Survey (RAMOS) and sisterhood methods.

Concerns such as these, and others related to the methodology itself, led to the decision to publish only aggregated regional and global estimates from these exercises because the individual country predictions were not deemed to be sufficiently sound for publication.

The widely quoted figure of 500,000 maternal deaths annually worldwide originates from this approach used in 1986 and again in 1991. The maternal mortality ratio declined very slightly between the two estimates, though the total number of deaths rose because there were more births in 1991. However, in view of the nature of the data, which were incomplete and covered a period of several years, these differences could not be considered to be indicative of any real secular trend. The 1991 estimate was considered the more reliable of the two simply because considerably more data had become available in the interval since the first estimates were made (World Health Organization 1991).

It is important to note that the starting point of the strategy adopted for both exercises was numbers of maternal deaths. An alternative strategy would have been to estimate the incidence of pregnancy-related complications and to apply case fatality rates for the major causes of maternal death in order to arrive at the number of deaths. This strategy was rejected simply on practical grounds. Not enough was known either about the incidence of complications or about case fatality rates, even for those complications that reached a facility let alone those that occurred at home. Interestingly, some 10 years on from the first modelling attempts, there remains considerable ignorance about both the incidence of complications and the likelihood they will end in death.

This strategy — starting with the numbers of maternal deaths — has again been followed in the preparation of estimates for the calculation of the global burden of disease. However, a new element has been added, namely the estimation of global and regional incidence rates for the major direct complications of pregnancy and delivery. Using these two pieces of information, we have calculated case fatality rates which turn out to be broadly in line with the, admittedly incomplete and biased, case fatality rates observed in a number of hospital studies (AbouZahr and Royston 1991)

Definition and measurement

Definition of maternal death

The Tenth Revision of the International Classification of Diseases (ICD-10) defines a maternal death as the death of a woman while pregnant or within 42 days of termination of pregnancy, irrespective of the duration and site of the pregnancy, from any cause related to or aggravated by the pregnancy or its management but not from accidental or incidental causes (World Health Organization 1992). This definition is unchanged from the Ninth Revision of the International Classification of Diseases (ICD-9).

There are two problems with this definition, one related to time of death, the second to cause of death. With regard to the first, historically, maternal mortality was defined as deaths occurring within six weeks of termination of pregnancy. This timing was sanctioned by a variety of practices, both religious (such as the churching of women in the Anglican church) and cultural (such as name-giving ceremonies in some Indonesian societies).

Modern life-sustaining procedures and technologies can, however, prolong dying and delay death. Even before the era of modern medicine it is likely that some maternal deaths took place beyond the six week interval but the proportion was probably very small. Medical procedures may increase that proportion but it is likely to remain fairly small though by no means negligible. For example, the Centers for Disease Control and Prevention report that 29 per cent of maternal deaths in Georgia over the period 1974–75 occurred after 42 days of pregnancy termination and 6 per cent occurred after 90 days postpartum (Koonin et al. 1988). For this reason, ICD-10 introduced a new category, namely the *late maternal death* which is defined as the *death of a woman from direct or indirect obstetric causes more than 42 days but less than one year after termination of pregnancy.*

The second problem with the definition of maternal death lies in the classification of cause of death. According to ICD-9 and ICD-10, maternal deaths should be divided into two groups:

Direct obstetric deaths are those resulting from obstetric complications of the pregnant state (pregnancy, labour and the puerperium), from interventions, omissions, incorrect treatment, or from a chain of events resulting from any of the above.

Indirect obstetric deaths are those resulting from previous existing disease or disease that developed during pregnancy and which was not due to direct obstetric causes, but was aggravated by physiologic effects of pregnancy.

The drawback of this definition is that maternal deaths can escape being so classified because the precise cause of death cannot be given even though the fact of the woman having been pregnant is known. Such under-registration is frequent in both developing and developed countries. Even in countries where all or most deaths are medically certified, maternity-related mortality can still be grossly underestimated. Record linking and other studies have shown misreporting of between 25 per cent and 70 per cent of maternal deaths (Bouvier-Colle et al. 1994, Smith 1984, Centers for Disease Control and Prevention 1991). The situation is even worse where the registration of death is complete but attribution of cause of death is inadequate, as is frequently the case.

Deaths from "accidental or incidental" causes have historically been excluded from maternal mortality. However, in practice, the distinction between incidental and indirect causes of death is difficult to make. Some deaths from external causes may be attributable to the pregnancy itself. It is likely that many homicides and suicides of pregnant or recently pregnant women are attributable in some way to the pregnancy — either because suicide is preferable to the shame of premarital pregnancy or, perhaps, because the pregnancy produced a child of the "wrong" sex (Fortney et al. 1984). Nor is the phenomenon confined to developing countries. A study in the United States found that several deaths of pregnant or recently pregnant women were the result of physical violence related to the fact of pregnancy and that had they been included as maternal deaths the overall maternal mortality ratio would have increased by 8 per cent (Chavkin and Allen 1993).

In countries where maternal mortality is high the bias introduced by the inclusion of accidental or incidental causes is usually low. In rural Bangladesh, for example, where the overall maternal mortality ratio is 570 per 100 000 live births, it was found that 90 per cent of the deaths of women who were pregnant or had been pregnant within the preceding 90 days, were due to direct and indirect maternal causes (Chen et al. 1974). In an area of Egypt, with a maternal mortality ratio of 263 per 100 000 live births, 87 per cent of deaths of pregnant women were due to maternal (direct and indirect) causes (Fortney et al. 1984).

To facilitate the identification of maternal deaths under circumstances where cause of death attribution is inadequate, ICD-10 introduced a new category, that of *pregnancy-related death,* which is defined as:

the death of a woman while pregnant or within 42 days of termination of pregnancy, irrespective of the cause of death.

In practice, different countries use different definitions and there is an ongoing need to clearly define the terminology used in any particular case. For example, in the United States, the term "pregnancy associated" is used instead of the ICD-10 term "pregnancy related" and the term "pregnancy associated and related" is used instead of the ICD-10 term "maternal". In New Zealand, the definition used is, in fact, "pregnancy-related" though it is reported as "maternal".

ICD-9 AND ICD-10 CODES FOR CLASSIFYING CAUSES OF MATERNAL DEATHS

The Ninth International Classification of Diseases (ICD-9) classified complications of pregnancy, childbirth and the puerperium into five broad classes, as follows:

pregnancy with abortive outcome (630-639), including hydatidiform mole, other abnormal products of conception, missed abortion, ectopic pregnancy, spontaneous abortion, legally induced abortion, illegally induced abortion, unspecified abortion, failed attempted abortion, and complications following abortion and ectopic and molar pregnancies;

complications mainly related to pregnancy (640-648), including haemorrhage in early pregnancy, antepartum haemorrhage, *abruptio placentae* and *placenta praevia*, hypertension complicating pregnancy, childbirth and the puerperium, such as pre-eclampsia and eclampsia, excessive vomiting in pregnancy, early or threatened labour, prolonged pregnancy and other complications of pregnancy not elsewhere classified, infective and parasitic conditions in the mother classifiable elsewhere but complicating pregnancy, childbirth and the puerperium, such as syphilis, gonorrhoea, tuberculosis, malaria, and other current conditions in the mother classifiable elsewhere but complicating pregnancy, childbirth and the puerperium, such as diabetes mellitus, thyroid dysfunction, anaemia, cardiovascular disorders;

normal delivery, and other indications for care in pregnancy, labour and delivery (650-659), including multiple gestation, malposition and malpresentation of fetus, disproportion, abnormality of organs and soft tissues of pelvis, known or suspected fetal abnormality affecting management of mother, other fetal and placental problems affecting management of mother, polyhydramnios, other problems associated with amniotic cavity and membranes, and other indications for care or intervention related to labour and delivery not elsewhere classified;

complications occurring mainly in the course of labour and delivery (660-669), including obstructed labour, abnormality of forces of labour, long labour, umbilical cord complications, trauma to perineum and vulva during delivery, other obstetrical trauma, such as rupture of uterus and uterine inversion, postpartum haemorrhage, retained placenta or membranes without haemorrhage, complications of the administration of anaesthetic or other sedation in labour and delivery, and other complications of labour and delivery not elsewhere classified;

complications of the puerperium (670-676), including major puerperal infection, venous complications in pregnancy and the puerperium, pyrexia of unknown origin during the puerperium, obstetrical pulmonary embolism, other and unspecified complications of the puerperium not elsewhere classified, infections of the breast and nipple associated with childbirth, and other disorders of the breast associated with childbirth, and disorders of lactation.

The Tenth International Statistical Classification of Diseases and Related Health Problems (ICD-10) subdivided pregnancy-related health problems into eight blocks, covering slightly different groups of diseases, as follows:

pregnancy with abortive outcome (O00-O08), including ectopic pregnancy, hydatidiform mole, other abnormal products of conception, spontaneous abortion, medical abortion, other abortion, unspecified abortion, failed attempted abortion, and complications following abortion and ectopic pregnancy;

oedema, proteinuria and hypertensive disorders in pregnancy, childbirth and the puerperium (O10-O16), which includes hypertensive complications previously classified under "complications relating mainly to pregnancy", namely, pre-existing hypertensive disorder with superimposed proteinuria, gestational oedema and proteinuria without hypertension, gestational hypertension with or without significant proteinuria, eclampsia and unspecified maternal hypertension;

other maternal disorders predominantly related to pregnancy (O20-O29) including haemorrhage in early pregnancy, excessive vomiting in pregnancy, venous complications, genitourinary tract infections, diabetes mellitus in pregnancy, malnutrition, maternal care for other conditions predominantly related to pregnancy, abnormal findings of prenatal screening and complications of anaesthesia during pregnancy;

maternal care related to the fetus and amniotic cavity and possible delivery problems (O30-O48), including multiple gestation, malpresentation of fetus, suspected disproportion, known or suspected abnormality of pelvic organs, fetal abnormality and damage, other suspected fetal problems, polyhydramnios, other disorders of amniotic fluid or membranes, premature rupture of membranes, placental disorders, *placenta praevia, abruptio placentae*, antepartum haemorrhage not elsewhere classified, false labour and prolonged pregnancy;

complications of labour and delivery (O60-O75) including preterm delivery, failed induction of labour, abnormality of the forces of labour, long labour, obstruction due to malposition and malpresentation of fetus, obstructed labour due to maternal pelvic deformity, labour and delivery complicated by intrapartum haemorrhage not elsewhere classified, labour and delivery complicated by fetal distress, umbilical cord complications, perineal laceration during delivery, other obstetric trauma, postpartum haemorrhage, retained placenta and membranes, complications of anaesthesia during labour and delivery and other complications of labour and delivery;

delivery (O80-O84) including single spontaneous delivery, single delivery by forceps and vacuum extractor, single delivery by caesarean section, other assisted single delivery, multiple delivery;

complications predominantly related to the puerperium (O85-O92) including puerperal sepsis, other puerperal infections, venous complications in the puerperium, obstetric embolism, complications of anaesthesia during the puerperium, other complications of the puerperium, infections of the breast associated with childbirth and other disorders of breast and lactation;

other obstetric complications not elsewhere classified (O95-O99) including maternal infectious and parasitic diseases classifiable elsewhere but complicating pregnancy, childbirth and the puerperium such as tuberculosis, syphilis, gonorrhoea, viral hepatitis, and other maternal diseases such as anaemia, endocrine, nutritional and metabolic diseases, mental disorders, diseases of the circulatory system and diseases of the digestive system.

The ICD reporting system assumes a single cause of death and gives clear definitions about the hierarchy of reporting of multiple causes. According to ICD, multiple causes of death are recorded in the sequence in which they occur and are classified as immediate, underlying or associated causes. In summary tabulations, only the single underlying cause of death is reported. A typical example for a maternal death would be antepartum haemorrhage, caused by abruptio placentae, caused by pre-eclampsia. The last condition quoted in this sequence — the first condition to occur — becomes the underlying cause of death and the cause to be reported in summary tables (World Health Organization 1995).

Concerns have been expressed that attribution of a single underlying cause is necessarily very subjective. The single-cause classification will tend to reflect the quality of cause of death ascertainment rather than a meaningful set of causes and there may be major problems of comparability between settings with different levels of cause of death ascertainment. Moreover, identifying a single cause of death masks the multifactorial nature of any death and the particular combinations of events that are relevant for the development of interventions. For example, a death from sepsis alone indicates the need for improved case management; sepsis in combination with obstructed labour indicates the need for primary prevention and detection of women at high risk of obstructed labour; and sepsis following abortion complications indicates a need for prevention and management of unsafe abortion.

The importance of analysing causes of death according to specific diagnostic categories has been stressed by researchers. For example, most studies report all haemorrhage deaths as a single group, with no differentiation into those caused by placenta praevia, placental abruption or postpartum haemorrhage. Yet the interventions needed to address these three types of haemorrhage-related deaths will be different. Similarly, it is increasingly important to distinguish sepsis-related deaths associated with caesarean section from those occurring following vaginal deliveries (Hoestermann et al. 1996).

In developing country settings where communicable diseases such as malaria and hepatitis are endemic, studies indicate that indirect causes account for 20 per cent or more of all maternal deaths. Official figures often underreport such indirect causes.

Such problems may not be confined to developing country settings. Very few industrialised countries officially report indirect causes of maternal death. A review of WHO maternal health databases found that of the 60 countries reporting vital registration figures for causes of maternal deaths over the period 1992–1993, over half (33 countries) reported no indirect deaths at all. Yet the most recent Confidential Enquiry in the United Kingdom found that 43 per cent of maternal deaths during the period 1991–1993 were due to indirect causes (Hibbard et al. 1996).

In both developed and developing countries, cardiac diseases are an important component of indirect causes of death. By contrast, indirect causes of maternal death in the industrialised world are mainly due to diseases of the endocrine or metabolic system, diseases of the central nervous system and other non-communicable diseases rather than to endemic tropical diseases such as malaria.

While the risks of perinatal transmission of HIV/AIDS during pregnancy, childbirth and lactation have been amply demonstrated, the impact of HIV and AIDS on maternal outcome remains unclear. There is no evidence of any short term effect of pregnancy on the progression of HIV/AIDS in the mother; the results of long-term follow-up are not yet available. Nor does HIV infection appear to have a direct effect on the outcome of pregnancy, though a recent prospective cohort study in Rwanda found that post-operative complications were more common among HIV positive women with the risk apparently higher among severely immuno-suppressed women. (Bulterys et al. 1996). However in developed countries there is a correlation between the risk factors for HIV infection and for adverse pregnancy outcomes, including poverty, lack of perinatal care, intravenous drug use and multiple sex partners. Further research is needed on the interactions between pregnancy-related complications and HIV infection in women.

The complexity of issues of attribution of cause of death was recognised in the ICD-10 which sought to clarify the relative hierarchy of chapters and to make it clear that the chapters "Pregnancy, childbirth and the puerperium" as well as "Certain conditions arising in the perinatal period" had priority over organ or system chapters. The extent to which this advice will be followed in the classification of maternal death remains to be seen.

Measures of maternal mortality

The ICD-10 does not address the issue of statistical measures, but the evolution of maternal mortality research has produced a need for at least two distinct measures. The most commonly used maternal mortality measure is the number of maternal deaths during a given time period per 100 000 live births during the same time period. This is not a true death rate in that it does not measure deaths per woman-year of exposure within a specified time period. Rather, it is a ratio which measures the obstetric risk. Although it has traditionally been called a rate this is actually a ratio and is now usually called such by researchers. However, for the sake of historical consistency, ICD-10 continues to use the term rate for this measure.

The appropriate denominator for the maternal mortality ratio would be the total number of pregnancies (live births, fetal deaths (stillbirths), induced and spontaneous abortions, ectopic and molar pregnancies). However, this figure is seldom available, either in developing countries where most of the world's births take place, or in developed countries. Hence the general use of live births in the denominator. Although the use of total pregnancies or total births is more accurate from an epidemiological point of view, in practice live births is used in the denominator simply for practical reasons. This mismatch between the population in the numerator and that in the denominator has a number of disadvantages. Some pregnancies result in multiple births and some in stillbirths, spontaneous or induced abortions, ectopic or molar pregnancies. Indeed, such pregnancy outcomes are particularly significant because they are associated with an increased risk of maternal death.

The maternal mortality *ratio* measures the risk of death once a women has become pregnant. By contrast, the maternal mortality *rate*, the number of maternal deaths in a given period per 100 000 women of reproductive age during the same time period, is a true death rate. It measures both the obstetric risk and the frequency with which women are exposed to this risk. There may be variations in the definition of women of reproductive age. WHO, generally uses the period 15–45 years, but it is not unusual to see the use of age ranges 15–49 or, particularly where early fertility is an issue, 10–45/49 years

Because of the confusion in the use of the terms ratio and rate, for the sake of clarity it is essential to specify the denominator used when referring to either of these measures of maternal mortality.

The ideal measure of maternal mortality would take into account both the probability of becoming pregnant and the probability of dying as a result of that pregnancy cumulated across a woman's reproductive years — the lifetime risk. This measure is becoming increasingly popular. In theory, the lifetime risk is a cohort measure but it is usually calculated with period measures for practical reasons. It can be approximated by multiplying the maternal mortality rate by the length of the reproductive period (around 35 years). Thus, the lifetime risk is calculated as:

$$1 - (1 - \mathrm{MMR})^{35}$$

where MMR is the maternal mortality rate (maternal deaths per 100 000 women of reproductive age) (Campbell and Graham 1990). (A raising factor of 30 has also been suggested , depending on whether the reproductive age range is considered to be 15–44 years or 15–49 years.) The lifetime risk can also be approximated by the product of the total fertility rate (TFR) and the maternal mortality ratio. An adjustment factor of 1.2 or 1.5 is included in order to compensate for pregnancy loss. Thus, the lifetime risk is 1/(1.2*TFR*MMR).

MEASURING MATERNAL MORTALITY

Issues related to definitions, rates and ratios apart, counting the number of maternal deaths itself is extremely difficult. Most official measures of maternal mortality are underestimates. The reasons for this vary according to certification practices and the degree of sophistication of the vital registration system. Although the definition of a maternal death in the International Classification of Diseases (ICD-9 and ICD-10) is scientifically incontrovertible, in practice maternal deaths often escape being so classified for two reasons: either because the precise cause of death cannot be given even though the fact of the woman having been pregnant is known; or because while the cause of death is known (for example kidney failure) the fact of the pregnancy may not have been noted on the death certificate.

There are three main types of sources of data on maternal deaths — vital registration, population-based enquiries and health service statistics.

Table 1 Countries reporting maternal deaths 1985–89

Region	*Number of countries*	*Number reporting maternal deaths*	*Per cent reporting maternal deaths*
Africa	51	2	4
North America/ Caribbean	18	11	61
South America	12	10	83
Asia	39	7	18
Europe	27	26	96
Oceania	4	3	75
World	151	59	39

Source: United Nations Demographic Yearbook 1992 and World Population Prospects 1990

Vital registration

Cause of death is routinely reported for only 78 countries or areas, covering a total population of 1800 million, or 35 per cent of the world's population. The United Nations Demographic Yearbook estimates that over the period 1985–89 only 59 out of 151 countries (of total population over 300 000) reported maternal mortality figures, and of these, most were in Europe and North America. Other countries that routinely report maternal deaths tend to have small populations and very few maternal deaths, for example, Singapore and Hong Kong (see Table 1).

It was to help those countries wishing to report maternal deaths but whose vital registration systems were unable adequately to attribute cause of death that ICD-10 introduced a new category of "pregnancy-related death". This is intended for use in countries that wish to count maternal deaths but where the cause of death cannot be identified precisely. This will however require that all death certificates include a question on pregnancy status of the deceased woman. Only a few countries do so at present.

Even with good vital registration systems, biases can arise, usually due to incorrect classification of the cause of death. Death certificates often fail to certify the cause of death, they may omit to note pregnancy status and deaths due to the sequelae of induced abortion are frequently omitted. There may be many social, religious, emotional or practical reasons for not classifying a maternal death as such. Deaths of unmarried women or those resulting from the complications of abortion, for example, may often be classed to another cause to avoid embarrassing the surviving family; this would be all the more likely if the abortion was illegal. The extent of this type of under reporting can be considerable. Another common cause for under reporting is a wish to avoid blame.

Active case-finding of maternal deaths

Because vital registration is essentially a passive system for maternal death reporting it cannot, by itself, be assumed to identify all maternal deaths.

Table 2 Under reporting of maternal deaths in official data — selected studies

Country	Date	Official deaths	Source of official data	Add'l deaths	Sources of add'l data	Total deaths identified	% of deaths missed
England & Wales[1]	1982-84	163	Mortality statistics	46	Confidential enquiries	209	22
United Kingdom[4]	1991-93	140	Mortaliy statistics	88	Confidential enquiries	228	39
United States[2]	1974-78	1,949	Vital statistics	606	Special study	2,555	24
France[3]	1988-89	24	Vital statistics	30	Manual review of death certificates	54	56
Puerto Rico[5]	1978-79	17	Vital statisics	45	Manual review of death certificates	62	73

1. Turnbull, A., Tindall, VR, Beard, RW, Robson, G, Dawson, IM, Cloake, EP, Ashley, JS and Botting B. Report on confidential enquiries into maternal deaths in England and Wales 1982-84. London HMSO
2. Smith, JC, Hugher, JM, Pekow, PS and Rochat, RW (1984) An assessment of the incidence of maternal mortality in the United States. American Journal of Public Health 74(8) 780-783
3. Bouvier-Colle et al. (1991)
4. Hibbard BM, Anderson MM, Drife JO, Tighe JR, Gordon G, Willatts S, de Swiet M, Shaw R, Thompson W, Lewis G, Botting B. Report on Confidential Enquiries into Maternal Deaths in the United Kingdom 1991-1993. HMSO London (1996)
5 Centers for Disease Control (1991)

More active case finding is needed to overcome the biases inherent in the vital registration system. Using a variety of methods to improve case finding, recent research has highlighted the extent of under reporting and misclassification of maternal deaths in countries with good vital registration (Atrash et al. 1995). Despite near universal coverage of vital events and medical certification of cause of death, significant proportions of maternal deaths are not classified as such in vital registration systems around the world (Table 2).

A recent review of maternal mortality in developed countries found that in the United States at least six different sources can be used to identify deaths related to pregnancy (Atrash et al. 1995) These include, in additional to published vital records:

- a manual review of death certificates to identify additional cases in which pregnancy has been indicated on the death certificate;
- using vital record linkage to match death certificates for women of reproductive age to certificates of reportable pregnancy outcomes (live births, still births, fetal deaths and, sometimes, abortion);
- review of autopsy reports;

- review of medical records;
- interviews with family members, health care providers etc.

No single source of information identifies all maternal deaths. Moreover, all such sources are oriented towards obstetric events with the result that a common shortcoming is the failure to record early pregnancy deaths which, in the United States for example, may account for up to 20 per cent of all maternal deaths (Atrash et al. 1995).

Different countries have tried different approaches for identifying all maternal deaths. Some have established task forces to undertake periodic reviews of deaths of women of reproductive age with active case-finding of maternal deaths. In Portugal this was done prospectively with the cooperation of hospitals (Da Purificacao 1988). In France, the review took place retrospectively and involved an analysis of all death certificates of women aged 15–44 years. (Bouvier-Colle et al. 1991).

In countries with very low levels of maternal mortality very few maternal deaths actually take place in obstetric departments of large hospitals because when life-threatening conditions such as acute renal failure arise the patient is usually transferred to another specialist department. If she dies there the death will be certified by a non-obstetric specialist and the cause of death appearing on the certificate may well not mention the obstetric condition which triggered the fatal sequence of events. There are other, more mundane sources of error. An enquiry in France found that 17 of the 41 deaths reported as being related to maternal conditions by the certifying doctor, were subsequently miscoded by the coding clerks. For example, cerebral haemorrhages were classified in "Diseases of the circulatory system" instead of "Complications of pregnancy, childbirth and the puerperium" (Bhatt 1989, Bouvier-Colle et al. 1994).

A study conducted in the United States by the New Jersey Health Department identified an additional 26 maternal deaths in that State during 1974–75 over and above the 30 deaths reported in the vital statistics (Ziskin et al. 1979). A Centers for Disease Control study found that the incidence of maternal mortality in the United States in 1974–78 was 12.1 per 100 000 live births rather than the reported rate of 9.6 (United States, Department of Health, Education and Welfare). Intensive surveillance through a review of death certificates and selected medical records in Puerto Rico in 1978 and 1979 revealed that only about 27 per cent of pregnancy-related deaths had been recorded through the registration system (Centers for Disease Control 1991). By linking death certificates of women in the childbearing ages with birth certificates of their offspring, researchers reported a 50 per cent increase in the number of known maternal deaths in Georgia in 1975 and 1976 compared with the figure obtained from vital registration (Rubin et al. 1981). A study in North Carolina which used computer-matching of birth and fetal death records with death certificates calculated a maternal mortality ratio of 24 per 100 000 live births compared with the 9.5 indicated by vital registration.

Only part of the discrepancy can be explained by the fact that the former counted maternal deaths occurring up to one year after termination of the pregnancy (May et al. 1991).

Confidential enquiries/medical audit

Another approach for improving the identification of maternal deaths is to establish a more formal procedure for bringing together information from different sources and analysing which deaths were, in fact, maternal. Maternal mortality committees, as they are often called, interact directly with civil registration and with other sources of information such as autopsy reports, increasing the information flow between different sources and thus helping to overcome problems of under reporting and misclassification. In the United Kingdom, this approach forms the basis for the regular Confidential Enquiries into maternal deaths.

The system of Confidential Enquiries into maternal deaths was first established in England and Wales in 1952, following on early enquiries initiated by the Ministry of Health in 1928 — a time of increasing concern about stagnant or rising levels of maternal mortality despite improvements in infant mortality and in environmental conditions. The system, which continues to this day, permits the health authorities to assess whether factors associated with maternal deaths were avoidable and to attribute responsibilities for these factors. The incidence of avoidable factors has been relatively steady, at around 50–60 per cent, though standards of assessment are increasingly high. Since 1979–81, the term "substandard care" has been used instead of avoidable factors, in order to take into account not only failures in clinical care but also other factors which might have adversely affected care, including shortages of resources for the provision of staff and administrative failures in the service or in the provision of backup services such as anaesthesia, radiology or pathology.

In recent years the enquiries have used more sophisticated statistical methodologies. They have, however, been handicapped by a relative lack of comprehensive morbidity data which makes it difficult to assess whether reductions of deaths from an individual cause has resulted from reduced frequency of the disorder or from better management of a similar number of cases (Department of Health 1989 and 1991). This problem is relevant to the discussion of causes of maternal deaths and to the estimation of long-term disabilities which follow in later chapters.

The confidential enquiry is not identical to the maternal death audit though both have a number of features in common. The death audit is often a routine procedure following a maternal death in a facility and is usually confined to a particular institutional setting. Audits are undertaken following other pregnancy-related events such as perinatal deaths or life-threatening complications or "near misses". The audit differs from the confidential enquiry largely in terms of coverage and in terms of who instigates and is responsible for the sustainability of the process. The confidential enquiry, as understood in the United Kingdom, is instigated by the public health authorities, brings together the information from all health facilities and consists of an audit of *all* providers of care. The report of the enquiry is then reviewed by independent assessors who add their comments and opinions regarding the cause of death and the contribution of substandard care. Reports presented to the assessors are made anonymous in order to ensure confidentiality.

It is this feature which permits the confidential enquiry to move from being simply a descriptive study of each maternal death to become a tool for improving quality of care. For example, the 1991–1993 Confidential Enquiry in the United Kingdom identified substandard care in 45 per cent of maternal deaths, with deficiencies in hospital care in 33 per cent of cases, in general practitioner care in 6 per cent and in patient compliance or actions in 11 per cent of cases (Hibbard et al. 1996). The report makes specific recommendations on better information and counselling for women, improvements in clinical services and staff deployment, availability of consultant care for the management of patients with existing diseases and on the use of standard management protocols for the management of particular problems such as sepsis and haemorrhage. Furthermore, the report comments on the importance of maintaining adequate records and recommends legislative changes to facilitate the reporting of maternal deaths by the introduction of a question related to pregnancy status on all death certificates.

Establishing and maintaining a system of confidential enquiries not only ensures that all maternal deaths are correctly classified as such but also permits a detailed analysis of the avoidable factors leading up to the death and identifies common problems in health care systems and practice that can be addressed. It also serves as a way of guarding against complacency. The very low levels of maternal mortality currently reported in many industrialised countries and the regular declines that have been registered over the past 20–30 years, have led many to assume that the "irreducible minimum" levels of maternal mortality are now being reached. The United Kingdom Confidential Enquiry cautions against this belief, pointing out that the continuing high proportion of deaths in which substandard care is a factor show that it is unjustified.

The medical audit can also become a mechanism for improving the quality of care if the identification of substandard care is accompanied by interventions to address the underlying reasons for it. Building a feedback component into the audit turns it from simply a descriptive tool to a more proactive, quality enhancing one. In countries where a comprehensive system of confidential enquiries is not an option on practical grounds, medical audit at the level of the individual facility is a useful way of enabling health personnel to make an honest appraisal of quality of maternal health care (Bhatt 1989).

Intermediate between countries with good vital registration and those where there is no or incomplete coverage of registration, there are many countries where the registration of deaths is fairly complete but registration of the cause of death is poor (World Health Organization 1993a). Maternal mortality figures based on data derived from such systems can be extremely misleading — in some countries as many as 63 per cent of women's deaths are without specified cause. In such settings, a system of epidemiological surveillance can be helpful in identifying maternal deaths that have been misclassified as non-maternal and in following up to determine causes and avoidable factors.

Population-based data

Where civil registration is incomplete or nonexistent, other sources of information and other methods have to be used. A variety of approaches has been tried with varying success; some of them are described below. Each method has its advantages and its drawbacks and not all approaches are feasible in all settings. It is possible to visualize a hierarchy of situations depending on the sort of records available and the degree of contact between the health system or other infrastructure and the population of childbearing women. These will range from countries such as Bangladesh, where some 95 per cent of the births are attended by untrained birth attendants or family members and no civil registration exists (Bangladesh, Ministry of Health and Population Control 1985) through countries like Niger, with good PHC records and poor civil registration (Thuriaux and Lamotte 1984) Brazil with 75 per cent coverage of civil registration (World Health Organization 1993a) and India, with a 1 per cent sample registration system (India, Ministry of Home Affairs 1981).

Household surveys

Maternal mortality can be measured by incorporating questions into ongoing (large-scale) household inquiries. It is possible to ask questions on pregnancy status and to make one or several repeat visits later to ascertain the pregnancy outcome (Greenwood et al. 1990). Alternatively, retrospective surveys ask questions about deaths of female household members during a specified time period and whether the death was associated with pregnancy or childbirth. Respondents can be husbands, parents, other family members, neighbours and community health workers. Such a survey in Addis Ababa was based on a sample of households to identify births, abortions and deaths over a defined period of time (Kwast et al. 1985). These were then followed up and details of care received, social and other characteristics of the women and households, as well as circumstances and causes of deaths were recorded.

A variant of the retrospective approach asks household members about possible maternal deaths occurring in other households and subsequently visits those households to interview relatives of the deceased women. This approach was used in Kenya where women interviewed in a child survival survey were asked whether they knew of any women who had died from maternal causes in the preceding year (Boerma and Mati 1989). The technique, known as networking, is promising for use in well defined geographic areas.

The problem with these approaches is the large number of households that have to be contacted in order to derive reliable estimates of maternal mortality. The Addis Ababa study interviewed more than 32 300 households to identify 45 deaths and an estimated maternal mortality ratio of 480. At the 95 per cent level of significance this gives a sampling error of about 30 per cent, i.e. the ratio could lie anywhere between 370 and 660. In another study in Indonesia, investigators visited 150 000 households, and recorded 15 000 births to identify 50 maternal deaths (Agoestina and Soejoenoes 1989). A prospective study in Gambia followed 672 women and identified 15 maternal deaths (Greenwood et al. 1987).

The problem with household surveys for studying maternal mortality is the very small numbers of deaths that are identified. This is inevitable because even in high mortality settings, maternal deaths are relatively rare events. For example, in a setting with a total population of 500 000, a crude birth rate of 35 per 1000 and an estimated maternal mortality ratio of 500 per 100 000 live births, only 88 maternal deaths would be expected in a given year. Assuming an average household size of 5, it would be necessary to visit 100 000 households to identify all the deaths.

One way around this problem is to increase the time period over which deaths are reported. The study in Addis Ababa used a two-year recall period. However, recall is likely to diminish over time; this could be a problem particularly if information is sought on the circumstances surrounding the death in order to identify it as maternal and to ascertain the cause of death.

Because of the small numbers of deaths reported, the analysis of the deaths becomes problematic also. Both the numbers of deaths and the ratios are likely to fluctuate widely from year to year and it is not possible to deduce anything about trends or about the effectiveness of interventions to reduce maternal mortality. Moreover, small numbers of deaths preclude the investigation of key differentials.

Another problem with such population-based enquiries is the simple omission of events. Respondents may be reluctant to talk about the death of a woman for a variety of emotional, social and cultural reasons. Because maternal deaths are comparatively rare, and because pregnancy and childbirth are surrounded by tradition and taboo in all countries, the reporting of maternal deaths is less accurate than the reporting of infant deaths. And in many settings, the loss of the mother may entail the break up of the family unit and render the reporting of the event extremely unlikely.

Sisterhood techniques

The major drawback of using household surveys is the expense involved. Household surveys are not a cost-effective way of measuring maternal mortality. However, it may be possible to add questions on maternal deaths on to demographic or household surveys. A recently developed technique which makes the most of the information so obtained is the *Sisterhood* method (Graham et al. 1989). The method uses the proportion of sisters who died from maternal causes to estimate a lifetime risk of maternal mortality and using additional information on fertility the maternal mortality ratio is estimated. The method is based on a number of assumptions about representativity of the respondents, age distribution of siblings and respondents and distribution of maternal deaths by age. This methodology offers a solution to the problem of precisely defining a population group about which a respondent can usually provide information while, at the same time, minimising the number of households which must be visited in order to obtain information on a large number of women.

The original indirect methodology asks all adults in a household survey questions about the survival of their sisters. Respondents are asked four questions:

- the number of sisters (born to the same mother) who have reached the age of 15 years and were ever married (or, where relevant, cohabiting);
- the number of those sisters who are still alive;
- the number of sisters who have died;
- the number of deceased sisters who died while they were pregnant, during childbirth or within six weeks of termination of pregnancy.

This information, along with the five-year age group of the respondent, provides the basic information for the calculation of life-time chances of dying from maternal causes and hence into estimates of maternal mortality by a series of mathematical calculations. Most sisterhood studies have restricted the respondents to women, probably on the grounds that they are more likely to recall pregnancy-related events that happen to their sisters than are brothers.

One practical feature of the method is that it does not require intensive efforts to eliminate double-counting because the sisterhood method is based on a proportional relationship. The number of living sisters who are counted more than once is, in practice, matched proportionately by repeat counting of sisters dying of maternal causes.

An interesting recent development in the use of the indirect sisterhood method is its application to a health facility-based sample. The results compare well with those derived from a household sample (Danel et al. 1996). This represents a low cost and efficient application of the method.

The sisterhood method assumes that contact between siblings is maintained throughout their lives. Where this is not, in fact, the case (for example, where women leave the maternal home on marriage and migrate to a different part of the country) there may be problems with its application. It also assumes that patterns of fertility for the appropriate period are known, relatively stable and high (total fertility rate of at least 3). An important weakness in the estimate derived using the sisterhood methodology is that it pertains to a point in time approximately 12 years prior to the survey. Furthermore, the mortality estimates are a weighted average of mortality conditions over a lengthy period of time and the degree to which they are an approximate reflection of current mortality levels is uncertain.

The Demographic and Health Surveys have been using a variant of the sisterhood approach termed the "direct approach" because no assumptions or models are used in the process for converting the collected data into estimates or mortality. The method requires more detailed data and necessitates a longer interview with each respondent than is needed for the indirect method (Rutenberg and Sullivan 1991).

The data collection procedure involves listing all siblings of the respondent and then obtaining information on:

- the survivorship of each;
- the ages of the survivors;
- the ages and dates of death of deceased siblings;
- whether the deaths of deceased sisters were due to maternal causes.

The direct estimation procedure involves computing the number of person-years of exposure to maternal mortality and the number of maternal deaths, then dividing the number of deaths by the person-years of exposure to calculate maternal mortality. The "direct" approach was seen as having a number of advantages over the original Graham and Brass indirect method. Because it involves taking sibling survivorship histories it requires fewer assumptions than the indirect method and is based on data that can be crossed-checked against other sources of information allowing for quality checks, particularly for completeness and plausibility. And because it includes information about the time period during which the sisters died it is possible to calculate maternal mortality rates and ratios for specific reference periods of interest, for example, for earlier or later periods. In theory, this would permit the method to be used to monitor changes over time.

An internal evaluation of experience in the use of the direct method is currently underway by DHS. This has brought to light some issues which need to be taken into account in interpreting the results (Stanton et al. 1996b). For example, an important assumption underlying the direct sisterhood approach is that respondents are able to accurately report the ages at death of their siblings and the time elapsed since death. In fact, it seems that in some DHS surveys a proportion of data relating to years since death is missing. There also appears to be heaping of the reported deaths (usually around the turn of a decade or quinquennium).

A more worrying feature of the direct approach relates to the way it has been used to generate estimates of maternal mortality for two sequential time periods, usually some 7–13 and 0–6 years preceding the survey date and the tendency of users to interpret the two figures as indicative of time trends in maternal mortality. An examination of data for selected countries shows that the ratios derived using the direct method for the two time periods appear to fluctuate in unexpected ways. In some cases, there is a pattern of increasing maternal mortality ratios for the later period compared with the earlier one. Some of the increases are of the order of 50 to 100 per cent. Although a real deterioration in maternal mortality rates in recent years cannot *a priori* be excluded, other explanations are possible and need to be examined before any conclusions are drawn. In any event, great care is needed in interpreting the data relating to the two time periods because of the relatively small sample sizes involved.

Sisterhood methods (indirect and direct) have been used in a variety of settings with varying degrees of success. The original approach by Graham and Brass was developed with rather specific intentions in mind. These included the desire to develop a methodology that would provide a rough estimate of the level of maternal mortality to serve as a stimulus for action and which was suitable for use in settings where no alternative methodology could be used. It was intended to be low-cost and suitable as an add-on to existing household surveys. It was never intended that it should be used to monitor developments over the short or even medium term. Nor was it thought of as a tool for producing a precise figure for maternal mortality.

Although the indirect methodology is relatively simple, care is, nonetheless, needed in its use. The data collection instrument needs careful pilot-testing in order to be sure that respondents have a true understanding of the term "sister" in the vernacular; in many settings the word "sister" is understood far more broadly than is generally the case in Europe and North America. Attention to translation, quality of interviewer training, the understanding that respondents have questions and their purpose, can make the difference between a maternal mortality estimate that is accepted and well received and one that is not considered credible by the local population — an important consideration when the estimate is needed for advocacy purposes (Filippi 1996). Moreover, the authors of the method have stressed that it should not be used in certain settings where the underlying assumptions used to convert the responses into estimates of mortality cannot be assumed to hold, for example in zones affected by war, high migration or other rapid health or demographic changes.

The direct method also has features which may limit its usefulness in some circumstances (Stanton et al. 1996b). The additional time needed to conduct each interview, though in theory modest (around 10 minutes) tends to come at the end of an already fairly lengthy questionnaire and may well tax the patience and understanding of interviewer and interviewee alike. For this reason, additional training and supervision of interviewers is needed. The considerable volume of information gathered using the direct method adds complexity to the data processing though it does permit data checking.

A final word of caution about all variants of the sisterhood method. Both direct and indirect methods will tend to underreport early pregnancy deaths, particularly those related to abortion or those that occur among unmarried women. These issues will always be difficult to address and under reporting of abortion-related mortality is common to all currently available methods for measuring maternal mortality.

A direct validation study of the indirect sisterhood method for data collection on maternal deaths was recently completed in the Matlab area of Bangladesh (Shahidullah 1995a). This area is unique in having had a Demographic Surveillance System (DSS) in operation since 1966. Reporting of maternal and non-maternal deaths of sisters by respondents was compared with DSS classification of deaths. Of the 384 maternal deaths for which siblings were interviewed, 305 deaths (79 per cent) were correctly reported, 16 (4 per cent) were not reported and 63 (16 per cent) were misreported as nonmaternal deaths. Misreporting was most likely for all women when induced abortion was the probable cause of death and for deaths to women who were unmarried when they became pregnant and died. It is probable that deaths related to direct obstetric causes have the best chance of being reported in a sisterhood survey (Shahidullah 1995b).

Questions remain about the possibility that sisterhood methods may underestimate female adult mortality and, by implication, maternal mortality as well. For example, in Egypt, the maternal mortality ratio using indirect estimation was 170 per 100 000 live births (Abdel-Azeem et al. 1993). This compares with 174 pe r 100 000 found in a recent nationwide survey (Ministry of Health, Child Survival Project, in cooperation with USAID, Egypt 1994). However, the former study refers to 1976 whereas the latter refers to 1992. Although 16 years separate the two estimates, the maternal mortality ratios are quite close. This is suggestive of underreporting of maternal deaths in the Egypt sisterhood survey, as infant mortality fell by 50 per cent over the period and fertility fell by 25 per cent.

Reproductive age mortality surveys (RAMOS)

Perhaps the most successful way of measuring the extent and causes of maternal mortality is to identify and investigate the causes of all deaths of women of reproductive age. This technique has been used successfully in countries as different as Guinea (Thonneau et al. 1992), Honduras (Castellanor et al. 1990) and Jamaica (Walker et al. 1986). In Honduras, the maternal mortality ratio was found to be four times that based on civil registration. How the deaths are identified differs according to the records and/or the types of knowledgeable informants available. All successful studies use multiple and varied sources of information —civil registers, hospitals and health centres, community leaders, schoolchildren, religious authorities, undertakers, cemetery officials etc. A general finding has been that no single source identifies all the deaths.

Where reasonable civil registration systems exist, death certificates alone are a useful starting point for identifying deaths of women of reproductive age. This was successful in some countries in Latin America in the 1960s and has lately been widely used elsewhere. A panel of medical specialists then establishes whether or not the death was pregnancy related from hospital records and/or from symptoms reported by the family of the deceased.

Complete recording of births is not very common in countries without registration systems. Nevertheless, a maternal death is a sufficiently memorable event for it to be possible to gather (numerator only) information on the number of maternal deaths occurring in a given area. In a study in Bangladesh (Rochat et al. 1981), specially trained interviewers visited health facilities (maternal and child health centers, family planning clinics, hospitals etc.) throughout Bangladesh to obtain reports about pregnancy-related deaths. Of the nearly 2000 deaths reported only 40 per cent were from hospitals. Family planning workers in rural clinics recalled more such deaths than did health workers in hospitals. Because family planning workers are most likely to know about reproductive health conditions they can be a very useful source of information. Even so, a comparison with the expected number of maternal deaths (using a previous estimate of the maternal mortality ratio for Bangladesh) showed considerable under-reporting of maternal deaths (Chen et al. 1974).

The latter study had used record matching of adult female death reports based on repeated household surveys coupled with live birth records to estimate maternal mortality patterns and levels in a rural area of Bangladesh. Admittedly, this type of study is only possible for relatively small populations subject to intense field surveillance of vital events. Nonetheless, inasmuch as the district (Matlab Thana) was thought to be reasonably representative of health conditions throughout the country, this form of sample vital registration yielded extremely useful information and the resulting estimate of 570 maternal deaths per 100 000 live births remained the definitive estimate for Bangladesh until more recent community studies (Khan et al. 1986) showed even this to be on the low side.

A similar approach using field interviews was used to investigate causes of death among women of reproductive age in Egypt and Indonesia, (Fortney et al. 1984) in India (Bhatia et al. 1988), in Jamaica (Walker et al. 1986) and in Bangladesh (Alauddin 1986, Khan et al. 1986). These studies differ from that done earlier in Bangladesh (Rochat et al. 1981) in one important aspect—non-medically trained persons were used to interview the families of the deceased. In the Indonesian study, family planning field workers were trained to carry out the interviews. In the Egyptian study, where vital registration of death in the reproductive ages is likely to be reasonably good (National Research Council Committee on Population Development and Demography 1981), deaths to women aged 15–50 in the study area of Menoufia were first identified through the vital registration system. Interviews with the family of the deceased (most often the husband) were conducted on average between 30 and 40 days after death to ascertain the symptoms. The interview schedules were then given to a panel of medical specialists for diagnosis. To estimate the maternal mortality ratio in the district, the annual number of live births was derived by applying estimated age-specific fertility ratios for Egypt as a whole to projections of the female population of Menoufia at these ages based on the latest available census results. The resulting estimate of maternal mortality was 263 per 100 000 live births, compared with the national ratio of maternal mortality, based on civil registration, of 79 three years earlier (United Nations, various years). Looked at another way, the "official" ratio was less than one third of that found in Menoufia, a relatively privileged area of Egypt. A more recent, nationwide study of all deaths of women of reproductive age in Egypt found a maternal mortality ratio of 174 per 100 000 live births (Ministry of Health, Child Survival Project 1994). This represents a ratio almost three times higher than the civil registration figure of 60 reported for 1987 (World Health Organization 1990).

In Indonesia family planning workers were asked to list all deaths in their villages during the previous month. This method proved less successful, as only about half the estimated number of deaths were traced; those taking place in remote areas being under-represented (Fortney et al. 1984). In the Bangladesh studies, which covered two rural areas, traditional midwives were asked to report all births and deaths of women of reproductive age. These were followed up by supervisors who interviewed close relatives to ascertain the circumstances surrounding the death, including menstrual history preceding the death (to identify cases of early pregnancy and abortion) (Alauddin 1986, Khan et al. 1986).

In Jamaica, multiple sources of information were used to identify deaths of women of reproductive age (hospitals, civil registers, schools, mortuaries etc.). Each death was then investigated to determine cases. A notable feature of these two studies was that no single source of information uncovered all the deaths (Walker et al. 1986).

All these inquiries used lay reporters and interviewers and a review panel who, after examining the lay reports (the symptoms leading to the death), assigned the cause of death to ICD categories. A similar procedure, but using health professionals as interviewers and tracing the deaths back through the health care system was used some 20 years earlier to investigate the causes of adult mortality in 12 cities in the United Kingdom, North and South America (Puffer and Griffith 1967). In every city it was found that maternal deaths had been under-enumerated. Overall, some 30 per cent of the final assignments to maternal causes had not originally been so classified. In eight cities the additions to maternal causes represented over 1/4 of the final assignments.

RAMOS-type studies are generally considered the "gold standard" for estimating maternal mortality. However, it has to be stressed that they can only be so when considerable efforts are expended on identifying *all* maternal deaths using multiple sources of information.

Health services data

Numerous community studies testify to the fact that good records at the primary care level can provide all the information necessary for computing infant mortality ratios for specific communities. Theoretically maternal mortality ratios can be calculated in the same way. The only difficulty is that of numbers. Even in countries with high maternal mortality ratios a maternal death is a relatively rare event and to establish a maternal mortality ratio of, for example, 300, correct to within 20 per cent (95 per cent confidence level), would require a sample size of 50 000 births!

In the absence of civil registration or other population-based data many researchers use hospital data to estimate maternal mortality. There are limitations to this approach and estimates calculated on hospital data alone tend to be unrepresentative. In general, the smaller the proportion of births taking place in hospital the greater the discrepancy between the true — usually unknown — community ratio and the hospital ratio. The reason for discrepancies between hospital and community mortality ratios is that either the numerator (the women who died), or the denominator (the women who gave birth in hospital), or both, are not a representative sample of all maternal deaths and of all women giving birth, respectively.

The bias found in ratios from hospitals is due to two factors. A large proportion of the women who die in hospitals are emergency admissions, women who had intended to give birth at home but who were transported to hospital when they developed a life-threatening condition. Often they arrive too late and their deaths swell the number of hospital deaths. Women who gave birth safely at home do not, of course, appear in the denominator. This phenomenon emerges very clearly when hospital data are divided into booked and unbooked patients. At the Black Lion Hospital in Addis Ababa, Ethiopia, for example, the overall maternal mortality ratio in 1980–81 was 960, but for booked patients it was 210 compared with 1050 for unbooked patients (Horvarth and Muletta 1982).

Bias also arises because of the way referral systems function. If a referral system is working efficiently most high-risk women — at least those who present themselves for prenatal care — are referred to the hospital for delivery. This means that among the women giving birth at the hospital there is a disproportionate number with obstetric complications, and hence of women who die there. It is not possible, therefore, to estimate the degree of bias introduced into the maternal mortality ratio as a result.

A third source of bias inherent in hospital ratios is that of socioeconomic selection. If a hospital is fee-paying or caters for patients with a certain type of insurance, e.g. private clinic, military hospital, it will attract economically advantaged women. Such hospitals may have a lower maternal mortality ratio then that prevailing in the community. Public, non fee-paying hospitals and charity institutions such as mission hospitals and clinics are likely to serve relatively poorer socioeconomic groups who may be less well-nourished, have more existing and untreated diseases, and make less effective use of medical services when problems arise during or after pregnancy and childbirth with resulting higher maternal mortality ratios.

Hospital data must be used cautiously for cause of death information. In general, emergency complications from which women die quickly (e.g. haemorrhage), will be under-represented because many women will not reach the hospital in time. A study in Bangladesh showed that only 1 of the 58 deaths identified took place in hospital, and this was from eclampsia whereas the majority of deaths at home were from haemorrhage (Bhatia 1988). Deaths occurring early in pregnancy, (e.g. abortions, ectopic pregnancies), may not be included because they occur in a different part of the hospital.

Hospital studies can, however, shed valuable light on avoidable factors, especially those related to quality of medical care. Several studies have used hospital deaths as a starting point in tracing back the path followed by the dead woman — her prenatal care, who attended the birth, problems encountered in transport, financial and social barriers to the use of services, as well as shortcomings in the health care system (Mbaye and Garenne 1987).

Computer matching of deaths of women with births and fetal deaths and then with their hospital records in the United States has, with the help of suitable controls, made it possible to evaluate the treatment they received (Centers for Disease Control, 1991).

Case-control studies for the study of the causes of maternal deaths require a very careful matching of controls, in the absence of which the study will only show the obvious — that the cases developed complications and the controls did not! — or that the cases were older, multiparous, poorer etc. Matching with women developing similar complications but who survived would yield much more useful results.

Table 3 summarizes the advantages and disadvantages of these various ways of measuring maternal mortality.

The burden of disease due to maternal deaths and disabilities

Maternal mortality

The difficulty of measuring maternal mortality has long been an impediment to progress in alerting health planners and others to the magnitude and causes of the problem and hence to effective interventions on an appropriate scale. In an attempt to fill the information gap the WHO Maternal Health and Safe Motherhood Programme has collected all available information and studies on maternal mortality for all countries and assembled the information in a computerized database. The database also covers related aspects of maternal health including coverage of maternity care; unsafe abortion incidence and mortality; anaemia in women; infertility; low birth weight; and perinatal mortality. Tabulations of the main indicators derived from the databases are issued periodically. A more comprehensive account of maternal mortality, causes of maternal deaths, avoidable factors and high risk groups was published in the form of country profiles in 1992 (AbouZahr and Royston 1991).

The data collected and analysed in the databases are by no means uniform in terms of quality or presentation. It is, therefore, difficult to make direct comparisons across time or between countries. Moreover, because the sources usually relate to sub-national levels, extrapolating to the national level is rarely possible.

Estimating maternal mortality

As already noted, the maternal health databases have served as the foundation for the development of model-based approaches to estimating maternal mortality. In 1994 WHO and UNICEF decided, in view of the increasing amounts of data now available from a series of sisterhood, household and other studies, to make a new attempt to develop estimates that could be used at both regional and global but also at national levels.

The model was developed in two stages. Initially, the approach used was similar to the earlier modelling strategy already described. Maternal mortality ratios for countries with no reliable national data were estimated using widely available predictor variables such as female life expectancy at birth, levels of contraceptive prevalence, coverage of prenatal and delivery care, percent GNP spent on health, and physicians per 100 000 population.

The problem with this approach was collinearity among the predictor variables. Once female life expectancy at birth was entered into the model none of the other process indicators remained significant. Thus, the model essentially predicted the maternal mortality ratio as a function of female life expectancy which is itself often modelled on the basis of estimates of child mortality!

The second approach was to model the proportion of maternal deaths among all deaths of women of reproductive age (15–49 years). Evidence from a number of community studies indicates that this proportion varies widely, from less than 1 per cent in industrialised countries to nearly 50 per cent in under served rural areas (Table 4). The model of the proportion of maternal deaths among women of reproductive age (PMDF) was estimated for countries with acceptable information on maternal mortality and the model was then used to predict the proportion of deaths of women of reproductive age that are maternal in countries without reliable national data.

The advantages of this approach are that the predicted proportion of deaths of women that are maternal can be applied to countries with complete death registration but incomplete attribution of cause. It also permits the use of the data derived from sisterhood studies.

The use of the maternal mortality ratio as the dependent variable in a model intended to predict values for countries lacking empirical observa-

Table 3 Methods of measuring maternal mortality - a comparison of strengths and weaknesses

Method	*Strengths*	*Weaknesses*
Vital registration		
	Complete coverage of births and deaths (>90%)	Coverage may be incomplete
	Cause of death attribution for all deaths	Cause of death attribution may be inadequate
	Data available on a regular basis (annually)	Pregnancy status may not be noted on death certificates
	Appropriate for monitoring indirect causes	ICD difficult to use for maternal deaths, particularly for indirect causes
	Serves as starting point for regular review of maternal deaths (confidential enquiries)	Tends to underreport maternal deaths because of misclassification
Household survey		
	Can be used where vital registration is non existent or inadequate	Large sample sizes needed for reliable estimates of maternal mortality
	Provides relatively current estimate	Expensive and time-consuming
	Can be used to gather information on causes, time and place of death, health-care seeking behaviour etc (with verbal autopsy)	Possible omission of deaths when recall period is long
		Not suitable for monitoring trends because confidence limits tend to be wide
Sisterhood method (indirect)		
	Four simple questions can be added to multipurpose surveys	Care needed in the use of the questions (translation, verification etc)
	Minimal sample size requirements compared with household surveys and other direct methods (all other things being equal and for same levels of precision, interviews needed with 5 500 households compared with 324 800 households for direct household survey)	Recall likely to be problematic when events took place many years earlier
		Provides retrospective not current estimate
		Not appropriate for use in populations with extensive migratory flows
		Adjustment factors may not always be appropriate in low fertility settings
	Simple calculations involved	Not appropriate for monitoring
	Additional useful information can be gathered on place/time/cause of death	
	Can be adapted for use at facilities	

Table 3 *(continued)*

Method	*Strengths*	*Weaknesses*
Sisterhood method (direct)	A few simple questions can be added to multipurpose surveys Smaller sample size requirements compared with household surveys Sibling survivorship information permits data quality checks Simple calculations involved Can be used to provide more recent estimates than the indirect sisterhood method No assumptions about patterns of fertility needed	Adds considerably to length of questionnaire Problems of recall, particularly of years elapsed since sister's death Separate time period estimates subject to wide standard errors Does not provide information about causes or other relevant circumstances Not appropriate for monitoring or for analysis of time trends
RAMOS	Can be used in a range of settings (where vital registration is incomplete or nonexistent) Provides information on cause of death, avoidable factors, high risk groups etc.	A range of different sources of information on reproductive age deaths needed to ensure complete coverage Time consuming and complex Not appropriate for regular monitoring
Facility data	Generally available even in countries with low levels of institutional infrastructure Individual facility data can be used as starting point for in-depth case reviews of maternal deaths and for audits Can be used to monitor progress in a particular facility on the assumption that there are no other changes that might affect levels of mortality (changes in catchment populations etc.) Can be used as starting point to stimulate improvements in quality of care	Not appropriate for calculation of ratios unless nearly 100% of births are registered Both numerator and denominator data will be biased and the direction of bias impossible to determine Medical records often poorly maintained and incomplete Unless "no name — no blame" philosophy widely accepted, there may be a tendency to misrepresent or alter medical records in an effort to avoid blame for any death Generally provides denominator data only

Table 4 Maternal deaths as a per cent of all deaths among women of reproductive age (PMDF); evidence from community studies

Setting	*Year of study*	*Maternal deaths as % of all deaths of women of age 15–49*	*Source*
Bangladesh, Matlab Thana	1976–52	37	Koenig et al. 1988
India, Andhra Prandesh Rural	1984–85	28	Bhatia 1988
India, Andhra Prandesh Urban	1984–85	38	Bhatia 1988
Indonesia, Bali	1980–82	23	Fortney et al. 1985
Egypt, Menoufia	1981–83	23	Gadalla 1984
Morocco	1980	29	DHS 1992
Guinea-Bissau	1989–90	41	Osterbaan and Barreto da Costa 1991
Honduras	1990	22	Pan American Health Organization 1995
United Kingdom	1992	0.7	World Health Organization 1994

tions could lead to the estimation of negative values. To avoid this possibility, a log transform of the dependent variable was used.

Two criteria were applied in the selection of independent variables, namely availability of the data for the majority of the countries for which predictions were needed, and some *a priori* association with maternal mortality. One obvious candidate for inclusion is an indicator of fertility: the more births there are each year, the higher the proportion of deaths of women of reproductive age that are related to pregnancy is likely to be, other things being equal. The fertility measure used was the general fertility rate — total births divided by the number of women of reproductive age. The more common indicator, total fertility rate, was not used because it is an age-standardised measure. General fertility rate, not being age standardised, corresponds better to the proportion maternal which is simply maternal deaths divided by total reproductive age deaths and is not age-standardised.

It was considered important to include among the independent variables, one indicative of health service access. The variable with the fewest missing values was the percentage of births assisted by a trained health worker (doctor, nurse, midwife). Reasonably good measures for this indicator are available for developing countries through Demographic and Health Surveys and similar exercises. These have been incorporated into the WHO database. However, doubts remain as to the quality of this indicator. For example, there is concern in some settings that the definition of trained attendant is poorly applied and that the indicator may, in practice, include traditional birth attendants with minimal training and who are unlikely to have the skills needed to detect and manage life-threatening obstetric complications.

A number of dummy variables were included in the model to control for possible sources of variation. The "Gold standard" dummy takes a value of 1 for estimates of the proportion maternal deemed most accurate (developed countries after adjustment by a factor of 1.5, sisterhood estimates and RAMOS studies). For all remaining counties this dummy takes a value of zero. Additional dummy variables were included to allow for a secular trend (a dummy variable set to 1 for all pre-1970 data) and region. One dummy variable was used to identify developing countries.

The final model of the proportion of maternal deaths among all deaths in women of reproductive age (PMDF) is as follows:

$$0.5*\ln(PMDF/(1\text{-}PMDF)) = \beta_0 + \beta_1\ln(GFR) + \beta_2 TRATT + \beta_3 GOLDSTAND + \beta_4 REGLDC + \beta_5 PRE70$$

where GFR is the general fertility rate, TRATT is the proportion of live births attended by trained health personnel (1983–93), GOLDSTAND is a data quality dummy variable taking a value of 1 for developed countries (after adjustment), sisterhood and RAMOS data, REGLDC is a dummy variable for an estimate from a developing country, PRE70 is a dummy variable for developed country estimates prior to 1970 (Stanton et al. 1996).

The observations for estimating the model, national level maternal mortality data, were taken from the WHO maternal health database. The selected data came from a variety of sources including Reproductive Age Mortality Surveys, DHS Sisterhood surveys, other sisterhood surveys, other sample surveys, and civil registration. Depending on the availability of data, maternal mortality estimates from civil registration data represent the average estimate for a three to five year period.

Because of concern about the accuracy of measures of maternal mortality derived from civil registration data, an adjustment factor was applied to all civil registration estimates. In theory, the size of the adjustment should vary according to an evaluation of the likely accuracy of the estimate. Studies in developed countries suggest that, even with good reporting, maternal mortality ratios are biased downwards by incorrect attribution of cause (see Table 2). Thus, an adjustment factor of 1.5 was applied to the civil registration estimates for the countries with good vital registration systems.

The results of the model are shown in Table 5.

The variables included in the model are all highly significant and all have the expected sign. Thus, the proportion of maternal deaths is higher where fertility is higher, lower if the proportion of births with a trained attendant is higher, higher in developing than in developed countries and higher prior to 1970 than more recently.

Table 5 Coefficients for model of PMDF

Independent variable	*Coefficient*	*Standard error*	*t*	*P-value*
ln(GFR)	0.5612	0.1320	4.25	0.000
% trained attendant	-0.0096	0.0025	-3.89	0.000
Gold standard	0.2455	0.0974	2.52	0.015
Pre-1970	0.6277	0.0984	6.38	0.000
Developing country	0.6976	0.1288	5.42	0.000
Constant	-4.0052	0.7066	-5.67	0.000

Dependent variable: ln(PMDF/(1-PMDF)), where PMDF is the proportion of maternal deaths of all deaths of females aged 15–49 years; Number of observations: 49; R^2= 0.939

The outcome of interest for prediction is not the proportion maternal itself, but rather the implied number of maternal deaths and the maternal mortality ratio. Predicted values for each country are obtained in one of five ways, depending on data availability and assumptions about data quality. The strategy adopted was one involving making best use of good, national data about maternal mortality and using predicted values only for countries without adequate national figures.

Maternal mortality estimates for individual countries thus fall into five groups:

A *Developed countries with complete vital registration systems and attribution of cause of death* — For these countries the maternal mortality ratio is the reported number adjusted by a factor of 1.5 to account for misclassification of maternal deaths. The 1.5 adjustment factor is based on evidence from several studies, e.g. Bouvier-Colle et al. 1991 and Atrash et al. 1995.

B *Developing countries with good death registration but poor or non-existent attribution of cause of death* — The model is used to predict the proportion of deaths of women of reproductive age that are maternal. This proportion is then applied to the deaths of women of reproductive age actually registered to obtain the number of maternal deaths and the maternal mortality ratio.

C *Countries with RAMOS type estimates of maternal mortality* — The maternal mortality ratio derived from the *RAMOS* study is used directly without any adjustments.

D *Countries with sisterhood estimates of maternal mortality* — The sisterhood method, in addition to providing an estimate of maternal mortality, also provides estimates of the *proportion* of all deaths of women of reproductive age that are maternal. Insofar as the *sisterhood method* identifies *all* pregnancy-related deaths which may include some due to fortuitous or accidental causes, it may over-estimate maternal mortality. However, the method is likely to miss some early maternal deaths such as those related to abortion or ectopic pregnancy. It has been assumed that the two biases cancel out. Therefore, for these countries, this *observed proportion* was applied to the total number of deaths of women of reproductive age generated by the United Nations Population Division's population projections (1994 Revision) for the year 1990 since these are believed to be better estimates of female adult mortality.

E *Countries with no estimates of maternal mortality* — For countries without accurate information on numbers of deaths and without direct or indirect estimates of maternal mortality, the model is used to predict the proportion maternal of all deaths of women of reproductive age and this proportion is applied to the 1990 United Nations projections of adult female deaths to derive the maternal mortality ratio.

Table 6 presents the number of maternal deaths and the predicted maternal mortality ratios for 1990 by United Nations regions.

A number of caveats are needed in using the results of this approach particularly when comparing countries.

- The model is estimated from data collected over a period of several years around the late 1980s and early 1990s, and the key programmatic variable included in the model (trained attendant at delivery) does not refer to a common time point.
- In most countries, the deaths of females of reproductive age are obtained from United Nations projections for 1990. This envelope of deaths may or may not be correct.
- The model is estimating the relationship between the proportion maternal and a set of predictor variables for a particular time period; there is no reason to suppose that this relationship is immutable over time.
- The standard errors associated with the predicted maternal mortality ratios are very large; they cannot, therefore, be used to monitor trends. The figures pertain to the year 1990 and should be seen as a recalculation of the earlier 1991 revision rather than as indicative of trends since then. For all of these reasons the individual country estimates should be treated with caution. The estimates provide orders of magnitude not precise values.

This new approach is primarily intended to be of use in countries with no estimates of maternal mortality or where there is concern about the adequacy of officially reported estimates. The intention was to draw attention to the existence and likely dimensions of the problem of maternal mortality. The estimates should be taken as indicating orders of magnitude rather than precise estimates and are not necessarily what governments consider most appropriate. The results for each country should serve

Table 6 Revised 1990 estimates of maternal mortality according to United Nations regions

	Maternal mortality ratio (maternal deaths per 100 000 live births)	*Number of maternal deaths*	*Lifetime risk of maternal death=1 in*
World total	430	585 000	60
More developed regions *	27	4 000	1800
Less developed regions	480	582 000	48
Africa	870	235 000	16
Eastern Africa	1060	97 000	12
Middle Africa	950	31 000	14
Northern Africa	340	16 000	55
Southern Africa	260	3 600	75
Western Africa	1020	87 000	12
Asia *	390	323 000	65
Eastern Asia	95	24 000	410
South-central Asia	560	227 000	35
South-eastern Asia	440	56 000	55
Western Asia	320	16 000	55
Europe	36	3 200	1400
Eastern Europe	62	2 500	730
Northern Europe	11	140	4000
Southern Europe	14	220	4000
Western Europe	17	350	3200
Latin America & the Caribbean	190	23 000	130
Caribbean	400	3 200	75
Central America	140	4 700	170
South America	200	15 000	140
Northern America	11	500	3700
Oceania *	680	1 400	26
Australia-New Zealand	10	40	3600
Melanesia	810	1 400	21

*Australia, New Zealand and Japan have been excluded from the regional totals but are included in the total for developed countries.

Editorial note: These estimates have not been subjected to the Global Burden of Disease validation algorithms (see Murray and Lopez 1996) and hence are not comparable to other mortality estimates for 1990 presented in this chapter.

as a stimulus to action and to help mobilize national and external resources to this end.

Calculation of maternal mortality estimates for the Global Burden of Disease Study

The revised estimates of maternal mortality described here were calculated using the United Nations estimates for deaths of women of reproductive age and live births. In calculating the total number of maternal deaths for the Global Burden of Disease Study different denominator data are used

Table 7 Proportion maternal of deaths of women reproductive age by World Bank region — WHO/UNICEF estimates for 1990

Region	*PMDF (%)*
Established Market Economies	0.7
Formerly Socialist Economies of Europe	2.9
India	23.3
China	5.0
Other Asia and Islands	20.8
Sub-Saharan Africa	29.1
Latin America and the Caribbean	9.9
Middle Eastern Crescent	23.6

and the model predictions have been adjusted accordingly. The proportion maternal of all deaths of women of reproductive age was calculated for World Bank regions (Table 7) and applied to World Bank estimates of total reproductive age deaths; maternal mortality ratios were calculated using World Bank estimates of live births for the year 1990.

In the Global Burden of Disease Study calculations, the epidemiological data on mortality was used by the authors to derive regional and global mortality estimates. When considered in conjunction with mortality estimates proposed by other authors for other diseases and injuries, the implied level of overall mortality usually exceeded the rate determined by various demographic methods. In order not to exceed this upper bound for mortality within each age -sex and broad cause group, an algorithm has been applied by the editors to reduce mortality estimates for specific causes so that their sum did not exceed the upper band.

There are important differences between the estimates of maternal mortality issued by the World Health Organization and those published in the context of the Global Burden of Disease Study. These result from several factors. First, as already noted, the World Bank regional groupings used in the Global Burden of Disease Study differ from the United Nations regional groups as do the estimates of the overall numbers of live births. In particular, the World Bank regional groups tend to result in higher weighting of births and maternal deaths in sub-Saharan Africa compared with Asia or Latin America and the Caribbean.

A second issue relates to the Global Burden of Disease Study (GBD) methodology itself which forces the attribution of cause of death to a single cause (Murray and Lopez 1996). This is problematic for the identification of maternal deaths which are often of multiple etiology, particularly in the case of indirect causes of maternal death. Deaths of pregnant women associated with malaria, hepatitis, anaemia and cardiovascular conditions — conditions that can occur at any time but which may be aggravated by pregnancy and its management — tend to be attributed to the disease rather than to maternal causes. It is likely, therefore, that the GBD methodology underestimates the contribution of indirect causes of maternal mortality. Furthermore, the GBD calculations focused on five direct pregnancy-realated complications, namely, postpartum haemorrhage, puerperal infections, hypertensive disorders of pregnancy, obstructed labour and unsafe abortion; estimates for other direct causes such as antepartum haemorrhage, ectopic pregnancy, embolisms and anaesthesia complications were not attempted because of lack of sufficient data. Estimates for specific indirect causes of maternal mortality and disability were also not made.

Incidence of, and mortality from specific obstetric complications

The WHO bibliographic reference databases include information about causes of maternal death. Unfortunately few studies collect information on cause of death in a standard format or follow the categories of causes of death defined in the International Classification of Diseases.

Nevertheless, subsequent chapters in this volume describe the estimated incidence of the five major obstetric complications, based on a combination of available epidemiological evidence and clinical judgement. The detailed references underpinning these estimates are described in the individuals chapters following. A summary of incidence of and mortality from the five major obstetric complications is given in Table 8.

It should be noted that the incidence of complications refers to cases, not women. Many women experience more than one complication during pregnancy. In these calculations, every effort has been made to avoid double counting. Thus it is assumed that the incidence of haemorrhage

Table 8 Estimated global incidence and mortality from main obstetric complications worldwide

Obstetric complications	Incidence (per 100 live births)	Number of cases (millions)	Number of deaths (000s)	% of all maternal deaths
Haemorrhage	10.0	14.5	114	25.1
Sepsis	8.4	12.0	68	15.0
Hypersensitive Disorders of Pregnancy	5.0	7.1	57	12.6
Obstructed labour	5.1	7.3	34	7.5
Unsafe abortion	13.9	19.8	61	13.4
Other maternal	12.0	17.1	121	26.4
Total		77.6	454	100

* estimated number of events, not women

Note: This is a global estimate and may vary in different settings. Figures may not add to totals due to rounding

Source: *Maternal Health and Safe Motherhood Programme*, Unpublished estimates, 1993

reflects only obstetric haemorrhage and excludes haemorrhage related to abortion and that the incidence of sepsis does not include abortion-related sepsis.

In calculating the global burden of disease it has been assumed that each complication is a discreet event, and therefore that complications arise in some 54 per cent of pregnancies ending in a live birth. The severity of the complication will, of course vary and WHO estimates that almost 15 per cent of all women develop complications serious enough to require rapid and skilled intervention if the woman is to survive without lifelong disabilities (World Health Organization 1995a). At country level, these estimates vary widely. In community-based studies in Guatemala and Indonesia between one quarter and one third of women reported complications (Bailey et al. 1994, Alisjahbona et al. 1995).

We have calculated mortality and morbidity only from the five major causes of maternal mortality in developing countries. However, we estimate that some 8 per cent of maternal deaths are related to other direct causes such as ectopic and molar pregnancies, anaesthetic complications, cerebrovascular accidents, and embolisms. Very little is known about the incidence of these complications and many of them have complex etiologies and multiple chains of causation.

Other considerations in calculating burden

The focus on five main causes of maternal mortality and the major morbidities associated with each (haemorrhage, infection, eclampsia, obstructed labour and unsafe abortion) means that no attempt has been made to include disability arising from other direct causes of maternal death (such as ectopic pregnancy) or from indirect causes (such as cardiovascular diseases or diabetes) with the exception of anaemia which has been included as an outcome of severe haemorrhage.

In the United States, ectopic pregnancy is an important cause of maternal mortality and morbidity during the first trimester: it accounted for 12 per cent of all such deaths from 1979–86 (Nederlof et al. 1990). Although case fatality rates in the United States have decreased by 90 per cent since 1970, incidence has increased fourfold from 4.5 to 16.8 ectopic pregnancies per 1 000 deliveries during the first 17 years of surveillance. These increases have also been observed in European countries, including the UK and Sweden. Data on ectopic pregnancy incidence in developing countries are limited: rates derived from hospital-based African studies have ranged from 4.8 to 23.2 ectopic pregnancies per 1 000 deliveries (Liskin 1992). Ectopic pregnancy is known to be associated with reproductive tract infection including sexually transmitted diseases, and postpartum or postabortal sepsis.

A comprehensive coverage of the burden of obstetric mortality and morbidity would need to address both direct and indirect causes of deaths and disabilities as well as at least a proportion of so called "fortuitous" causes and psychological conditions related to pregnancy and childbirth.

Direct conditions would include temporary, mild or severe conditions which occur during pregnancy and within 42 days of delivery (such as haemorrhage, eclampsia or sepsis) or permanent/chronic conditions that persist beyond the puerperium (such as obstetric fistula, urinary or faecal incontinence, scarred uterus, pelvic inflammatory disease, palsy, Sheehan's syndrome). Urinary and foecal incontinence following childbirth appear to be far more common than suspected hitherto, with studies finding some 6 per cent of postpartum women affected by urinary stress incontinece (Dimpfi et al. 1992) and 4 per cent by foecal incontinence (MacArthur et al. 1997). Some chronic conditions such as hypertension can be caused or aggravated by pregnancy and delivery, but may have other causes too.

Indirect conditions result from existing disease (such as anaemia, malaria, hepatitis, tuberculosis, cardiovascular disease) that is aggravated by the physiologic effects of pregnancy. Indirect obstetric morbidity may occur at any time and continue beyond the reproductive period. For example, to the extent that breast cancer progresses more rapidly during pregnancy, it should also be included here.

In the past, mortality and morbidity arising from "fortuitous" or "accidental" causes were not included under pregnancy-related causes of death or disability. More recently, because of the difficulty in distinguishing between conditions that are exacerbated by pregnancy and those which are not, and in determining whether external causes (suicide, violence) are pregnancy-related, it is proposed that this category be included under maternal mortality and morbidity.

Psychological obstetric morbidity includes puerperal psychoses, postpartum depression ("baby blues"), suicide or strong fear of pregnancy and childbirth that may be the result of obstetric complications, interventions or cultural practices.

The severity weights assigned to time spent in different health states for the Global Burden of Disease Study are based on preference measurement exercises in which the participants are asked to take into consideration the average level of disability that stems from a condition. The decision to assess the severity of health states based on a global average level of disability arose out of a desire to treat like outcomes as like, regardless of the setting in which they arise or of the circumstances of the individual concerned. While it was made on the grounds of equity, the result is to downplay factors that may weigh heaviest on those unable to take effective measures to mitigate the effects of disability. Where the social consequences of a disability are much greater than the global average, for example infertility in societies where women are valued largely in terms of their fertility, the GBD calculations may underestimate the burden of a condition.

Similarly, a vaginal discharge may not cause handicap in most societies; however, in societies with stringent rules about "purity" and "cleanliness" and regulations surrounding what women can and cannot do at different times during the menstrual cycle, a vaginal discharge or intermittent bleeding can cause major problems. In some cultures, women are barred from the preparation of food during menstruation or during periods of "uncleanliness" such as when there is a vaginal discharge. Vaginal discharge in women may be interpreted as due to sexually transmitted disease and viewed as a sign of infidelity. This leads women to hide the symptoms and inhibit them from seeking treatment.

PREGNANCY AS A RISK FACTOR FOR OTHER DISEASES

Pregnancy aggravate other diseases such as malaria, anaemia, jaundice, tuberculosis or heart disease. If the woman dies as a result, the death is classified as an indirect maternal death. Sometimes, more than one disease or condition is involved. For example, both anaemia and malaria worsen during pregnancy and malaria itself may cause anaemia or aggravate an existing anaemic condition.

Severe anaemia in pregnancy is a major obstetric problem in malaria endemic areas. Where stable transmission of *P. Falciparum* is the rule, women of childbearing age have generally acquired a relatively high degree of immunity to the parasite through repeated exposure. During pregnancy, particularly first pregnancy, through mechanisms that are not fully understood, women have an increased susceptibility to *P. Falciparum* and experience a higher frequency and density of parasitaemia. Because the incidence of malaria is often seasonal, complications during pregnancy will tend to cluster during certain times of the year.

Another contributor to anaemia during pregnancy is hookworm. While the helminth itself is unlikely to cause death, it further aggravates existing anaemia which is seriously debilitating and can be fatal for pregnant women.

The early stages of anaemia in pregnancy are often symptomless. However, as haemoglobin concentration falls, oxygen supply to the vital organs declines and the expectant mother begins to feel weak, tired and dizzy. Pallor of the skin and mucous membranes as well as of the nail beds and tongue, is not usually apparent until haemoglobin falls to 70 g/l or lower. As haemoglobin falls further most tissues of the body become starved of oxygen and the effect is most marked on the heart muscles which may fail altogether. Death from anaemia is the result of heart failure, shock or infection exacerbated by the patient's impaired resistance.

While less severe anaemia may not cause death directly, it can contribute towards death from other causes. Anaemic women do not tolerate blood loss to the same extent as healthy women. During childbirth, blood loss of up to one litre will not kill a healthy woman, but in an anaemic woman, much smaller loss can be fatal. Anaemic women are poor anaesthetic and operative risks. Following surgery, wounds may fail to heal promptly.

Viral hepatitis is another disease to which pregnant women seem particularly susceptible. Studies from Ethiopia and the Islamic Republic of Iran, for example, have found that the incidence of viral hepatitis in pregnant women is twice that in non-pregnant women (Tsega 1976, Borhanmanesh et al. 1973). Pregnant women are also more seriously ill and more likely to die. Case-fatality rates are up to 3.5 times higher than in non-pregnant women (Tsega 1976, Borhanmanesh et al. 1973). Viral hepatitis is an epidemic disease. In 1983 in Addis Ababa, Ethiopia, it was the third most important cause of maternal deaths (Kwast and Stevens 1987).

Viral hepatitis in the fulminating form occurs most commonly during the third trimester of pregnancy. Premature labour, liver failure and severe haemorrhage commonly complicate this form of the disease and the infant is unlikely to survive. Fatal haemorrhage is triggered by acute liver failure. In this condition, the blood loses its ability to clot, and bleeding occurs not only through the genital tract but also into other sites such as the stomach, intestines, mucous membranes and injection sites in the skin and muscle.

In expectant mothers with sickle cell disease, the last four weeks of pregnancy, labour and the first week after delivery are particularly dangerous. Deaths result from the effects of embolism, anaemia and bacterial infections.

Sexually transmitted diseases during pregnancy are risk factors for certain complications, particularly for sepsis. Infection with HIV and AIDS is associated with both increased incidence of sepsis and also with higher case-fatality rates. Anecdotal evidence from a number of countries indicates that antibiotic-resistant sepsis is common in HIV positive women, and that post-caesarean section infections are more common in HIV positive women (Semprini et al. 1995).

There is evidence from a number of studies that pregnancy is associated with an increased incidence of domestic violence. In some cases, violence against women, including homicide, is related to the fact of the pregnancy being unwanted because the woman is not married or is suspected of having an extra-marital relationship (Fortney 1984). Studies in India and China have found that women are at increased risk of violence if they produce a child of the "wrong" sex, that is a girl. In Matlab Thana, Bangladesh, homicide and suicide motivated by the stigma of rape, pregnancy outside marriage, or dowry problems accounted for 6 per cent of 1139 maternal deaths between 1976 and 1986 (Fauveau and Blanchet 1989). The figure rises to 21.5 per cent if deaths due to unsafe abortions are included, many of which are also related to shame over extra-marital pregnancies.

Intentional injury was also found to be a significant cause of maternal deaths among women in Chicago, Illinois, United States. Trauma accounted for 46 per cent of maternal deaths between 1986 and 1989, of which 57 per cent were due to homicide and 9 per cent to suicide (Fildes et al. 1992). A random sample of 342 women living near Mexico City revealed that 20 per cent of those battered reported blows to the stomach during pregnancy (Shrader and Caldez 1992).

Pregnancy — particularly unwanted pregnancy — is also a risk factor for mental illness, particularly depression, and for suicide. Motherhood represents a major change in the life course and there is growing evidence that many women suffer considerable psychological distress in the 12 months after childbirth. The relative risk for a woman to be admitted to a psychiatric hospital with a psychotic illness in the first month after childbirth is about 22 times greater than in any of the 24 months preceding delivery; such an admission is 35 times more likely after the first baby (Kendell et al. 1989).

The increased incidence, coupled with the short delay between childbirth and the onset of illness, and the early symptoms of perplexity and confusion suggestive of an organic disturbance, add weight to the primary etiology being physiological with psychological and social factors of secondary importance (Dennerstein et al. 1993).

Postpartum psychological disorders include postpartum "blues," postpartum psychoses, postpartum depression and disorders of the mother-infant interaction. The reported incidence of postpartum blues has ranged from 15 per cent to 84 per cent in various studies (Oakley and Chamberlain 1981). Most authors have concluded that the condition is a benign and transient disturbance. Postpartum psychosis, by contrast, is a more severe disturbance which may occur with a frequency of 1–2 per 1 000 births. The condition is reported from countries as diverse as Saudi Arabia, Tanzania, Nigeria, Senegal, United Kingdom and the United States (Dennerstein et al. 1993).

Impact of interventions on disease burden

Historical evidence permits an assessment of the impact of interventions on the burden of disease due to pregnancy-related conditions. Data from the United Kingdom, for example, indicate that substantial reductions in maternal mortality were not achieved until the late 1930s, although general living standards and nutrition had been improving for several decades previously. At the turn of the century, maternal mortality ranged from 400–600 per 100 000 live births. Substantial and sustained reductions in maternal mortality became possible following the application of measures to prevent infection, the availability of sulphonamides, the advent of antibiotics, safe blood transfusions and caesarean deliveries, and better management of eclampsia. Until 1935, maternal mortality ratios in England and Wales remained at some 400 per 100 000 live births (MacFarlane and Mugford 1984).

Further back in time, ratios as high as 1 000 per 100 000 appear to have been common. In eighteenth century France and Sweden the ratio was over 1 000 per 100 000 births (Gutierrez and Houdaille 1983, Hogberg 1985).

The earliest documented reports of a decline are from Sweden where maternal mortality fell significantly from over 400 per 100 000 births during the 1860s to under 200 per 100 000 by the early 1900s following improvements in midwifery practice.

More recently, Sri Lanka witnessed significant decreases in maternal mortality in a relatively short period. From levels of over 1 500 in 1940–45 and 555 per 100 000 live births in 1950–55, maternal mortality fell to 239 per 100 000 ten years later and to 95 per 100 000 in 1980 (Nadarajah 1983, Ministry of Plan Implementation 1981). These declines followed the introduction of a system of health centres around the country accompanied by the expansion of midwifery skills and the spread of family planning. During the 1950s most births in Sri Lanka took place at home with the assistance of untrained birth attendants. By the end of the 1980s, only 30 years later, over 85 per cent of all births were attended by trained people and 76 per cent took place in an institutional setting.

An analysis of causes of maternal death in Sri Lanka over the period 1953 to 1968 shows that the decline was most rapid among sepsis deaths. At the beginning of the period one-quarter of all non-abortion deaths were due to sepsis. By the end of the period the proportion had fallen to 10 per cent (Vidyasagara 1985). Unlike the rapid decline in deaths from sepsis, deaths from haemorrhage declined more slowly, particularly in the early years. Haemorrhage as a cause of death is less easy to prevent because of the short time between the onset of serious bleeding and death.

Similar evidence for the effectiveness of health care interventions is available from Cuba and China. Both countries established community-based maternal health care systems comprising prenatal, delivery and postpartum care and a referral system for complications. Cuba set up maternity waiting homes where pregnant women who lived far from a health facility could await delivery close to a health centre or hospital (Ministerio de Salud Publica 1990). In China, a widespread campaign to raise awareness about the need for clean delivery resulted in a massive fall in sepsis-related mortality. Haemorrhage continues, however, to present problems in rural areas with scattered populations where access to health care is difficult (Zhang and Ding 1986).

The evidence from the historical record and from developing countries today indicates that health care is the critical factor in reducing maternal mortality. However, in both instances other changes were taking place that almost certainly helped to improve maternal health and increase the chances of survival. These include better nutrition, increasing education, improved status of women and substantial reductions in fertility.

Fertility reduction is an important component of all efforts to reduce maternal mortality. Increased contraceptive prevalence helps reduce maternal deaths in two ways. First it results in a reduction in the numbers of pregnancies with at least an equivalent reduction in maternal deaths. Second, it can help to limit high risk pregnancies that are particularly associated with risk of mortality — those among very young women, women of high parity and women whose pregnancies are unwanted. However, fertility reduction cannot by itself reduce the risk of death once a woman is pregnant. The maternal mortality ratio — which represent a pregnancy-related risk — can remain high even though the number of maternal deaths falls because there are fewer pregnancies. This was well-illustrated by the experience in Matlab, Bangladesh, where a major family planning programme led to a decrease in the maternal mortality rate (deaths per number of women of reproductive age) and in the number of maternal deaths, but where the maternal mortality ratio (deaths per live births) fluctuated from year to year and there was no evidence of a real decline (Chen et al. 1974, Fauveau et al. 1988).

The Matlab study highlights the importance of health care in reducing the maternal mortality ratio. Another study, though based on very small numbers, illustrates the point in a different way. Among women members of a religious group in the United States which rejected all medical care — prenatal, delivery, postpartum or for treatment of emergencies — but whose members were otherwise of similar social and economic status to others living in the same area, the maternal mortality ratio — 870 per 100 000 live births — was comparable to many developing areas today (Kaunitz et al. 1984).

Such evidence indicates the need to make maternity care accessible to all pregnant women. However, at present only 53 per cent of women in developing countries deliver with the help of a trained person. Many are assisted only by relatives or by traditional birth attendants. Only 40 per cent of women in developing countries deliver in an institutional setting (World Health Organization 1993).

These figures tell only part of the story. Internationally collected data do not clearly define what is meant by a "trained attendant" and in practice the category can cover a range of attendants from specialist obstetricians to auxiliary medical personnel with limited midwifery training. What matters is the availability to the pregnant woman and to the woman in labour of the skills to prevent, detect and manage the major obstetric complications together with the equipment, drugs and supplies to treat them effectively. In the absence of more detailed information as to the quality of the assistance, it cannot be assumed that all women who delivered with a "trained" attendant had effective access to quality obstetric care (World Health Organization 1993b).

Some 65 per cent of pregnant women in developing countries have prenatal care but again, little is known about the quality of prenatal care received. At its best, prenatal care represents an opportunity for the health care provider to treat any diseases, prevent certain conditions common during pregnancy such as anaemia and, most critically, to detect complications early and refer to the appropriate level of care for management.

In practice, much prenatal care in developing countries cannot serve these vital preventive and treatment functions. All too often, the necessary drugs and equipment are absent or only intermittently available. And

Table 9 Maternal mortality, coverage of delivery care and national wealth (selected countries)

Country	*GDP per capita (1992)**	*Trained attendant at delivery (around 1990) (%)***	*Maternal mortality ratio (Maternal deaths per 100,000 live births) (1990)****
Afghanistan	819	8	1700
Guinea Bissau	820	30	910
Somalia	1 001	2	1600
China	1 950	85	95
Honduras	2 000	47	220
Sri Lanka	2 850	94	140
Brazil	5 240	81	220
Costa Rica	5 480	98	55
Mexico	7 300	69	110
Singapore	18 330	100	10
United Arab Emirates	21 830	96	25

* UNDP Human Development Report

** World Health Organization 1993

***WHO and UNICEF 1996

often, time and energy is dissipated in tests and treatments that are of limited effectiveness rather than in those known to work. Because so little information is available on the quality of prenatal care or on the effective skills of so called "trained" birth attendants, it is not possible to assert unequivocally what proportion of pregnant women in the world have access to effective pregnancy management.

On the basis of the evidence available, we have developed a conceptual model illustrating the impact of maternity care on maternal mortality. The model comprises four scenarios (Figure 1 and Table 9).

The first, "best case" scenario assumes near universal access to quality maternity care in socio-economically developed areas such as Europe, North America, Singapore or the United Arab Emirates. In such settings maternal mortality is around 10–25 per 100 000 live births.

The alternative "worst case" scenario assumes a total absence of health care in a poor socio-economic setting (e.g. Afghanistan, Somalia). Here we can expect to find maternal mortality ratios of the order of 1000 per 100 000 live births — ratios found in studies from several parts of Africa, Asia and Latin America (Preserm 1992, de Groof et al. 1993, Koblinsky 1991).

An intermediate scenario is one in which socio-economic indicators are relatively poor but where access to essential health care is available, for example, Sri Lanka (Ministry of Health, Sri Lanka 1987), Jamaica

Figure 1 Maternal mortality at different levels of care

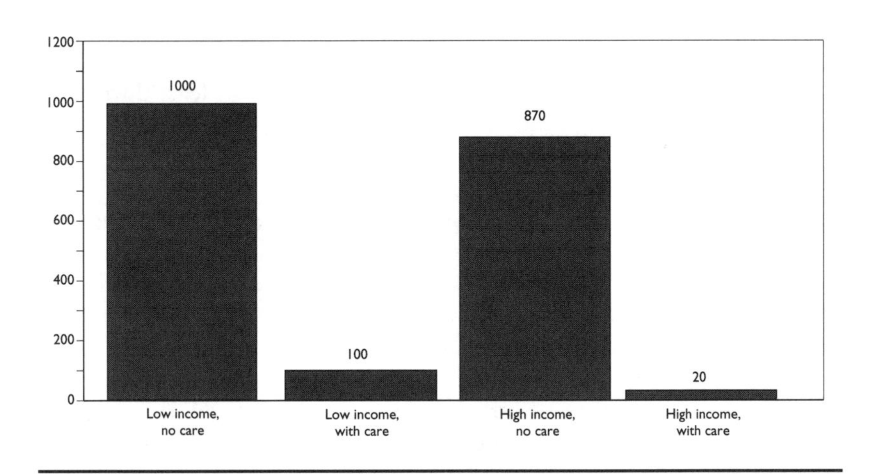

(Golding et al. 1989) and China (Hua 1993). Here, maternal mortality ratios range between 80 and 200 per 100 000 live births.

The fourth scenario assumes high socio-economic development but absent health care (as among the religious group described earlier). Maternal mortality ratios in such as setting appear to be very high at around 850–900 per 100 000 live births.

Conclusions

Estimating deaths and disabilities due to pregnancy-related complications is difficult. Calculation of maternal mortality requires the existence of comprehensive vital registration systems and careful monitoring of both numbers and causes of death. In the absence of such systems, a variety of alternative methodologies has been developed to estimate maternal mortality but these tend to be expensive and time-consuming and remain beyond the material capabilities of most developing countries.

Because of this difficulty, maternal mortality remains a neglected issue. Even where maternal mortality ratios are high, maternal deaths are relatively rare compared with, for example, infant deaths. Such rare events can easily go unnoticed or pass for accidents of fate rather than as symptoms of a neglect of women's health. The process of giving birth was long viewed as a risky affair not amenable to external assistance. This view continues in many parts of the world today and is compounded by a general neglect of conditions that affect women. Where women's status is low, they are often viewed primarily as vehicles for childbearing and their own fate rarely taken into consideration.

The rarity of maternal deaths does not mean that their contribution to the global burden of disease is negligible. While maternal deaths may be relatively infrequent, maternal disabilities are much less so. The calculations presented in the following chapters indicate that for every woman who dies following a pregnancy-related complication, at least thirty suffer disabilities of varying degrees of severity, ranging from anaemia, to reproductive tract infections, infertility and obstetric fistulae.

Moreover, maternal mortality and morbidity have pronounced intergenerational effects. The complications that cause the deaths and disabilities of mothers also damage the infants they are carrying. Of nearly 8 million infant deaths each year, around two-thirds occur during the neonatal period, before the baby is one month old. Every year there are 5 million neonatal deaths of which 3.4 million occur within the first week of life and are largely a consequence of inadequate or inappropriate care during pregnancy, delivery or the first critical hours after birth. And for every newborn death at least one other infant is stillborn. These perinatal and neonatal deaths need to be considered in addition to maternal deaths in estimating the global burden of disease due to pregnancy-related conditions because the conditions that cause the deaths and disabilities of these infants are the same that cause maternal mortality and morbidity (see Table 10). However, the methodology employed by the GBD in the calculation of Disability Adjusted Life Years (DALYs) imputes no healthy year of life lost for stillbirths because counting can start only at birth by definition. Thus, the burden of disease due to perinatal causes does not include late fetal or intrapartum death.

The impact of maternal health status and care may affect the infant well beyond infancy. Birth asphyxia can result in brain damage though further research is needed to quantify the effect of birth asphyxia on cognitive development in later life. There is evidence that poor health status at birth may have long-term physical consequences. Analysis of historical records indicates that retarded fetal growth is associated with an increased risk of mortality from cardiovascular and cerebrovascular diseases in adulthood. The relation between impaired growth in early life and *in utero* is probably due to long term effects on physiology and metabolism imposed by an adverse environment during critical periods of development (Marker and Osmond 1992).

A study of geographical differences in maternal mortality in England and Wales during 1911–14 found that they correlate closely with death rates from stroke in the generation born around that time. "The geographical distribution of stroke is more closely related to past maternal mortality than to any other leading cause of death, past or present, except ischaemic heart disease, for which correlation coefficients with stroke are similar."(Marker and Osmond 1992)

The relationship is restricted to maternal death from causes other than puerperal sepsis which is determined largely by midwifery practices. Other causes of maternal deaths — hypertensive disorders, haemorrhage, ob-

Table 10 How complications affect mother and baby

Problem or complication	*Most serious effects on mother's health*	*Most serious effects on newborn baby/fetus*
Severe anaemia	Cardiac failure	Low birth weight, asphyxia, stillbirth
Haemorrhage	Shock, cardiac failure, infection	Asphyxia, stillbirth
Hypertensive disorders of pregnancy	Eclampsia, cerebrovascular accidents	Low birth weight, asphyxia, stillbirth
Puerperal sepsis	Septicaemia, shock	Neonatal sepsis
Obstructed labour	Fistulae, uterine rupture, prolapse, amnionitis, sepsis	Stillbirth, asphyxia, sepsis, birth trauma, handicap
Infection during pregnancy, sexually transmitted diseases (including HIV)	Premature onset of labour, ectopic pregnancy, pelvic inflammatory disease, infertility	Premature delivery, neonatal eye infection, blindness, pneumonia, stillbirth, congenital syphilis, HIV infection
Hepatitis	Postpartum haemorrhage, liver failure	Hepatitis
Malaria	Severe anaemia, cerebral thrombosis	Prematurity, intrauterine growth retardation
Unwanted pregnancy	Unsafe abortion, infection, pelvic inflammatory disease, haemorrhage, infertility	Increased risk of morbidity, mortality; child abuse, neglect, abandonment
Unclean delivery	Infection, maternal tetanus	Neonatal tetanus, sepsis

structed labour and other accidents of childbirth — are more clearly related to the poor health status of mothers. In the early years of the 19th century poor nutrition and ill-health was common among girls as a result of poverty, the industrial employment of children and inadequate diet. Poor living standards, which accompanied industrialization or economic depression in many areas, adversely affected the development of adolescent girls and impaired their subsequent reproductive performance. Hypertension is one of the possible links between maternal health and stroke in the subsequent generation. A parental history of hypertension increases the risk of hypertension in the offspring and hypertension is a risk factor for stroke.

Research is needed on the complex interactions between maternal health status, care during pregnancy and child birth and long term prognosis in terms of death and disability for the infant. In the absence of adequate evidence, the effects of such linkages have not been incorporated into the calculations for the global burden of disease due to maternal causes. The are, however, likely to be significant.

Aside from considerations of the numbers of deaths and disabilities, there is also the issue of the nature of a maternal death. The mothers who die are in the prime of life, at the summit of their social and economic productivity. They leave behind them families, many with young children, who must now survive without the support of the prime care-giver, producer of food and, possibly, generator of income. Babies who survive the death of the mother seldom reach their first birthday (Boerma and Mati 1989). Older children may have to halt their schooling to look for paid employment or, if they are girls, to care for the rest of the family. A recent study in Kenya, found that of the infants from the pregnancy which led to the death of the mother, only one third were alive and well within a year. Nearly one-quarter of the infants died undelivered and a 15 per cent were dead within a few months of delivery. The remainder of the infants survived but were considered "sickly." (University of Nairobi 1996).

Maternal mortality is an important component of the wider problem of reproductive ill-health, particularly for women. In many developing countries women of reproductive age spend around 60 per cent of their lives either pregnant or lactating. Their health during this prolonged period will affect their health in old age, the health of their children and the well-being of their whole families.

Notes

1 The author wishes to express particular thanks to Elisabeth Åhman who provided invaluable assistance in the preparation of this chapter.

References

Abdel-Azeem F et al. (1993) Egupt maternal and child health survey 1991. *Pan Arab Project for Child Development.*

AbouZahr C, Royston E (1991) *Maternal Mortality: A Global Factbook*. World Health Organization. WHO/MCH/MSM/91.3. Geneva.

Agoestina T, Soejoenoes A (1989) *Technical report on the study of maternal and perinatal mortality, Central Java Province*. Republic of Indonesia, BKS PENFIN/ Ministry of Health.

Alauddin M (1986) Maternal mortality in Rural Bangladesh: The Tangail District. *Studies in Family Planning*. 17:(1)13–21.

Alisjahbana A et al. (1995) An integrated village maternity service to improve referral patterns in a rural area in West Jaun. *International Journal of Gynecology and Obstetrics* 48(suppl):583–594.

Atrash H, Alexander S and Berg C (1995) Maternal mortality in developed countries: Not just a concern of the past. *Obstetrics and Gynecology*. 86(4) (II).

Bailey PE et al. (1994) *Analysis of the vital events reporting system of the maternal and neonatal health project: Quetzalanongo, Guatemala*. Mother Care Working Paper #3. John Snow Inc, Washington, D.C., United States.

Bangladesh, Ministry of Health and Population Control (1985) MCH Task Force. *National Strategy for a comprehensive MCH programme*. Dhaka, Bangladesh.

Bhatia JC (1988) A study of maternal mortality in Anantapur District. *Indian Institute of Management*.

Bhatia JC (1991) Maternal morality: a South Indian Study. In Kessel E et al, eds. *Maternal and infant mortality — closing gap between perinatal health services. Bandung, Indonesia, Proceedings of the 4th International Congress for Maternal and Neonatal Health*.

Bhatt RV (1989) Professional responsibility in maternity care: role of medical audit. *International Journal of Gynecology and Obstetrics*. 30:47–50.

Boerma JT, Mati JKG (1989) Identifying maternal mortality through networking: results from coastal Kenya. *Studies in Family Planning*. 20:245–253.

Borhanmanesh F et al. (1973) Viral hepatitis during pregnancy. *Gastroenterology*. 64.

Bouvier-Colle M-H et al. (1991) Reasons for the underreporting of maternal mortality in France, as indicated by a survey of all deaths of women of childbearing age. *International Journal of Epidemiology*. 20:717-721.

Bouvier-Colle M-H et al. (1994) Les morts maternelles en France. *Les éditions INSERM*. 1994.

Bulterys M et al. (1996) Fatal complications after Caesarean section in HIV-infected women (letter) *AIDS* 10(8):923–924.

Cambell OMA, Graham WJ (1990) *Measuring maternal mortailyut and morbidity: levels and trends*. Maternal and Child Epidemiological Unit, London School of Medicine and Tropical medicine.

Castellanor M et al. (1990) *Mortalidad materna. Investigación sobre mortalidad de mujeres en edad reproductiva con énfasis en mortalidad materna*. Honduras.

Centers for Disease Control (1991) Enhanced maternal mortality surveillance—North Carolina, 1988 and 1989. *Mortality and Morbidity Weekly Report*, 40:469–471.

Centers for Disease Control (1991b) Maternal mortality surveillance —Puerto Rico 1989 *Mortality and Morbidity Weekly Report*. 40:521–523.

Centers for Disease Control (1991c) *National pregnancy mortality surveillance*. Surveillance Unit. Division of Reproductive Health, National Center for Chronic Disease Prevention and Health Promotion, Atlanta, United States.

Chavkin W, Allen M (1993) Questionable category of non-maternal death. *American Journal of Obstetrics and Gynecology*. 168(5):1640–1641.

Chen LC et al. (1974) Maternal mortality in rural Bangladesh. *Studies in Family Planning*. 5(1):334–341.

Da Purificacao Araujo M. (1988) Necessidades nao satisfeutas em saude materna e planeamento familiar, relatorio de um estudo de colaboracao OMS? Portugal. Lisboa, Portugal: Direccao-general de Saude Primarios.

Danel I et al. (1996) Applying the sisterhood method for estimating maternal morbidity to a health facility-based sample: a comparison with results from a household-based sample. *International Journal of Epidemiology*. 26(5):1017–1022.

de Groof D et al. (1993) Estimation de la mortalité maternelle en zone rurale au Niger: utilisation de la méthode indirecte des soeurs. *Annales de la Société Belge de Médicine Tropicale*. 73(4):279–285.

Demographic and Health Surveys (1992) Enquete nationale sur la population et la sante en Maroc (EPNS-II) Ministere de la Sante Publique and DHS (Macro International Inc).

Dennerstein L et al. (1993) *Psychosocial and mental health aspects of women's health* Division of Family Health, World Health Organization, WHO/FHE/MNH/93.1, 1993.

Department of Health (1989, 1991) *Report on Confidential Enquiries into Maternal Deaths in England and Wales 1982–1984 and 1985–1987*, Her Majesty's Stationary Office, London.

Dimpfl T et al. (1992) Incidence and cause of postpartum urinary stress incontinence. *European Journal of Obstetrics, Gynecology and Reproductive Biology*. 43:29–33.

Fauveau V and Blanchet T (1989) Deaths from injuries and induced abortion among rural Bangladeshi women *Social Science and Medicine*, 29(9).

Fauveau V et al. (1988) Impact of a family planning and health services programme on adult female mortality. Health Policy and Planning 3(4):271–279.

Fildes J et al. (1992) Trauma: The leading cause of maternal death, *Journal of Trauma*, 32.

Filippi V (1996) Personal communication.

Fortney JA et al. (1984) *Causes of death to women of reproductive age in Egypt*. Michigan State University Working Paper No. 49.

Fortney JA et al. (1985) *Maternal mortality in Indonesia and Egypt in interregional meeting on the prevention of maternal mortality, Geneva 11-15 November 1985*. Unpublished WHO document FHE/PMM/85.9.13.

Franks AL et al. (1992) Hospitalization for pregnancy complications, United States, 1986 and 1987. *American Journal of Obstetrics and Gynecology*. 166:1339–44.

Gadalla S (1984) Reproductive age mortality survey (unpublished data).

Golding J et al. (1989) Maternal mortality in Jamaica. Socioeconomic factors. *Acta Obstetrica et Gynecologica Scandinavica*. 68(7):581–587.

Graham W, Brass W and Snow RW (1989) Estimating maternal mortality: the sisterhood method. *Studies in Family Planning*, 20:125–135.

Greenwood AM et al. (1987) *A prospective study of the outcome of pregnancy in a rural area of the Gambia*. World Health Organization. 65(5): 635–643.

Greenwood AM et al. (1990) Evaluation of a primary health care programme in The Gambia. I The impact of trained traditional birth attendants on the outcome of pregnancy. *Journal of Tropical Medicine and Hygiene*. 93:58–66.

Gutierrez H, Houdaille J (1983) La mortalité maternelle en France au XVIIIe siècle. *Population*, 6.

Heise LL (1994) *Violence against women: the hidden health burden,* World Bank Discussion Papers 255.

Hibbard BM et al. (1996) *Report on confidential enquiries into maternal deaths in the United Kingdom 1991–1993.* HMSO London.

Hoestermann CFL et al. (1996) Maternal Mortality in the main referral hospital in the Gambia, West Africa. *Tropical Medicine and International Health*; 1(5):710–717.

Hogberg U (1985) *Maternal mortality in Sweden.* Umea Sweden, Umea University.

Horvarth B, Muletta E (1982) *Maternal Mortality in Black Lion Hospital.* Addis Ababa, Department of Gynaecology and Obstetrics, Faculty of Medicine. Unpublished document.

Hua JZ (1993) Chung hua fu chan ko tsa chih. [Women's health care in China.] *Chinese Journal of Obstetrics and Gynecology.* 28(8):453–456.

India, Ministry of Home Affairs, Office of Registrar General (1981) *Vital Statistics of India 1976, (16th Issue).*

Kaunitz AM et al. (1984) Perinatal and maternal mortality in a religious group avoiding obstetric care. *American Journal of Obstetrics and Gynecology.* 150(7).

Kendell RE, Chalmers JC and Platz C (1989) Epidemiology of puerperal psychoses *British Journal of Psychiatry*, 150.

Khan AR et al. (1986) Maternal mortality in Rural Bangladesh: The Jamalpur District. *Studies in Family Planning* 17:(1)7–12.

Koblinsky M (1991) *Inquisvi study, Bolivia.* MotherCare. John Snow Inc.

Koenig MA et al. (1988) Maternal mortality in Matlab, Bangladesh *Studies in family planning*, 19(2):31–21.

Koonin LM et al. (1988) Maternal mortality surveillance, United States, 1980–1985. *Mortality and morbidity weekly reports.* 37(SS5):19–29.

Kwast BE et al. (1985) Epidemiology of maternal mortality in Addis Ababa: a community-based study. *Ethiopian Medical Journal.* 23:7–16.

Kwast BE, Stevens JA (1987) Viral hepatitis as a major cause of maternal mortality in Addis Ababa, Ethiopia. *International Journal of Gynaecology and Obstetrics.* 25.

Liskin LS (1992) Maternal morbidity in developing countries: a review and comments. International journal of gynaecology and obstetrics. 37:77–87.

MacArthur C et al. (1997) Faecal incontinece after childbirth. *British Journal of Obstetrics and Gynaecology.* 104:46–50.

MacFarlane A, Mugford M (1984) *Birth counts: statistics of pregnancy and childbirth.* HMSO London.

Marker DJP and Osmond C (1992) Death rates from stroke in England and Wales predicted from past maternal mortality. In Barker D.J.P. (ed.) *Fetal and infant origins of adult disease*, British Medical Journal, London.

May WJ et al. (1991) Enhanced maternal mortality surveillance. North Carolina, 1988 and 1989. *Mortality and Morbidity Weekly Report* 40(28):469–71.

Mbaye K, Garenne M (1987) *Determinants de la mortalité maternelle à Dakar. Analyse et principaux résultats d'une étude hospitalière.* Unpublished report to the Maternal Health and Safe Motherhood Programme, WHO, Geneva.

Ministerio de Salud Publica (1990) ISCM_H. Facultad de Ciencias Medicas "Julio Trigo" Contribucion de los hogares maternos de Cuba a la maternidad sinriesgo.

Ministry of Plan Implementation, Sri Lanka (1981) Bulletin of Vital Statistics 1979 Department of Census and Statistics, Colombo.

Ministry of Health, Egypt (1994) Child Survival Project, in cooperation with USAID. *National Maternal Mortality Study. Findings and Conclusions. Egypt, 1992–1993.*

Ministry of Health, Sri Lanka (1987) *Maternal Mortality Statistics.* 1987.

Murray CJL, Lopez AD (1996) *The Global Burden of Disease: a comprehensive assessment of mortality and disability from diseases, injuries, and risk factors in 1990 and projected to 2020.* Cambridge, Harvard University Press.

Nadarajah T (1983) The transition from higher female to higher male morlaity in Sri Lanka. *Population and Development Review*; 9(2):317–325.

Nadarajah T (1983) and Minsitry of Plan Implementation (1981).

National Research Council Committee on Population Development and Demography (1981) The estimation of recent trends in fertility and mortality in Egypt. *Research Report. No. 9.* Washington Academy Press.

Nederlof KP et al. (1980) Ectopic pregnancy surveillance. United States, 1970-1987. Morbidity and mortality weekly report. 39(554):9–17.

Oakley A and Chamberlain G (1981) Medical and social factors in postpartum depression, *Journal of obstetrics and gynaecology*, 1.

Osterbaan M, Barreto da Costa MV (1991) A mortalidad materna na Guinea-bissau (unpublished report to the Maternal Health and Safe Motherhood Programme) World Health Organization.

Pan American Health Organization (1995) Evaluacion del plan regional para la deuccion de la mortalidad materna en las america. Informes de lss paises. Washington DC.

Piper JM (1992) Maternal morbidity following childbirth in the Tennessee Medicaid Population. Vanderbilt University School of Medicine (study protocol submitted to CDC Atlanta).

Preserm C (1992) Maternal mortality in Nepal. *Nursing Times.* 88(9):64.65.

Puffer RR, Griffith GW (1967) Patterns of Urban Mortality. *Pan American Health Organization Scientific Publication No. 151.*

Rochat RW et al. (1981) Maternal and abortion related deaths in Bangladesh, 1978-1979. *International Journal of Gynaecology and Obstetrics.* 19:155–164.

Rubin G et al. (1981) The risk of childbearing re-evaluated. *American Journal of Public Health.* 71(7):712–716.

Rutenberg N, Sullivan JM (1991) Direct and indirect estimates of maternal mortality from the sisterhood method. *Demographic and Health Surveys World Conference Proceedings III*. Washington.

Semprini AE et al. (1995) The incidence of complications after caesarean section in 150 HIV positive women. *AIDS* 9(8): 913–917.

Shahidullah M (1995a) The sisterhood method of estimating maternal mortality; the Matlab experience. *Studies in Family Planning*. 26(2):101–106.

Shahidullah M (1995b) A comparison of sisterhood information on causes of maternal death with the registration causes of maternal death in Matlab, Bangladesh. International Journal of Epidemiology; 24:937–942.

Shrader Cox E and Caldez Santiago R. *La violencia hacia la mujer Mexicana como problema de salud pública: La incidencia de la violencia doméstica en una microregion de Cuidad Nexahualcoyotl,* Centro de Investigación y Lucha Contra la Violencia Doméstica (CECOVID), Mexico City, 1992.

Stanton C (1996b) DHS comparative report-preliminary unpublished information and personal communication.

Stanton C et al. (1996a) *Modelling maternal mortality in the developing world* (unpublished).

Thonneau P et al. (1992) Risk factors for maternal mortality: results of a case-control study conducted in Conakry (Guinea). *International Journal of Gynecology and Obstetrics*. 39:87–92.

Thuriaux MC, Lamotte JM (1984) Maternal mortality in developing countries: a note on the choice of a denominator. *International Journal of Epidemiology*. 13(2):246–247.

Tsega E (1976) Viral hepatitis during pregnancy in Ethiopia. *East African Medical Journal*. 53(5).

United Nations. *Demographic Year Book*. Various years.

United States, Department of Health, Education and Welfare. *Methodology for intensive surveillance of pregnancy-related deaths, Puerto Rico, 1978–79*. Atlanta, Centers for Disease Control (undated).

University of Nairobi (1996) Kenya Maternal Mortality Baseline Survey Population Studies and Research Institute, Nairobi, Kenya.

Vidyasagara NW (1985) *Maternal Services in Sri Lanka*. Unpublished paper presented at the Tenth Asian and Oceanic Congress of Obstetrics and Gynaecology. Colombo.

Walker GJ et al. (1986) Maternal mortality in Jamaica. *Lancet* 1(8479):486–488.

World Health Organization (1975) *International Statistical Classification of Diseases. Ninth Revision*. Geneva, World Health Organization.

World Health Organization (1991) Maternal mortality ratios and rates: a tabulation of available information. WHO/MCH/MSM/91.6.

World Health Organization (1992) *International Statistical Classification of Diseases and Related Health Problems. Tenth Revision*. Geneva, World Health Organization.

World Health Organization (1995) Verbal autopsies for maternal deaths. WHO/FHE/MSM/95.15. Geneva.

World Health Organization (1993a) Cause of death statistics and vital rates, civil registration systems and alternative sources of information. *World Health Statistics Annual 1990 and 1993.*

World Health Organization (1993b) Maternal Health and Safe Motherhood Programme. *Coverage of maternity care: A tabulation of available information. Third edition.* WHO/FHE/MSM/93.7. Geneva.

World Health Organization (1994) Maternal Health and Safe Motherhood Programme. *The Mother-Baby Package: implementing safe motherhood in countries.* WHO/FHE/MSM/94.11. Geneva, 1995.

World Health Organization and United Nations Children's Fund (1996) Revised 1990 estimates of maternal mortality.

World Health Organization Statitistics Annual (1994) World Health Statistics Annual.

Zhang L, Ding H (1986) Analysis of cause and rate of maternal death in 21 provinces, municipalities and autonomous regions. *Chinese Journal of Obstetrics and Gynaecology.* 21(4).

Ziskin LZ et al. (1979) Improved surveillance of maternal deaths. *International Journal of Gynecology and Obstetrics.* 16:282–286.

Chapter 4

Antepartum and Postpartum Haemorrhage

Carla AbouZahr

Introduction

Pregnancy-related haemorrhage can occur during pregnancy (antepartum) or after the delivery of the infant (postpartum). Although in developed countries antepartum haemorrhage is no longer a leading cause of maternal death, it continues to be a major cause of both maternal and perinatal morbidity. By contrast, postpartum haemorrhage is a significant feature in maternal deaths in developing and industrialized countries alike.

Both antepartum and postpartum haemorrhage are unpredictable. Although antepartum haemorrhage due to placental abruption has been associated with chronic or pregnancy-induced maternal hypertension this has been disputed in the literature (Fraser and Watson 1989). Antepartum haemorrhage associated with placenta praevia is more common with high parity and among women with previous caesarean deliveries (Barron 1989).

Haemorrhage — particularly postpartum haemorrhage caused by uterine atony — is rapidly fatal unless treatment is instituted rapidly. In many parts of the world where institutional deliveries are the norm, the incidence of postpartum haemorrhage has been reduced as a result of the active management of the third stage of labour, including use of oxytocic drugs. Postpartum haemorrhage, however, remains a serious problem where such drugs are not available. Fatality rates due to haemorrhage are increased where anaemia in pregnant women is widespread. Anaemic women cannot tolerate blood loss and where blood for transfusion is not readily available their condition may rapidly deteriorate. In the absence of screening of blood, there are also serious risks to the woman of transmission of hepatitis and HIV infection.

Definition and Measurement

In the Tenth Revision of the International Classification of Diseases (ICD-10), antepartum and postpartum haemorrhage may be associated with the following categories:

O44 Placenta praevia with haemorrhage.
O45 Premature separation of placenta [abruptio placentae]
O46 Antepartum haemorrhage, not elsewhere classified
  O46.0 Antepartum haemorrhage with coagulation defect
  O46.8 Other antepartum haemorrhage
  O46.9 Antepartum haemorrhage, unspecified
O67 Labour and delivery complicated by intrapartum haemorrhage, not elsewhere classified (including coagulation defects).
O72 Postpartum haemorrhage (associated with retained placenta and retained products of conception and including postpartum coagulation defects)

Postpartum haemorrhage may also be associated with other conditions that may be coded to the following:

O70 Perineal laceration during delivery
O71 Other obstetric trauma (including rupture of the uterus)

The coding system employed in the Tenth Revision of the ICD is quite different from previous ones. More specifically, in the Ninth Revision of the ICD, antepartum and postpartum haemorrhage were classified as follows:

640 Haemorrhage in early pregnancy
641 Antepartum haemorrhage, abruptio placentae, and placenta praevia
  641.0 Placenta praevia without haemorrhage
  641.1 Haemorrhage from placenta praevia
  641.2 Premature separation of placenta
  641.3 Antepartum haemorrhage associated with coagulation defects
  641.8 Other antepartum haemorrhage
  641.9 Unspecified antepartum haemorrhage
666 Postpartum haemorrhage
  666.0 Third-stage haemorrhage
  666.1 Other immediate postpartum haemorrhage
  666.2 Delayed and secondary postpartum haemorrhage
  666.3 Postpartum coagulation defects

As with ICD-10, postpartum haemorrhage may be associated with the following ICD-9 codes:

664 Trauma to perineum and vulva during delivery
665 Other obstetrical trauma

The Eighth Revision of the ICD was less specific than the Ninth and used the following as reference codes:

651 Delivery complicated by placenta praevia or antepartum haemorrhage
652 Delivery complicated by retained placenta
653 Delivery complicated by other postpartum haemorrhage

Antepartum Haemorrhage

Antepartum haemorrhage is bleeding from the genital tract before labour but after early pregnancy. The time boundary between the definition of antepartum haemorrhage and bleeding in early pregnancy was traditionally the 28th week of pregnancy but changes in the concept of viability have tended to move the boundary to earlier in the pregnancy (Barron 1989).

The frequency of antepartum haemorrhage is difficult to assess at the population level, particularly in developing countries as there are no widely accepted diagnostic criteria and ascertainment rates depend on the quality and availability of prenatal care. Low reported incidence may simply mean that some episodes of bleeding, judged by the woman or her attendant to be trivial, do not come to the attention of clinicians and are, therefore, not reported. On the other hand, high reported incidence from some hospitals may be biased by the fact that women with bleeding are more likely to be sent to a referral centre than women without complications. Two community studies carried out in the United Kingdom and the United States some 30 years ago reported an incidence of 3–4.8 per cent (Paintin 1962, Roberts 1970).

Approximately half the cases of antepartum haemorrhage are due to either placental abruption (ICD-10 O44) or placenta praevia (ICD-10 O45). In the other half of cases no precise cause can be identified and the haemorrhage is considered to be of uncertain or indeterminate origin (ICD-10 O46). In some cases the bleeding arises from the lower genital tract and is rarely serious as far as the pregnancy is concerned.

Placental abruption or retroplacental haemorrhage is a major contributor to perinatal mortality. Although associated maternal deaths are rare in developed countries it is thought that they are likely to be high in the developing world where antenatal care is less accessible and often of poor quality and where referral for complications is difficult. In both developed and developing countries placental abruption is a major contributor to maternal morbidity in the form of haemorrhage, shock, disseminated intravascular coagulation and renal failure. Comparable data on the incidence of placental abruption are not available. In the United Kingdom it was found to occur in about 1 per cent of pregnancies (Chamberlain et al 1978). The etiology remains obscure though direct trauma to the uterus is the causative factor in some cases. The risk of placental abruption is significantly higher among smokers.

Placenta praevia is defined as a placenta which is situated wholly or partly in the lower uterine segment. The overall incidence of placenta praevia, calculated from developed country series is 0.55 per 100 pregnancies, ranging from 0.29 to 1.24 per cent of pregnancies (Fraser and Watson 1989). Variations in the reported prevalence are due to differences in definition, the duration of the pregnancy at the time of diagnosis, and the sociomedical characteristics of the population being studied. Maternal mortality associated with placenta praevia is low in developed countries but very little is known about either incidence or mortality in the developing world. A study carried out in the United States from 1979 through 1987 (Iyasu et al. 1993) found that placenta praevia complicated 4.8 per 1000 deliveries annually and was fatal in 0.03 per cent of cases. Both incidence and case fatality rates were higher among black and other minority women and case fatality increased significantly with age and parity.

The characteristic feature of placenta praevia is painless bleeding, usually in the third trimester. In developed country settings where routine ultrasound screening is practiced, many cases of placenta praevia are identified before the occurrence of signs and symptoms. This is unlikely to be the case in most developing countries. Although the first episode of bleeding is often minor, immediate referral is always recommended. Vaginal examination should never be attempted when a placental praevia is suspected as it may provoke serious bleeding.

Postpartum Haemorrhage

Postpartum haemorrhage is usually defined as bleeding from the genital tract of 500 ml or more following delivery of the baby. The choice of 500 ml as the level of blood loss defining postpartum haemorrhage, while arbitrary, is internationally accepted. Often, the loss of 500 ml is not always of great clinical significance. Clinical estimates of the amount of blood lost, however, tend to underestimate the actual blood loss by between 34 and 50 percent (Prendiville and Elbourne 1989). It has been noted that the most common preventable factor in deaths from obstetric haemorrhage is underestimation of blood loss (Boes 1987). One study found that the greater the blood loss, the greater the tendency to underestimate the true amount and the authors suggested that all estimates of blood loss over 500 ml be doubled in order to give more accurate assessments (Levy and Moore 1985).

Clinicians may decide that a lower level of blood loss should be the cutoff point for the institution of therapeutic action, especially where anaemia is prevalent or there are other complicating medical conditions in the mother such as cardiac disease.

Primary postpartum haemorrhage includes all episodes of bleeding occurring within the first 24 hours of the delivery of the baby. Secondary postpartum haemorrhage includes all cases of bleeding occurring more than 24 hours but less than 6 weeks from the delivery.

Table 1 Risk factors for postpartum haemorrhage

Predating pregnancy	*Arising antenatally*	*Arising during labour*
Primigravidity	Placenta praevia	Induced labour
Grand multiparity (5+)	Placenta praevia with previous caesarean section*	Prolonged/obstructed labour
Fibroids		Precipitate labour
Idiopathic thrombocytopenia purpura*	Abruptio placentae	Forceps delivery
	Polyhydramnios	Caesarean section
Von Willebrand's disease*	Multiple pregnancy	General/epidural anaesthesia
Anaemia	Previous third stage complication	Chorioamnionitis*
	Intra-uterine death*	Disseminated intravascular coagulation*
	Eclampsia	
	Hepatitis	

* Associated with high case fatality rate

Source: World Health Organization (1989).

ETIOLOGY

While there are many causes of postpartum haemorrhage, the most frequent are retained placenta, which is associated with between one third and half of all maternal deaths from postpartum haemorrhage, and uterine atony. Retained placenta occurs relatively frequently and has a high case fatality rate. Uterine atony is less frequent but also has a high case fatality rate. Coagulation defects and uterine inversion have high case fatality rates but are relatively rare occurrences. Genital tract injury such as episiotomy, vulval haematoma and "gishiri cuts" carried out by traditional practitioners in some parts of Africa, are more common and may exacerbate bleeding from other causes but alone are rarely causes of severe postpartum haemorrhage. Secondary postpartum haemorrhage may also be caused by chorioamnionitis or retained fragments of placental membranes (World Health Organization 1989).

By definition, blood loss at caesarean section should also be included as cases of postpartum haemorrhage since the amount of blood lost is frequently more than 500 ml. However, most studies of maternal morbidity and mortality conventionally separate the risks and complications of caesarean section from those of vaginal deliveries.

Both the frequency and the case-fatality rate of postpartum haemorrhage are increased among women with certain conditions such as intrauterine death (see Table 1). However, the predictive value of antenatal factors is generally low and only a minority of postpartum haemorrhages have a predisposing factor identifiable in the antenatal period. Some factors, such as primigravidity and grand multiparity are very common and therefore not highly specific when used in screening. On the other hand, comparatively rare conditions such as placenta praevia and/or previous caesarean section, or intrauterine death are very likely to be accompanied by postpartum haemorrhage. The most predictive risk factor is a history of a previous third stage complication for which the risk of postpartum haemorrhage is increased two or three times. Up to one-quarter of multiparae who experience a postpartum haemorrhage have had one in a previous pregnancy.

A number of conditions and characteristics of women which do not affect the incidence of postpartum haemorrhage are known to increase the serious sequelae of haemorrhage. These factors include age over 35 years, anaemia, uterine sepsis and associated medical conditions such as cardiac disease and diabetes mellitus.

Incidence, mortality and disability due to postpartum haemorrhage

Incidence of postpartum haemorrhage

Little information is available from developing countries on the incidence of postpartum haemorrhage. The few studies available indicate substantial variations in incidence, generally due to differences in definitions and in measurement of blood loss. As already observed, even within an institutional setting, underestimation of blood loss is very common. In parts of the world where a large proportion of deliveries takes place in the home with the assistance of family members or traditional birth attendants (TBAs), such underestimation is likely to be even greater. Indeed, many cultural beliefs welcome major postpartum blood loss as a form of cleansing and purification. In such circumstances, there will be long delays before women and their attendants seek skilled assistance (Mutambirwa 1984, Ryan 1981, Thompson 1996). It has been estimated that the time between onset of haemorrhage and death, however, can be as little as two hours, as shown in Table 2 (Maine 1992).

Where many deliveries do not take place in institutional settings, hospital studies of the incidence of haemorrhage are likely to seriously underestimate the true incidence. On the other hand, they will overestimate the incidence of complications that are slower to be fatal and which are, therefore, over-represented in admissions statistics simply because women reached the hospital in time. Thus incidence rates of postpartum haemorrhage derived from hospital studies in such settings are a poor guide to true incidence.

Several studies have been undertaken in developed country settings to ascertain the incidence of postpartum haemorrhage. Because these have been carried out in areas where almost all deliveries take place in a health facility or with the close supervision of a highly skilled midwifery attendant, they do not suffer from this kind of under-reporting. However, the problem of accurate measurement of blood loss has proved to be immensely difficult to deal with. Nonetheless, two studies, one in the United Kingdom and one in Australia, which used a variety of techniques to ac-

Table 2 Estimated average interval from onset to death for major obstetric complications

Complication		*Hours*	*Days*
Haemorrhage	— Postpartum	2	
	— Antepartum	12	
Ruptured uterus			1
Eclampsia			2
Obstructed labour			3
Infection			6

Source: Maine 1992.

curately calculate blood loss, provide good indications of the true incidence of postpartum haemorrhage (McDonald et al. 1993, Prendiville 1988)

The latter study is of particular interest as it made very accurate calculations of blood loss and found that 17 per cent of women experience a blood loss of 500 cc or more and that 4 per cent lost one litre or more. A recent World Health Organization technical working group concluded that around 5 per cent of women delivering vaginally loose more than 1000cc of blood (Table 3) (World Health Organization 1996). The study by McDonald et al. (1993) found a lower incidence of postpartum haemorrhage (loss of 500 cc or more) of 12 per 100 deliveries. A study in Malawi, where women were delivered by TBAs, found a lower incidence of postpartum haemorrhage at 8 per cent (Bullogh et al. 1989). There are two possible explanations. Either the measurement of the amount of blood loss underestimated the true figure or the nature of the delivery was such that blood loss was lower in the Malawi study. A recently completed study in the Philippines found that 8 per cent of women self-reported an incident of severe postpartum bleeding (Demographic and Health Surveys 1994). The questions used to elicit responses on haemorrhage were very specific, referring to episodes of fainting and to uncontrolled bleeding. Taking a weighted average of these results gives an incidence of 10.6 per cent.

More research is needed on whether the incidence of postpartum haemorrhage varies between regions and population groups or by type of delivery. In the absence of evidence of differences in blood loss among different populations, the findings of these studies have been applied to all obstetric populations. For the purposes of these calculations, the estimate of 10 per cent was applied to all live births. It should be noted that the calculations are based on live births rather than deliveries and that this may bias the estimates of the incidence of postpartum haemorrhage downwards because still births are associated with a higher incidence of postpartum haemorrhage.

Table 3 Postpartum blood loss reported in five studies

Country		*Women with Blood loss >500 ml %*		*Study year*
		%	*Number*	
United Kingdom[1]	Active management	*5.9	846	1986
	Physiological management	*17.9	849	1986
Malawi[2]		8.4	2123	1987-88
Australia[3]		17.3	3483	1990-91
Philippines[4]		**7.7	3846	1990-93
El Salvador[5]		**5.8	1830	1991-93
Weighted Average		10.6	12977	

* Management of third stage of labour.
** Self-reported in survey using stringent criteria of severe blood loss.

Sources:
1. Prendiville et al. (1988).
2. Bullough et al. (1989).
3. McDonald et al. (1993).
4. Demographic and Health Surveys (1994).
5. Asociación Demográfica Salvadoreña (ADS) et al. (1994).

MORTALITY FROM POSTPARTUM HAEMORRHAGE

Although little is known about the incidence of postpartum haemorrhage, data on the proportion of maternal deaths due to postpartum haemorrhage are available from a number of community and hospital studies. It is advisable to use community-based data for this purpose where possible because, as already observed, haemorrhage is swift to kill and in countries where access to health facilities is poor, few haemorrhage deaths will take place in the hospital. Both hospital and community studies, however, do indicate a relatively uniform pattern around the world, with haemorrhage being the main cause of maternal deaths in countries as varied as Angola (Ministry of Health, Angola 1990, Rita 1988); Botswana (Botswana Country Team 1990, Gongoro 1988, UN Children's Fund 1989); China (Ni and Rossignol 1994, Wenzhen 1991, Zhang 1991); Egypt (Ministry of Health 1993); Honduras (Castellanos et al. 1991); Indonesia (Agoestina and Soejoenes 1989, Fortney et al. 1985); Paraguay (World Health Organization 1990); Sri Lanka (World Health Organization 1986); and the United States (Berg et al. 1996). On the basis of the community studies it has been estimated that at least 25 per cent of maternal deaths are due to haemorrhage — the majority due to postpartum haemorrhage (Table 4). In view of the paucity of available information it was decided not to attempt to calculate global incidence or mortality from antepartum haemorrhage. The studies conducted on postpartum haemorrhage are presented in Tables 4 and 5.

Epidemiological data on mortality have been used by the author to derive a first set of regional mortality estimates. When considered in conjunction with mortality estimates proposed by other authors for other diseases and injuries in the Global Burden of Disease Study, the implied level of overall mortality usually exceeded the rate estimated by various demographic methods. In order not to exceed this upper bound for mortality within each age-sex and broad-cause group, an algorithm has been applied by the editors to reduce mortality estimates for specific conditions so that their sum did not exceed this upper bound. The algorithm has been described in more detail in *The Global Burden of Disease* (Murray and Lopez 1996a).

Disability following maternal haemorrhage

The two major disabling sequelae resulting from maternal haemorrhage are Sheehan's syndrome and severe anaemia. Table 6 presents the disability weights used in the calculation of Years Lived with Disability (YLDs) and Disability-Adjusted Life Years (DALYs) due to Sheehan's syndrome and severe anaemia. As there is no effective treatment for conditions resulting from maternal haemorrhage, the disability weights used for treated and untreated forms of Sheehan's syndrome and severe anaemia are identical. The distribution of maternal haemorrhage episodes, as well as cases of Sheehan's syndrome and severe anaemia, across the seven disability classes used in the Global Burden of Disease Study are shown in Table 7.

The major disability resulting from non-fatal haemorrhage is Sheehan's syndrome, postpartum pituitary necrosis following obstetric shock. The clinical symptoms include chronic weakness, premature old age, amenorrhoea, loss of pubic hair and mental changes including apathy and confusion. The symptoms may never be severe and may be delayed for several years after the pregnancy. Because of the apathy induced by the disease, few women consult a doctor with such symptoms and the only way to estimate its extent would be to conduct detailed community-based studies. Sheehan, who first identified the syndrome, followed up a series of obstetric patients who had haemorrhage or shock at delivery to find out what percentage actually showed evidence of pituitary insufficiency in the following years. The findings are shown in Table 8. From these data it would appear that some 15 per cent of the survivors from moderate obstetric haemorrhage and about 40 per cent of the survivors from severe or very severe haemorrhage had subsequent hypopituitarism. Of all those with some degree of hypopituitarism, 60 per cent had a severe form (Sheehan 1954).

These figures must, however, be interpreted with great caution. The study did not provide any objective measure of "moderate" or "severe" blood loss. Mention has already been made of the difficulty of accurately estimating blood loss following delivery. The investigation was undertaken before Sheehan's syndrome had been so classified and the true syndrome had to be defined during the course of the study. A more serious consid-

Table 4 Per cent of maternal deaths due to haemorrhage

Region/Country	*No. of Studies*	*No. of Maternal Deaths*	*% Due to Haemorrhage*
India	15	7841	16
China	8	8567	16
Other Asia and Islands			
Bangladesh	5	563	21
Fiji	1	164	37
Hong Kong	3	355	30
Indonesia	4	479	43
Malaysia	4	937	44
Papua New Guinea	3	1 341	25
Philippines	3	3 613	53
Republic of Korea	1	114	20
Sri Lanka	3	2 421	35
Thailand	2	452	16
Sub-Saharan Africa			
Benin	2	319	22
Burkina Faso	1	384	59
Congo	1	120	13
Ivory Coast	3	297	37
Ethiopia	5	446	10
Ghana	2	447	16
Guinea	1	212	43
Kenya	3	284	16
Malawi	3	351	16
Niger	2	330	29
Nigeria	18	2 570	20
Senegal	1	152	21
Sierra Leone	2	134	23
South Africa	3	936	15
Sudan	8	565	18
Togo	2	251	19
Uganda	3	1 048	18
Tanzania	11	1 506	19
Zambia	4	376	16

eration is the extent to which the cases studied were representative of the group originally collected for follow-up. It was not possible to trace all the survivors and no indication is given as to the proportion of women lost to follow-up. Nevertheless, this series is the only such study of survivors currently available. A few studies in Africa have reported cases of Sheehan's syndrome but all have been hospital-based (Bahemuka and Rees 1981, Cenac et al. 1991, Correa et al. 1975, Dano et al. 1982, Ducloux et al. 1976, Famuyiwa et al. 1992, Sankale et al. 1978).

On the basis of these data, we hypothesize an incidence of 2 per cent severe and 2 per cent moderate hypopituitarism following postpartum haemorrhage of 800 cc or more. Assuming a 4 per cent incidence of severe blood loss this would imply a total of over 228 000 cases annually world-wide.

Table 4 *(continued)*

Region/Country	*No. of Studies*	*No. of Maternal Deaths*	*% Due to Haemorrhage*
Latin America and the Caribbean			
Brazil	6	750	20
Chile	4	744	10
Colombia	7	3372	17
Cuba	5	603	6
Ecuador	3	1204	20
El Salvador	2	414	18
Guatemala	2	838	2
Honduras	1	381	33
Jamaica	3	269	20
Mexico	2	1821	24
Paraguay	1	140	31
Venezuela	3	423	17
Middle Easern Crescent			
Algeria	3	383	27
Egypt	9	1541	32
Iraq	2	125	8
Morocco	2	214	29
Pakistan	6	680	23
Tunisia	5	363	29
Turkey	2	661	9

Source: World Health Organization (1991).

Table 5 Maternal mortality due to haemorrhage—community studies (Selected countries, Latest available data)

Country/region	*% of maternal deaths*	*Year of study*	*Reference*
China, 30 provinces	49	1989	Ni and Rossignol 1994
Sichuan province	60	1989-90	
Egypt, National	32	1992-93	Ministry of Health, Egypt 1993
Honduras, National	33	1989-90	Castellanos et al. 1991
Indonesia, Bali	42	1980-82	Fortney et al. 1985
Central Java	46	1986-87	Agoestina and Soejoenoes 1989
Sri Lanka, National*	32	1985	Sri Lanka, Ministry of Health 1987

* civil registration

Table 6 Disability weights used to calculate the burden from obstructed labour, treated and untreated forms.

Disability Weights	*0-4*	*5-14*	*15-44*	*45-59*	*60+*
Sheehan's syndrome	–	–	0.093	0.090	0.087
Severe anaemia	–	–	0.065	0.065	0.065

Table 7 Distribution of episodes of obstructed labour and cases of severe anaemia and Sheehan's syndrome resulting from haemorrhage across the seven classes of disability by age group, females, 1990.

	Disability class						
	I	**II**	**III**	**IV**	**V**	**VI**	**VII**
				Episodes			
0-4	0	0	0	0	0	0	0
5-14	0	0	0	0	0	0	0
15-44	0	0	100	0	0	0	0
45-59	0	0	0	0	0	0	0
60+	0	0	0	0	0	0	0
				Sheehan's syndrome			
0-4	0	0	0	0	0	0	0
5-14	0	0	0	0	0	0	0
15-44	27.50	45.63	9.63	3.50	0.63	0	0
45-59	27.50	45.63	9.63	3.50	0.63	0	0
60+	27.50	45.63	9.63	3.50	0.63	0	0
				Severe anaemia			
0-4	0	0	0	0	0	0	0
5-14	0	0	0	0	0	0	0
15-44	2.50	78.13	16.88	2.50	0	0	0
45-59	2.50	80.63	14.38	2.50	0	0	0
60+	2.50	83.13	11.88	2.50	0	0	0

Table 8 Incidence of symptoms of hypopituitarism in live patients some years after delivery.

Degree of haemorrhage and/or shock at delivery	*Subsequent clinical hypopituitarism*		
	None	**Partial**	**Severe**
None or trivial	90	0	0
Moderate	52	7	2
Severe or very severe	24	11	6

Source: Sheehan et al. 1994

Endocrinologists are likely to be sceptical about such a high figure since patients with hypopituitarism are rarely seen in clinics. Part of the problem is that the very nature of the disease inhibits health care seeking behaviour. Many cases undoubtedly go undiagnosed or misdiagnosed as myxoedema, premature menopause, anaemia or other conditions. To quote: "Some workers believe that postpartum hypopituitarism is rare since few such patients attend gynaecological or endocrine clinics; but Sheehan points out that the patients are not worried about their amenorrhoea and that they rarely consult a doctor, because they are deterred by the apathy and inertia of the disease. Questionnaires are not answered for the same reason. Pituitary cripples have to be looked for at home, especially among women with a history of severe circulatory collapse after postpartum haemorrhage, if the frequency is to be truly assessed." (Lancet editorial 1965)

Certainly it is true that the estimates are based on weak data. The incidence of moderate or severe hypopituitarism could well be half that described by Sheehan. Alternatively, the incidence of severe postpartum blood loss could be lower than the 4 per cent assumed here. We decided to retain the incidence estimated by Sheehan, but to assume that the blood loss involved in Sheehan's syndrome was probably greater than 800 cc. We therefore calculated the incidence of Sheehan's on the basis of an incidence of severe postpartum haemorrhage of 2 per cent, implying some 114 000 cases annually world-wide.

A more common complication of haemorrhage is anaemia. A woman with a normal haemoglobin level at the end of pregnancy who suffers even a normal blood loss (less than 500 cc), will need to make good the loss subsequently if she is to avoid becoming anaemic. (This is in addition to the extra demands for iron imposed by lactation). Where pregnant women are already anaemic, postpartum haemorrhage is likely to aggravate the anaemia and may even be fatal. Of the 14 million cases of postpartum haemorrhage which occur every year, it is reasonable to assume that half will occur to women who are already anaemic (since over half of all pregnant women are anaemic). Thus, a total of 7 million cases of moderate or severe anaemia will occur each year. With each subsequent pregnancy these women are exposed to an ever increasing risk of serious disability or death. Unfortunately, little is known about the complex and interrelated epidemiology and etiology of haemorrhage and anaemia and there is a need for further studies elucidating the relationships. The high incidence of haemorrhage and high case-fatality rates, coupled with the relative frequency of long-term disabilities make haemorrhage — particularly postpartum haemorrhage — a major contributor to the global burden of maternal mortality and disability.

Depending on the condition under study, epidemiological data may be available for incidence, prevalence, case-fatality or mortality. Where data on more than one of these parameters are available, estimates of each of the epidemiological parameters derived from the data may not be internally consistent or consistent with the adjusted mortality rates described above. To ensure that all epidemiological information concerning a given condition is internally consistent, the editors have undertaken extensive analyses using computer models of the natural history of disease described in Murray and Lopez (1996b). The incidence, prevalence, and duration estimates have consequently been revised where necessary. In view of these adjustments to the basic epidemiological estimates originally provided for the Global Burden of Disease Study, the data (presented in the following tables) which have undergone the GBD validation process are the joint responsibility of the authors and the editors.

The estimates of number of deaths, Years of Life Lost (YLLs), YLDs and DALYs from maternal haemorrhage episodes, Sheehan's syndrome and severe anaemia are presented in Tables 9–12.

Impact of interventions on the burden of maternal haemorrhage

Haemorrhage (antepartum and postpartum) is globally the major cause of maternal death and most haemorrhage deaths are due to postpartum haemorrhage which is difficult to predict, prevent and treat. Maternal mortality from haemorrhage continues to be a problem even in countries with good systems of antenatal and delivery care (Bouvier-Colle et al. 1994). Postpartum haemorrhage is unpredictable and often swift to kill. It requires rapid intervention by a skilled health care provider. For this reason, it tends to remain one of the slowest causes of death to respond to maternal care interventions. In both Sri Lanka and China, where a system of primary health care including antenatal and delivery care for pregnant women, has been in place for many years, haemorrhage is still an outstanding problem (Figure 1).

Even in developed countries where the overwhelming majority of births occur in institutional setting with highly trained birth attendants, haemorrhage is one of the leading causes of maternal deaths (Berg et al. 1996). In recent years, significant progress has been made in increasing the availability of life saving management of haemorrhage at the community level. Increased availability of oxytocic drugs is being promoted by many national safe motherhood programs, along with access to modern transport and communications (World Health Organization 1992). Research is underway on the feasibility of delivery of oxytocic drugs at the periphery. While better obstetric care and more timely referral for emergencies will contribute to a reduction in such deaths, a realistic assumption given the current status of maternal care in developing countries is that it will not be possible to reduce haemorrhage-related mortality by more than about 55 per cent by the end of this century (World Health Organization 1994).

Conclusions

Haemorrhage, particularly postpartum haemorrhage, is the leading cause of maternal mortality in both developing and industrialized countries. It also causes significant maternal morbidity and is a major contributor to high levels of anaemia in women of reproductive age. It is difficult to

Figure 1 Maternal deaths by cause (%) in Sri Lanka, 1984

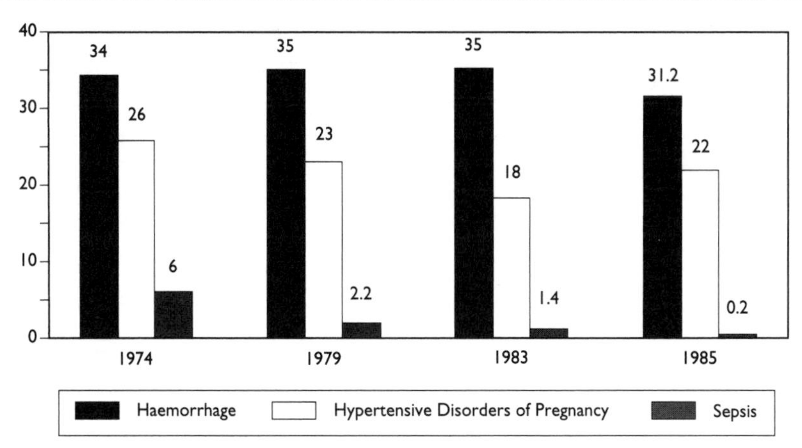

Source: Sri Lanka, Ministry of Health.

predict and generally requires rapid treatment at a health facility which is able to provide blood transfusions and other clinical measures if the woman's life is to be saved. Where many deliveries take place at home and transport to a health care facility is likely to take some time, the risk of death following postpartum haemorrhage is particularly high. WHO advises that all health care workers at the periphery be able to provide obstetric first aid to manage life-threatening obstetric haemorrhage. Simple techniques that are possible with limited training and skills include uterine massage and elevation of the limbs and, where supplies can be made available, the use of oxytocic drugs to contract the uterus. In addition, the use of plasma expanders at the level of the health centre where blood transfusion is not available should also be explored. Prevention of many cases of postpartum haemorrhage is possible in settings where active management of the third stage of labour is available. However, this requires a level of competency that is not generally available in peripheral health care facilities.

Table 9 Epidemiological estimates of episodes of maternal haemorrhage, females, 1990.

Age group (years)	*Incidence* Number ('000s)	Rate per100 000	*Avg. age at onset* (years)	*Deaths* Number ('000s)	Rate per100 000	*YLLs* Number ('000s)	Rate per100 000
Established Market Economies							
0-4	0	0	–	0	0.00	0	0.00
5-14	0	0	–	0	0.00	0	0.00
15-44	1 040	580	30.00	0	0.10	4	2.23
45-59	0	0	–	0	0.00	0	0.00
60+	0	0	–	0	0.00	0	0.00
All Ages	*1 040*	*255*	*30.00*	*0*	*0.00*	*4*	*0.98*
Formerly Socialist Economies of Europe							
0-4	0	0	–	0	0.00	0	0.00
5-14	0	0	–	0	0.00	0	0.00
15-44	529	706	29.90	0	0.30	6	8.00
45-59	5	17	52.40	0	0.00	0	0.00
60+	0	0	–	0	0.00	0	0.00
All Ages	*534*	*295*	*30.10*	*0*	*0.10*	*6*	*2.47*
India							
0-4	0	0	–	0	0.00	0	0.00
5-14	0	0	–	0	0.00	0	0.00
15-44	2 581	1 409	29.80	27	14.50	785	428.40
45-59	84	183	52.40	1	1.90	14	30.43
60+	0	0	–	0	0.00	0	0.00
All Ages	*2 665*	*650*	*30.50*	*28*	*6.70*	*799*	*194.82*
China							
0-4	0	0	–	0	0.00	0	0.00
5-14	0	0	–	0	0.00	0	0.00
15-44	2 513	885	29.90	11	3.90	346	121.80
45-59	159	246	52.40	1	1.10	11	17.08
60+	0	0	–	0	0.00	0	0.00
All Ages	*2672*	*487*	*31.20*	*12*	*2.20*	*357*	*65.09*
Other Asia and Islands							
0-4	0	0	–	0	0.00	0	0.00
5-14	0	0	–	0	0.00	0	0.00
15-44	1 887	1 182	29.40	12	7.50	351	219.91
45-59	79	224	52.20	1	1.40	8	22.80
60+	0	0	–	0	0.00	0	0.00
All Ages	*1 966*	*579*	*30.30*	*13*	*3.70*	*359*	*105.72*
Sub-Saharan Africa							
0-4	0	0	–	0	0.00	0	0.00
5-14	142	204	10.00	2	3.40	90	128.91
15-44	2 518	2 370	29.50	42	39.80	1 236	1 163.22
45-59	5	25	52.20	0	0.40	1	4.52
60+	0	0	–	0	0.00	0	0.00
All Ages	*2 666*	*1033*	*28.50*	*45*	*17.30*	*1 327*	*514.44*

Table 9 *(continued)*

Age group (years)	*Incidence* Number ('000s)	Rate per100 000	*Avg. age at onset (years)*	*Deaths* Number ('000s)	Rate per100 000	*YLLs* Number ('000s)	Rate per100 000
Latin America and the Caribbean							
0-4	0	0	–	0	0.00	0	0.00
5-14	9	18	10.00	0	0.10	1	1.97
15-44	1 246	1 197	29.90	5	4.40	139	133.54
45-59	8	35	52.40	0	0.10	0	0.00
60+	0	0	–	0	0.00	0	0.00
All Ages	*1 263*	*567*	*29.90*	*5*	*2.10*	*140*	*62.87*
Middle Eastern Crescent							
0-4	0	0	–	0	0.00	0	0.00
5-14	2	4	10.00	0	0.00	1	1.61
15-44	1 958	1 826	29.80	11	10.40	324	302.21
45-59	125	562	52.30	1	3.20	11	49.35
60+	0	0	–	0	0.00	0	0.00
All Ages	*2 086*	*846*	*31.10*	*12*	*4.80*	*336*	*136.21*
Developed Regions							
0-4	0	0	–	0	0.00	0	0.00
5-14	0	0	–	0	0.00	0	0.00
15-44	1 569	617	29.97	0	0.00	10	3.93
45-59	5	5	52.4	0	0.00	0	0.00
60+	0	0	–	0	0.00	0	0.00
All Ages	*1 574*	*242*	*30.0*	*0*	*0.00*	*10*	*1.54*
Developing Regions							
0-4	0	0	–	0	0.00	0	0.00
5-14	153	34	10	2	0.45	92	20.52
15-44	12 703	1 345	30	108	11.43	3 181	336.80
45-59	460	216	52	4	1.88	45	21.10
60+	0	0	–	0	0.00	0	0.00
All Ages	*13 316*	*657*	*30.3*	*114*	*5.63*	*3 318*	*163.81*
World							
0-4	0	0	–	0	0.00	0	0.00
5-14	153	29	10.0	2	0.38	92	17.51
15-44	14 272	1 191	29.74	108	9.01	3 191	266.22
45-59	465	149	52.3	4	1.29	45	14.47
60+	0	0	–	0	0.00	0	0.00
All Ages	*14 890*	*570*	*30.2*	*114*	*4.36*	*3 328*	*127.33*

Table 10 Epidemiological estimates of Sheehan's syndrome resulting from maternal haemorrhage, females, 1990.

Age group (years)	*Incidence* Number ('000s)	Rate per100 000	*Prevalence* Number ('000s)	Rate per100 000	*Avg. age at onset* (years)	*Avg. duration* (years)	*YLDs* Number ('000s)	Rate per100 000
Established Market Economies								
0-4	0	0.00	0	0	–	–	0	0
5-14	0	0.00	0	0	–	–	0	0
15-44	8	4.50	120	67.00	30.00	50.00	9	5
45-59	0	0.00	91	134.00	–	–	4	6
60+	0	0.00	113	134.00	–	–	2	3
All Ages	*8*	*2*	*324*	*79*	*30.00*	*50.00*	*15*	*4*
Formerly Socialist Economies of Europe								
0-4	0	0.00	0	0	–	–	0	0
5-14	0	0.00	0	0	–	–	0	0
15-44	4	5.30	60	80.00	29.90	46.80	4	6
45-59	0	0.00	48	160.00	–	–	2	7
60+	0	0.00	58	160.00	–	–	1	3
All Ages	*4*	*2.2*	*166*	*92*	*29.90*	*46.80*	*8*	*3*
India								
0-4	0	0.00	0	0	–	–	0	0
5-14	0	0.00	0	0	–	–	0	0
15-44	21	11.40	310	169.00	29.80	41.70	23	13
45-59	0	0.00	158	343.00	–	–	11	25
60+	0	0.00	99	343.00	–	–	4	15
All Ages	*21*	*5.1*	*567*	*138*	*29.80*	*41.70*	*39*	*9*
China								
0-4	0	0.00	0	0	–	–	0	0
5-14	0	0.00	0	0	–	–	0	0
15-44	20	7.00	298	105.00	29.90	44.20	22	8
45-59	0	0.00	136	221.00	–	–	11	17
60+	0	0.00	109	221.00	–	–	5	9
All Ages	*20*	*3.6*	*543*	*99*	*29.90*	*44.20*	*37*	*7*
Other Asia and Islands								
0-4	0	0.00	0	0	–	–	0	0
5-14	0	0.00	0	0	–	–	0	0
15-44	15	9.40	222	139.00	29.40	41.50	17	11
45-59	0	0.00	99	282.00	–	–	8	23
60+	0	0.00	64	828.00	–	–	3	13
All Ages	*15*	*4.4*	*384*	*113*	*29.40*	*41.50*	*28*	*8*
Sub-Saharan Africa								
0-4	0	0.00	0	0	–	–	0	0
5-14	0	0.00	0	0	–	–	0	0
15-44	20	190.00	289	272.00	29.50	37.20	23	21
45-59	0	0.00	125	563.00	–	–	11	49
60+	0	0.00	72	563.00	–	–	3	21
All Ages	*20*	*7.8*	*486*	*188*	*29.50*	*37.20*	*36*	*14*

Table 10 *(continued)*

Age group (years)	Incidence Number ('000s)	Incidence Rate per100 000	Prevalence Number ('000s)	Prevalence Rate per100 000	Avg. age at onset (years)	Avg. duration (years)	YLDs Number ('000s)	YLDs Rate per100 000
Latin America and the Caribbean								
0-4	0	0.00	0	0	–	–	0	0
5-14	0	0.00	0	0	–	–	0	0
15-44	10	9.60	149	143.00	29.90	44.60	11	11
45-59	0	0.00	67	228.00	–	–	5	23
60+	0	0.00	48	288.00	–	–	2	14
All Ages	*10*	*4.5*	*265*	*119*	*29.90*	*44.60*	*19*	*8*
Middle Eastern Crescent								
0-4	0	0.00	0	0	–	–	0	0
5-14	0	0.00	0	0	–	–	0	0
15-44	16	14.90	237	221.00	29.80	42.60	18	16
45-59	0	0.00	100	447.00	–	–	9	39
60+	0	0.00	69	447.00	–	–	3	22
All Ages	*16*	*6.5*	*406*	*165*	*29.80*	*42.60*	*30*	*12*
Developed Regions								
0-4	0	0.00	0	0.00	–	–	0	0
5-14	0	0.00	0	0.00	–	–	0	0
15-44	12	4.72	180	70.82	29.97	44.15	13	5
45-59	0	0.00	139	142.12	–	–	6	7
60+	0	0.00	171	141.37	–	–	3	3
All Ages	*12*	*1.85*	*490*	*75.38*	*30.0*	*44.2*	*23*	*4*
Developing Regions								
0-4	0	0.00	0	0.00	–	–	0	0
5-14	0	0.00	0	0.00	–	–	0	0
15-44	102	10.80	1 505	159.35	30	42	114	12
45-59	0	0.00	685	321.20	–	–	55	26
60+	0	0.00	461	310.95	–	–	20	14
All Ages	*102*	*5.04*	*2 651*	*130.88*	*29.7*	*41.7*	*189*	*9*
World								
0-4	0	0.00	0	0.00	–	–	0	0
5-14	0	0.00	0	0.00	–	–	0	0
15-44	114	9.51	1 685	140.58	29.74	42.45	127	11
45-59	0	0.00	824	264.89	–	–	61	20
60+	0	0.00	632	234.76	–	–	24	9
All Ages	*114*	*4.36*	*3 141*	*120.17*	*29.7*	*42.4*	*212*	*8*

Table 11 Epidemiological estimates for severe anaemia resulting from maternal haemorrhage, females, 1990.

Age group (years)	Incidence Number ('000s)	Incidence Rate per100 000	Prevalence Number ('000s)	Prevalence Rate per100 000	Avg. age at onset (years)	Avg. duration (years)	YLDs Number ('000s)	YLDs Rate per100 000
Established Market Economies								
0-4	0	0.00	0	0.00	–	–	0	0
5-14	0	0.00	0	0.00	–	–	0	0
15-44	10	5.60	5	2.80	30.00	0.50	1	0
45-59	0	0.00	0	0.00	–	–	0	0
60+	0	0.00	0	0.00	–	–	0	0
All Ages	*10*	*2.5*	*5*	*1.2*	*30.00*	*0.50*	*1*	*0*
Formerly Socialist Economies of Europe								
0-4	0	0.00	0	0.00	–	–	0	0
5-14	0	0.00	0	0.00	–	–	0	0
15-44	5	6.70	2	3.30	29.90	0.50	0	0
45-59	0	0.00	0	0.00	–	–	0	0
60+	0	0.00	0	0.00	–	–	0	0
All Ages	*5*	*2.8*	*2*	*1.4*	*29.90*	*0.50*	*0*	*0*
India								
0-4	0	0.00	0	0.00	–	–	0	0
5-14	0	0.00	0	0.00	–	–	0	0
15-44	26	14.20	65	35.50	29.80	2.50	9	5
45-59	0	0.00	0	0.00	–	–	0	0
60+	0	0.00	0	0.00	–	–	0	0
All Ages	*26*	*6.3*	*65*	*15.8*	*29.80*	*2.50*	*9*	*2*
China								
0-4	0	0.00	0	0.00	–	–	0	0
5-14	0	0.00	0	0.00	–	–	0	0
15-44	25	8.80	13	4.40	29.90	0.50	2	1
45-59	0	0.00	0	0.00	–	–	0	0
60+	0	0.00	0	0.00	–	–	0	0
All Ages	*25*	*4.6*	*13*	*2.3*	*29.90*	*0.50*	*2*	*0*
Other Asia and Islands								
0-4	0	0.00	0	0.00	–	–	0	0
5-14	0	0.00	0	0.00	–	–	0	0
15-44	19	11.90	14	8.90	29.40	0.75	2	1
45-59	0	0.00	0	0.00	–	–	0	0
60+	0	0.00	0	0.00	–	–	0	0
All Ages	*19*	*5.6*	*14*	*4.2*	*29.40*	*0.75*	*2*	*1*
Sub-Saharan Africa								
0-4	0	0.00	0	0	–	–	0	0
5-14	142	204.00	0	0	10.00	–	0	0
15-44	25	23.50	63	59.00	29.50	2.50	8	8
45-59	0	0.00	0	0.00	–	–	0	0
60+	0	0.00	0	0.00	–	–	0	0
All Ages	*25*	*9.7*	*63*	*24*	*29.50*	*2.50*	*8*	*3*

Table 11 *(continued)*

Age group (years)	Incidence Number ('000s)	Incidence Rate per100 000	Prevalence Number ('000s)	Prevalence Rate per100 000	Avg. age at onset (years)	Avg. duration (years)	YLDs Number ('000s)	YLDs Rate per100 000
Latin America and the Caribbean								
0-4	0	0.00	0	0.00	–	–	0	0
5-14	9	18.00	0	0.00	10.00	–	0	0
15-44	12	11.50	9	8.60	29.90	0.75	1	1
45-59	0	0.00	0	0.00	–	–	0	0
60+	0	0.00	0	0.00	–	–	0	0
All Ages	*12*	*5.4*	*9*	*4*	*29.90*	*0.75*	*1*	*1*
Middle Eastern Crescent								
0-4	0	0.00	0	0.00	–	–	0	0
5-14	2	4.00	0	0.00	10.00	–	0	0
15-44	20	18.70	15	14.00	29.80	0.75	2	2
45-59	0	0.00	0	0.00	–	–	0	0
60+	0	0.00	0	0.00	–	–	0	0
All Ages	*20*	*8.1*	*15*	*6.1*	*29.80*	*0.75*	*2*	*1*
Developed Regions								
0-4	0	0.00	0	0.00	–	–	0	0
5-14	0	0.00	0	0.00	–	–	0	0
15-44	15	5.90	7	2.75	29.97	0.45	1	0
45-59	0	0.00	0	0.00	–	–	0	0
60+	0	0.00	0	0.00	–	–	0	0
All Ages	*15*	*2.31*	*7*	*1.08*	*30.0*	*0.4*	*1*	*0*
Developing Regions								
0-4	0	0.00	0	0.00	–	–	0	0
5-14	153	34.12	0	0.00	10	0	0	0
15-44	127	13.45	179	18.95	30	1	24	3
45-59	0	0.00	0	0.00	–	–	0	0
60+	0	0.00	0	0.00	–	–	0	0
All Ages	*280*	*13.82*	*179*	*8.84*	*18.9*	*0.6*	*24*	*1*
World								
0-4	0	0.00	0	0.00	–	–	0	0
5-14	153	29.11	0	0.00	10.0	0.0	0	0
15-44	142	11.85	186	15.52	29.74	1.30	25	2
45-59	0	0.00	0	0.00	–	–	0	0
60+	0	0.00	0	0.00	–	–	0	0
All Ages	*295*	*11.29*	*186*	*7.12*	*19.5*	*0.6*	*25*	*1*

Table 12 Summary table of epidemiological estimates for maternal haemorrhage, females, 1990.

Age group (years)	Incidence Number ('000s)	Incidence Rate per100 000	Prevalence Number ('000s)	Prevalence Rate per100 000	Deaths Number ('000s)	Deaths Rate per100 000	YLLs Number ('000s)	YLLs Rate per100 000	YLDs Number ('000s)	YLDs Rate per100 000	DALYs Number ('000s)	DALYs Rate per100 000
Established Market Economies												
0-4	0	0.00	0	0.00	0	0.00	0	0	0	0	0	0
5-14	0	0.00	0	0.00	0	0.00	0	0	0	0	0	0
15-44	18	10.04	125	69.75	0	0.00	4	2	9	5	13	8
45-59	0	0.00	91	134.22	0	0.00	0	0	4	6	4	6
60+	0	0.00	113	133.63	0	0.00	0	0	2	3	2	3
All Ages	*18*	*4.42*	*329*	*80.77*	*0*	*0.00*	*4*	*1*	*16*	*4*	*20*	*5*
Formerly Socialist Economies of Europe												
0-4	0	0.00	0	0.00	0	0.00	0	0	0	0	0	0
5-14	0	0.00	0	0.00	0	0.00	0	0	0	0	0	0
15-44	9	12.01	62	82.71	0	0.00	6	8	5	6	11	14
45-59	0	0.00	48	159.97	0	0.00	0	0	2	7	2	7
60+	0	0.00	58	159.37	0	0.00	0	0	1	3	1	3
All Ages	*9*	*3.71*	*168*	*69.21*	*0*	*0.00*	*6*	*2*	*8*	*3*	*14*	*6*
India												
0-4	0	0.00	0	0.00	0	0.00	0	0	0	0	0	0
5-14	0	0.00	0	0.00	0	0.00	0	0	0	0	0	0
15-44	47	25.65	375	204.65	27	14.73	785	428	32	17	817	446
45-59	0	0.00	158	343.44	1	2.17	14	30	11	25	25	55
60+	0	0.00	99	342.28	0	0.00	0	0	4	15	4	15
All Ages	*47*	*11.46*	*632*	*154.10*	*28*	*6.83*	*799*	*195*	*47*	*12*	*846*	*206*
China												
0-4	0	0.00	0	0.00	0	0.00	0	0	0	0	0	0
5-14	0	0.00	0	0.00	0	0.00	0	0	0	0	0	0
15-44	45	15.84	311	109.48	11	3.87	346	122	24	8	370	130
45-59	0	0.00	136	211.17	1	1.55	11	17	11	17	22	34
60+	0	0.00	109	210.97	0	0.00	0	0	5	9	5	9
All Ages	*45*	*8.20*	*556*	*101.37*	*12*	*2.19*	*357*	*65*	*39*	*7*	*396*	*72*
Other Asia and Islands												
0-4	0	0.00	0	0.00	0	0.00	0	0	0	0	0	0
5-14	0	0.00	0	0.00	0	0.00	0	0	0	0	0	0
15-44	34	21.30	236	147.86	12	7.52	351	220	19	12	370	232
45-59	0	0.00	99	282.13	1	2.85	8	23	8	23	16	46
60+	0	0.00	64	282.41	0	0.00	0	0	3	13	3	13
All Ages	*34*	*10.01*	*399*	*117.50*	*13*	*3.83*	*359*	*106*	*30*	*9*	*389*	*114*
Sub-Saharan Africa												
0-4	0	0.00	0	0.00	0	0.00	0	0	0	0	0	0
5-14	142	203.39	0	0.00	2	2.86	90	129	0	0	90	129
15-44	45	42.35	352	331.27	42	39.53	1236	1163	31	29	1 267	1 192
45-59	0	0.00	125	565.18	0	0.00	1	5	11	49	12	53
60+	0	0.00	72	565.59	0	0.00	0	0	3	21	3	21
All Ages	*187*	*72.49*	*549*	*212.83*	*44*	*17.06*	*1327*	*514*	*45*	*17*	*1 372*	*532*

Table 12 *(continued)*

Age group (years)	*Incidence* Number ('000s)	Rate per100 000	*Prevalence* Number ('000s)	Rate per100 000	*Deaths* Number ('000s)	Rate per100 000	*YLLs* Number ('000s)	Rate per100 000	*YLDs* Number ('000s)	Rate per100 000	*DALYs* Number ('000s)	Rate per100 000
Latin America and the Caribbean												
0-4	0	0.00	0	0.00	0	0.00	0	0	0	0	0	0
5-14	9	17.74	0	0.00	0	0.00	1	2	0	0	1	2
15-44	22	21.14	158	151.80	5	4.80	139	134	12	12	151	145
45-59	0	0.00	67	286.88	0	0.00	0	0	5	23	5	23
60+	0	0.00	48	285.31	0	0.00	0	0	2	14	2	14
All Ages	*31*	*13.92*	*273*	*122.60*	*5*	*2.25*	*140*	*63*	*20*	*9*	*160*	*72*
Middle Eastern Crescent												
0-4	0	0.00	0	0.00	0	0.00	0	0	0	0	0	0
5-14	2	3.23	0	0.00	0	0.00	1	2	0	0	1	2
15-44	36	33.58	252	235.05	11	10.26	324	302	20	18	344	321
45-59	0	0.00	100	448.59	1	4.49	11	49	9	39	20	88
60+	0	0.00	69	446.60	0	0.00	0	0	3	22	3	22
All Ages	*38*	*15.40*	*421*	*170.66*	*12*	*4.86*	*336*	*136*	*32*	*13*	*368*	*149*
Developed Regions												
0-4	0	0.00	0	0.00	0	0.00	0	0	0	0	0	0
5-14	0	0.00	0	0.00	0	0.00	0	0	0	0	0	0
15-44	27	10.62	187	73.58	0	0.00	10	4	14	6	24	10
45-59	0	0.00	139	142.12	0	0.00	0	0	6	7	6	7
60+	0	0.00	171	141.37	0	0.00	0	0	3	3	3	3
All Ages	*27*	*4.15*	*497*	*76.46*	*0*	*0.00*	*10*	*2*	*24*	*4*	*34*	*5*
Developing Regions												
0-4	0	0.00	0	0.00	0	0.00	0	0	0	0	0	0
5-14	153	34.12	0	0.00	2	0.45	92	21	0	0	92	21
15-44	229	24.25	1 684	178.30	108	11.43	3181	337	138	15	3 319	351
45-59	0	0.00	685	321.20	4	1.88	45	21	55	26	100	47
60+	0	0.00	461	310.95	0	0.00	0	0	20	14	20	14
All Ages	*382*	*18.86*	*2 830*	*139.72*	*114*	*5.63*	*3318*	*164*	*213*	*11*	*3 531*	*174*
World												
0-4	0	0.00	0	0.00	0	0.00	0	0	0	0	0	0
5-14	153	29.11	0	0.00	2	0.38	92	18	0	0	92	18
15-44	256	21.36	1 871	156.09	108	9.01	3191	266	152	13	3 343	279
45-59	0	0.00	824	264.89	4	1.29	45	14	61	20	106	34
60+	0	0.00	632	234.76	0	0.00	0	0	24	9	24	9
All Ages	*409*	*15.65*	*3 327*	*127.29*	*114*	*4.36*	*3328*	*127*	*237*	*9*	*3 565*	*136*

References

Agoestina T and Soejoenoes A (1989) *Technical report on the study of maternal and perinatal mortality,* Central Java Province, Republic of Indonesia.

Angola, Ministry of Health (1990) *Information from the Angolan delegation to the Safe Motherhood Conference,* Harare, Zimbabwe.

Asociación Demográfica Salvadoreña (ADS) et al. (1994) Encuesta nacional de salud familiar. FESAL-93. [National family health survey.] ADS.

Bahemuka M, Rees PH (1981) Sheehan's syndrome presenting with psychosis. *East African Medical Journal,* 58(5):324–329.

Barron Sl (1989) Antepartum haemorrhage in Turnbull A and Chamberlain G. *Obstetrics,* Churchill Livingston.

Berg CJ et al. (1996) Pregnancy-related mortality in the United States, 1987-1990. *Obstetrics and Gynaecology.* 88(2): 161-7.

Boes EGM (1987) Maternal mortality in southern Africa 1980-1982. Part II — Causes of maternal death. *South African Medical Journal,* 71:160–161.

Botswana Country Team (1990) *Botswana country paper prepared for the Safe Motherhood Conference, 29 October – 1 November 1990.*

Bouvier-Colle MH, Varnoux N, Breart G (1994) *Les Morts maternelles en France.* Les editions INSERM. Paris.

Bullogh CHW et al. (1989) Early suckling and postpartum haemorrhage: controlled trial in deliveries by traditional birth attendants. *The Lancet.* 2(8622): 522–525.

Castellanos M de J et al. (1991) *Mortalidad materna — Honduras 1990.* UNAH, MSP, OPS, UNFPA, MSH.

Cénac A et al. (1991) Le syndrome de Sheehan en Afrique Soudano-Sahélienne. 40 observations. *Bulletin de la Société de Pathologie exotique et de ses Filiales.* 84(5/5):686–692.

Chamberlain GVP, Phillips E, Howlett B, Mastersk (1978) *British births,* Heinman, London.

Correa P et al. (1975) Le syndrome de Sheehan chez l'Africaine. *Afrique médicale.* 14(126):27–32.

Dano P et al. (1982) Le syndrome de Sheehan (a propos de 5 cas en Afrique). *Dakar Medical.* 27(3):323–330.

Demographic and Health Surveys (1994) *Philippines National Safe Motherhood Survey 1993.* Calverton, MD, USA Macro International Inc.

Ducloux M et al. (1976) Panhypopituitarisme du post partum chez une Senegalaise (syndrome de Sheehan). *Bulletin de la Société médicale d'Afrique noire de Langue française.*

Editorial (1965) Hypopituitarism after childbirth. *Lancet.* 5/6:1204–05.

Famuyiwa OO et al. (1992) Sheehan's syndrome in a developing country, Nigeria: a rare disease or problem of diagnosis? *East African Medical Journal,* 69(1):40–43.

Fortney JA et al. (1985) Maternal mortality in Indonesia and Egypt. In *Proceedings of the Interregional meeting on the prevention of maternal mortality, Geneva, 11–15 November 1985*. WHO/FHE/PMM/85.9.13.

Fraser R, Watson R (1989) Bleeding during the latter half of pregnancy. In Chalmers I. et al. (eds.) *Effective care in pregnancy and childbirth*, Oxford University Press.

Gongoro H (1988) Maternal mortality in Botswana 1982–1986. *Journal of the Medical and Dental Association of Botswana,* 18(3–4): 49–61.

Iyàsu S et al. (1993) The epidemiology of placenta praevia in the United States, 1979 through 1987. *American Journal of Obstetrics and Gynecology*, 168:(5) 1424–9.

Levy V, Moore J (1985) The midwife's management of the third stage of labour. *Nursing Times*, 81(5):47–50.

Maine D. (1992) *Safe Motherhood Programs: Options and Issues*. Center for Population and Family Health, Faculty of Medicine, Columbia University, New York.

McDonald SJ et al. (1993) Randomised controlled trial of oxytocin alone versus oxytocin and ergometrine in active management of third stage of labour. *British Medical Journal*, 307:1167–1171.

Ministry of Health, Egypt (1993) Child Survival Project. *National Maternal Mortality Study. Findings and Conclusions.*

Ministry of Health, Sri Lanka (1987) Maternal mortality statistics.

Ministry of Plan Implementation. (1981) Bulletin of vital statistics 1979:6th issue. Colombo, Department of Census and Statistics.

Murray CJL and Lopez AD (1996a) Estimating causes of death: new methods and global and regional applications for 1990. In: Murray CJL and Lopez AD, eds. *The global burden of disease: a comprehensive assessment of mortality and disability from diseases, injuries, and risk factors in 1990 and projected to 2020.* Cambridge, Harvard University Press.

Murray CJL and Lopez AD (1996b) Global and regional descriptive epidemiology of disability: incidence, prevalence, health expectancies and Years lived with Disability. In: Murray CJL and Lopez AD, eds. *The global burden of disease: a comprehensive assessment of mortality and disability from diseases, injuries, and risk factors in 1990 and projected to 2020.* Cambridge, Harvard University Press.

Mutambirwa J (1984) *Appropriate technology for management of the third stage of labour and cord core.* Paper presented to WHO First Meeting of the Steering Committee of the Task Force on appropriate technology for pregnancy and perinatal care, Oxford (mimeographed document).

Ni H and Rossignol AM (1994) Maternal deaths among women with pregnancies outside of family planning in Sichuan, China. *Epidemiology*, 4(5):490–494.

Paintin DB (1962) The epidemiology of ante-partum haemorrhage: A study of all births in a community. *Journal of Obstetrics and Gynecology of British Commonwealth* 69:16–25.

Prendiville WJ et al. (1988) The Bristol third stage trial: active versus physiological management of the third stage of labour. *British Medical Journal* 297:1295–1300.

Prendiville W, Elbourne D (1989) Care during the third stage of labour. In Chalmers I et al. (eds.) *Effective care in pregnancy and childbirth.* Oxford, Oxford Medical Publications.

Prendiville WJ et al. (1988) The Bristol third stage trial: active versus physiological management of third stage of labour. *British Medical Journal,* 297:1295–1300.

Rita M (1988) Estudo de mortalidade materna hospitalar em 1987 em Luanda. [Study of maternal mortality in a hospital in 1987 in Luanda.] *Acta Medica Angolana, 7:31–40.*

Roberts G (1970) Unclassified ante-partum haemorrhage. Incidence and perinatal mortalilty in a community. *Journal of Obstetrics and Gynaecology of the British Commonwealth* 77:492–495.

Ryan M (1981) Childbirth in remote Papua New Guinea. *Austalian Nurses' Journa*l 10/11: 44–45.

Sankale M et al. (1978) Le syndrome de Sheehan en Afrique noire (a props de neuf cas, dont cinq personnels). [Sheehan's syndrome in Africa (on nine cases, in which five are personal.] *African Journal of Medicine and Medical Sciences,* 7:65–69.

Sheehan HL (1954) The incidence of postpartum hypopituitarism. *American Journal of Obstetrics and Gynaecology,* 68(1).

Thompson A (1996) Personal Communication.

United Nations Children's Fund. (1989) Children, women and development in Botswana: a situation analysis. Consultant's report compiled for the Joint GOB/ UN UNICEF.

Wenzhen C (1991) Annual Report 1990. WHO Collaborating Centre for Research and Training on Perinatal Care.

World Health Organization (1986) *World Health Statistics Annual — Vital Statistics and Causes of Death.* Geneva.

World Health Organization (1989) The prevention and management of post partum haemorrhage: report of a technical working group. WHO/MCH/90.7 Geneva.

World Health Organization (1992) What can be done at different levels of the health care system. *Safe Motherhood Newsletter* 9.

World Health Organization (1994) Maternal Health and Safe Motherhood Programme. *The Mother-Baby Package. Implementing Safe Motherhood in Countries.* Geneva.

World Health Organization (1996) Care in normal birth: a practical guide. WHO/ FRH/MSM96.24, Geneva.

World Health Organization Pan American Health Organization (1990). Las condiciones de salud en las Americas. Washington, *PAHO Publicacion Cientifica No. 524.*

Zhang Lingmei (1991) Analysis of Surveillance results on maternal death in 30 provinces, municipalities and autonomous regions of China. Unpublished: Beijing Municipal Maternal Health Institute.

Chapter 5

Puerperal Sepsis and Other Puerperal Infections

Carla AbouZahr,[1] Elisabeth Åhman,
Richard Guidotti

Introduction

Historically, puerperal sepsis, or childbed fever was a common occurrence, greatly feared by women and their practitioners alike. Before the mechanism of contagion was fully understood and accepted by the medical community, puerperal sepsis often led to inevitable obstetric shock and death. The disease took on epidemic proportions, and was most evident in the lying-in hospitals in Europe (Gordon 1795, Semmelweis 1861). Transmission from patient to patient was predominantly carried by attending physicians and nurses, who tragically remained ignorant of their role as "vectors". Due to the vigilant observations of some investigators in recognizing how the disease spread and following their insistence in adopting clean delivery practices, the epidemic of puerperal sepsis came under control.

Semmelweis in Vienna, Austria and Holmes in Boston, USA are the two individuals who did the most to further the understanding of how sepsis spread and how it could be prevented. Both understood that puerperal sepsis was essentially an iatrogenic infection and that prevention required careful attention to hygiene, particularly among doctors who attended autopsies and treated obstetric patients. Holmes recommended that obstretric physicians should not perform autopsies on women who had died of puerperal sepsis and should refrain from providing any obstetrical care for a specified time after attending an autopsy for puerperal fever, or if two or more of their patients were infected (Charles and Larsen 1989). These efforts were followed by striking decreases in maternal mortality. In Vienna, Semmelweis achieved reduction in maternal mortality from 5 per cent to 1.3 per cent of deliveries (Semmelweis 1861).

With the introduction of antibiotics, puerperal sepsis declined further in industrialized countries. However, nosocomial infections remain a problem, particularly for operative deliveries, and increasing antibiotic resistance is noted regularly. The advent of the AIDS pandemic has been associated with an increased number of cases of antibiotic-resistant sepsis and of increased incidence of post-caesarean infection (Semprini et al. 1995).

In developing countries puerperal sepsis is still prevalent and continues to present a significant risk of obstetric morbidity and mortality to women in Africa, Latin America, Asia, and the Middle East. The study of puerperal sepsis and other puerperal infections is hampered by the lack of up-to-date population-based data for out-of-hospital births. The proportionate role that these infections play in maternal death varies greatly, but puerperal sepsis figures prominently in nearly every report on maternal mortality. In this chapter we deal with both puerperal sepsis (endometritis, peritonitis, setacemia) and other puerperal infections (of surgical wounds, genital and urinary tract) as well as with infections of the breast associated with childbirth.

Classification of Puerperal Infections

Puerperal infections are a general term and include not only infections due to puerperal sepsis — infection of the reproductive tract — but also extra-genital infections and incidental infections occurring during labour, delivery or the puerperium.

The International Classification of Diseases and Injuries (ICD) classifies puerperal sepsis and other puerperal infections under the heading of "Complications predominately related to the puerperium." The Tenth Revision of the ICD provides the following breakdown:

O85 Puerperal Sepsis
including puerperal endometritis, puerperal fever, puerperal peritonitis and puerperal septicaemia, but excluding obstetric pyaemic, septic embolism and septicaemia during labour; and

O86 Other puerperal infections (excluding infection during labour) including:

O86.0 infection of obstetric surgical wound (caesarean wound, perineal repair;

O86.1 other infection of genital tract following delivery (cervicitis, vaginitis);

O86.2 urinary tract infection following delivery;

O86.3 other genitourinary tract infections following delivery;

O86.4 pyrexia of unknown origin following delivery;

O86.8 and other specified puerperal infections

The main difference between the Ninth Revision (1975) and the Tenth Revision of the ICD (1992) is that the later version provides a coding scheme for cross reference with the infectious agents. Otherwise for practical purposes the two classifications are similar. Excluded from puerperal sepsis are: septic emboli, septicaemia during labour, and obstetrical tetanus.

In ICD-9 Puerperal infection is listed under Complications of the Puerperium and primarily includes:

670 Major puerperal infection
including puerperal endometritis, puerperal fever, puerperal pelvic cellulitis, puerperal pelvic sepsis, puerperal peritonitis but excluding infection following abortion, minor genital tract infection following delivery and urinary tract infection following delivery;

Associated codes that correspond to the codes includes in ICD-10 O86 include:

672 Pyrexia of unknown origin during the puerperium
including puerperal pyrexia NOS; and

675 Infections of the breast and nipple associated with childbirth
including Infections of nipple — abscess of nipple, abscess of breast — mammary abscess, purulent mastitis and subareolar abscess.

Etiology

It is thought that nosocomial infections with group A streptococci accounted for the majority of cases of puerperal sepsis in the 19th century. Even before antibiotics became available, major epidemics of puerperal sepsis were largely under control, probably because of better medical standards of care but also due, in part, to a decline in the virulence of the microorganism (Charles and Larsen 1989).

Fever is frequently the main clinical sign of puerperal infection though not all women with postpartum fever have a uterine infection. However, fever does not identify the site of infection. In developed country settings it has been postulated that some 5–10 per cent of women with postpartum fever either have no infection or have an infection at a site other than the genital tract. Infections can occur in the endometrium, at the site of the wound, in the breast and in the urinary tract (Table 1). Different microorganisms are found typically at each site of infection and can be identified only by culture. The predominant organisms will depend on the patient population and the place of delivery.

Uterine infections and their complications are responsible for the majority of deaths from puerperal infection. Many of the microorganisms that cause uterine infections are endogenous inhabitants of the lower genital tract, including one or more potentially pathogenic anaerobic bacteria, as well as, aerobic organisms. The microorganisms responsible for puerperal infection are often found to inhabit the lower genital tract, including one or more potentially pathogenic anaerobic bacteria, as well as aerobic organisms. The anaerobic bacteria may include species of bacteriodes, peptococcus, peptostreptococci, fusobacterium, and clostridia. The aerobic bacteria may include Group A, B & D streptococci, enterococcus, escherichia coli, klebsiella and proteus. Others include, mycoplasm hominis and Chlamydia trachomatis. These organisms, the so called mixed flora of the cervix and vagina, may ascend into the uterus (following rup-

Table 1 Table of postpartum infections and typical responsible micro-organisms.

Site of Infection	*Typical micro-organisms*
Endometritis	Mixed flora from cervix/vagina
Postpartum	Occasionally group B or group A
Post caesarean delivery	streptococci
Postabortal, spontaneous	Mixed flora from cervix/vagina
Postabortal, induced	*Clostridium spp*
Wound infection	
Wound cellulitis	Saphylococci
Wound abscess	*Escherichia coli*
Abdominal incision, episiotomy, vaginal,	Mixed anaerobes
cervical laceraion	Streptococci
Becritusubg fascitis	Staphylococci and anaerobic streptococci
Septicaemia	Group A or group B streptococci *Bacteroides* spp.
Septic pelvic thrombophlebitis	*Escherichia coli* *Bacteroides* spp Anaerobic cocci *Proteus*
Urinary infection	
Cystitis	*Escherichia coli*
Pyelonephritis	Group B, D streptococci *Proteus* spp, *Klebsiella* spp, *Enterobacter* spp, *Pseudomonas* spp
Breast infection	
Puerperal mastitis	*Staphylococcus aureus*
Breast abscess	

Source: Charles and Larsen 1989

ture of the membranes) during labour or may be pushed through the cervical canal by the examining finger during the pelvic examination. These organisms may then become pathogenic in the presence of traumatized, devitalized tissue or when the host defense mechanisms are weakened as in anaemic, malnourished or diabetic patients.

Uterine infections are also caused by exogenously introduced bacteria such as staphylococci (which are normal inhabitants of skin, nostrils and perineum), clostridium tetani, *pseudomonas.* These bacteria are introduced into the uterus by contaminated instruments and examining fingers, or by insertion of foreign objects into the vagina such as herbs, cow dung, or cloths, traditional practices in some developing countries.

The organisms primarily responsible for infection may vary from population to population. For example in many regions, sexually transmitted diseases (such as gonorrhoea or chlamydial infections) are highly prevalent and may contribute to a substantial proportion of uterine infections in the postpartum period. These organisms may initiate the infection process and be substituted by more virulent species.

Before delivery, prolonged rupture of membranes allows bacteria to ascend through the cervical canal into the amniotic cavity. On occasion, bacteria may migrate across the intact amniotic membranes during labour. The resulting chorioamnionitis may develop into a postpartum uterine infection.

After delivery, the area of placental attachment is similar to a wound and is an excellent culture medium for bacteria. In addition, blood clots, tissue or placental fragments may be present and these easily become infected. Following this initial invasion the infection can spread rapidly to involve the entire endometrium. If untreated, the infection may then spread to other layers of the uterus and adjacent structures, resulting in myometritis, parametritis or salpingitis. Pelvic abscesses, peritonitis, septic thrombophlebitis, septicaemia and septic shock may complicate the illness.

Studies have found that infection following a laparotomy for caesarean section is 10–20 times more common than that following vaginal deliveries, and the risk of death from sepsis is thirteen times greater (Department of Health and Social Security 1980). The risk of postpartum infection is related to the extent of bacterial contamination at the time of surgery and to the woman's general health status. Staphylococci are primarily responsible for surgical wounds involving sutures.

Lacerations of the cervix or vagina, episiotomies, and traditional practices such as "gishiri" cuts of the cervix, provide ready sites for bacterial invasion from both endogenous or exogenous sources (Eschenbach and Wager 1980). In obstructed labour, pressure necrosis of the bladder, urethra or rectum may lead to infection and formation of fistulae from the vagina to one or more of these sites.

The urinary tract is another common cause of puerperal infections. During the postpartum period, the urinary tract is particularly vulnerable to infection. Bladder and urethral trauma can occur during labour and delivery, and bacteria may be introduced when the urethra is catheterized. Between 1 and 5 per cent of patients with single, short term catheterizations and 50 per cent of patients with intermittent catheterization develop bacteruria (Charles and Larsen 1989). Moreover, the bladder remains enlarged from the pregnancy and the presence of residual urine due to decreased bladder tone increases the risk of a postpartum urinary tract infection, resulting in cystitis or pyelonephritis. Studies have shown that women with asymptomatic bacteriuria during pregnancy have a greater risk of developing pyelonephritis in the postpartum period.

Septic thrombophlebitis in the legs due to increased coagulability of the blood and circulatory stasis may occasionally complicate the puerperium. The picture may be confusing; classically there is marked fluctuation in temperature from recurring dispersion of septic emboli throughout the body. Temperatures may reach 39.5 – 40.5°C with rigours although the patient may not appear as ill as the temperature chart suggests. Before antibiotics, septic thrombophlebitis and septic pulmonary emboli were frequently noted at autopsy in patients who died from fulminating puerperal sepsis.

Acute mastitis and breast abscess produce painful symptoms in lactating women. Breast infection can occur in sporadic and epidemic forms (Charles and Larsen 1989). Sporadic mastitis results from poor nursing technique, breast engorgement and milk stagnation, caused by trauma to the nipple, opening fissures into which micro-organisms migrate. Epidemic mastitis usually occurs without cracked nipples and is often acquired in hospital. Both types are often caused by *staphylcoccus aureus.*

Infections which are unrelated to the birth process may occur in the puerperium and these may include respiratory and gastrointestinal tract infections, influenza, malaria, other tropical diseases, typhoid, and AIDS-related infections to name a few. The main challenge to health workers is to accurately make the correct diagnosis, in order to separate life threatening conditions from the more benign ones.

Risk factors for puerperal sepsis

The epidemics of puerperal sepsis of the late 19th century were usually caused by the virulent group A beta-haemolytic streptococcus. Nowadays, it is thought that in the industrialized world most puerperal infections involve less virulent organisms, partly because modern obstetrics use procedures to prevent infections with exogenous micro-organisms and partly because the virulence of the group A streptococcus has declined (Kass 1971). Infection therefore depends on the interplay between the virulence of endogenous micro-organisms and the defences of the host (Charles and Larsen 1989). Following childbirth, the uterus offers an excellent microbial culture medium and the normal defenses are reduced.

It is unclear to what extent this decline in the virulence of group A streptococcus has also occurred in the developing country settings. In any event, in industrialized and developing countries alike, certain obstetric procedures, such as frequent vaginal examination, particularly when associated with premature rupture of the fetal membranes and caesarean section may increase susceptibility to infection. Some researchers have postulated that complications following caesarean section particularly infection, are higher in HIV-infected women with the risk highest among severely immuno-suppressed women (Charles and Larsen 1989). The high risk of post-caesarean infection has important implications for obstetric care, especially in the developing world where standards of hygiene during operative procedures may be difficult to maintain and where women's general health status is already compromised. Rates of caesarean delivery are increasing generally in developing countries. Recent evidence from China shows that the rate of caesarean delivery in Shanghai increased from around 10 per cent in the 1980's to reach 32 per cent in 1990 (Guo et al. 1995).

In the developing world, predisposing factors for puerperal sepsis include: pre-existing sexually transmitted infections and other vaginal infec-

Table 2 Risk factors for puerperal infection in vaginal and caesarean section deliveries, Ghana, 1992

	Vaginal			*Caesarean section*		
	Infected (n=15)	**Non-infected (n=1248)**		**Infected (n=27)**	**Non-infected (n=18)**	
1. Referred	1	39	p=.385	11	6	p=.851
2. Prolonged labour (>24 hours)	2	17	p=.037*	7	6	p=.417
3. Obstructed labour	0	9	p=.896	16	10	p=.951
4. Premature rupture of membranes	8	82	p<.0001*	17	11	p=.977
5. Foul smelling amniotic fluid	4	35	p<.0001*	10	4	p=.237
6. Frequent pelvic examinations (>1)	3	192	p-.417	17	11	p=.977
7. Inadequate prenatal care (less than 7 visits)	14	1026	p=.239	21	14	p=.647
8. Anaemia	6**	682**	p=.384	26	13	p=.031
9. Cephalo-pelvic disproportion	0	1	p=.988	16	12	p=.851
10. Vaginal herb insertion prior to delivery	1	3	p=.046*	1	1	p=.668
11. Emergency caesarean section	NA	NA		21	5	p=.001*
12. Episiotomy	1	45	p=.455	NA	NA	

* Significant by Chi square or Fishers exact test

** Among vaginal deliveries, ten women who became infected and 991 who were not were tested for % haemoglobin.

The 96 women not tested are not represented in this analysis.

Source: Report on a baseline survey for the reduction of maternal infection and related mortality in Ghana, 1992

tions; prolonged rupture of membranes; retained products of conception; diabetes; caesarean delivery (especially if done as an emergency) and other operative deliveries; postpartum haemorrhage; history of previous complications of labour; anaemia and malnutrition and poor infection control practices (Table 2).

Community factors which increase a woman's risk of developing puerperal sepsis and of dying from it, include: delivery by an untrained traditional birth attendant; traditional practices such as the insertion of foreign objects and substances into the vagina; lack of transportation and resources; the great distance from a women's home to a health facility; the inadequacy of health facilities which are often ill-equipped and ill-staffed; cultural factors which delay care-seeking behaviour; the low status of women which contributes to their poor health in general and deprives them of adequate medical care and resources; the lack of knowledge about signs and symptoms of puerperal sepsis and of its risk factors; and the lack of postnatal care.

The picture is complicated by the close interrelationships between sexually transmitted diseases (STDs) and puerperal sepsis. A hospital study in Nairobi of 728 consecutive vaginal deliveries found that at the seventh day postpartum, 18 per cent of the women had developed an upper reproductive tract infection of which 44 per cent were attributable to an underlying sexually transmitted disease whereas the remainder were associated with other vaginal infections and iatrogenic infections. However, STDs alone cannot explain the very high prevalence of reproductive tract infections (RTIs) found in several community studies. For example, a study in Egypt found relatively low rates of STDs coupled with high levels of RTIs including cervicitis and vaginitis (Younis 1993).

Definition and Measurement

The classical definition of puerperal sepsis consists of the following essential elements:

1. Fever equal to or greater than 38.0 C (100.4 F).
2. Fever must be present on any two of the first ten days of the postpartum period (exclusive of the first 24 hours).

A WHO Technical Working Group on puerperal sepsis convened in 1993 suggested the following definition for use in developing countries, and stated that a diagnosis can be made when two or more of the following conditions are present. (World Health Organization 1996)

- Fever, oral temperature 38.5°C (101.3°F) or higher on any occasion.
- Pelvic pain.
- Abnormal vaginal discharge, e.g. presence of pus.
- Abnormal smell/foul odour of discharge.
- Delay in the rate of reduction of the size of the uterus (<2 cm/day during first 8 days).

These symptoms could occur at any time between the onset of ruptured membranes or labour and the 42nd day postpartum.

The main differences between this diagnosis and the classical definition are the recommendation that recorded temperature should be one half of a degree Centigrade more than the classical definition and the addition of presence of pelvic pain, abnormal vaginal discharge and foul odour. The group also felt that the rate of the reduction of the size of the uterus was an important clinical sign. Finally, the group broadened the time period in which the symptoms could occur to include the period from the onset of ruptured membranes or labour until the 42nd day postpartum. It is important to note that not all postpartum infections result in fever; a proportion of women are infected several days before their temperature rises (Charles and Larsen 1989).

Mortality and Disabilities Due to Puerperal Infections and Sepsis

Incidence of puerperal infections

As previously mentioned puerperal infections are an important cause of morbidity and mortality for mothers in developing nations. The infected mother, in acute stages, suffers pain and illness. Her condition may eventually result in infertility, chronic debilitation, or death.

The incidence of puerperal infections in developing countries is not accurately known. The numbers may be vast. For the most part, data on morbidity come from industrialized nations. In the United States, from 1–7 per cent of postpartum women develop a puerperal infection. (Eschenbach and Wager 1980) Sweet and Ledger's (1973) prospective surveillance study of over 6000 postpartum women indicated an infection rate of nearly 6 per cent. The rate of postpartum endometritis in the United States appears to be 2–3 per cent (Gibbs and Weinstein 1976). A recent study from Zaria, Nigeria (Harrison and Rossiter 1985) reported a rate of postpartum genital sepsis at 7.9 per cent. However, the rate rose to 14.9 per cent among women who delivered at home. Some studies have reported even higher rates of morbidity due to genital sepsis. In a maternity hospital in Nairobi, Kenya, 20 per cent of women developed a postpartum upper genital tract infection (Plummer et al. 1987). On the other hand, in the Philippines study on obstetric morbidity (Demographic and Health Surveys 1993) self reported symptoms of sepsis were remarkably low at 2 per cent. This study did not include any postpartum physical examination however. Various reports have indicated considerably higher rates of infection following caesarean section compared with vaginal delivery. In the United States, incidence was 0.26 per cent among women delivered vaginally and 36 per cent among those who had caesarean deliveries (Sweet and Ledger 1973). A report from the Congo found that post-caesarean infection caused one third of all maternal deaths in two urban areas (Locko-Mafouta 1988). A study in Ghana found that infection occurred in 60 per cent of women who had caesarean deliveries compared with less than 2 per cent of women with vaginal deliveries (Table 2).

Based on the available information (which is limited) the rates of incidence of puerperal sepsis have been estimated to range from a high of 10 per cent in sub-Saharan Africa to a low of 5 per cent in Established Market Economies. However, such data represent educated guesses rather than informed opinion. In most parts of sub-Saharan Africa, and Asia postpartum follow-up of women after delivery is virtually non-existent. Even hospital deliveries are routinely discharged within 24 hours and there is rarely any contact with the woman until she presents with the infant for immunization and/or for a six week postpartum check-up. At six weeks, postpartum signs and symptoms of sepsis are no longer likely to be clinically manifest with many infections rising to the upper genital tract. Some

Table 3 Per cent of infection-related maternal deaths by outcome of pregnancy, United States, 1987-1990.

	Live birth	*Stillbirth*	*Ectopic*	*Abortion*	*Undelivered*	*Unknown*	*Total*
Infection	12.2	19.4	1.3	49.4	12.5	9.1	13.1

Source: Berg et al. 1996

women will have died following severe sepsis. Women whose infants have died may not present for postpartum check-ups and will not be found through immunization programmes.

It is not possible to compare the incidence of sepsis in institutional and home deliveries. Incidence is likely to be high in the former as a result of nocosomial factors. On the other hand, certain traditional practices such as insertion of substances into the vagina, are likely to foster the development of sepsis in home deliveries.

Mortality from puerperal sepsis

The role that infection plays in maternal death varies greatly. Even so, obstetric sepsis, particularly puerperal sepsis, figures prominently in nearly every report. The risk of obstetric sepsis is lowest in industrialized nations. Nevertheless, a substantial risk still exists. In the United States, for example, infection accounted for under 8 per cent of maternal deaths over the period 1979–86 (Atrash 1990). Eighteen per cent of the infections were in the genital tract, 15 per cent were attributed to chorioamnionitis, and 32 per cent were due to septicaemia. The proportion of maternal deaths associated with obstetric sepsis represents a decline from just a few decades ago. The two major reasons for the decline were the legalization of abortion and the use of broader spectrum antibiotics (Sachs et al. 1988). More recent data from the United States show that just over 13 per cent of maternal deaths were due to infection, with the majority caused by general septicaemia. Infection accounted for slightly more than 12 per cent of maternal deaths following a live birth, 19.4 per cent of deaths following a stillbirth and nearly 50 per cent of deaths following legally and illegally induced and spontaneous abortion (Table 3) (Berg et al. 1996).

The reported number of maternal deaths due to sepsis is presented in Table 4 by region. More than 100 countries are included. The figures for most countries are based on "sepsis" as a cause of death and should correspond ICD-9 code 670 and ICD-10 code O85. However, many of the reports quoted in the literature do not clearly describe the ICD codes covered under the general heading "sepsis." In some studies, the more general category of "complications during the puerperium" was listed, and used only if "sepsis" was not listed at all. In cases where both "sepsis" and "complications during the puerperium" are listed as causes of death then only the former was tabulated.

Epidemiological data on mortality have been used by the authors to derive a first set of regional mortality estimates. When considered in conjunction with mortality estimates proposed by other authors for other diseases and injuries in the Global Burden of Disease Study, the implied level of overall mortality usually exceeded the rate estimated by various demographic methods. In order not to exceed this upper bound for mortality within each age-sex and broad-cause group, an algorithm has been applied by the editors to reduce mortality estimates for specific conditions so that their sum did not exceed this upper bound. The algorithm has been described in more detail in *The Global Burden of Disease* (Murray and Lopez 1996a).

Disability due to sepsis

Global information about the long-term sequalae of puerperal sepsis and its associated complications is scarce. However, it is known that puerperal infection may lead directly to conditions such as ectopic pregnancy, chronic pelvic pain and infertility. Chronic or acute pelvic inflammatory disease (PID) is caused when the infection spreads upwards through the genital tract causing damage to fallopian tubes and ovaries. The condition causes pain and discomfort which affects the lives of sufferers continuously. If left untreated it can result in chronic pelvic pain, bilateral tubal occlusion and infertility. Scars and adhesions that form around the uterus as a result of infection may cause it to change position, adding to the range of symptoms experienced. Pain is the dominant symptom, and in severe cases of PID occurs during defecation, when passing urine, during sexual intercourse and at and around menstruation. Low backache is common and the menstrual periods may become irregular and very heavy. Widespread damage to the reproductive system caused by chronic PID often leads to irreversible infertility. Uterine infection may spread by way of lymphatics to reach the abdominal cavity and cause peritonitis. Purulent exudate between the loops of bowel, or between bowel and other organs, may cause intestinal kinking, following which systems of mechanical bowel construction can occur. This condition can be fatal if left untreated.

Women whose fallopian tubes are damaged by infection are more at risk of a second tubal infection and are more likely to become infertile when a further episode of pelvic inflammatory disease occurs. In a Swedish follow up study of women with PID, infertility due to occlusion following scarring obstruction was found in 11 per cent after one episode of infection, 23 per cent after two, and 54 per cent after three episodes (Westrom 1980). In women who had only one episode of salpingitis (inflammation due to infection of fallopian tubes), the infertility rate increased with the severity of inflammation (Westrom 1980). However, in the pre-antibiotic era rates of infertility between 60 and 75 per cent were observed following acute PID, conditions comparable to the current reality in many developing countries where treatment is frequently unavailable or delayed (Westrom and Mard 1990).

Table 4 Reported maternal deaths due to sepsis as a per cent of total maternal deaths in developing countries, 1960-1990

Country	*Number of studies*	*Number of maternal deaths*	*% of deaths due to sepsis*
India	15	7841	11.5
China	7	8613	4.9
Other Asia and Islands			
Bangladesh	5	563	6.6
Fiji	1	164	4.9
Hong Kong	3	355	5.1
Indonesia	4	479	15.7
Malaysia	5	950	8.5
Papua New Guinea	3	1341	26.4
Philippines	3	3613	6.3
Republic of Korea	1	114	37.7*
Sri Lanka	3	2421	5.7
Thailand	3	478	10.0
Sub-Saharan Africa			
Burkina Faso	1	384	14.8
Ethiopia	5	446	14.1
Ghana	2	447	7.6
Guinea	1	212	20.0
Ivory Coast	3	297	32.7
Kenya	3	284	19.0
Malawi	3	420	12.9
Niger	2	330	25.1
Nigeria	18	2570	8.2
Senegal	1	152	24.3
Sierra Leone	2	134	8.2
South Africa	3	936	17.2
Sudan	8	565	20.0
Tanzania	10	1514	14.6
Togo	2	251	22.7
Tunisia	5	363	4.4
Uganda	3	1048	20.0
Zambia	4	376	20.0
Latin America and Caribbean			
Chile	4	744	24.6*
Columbia	7	3372	8.8*
Cuba	5	603	9.6*
Ecuador	3	1204	10.4*
El Salvador	2	414	21.0*
Guatemala	2	838	8.9*
Honduras	1	381	20.7*
Jamaica	3	269	9.7
Mexico	2	1821	9.7*
Paraguay	1	140	17.0*
Peru	2	706	14.9*
Venezuela	3	423	12.1*

Table 4 *(continued)*

Country	*Number of studies*	*Number of maternal deaths*	*% of deaths due to sepsis*
Middle Eastern Crescent			
Algeria	3	383	15.4
Egypt	9	1541	13.3
Iraq	2	125	16.8
Morocco	2	214	15.4
Pakistan	6	680	20.6
Turkey	2	661	2.3

* Reported as "complications of the puerperium"
Source: World Health Organization (1991a).

Women who have suffered from puerperal sepsis—particularly those who have not received adequate treatment for the condition—may be at a higher risk of subsequent abdominal surgery (caesarean section, appendectomy, ectopic pregnancy, etc.) due to adhesions within the abdominal cavity.

Although PID associated with puerperal or post-abortal infection is a known cause of tubal damage leading to infertility, sexually transmitted diseases can have the same effect, and reports of tubal infertility often do not distinguish between the two causes. However, high rates of secondary infertility (failure to conceive again after a previous conception) may indicate that complications of pregnancy and delivery have played a role. A recent study of 758 women in a rural community in Nigeria found that the prevalence of infertility was 30 per cent but that only 23 per cent of the total was attributable to a history of sexually transmitted disease, the remainder presumably due to postpartum or post-abortion infections and pelvic inflammatory disease (Adetoro and Ebomoyi 1991).

Few community-based studies in developing countries have examined the prevalence of reproductive tract infections and associated infertility. A rare study in rural Egypt found that 51 per cent of the women had reproductive tract infections, and pelvic inflammatory disease was suspected in 20 per cent (Younis et al. 1993). A similar study in Lahore, Pakistan, found an incidence of 3 per cent of pelvic inflammatory disease and 5 per cent of infertility (Awan et al. 1994). In rural India, the prevalence of reproductive tract infections was found to be 46 per cent and of pelvic inflammatory disease 24 per cent (Bang et al. 1989). A study in rural Nigeria found a prevalence of reproductive tract infections in women aged 20 years or older of 23 per cent and the prevalence of pelvic inflammatory disease of 9 per cent. Among adolescents in this study, the prevalence was 40 per cent and 4 per cent respectively (Brabin et al. 1995).

In an attempt to cross-validate the estimates of infertility from puerperal sepsis and post-abortion sepsis, Table 5 summarizes the combined effect of these two conditions on long-term reproductive tract infections and infertility over a cumulative period of 20 years, corresponding to an average number of childbearing years in a population in a low or non-

Table 5 Prevalence, estimated as per cent of all women aged 15–49, of long-term reproductive tract infection and secondary infertility caused by puerperal infection and by septic abortion

	Prevalence of Infertility by cause			*Prevalence of long-term RTI by cause*		
	Puerperal infection	**Abortion**	**Both**	**Puerperal infection**	**Abortion**	**Both**
Established Market Economies	0.3	< 0.05	0.3	1	0.2	1
Formerly Socialist Economies of Europe	1	2	2	4	6	10
India	3	5	8	11	8	19
China	1	–	1	4	–	4
Other Asia & Islands	2	3	5	8	8	17
Sub-Saharan Africa	6	8	13	24	12	35
Latin America & the Caribbean	1	3	4	7	11	17
Middle Eastern Crescent	3	2	5	15	8	23
World	2	2	4	8	5	14

contracepting environment, using a simplified method that assumes an annual constant addition of cases. This was done by multiplying the yearly caseload by 20, and dividing by the current number of women of reproductive age. For a number of reasons this calculation is not precise, but serves to illustrate the magnitude of the problem. In effect, using the yearly caseload in the numerator would imply that each infection affects a different woman, whereas the same woman may actually acquire several long-term reproductive tract infections during her life. This assumption, therefore, may contribute to an overestimation of the prevalence which is expressed here as a per cent of all women aged 15–49 years.

These estimates may be compared with estimates of secondary infertility in Table 6. Primary infertility is determined by the proportions of women in the oldest childbearing age groups — usually 40–44 or 45–49 years — who have had no live birth, i.e. who are childless. Secondary infertility is less straightforward to estimate than primary infertility. It requires judgment regarding how much elapsed time after a birth constitutes an extraordinary birth interval or what are unexpectedly low age-specific parities. Both of these determinations will be influenced by other factors, such as overall levels and ranges of fertility in a society, and other determinants of fertility, such as levels of practice of contraception and levels of sterilization, estimates of voluntary pregnancy termination, self-reported fecundity status, and so on. Consequently, there is no agreement on a standard means to estimate secondary infertility.

Table 6 Estimates of primary and secondary infertility prevalence, women aged 40–44 or 45–49 years.

	Primary infertility (%)	*Estimated range of secondary infertility (%)*
North America	6	7 – 17
Caribbean	6.5	7 – 19
South America	3.1	4 – 9
Europe	5.4	7 – 15
Middle East	3	4 – 9
Sub-Saharan Africa	10.1	12 – 29
Asia and Oceania	4.8	6 – 14

Sources: Primary infertility estimates for major world regions are from Frank (1993)
Secondary infertility calculated on the basis of Cantrelle and Ferry (1979) and Frank (1983).

It is possible, however, to estimate secondary infertility in populations that manifest "natural" fertility, which is fertility that is not influenced — or influenced little — by behavioural limitations such as contraceptive practice. This has been the case for some African populations. Estimates of infertility for these populations suggest two generalizations: everywhere, secondary infertility affects more women and accounts for a larger part of overall infertility than does primary infertility; and the range in the proportion of women with primary infertility to total infertility (the total number of women at the oldest childbearing ages of parity zero, one or two) is narrow enough — between 25 and 45 per cent — to warrant estimation of secondary infertility on the basis of measurement of primary infertility.

Accordingly, the estimates of secondary infertility in Table 6 are based on an assumed relationship between levels of primary infertility and levels of secondary infertility whereby the proportion of childless women represents between 26 and 45 per cent of all women who are infertile. The estimates of secondary infertility are similarly expressed as a possible range.

Depending on the condition under study, epidemiological data may be available for incidence, prevalence, case-fatality or mortality. Where data on more than one of these parameters are available, estimates of each of the epidemiological parameters derived from the data may not be internally consistent or consistent with the adjusted mortality rates described above. To ensure that all epidemiological information concerning a given condition is internally consistent, the editors have undertaken extensive analyses using computer models of the natural history of disease described in Murray and Lopez (1996b). The incidence, prevalence, and duration estimates have consequently been revised where necessary. In view of these adjustments to the basic epidemiological estimates originally provided for the Global Burden of Disease Study, the data which have undergone the GBD validation process are the joint responsibility of the authors and the editors.

The estimates of number of deaths, Years of Life Lost (YLLs), YLDs and DALYs from maternal sepsis episodes and infertility following puerperal infections are presented in Tables 7, 8 and 10. All episodes of maternal sepsis and all cases of subsequent infertility were classified as a class III disability and assigned a disability weight of 0.18; as there is no effective treatment, the disability weight was the same for treated and untreated form of infertility induced sepsis. The disability from sepsis-induced reproductive tract infections and pelvic inflammatory disease was not counted in the calculation of YLDs for sepsis for the Global Burden of Disease Study; instead it was taken into account in the sexually transmitted diseases calculations. However, we are showing the incidence, prevalence and YLDs from these sequelae in Table 9 in this chapter.

Puerperal Infection as a Risk Factor for Other Diseases

Both puerperal uterine infection and sexually transmitted diseases may cause ectopic pregnancy — a pregnancy where the fertilized ovum develops outside the uterus, usually in the Fallopian tube (see Chapter 7 in this volume). Left untreated, ectopic pregnancy can be fatal. Such deaths are rarely reported as maternal deaths, however, because in many instances the fact of the pregnancy was not known, even by the woman herself. It is probable that many hospital admissions of women of reproductive age classified as "acute abdomen" are, in fact, cases of ectopic pregnancy.

When uterine infection occurs during labour or after the rupture of the membranes, it may affect the newborn. Chorioamnionitis can cause neonatal infection which is evident at birth, or within a few hours of delivery manifesting as septicaemia, respiratory distress syndrome and pneumonia, with symptoms being more severe in pre-term infants. Choriamnionitis is also associated with an increased likelihood of premature birth which, in itself, is a risk factor for neonatal morbidity and mortality.

Gonococcal or chlamydia vaginal infections, although not strictly limited to this time period, may lead to uterine puerperal infections and can cause gonococcal infection or chlamydia ophthalmia in the newborn. This may occur during the infant's passage through the infected birth canal. Sexually transmitted infections are also associated with stillbirths, premature labours, intrauterine growth retardation and congenital disease.

Asymptomatic bacteriuria during pregnancy, although not a puerperal infection per se, can often lead to urinary tract infections which are associated with premature birth, low birth weight, and neonatal morbidity or mortality.

When puerperal infections occur intrapartum they may affect the newborn. Chorioamnionitis can cause neonatal infection which is evident at birth, or within a few hours of delivery manifesting as septicaemia, respiratory distress syndrome and pneumonia, with symptoms being more severe in pre-term infants. Chorioamnionitis is also associated with an increased likelihood of premature birth which, in itself, is a risk factor for neonatal morbidity and mortality.

Tetanus neonatorum is not acquired from the mother but is caused by the same factor as puerperal tetanus, namely: unclean delivery.

Further work is necessary to elucidate the complex interactions between the incidence, mortality and disabilities associated with puerperal sepsis. For the purposes of these calculations it has been calculated that 41.2 per cent of all cases of sepsis will result in long-term reproductive tract infections and 9.5 per cent in infertility. In effect, it is estimated that, on the average, every second woman will experience long term consequences following puerperal infection.

IMPACT OF INTERVENTIONS ON THE BURDEN

Sepsis is rare if delivery is straightforward, normal and spontaneous and so long as nothing is introduced into the vagina during labour. It continues to account for a substantial proportion of maternal deaths largely because of iatrogenic factors such as lack of hygiene during labour and childbirth and inappropriate and unnecessary procedures such as frequent vaginal examinations. Incidence of infection can be greatly reduced through improved cleanliness during delivery whether delivery occurs at home or within a health facility and deaths can be prevented through early detection of postpartum infections and timely use of antibiotics.

Sepsis is usually the first cause of death to decline as the overall level of maternal mortality falls, particularly where the ratio was originally very high. The historical record from England and Wales shows rapid declines in puerperal sepsis deaths compared with those from haemorrhage and hypertensive disorders (Figure 1). In Sri Lanka, the proportion of mater-

Figure 1 Declines in cause-specific maternal mortality, England & Wales, 1931–1978 (maternal deaths per 100 000 total births)

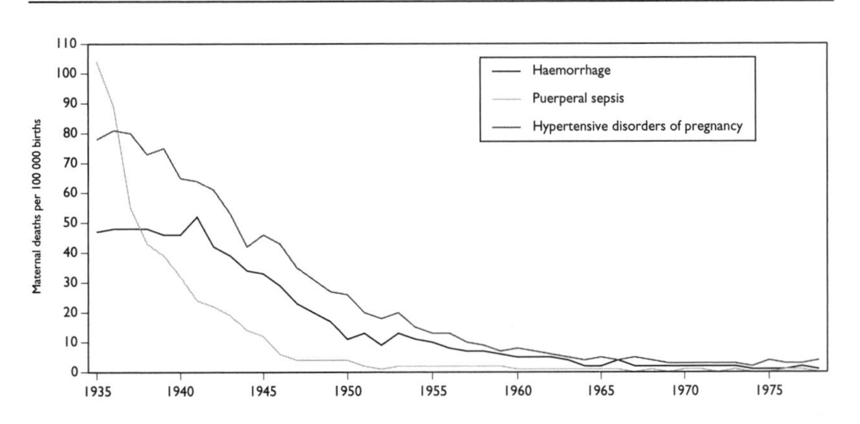

Source: MacFarlane and Mugford (1984)

Table 7 Epidemiological estimates for episodes of maternal sepsis, females, 1990.

Age group (years)	*Incidence* Number ('000s)	Rate per100 000	*Avg. age at onset* (years)	*Deaths* Number ('000s)	Rate per100 000	*YLLs* Number ('000s)	Rate per100 000
Established Market Economies							
0-4	0	0	–	0	0	0	0
5-14	0	0	–	0	0	0	0
15-44	520	290	25	0	0	2	1
45-59	0	0	–	0	0	0	0
60+	0	0	–	0	0	0	0
All Ages	*520*	*128*	*25*	*0*	*0*	*2*	*0*
Formerly Socialist Economies of Europe							
0-4	0	0	–	0	0	0	0
5-14	0	0	–	0	0	0	0
15-44	370	494	25	0	0	6	8
45-59	0	0	–	0	0	0	0
60+	0	0	–	0	0	0	0
All Ages	*370*	*205*	*25*	*0*	*0*	*6*	*2*
India							
0-4	0	0	–	0	0	0	0
5-14	0	0	–	0	0	0	0
15-44	2 581	1 409	25	18	10	523	285
45-59	84	183	52	1	1	9	20
60+	0	0	–	0	0	0	0
All Ages	*2 665*	*650*	*26*	*18*	*5*	*532*	*130*
China							
0-4	0	0	–	0	0	0	0
5-14	0	0	–	0	0	0	0
15-44	1 509	531	25	1	1	42	15
45-59	95	148	52	0	0	1	2
60+	0	0	–	0	0	0	0
All Ages	*1 604*	*292*	*27*	*1*	*0*	*43*	*8*
Other Asia and Islands							
0-4	0	0	–	0	0	0	0
5-14	0	0	–	0	0	0	0
15-44	1 672	1 048	25	8	5	234	147
45-59	70	199	52	0	1	5	14
60+	0	0	–	0	0	0	0
All Ages	*1 742*	*513*	*26*	*8*	*3*	*239*	*70*
Sub-Saharan Africa							
0-4	0	0	–	0	0	0	0
5-14	142	204	10	2	2	60	86
15-44	2 518	2 370	25	28	27	823	775
45-59	5	25	52	0	0	1	5
60+	0	0	–	0	0	0	0
All Ages	*2 666*	*1 033*	*24*	*30*	*12*	*884*	*343*

Table 7 *(continued)*

Age group (years)	Incidence Number ('000s)	Incidence Rate per100 000	Avg. age at onset (years)	Deaths Number ('000s)	Deaths Rate per100 000	YLLs Number ('000s)	YLLs Rate per100 000
Latin America and the Caribbean							
0-4	0	0	–	0	0	0	0
5-14	6	12	10	0	0	0	0
15-44	872	838	25	2	2	47	45
45-59	6	24	52	0	0	0	0
60+	0	0	–	0	0	0	0
All Ages	*884*	*397*	*25*	*0*	*1*	*47*	*21*
Middle Eastern Crescent							
0-4	0	0	–	0	0	0	0
5-14	2	4	10	0	0	0	0
15-44	1 958	1 826	25	8	7	217	202
45-59	125	562	52	0	2	7	31
60+	0	0	–	0	0	0	0
All Ages	*2 086*	*846*	*27*	*8*	*3*	*224*	*91*
Developed Regions							
0-4	0	0	–	0	0	0	0
5-14	0	0	–	0	0	0	0
15-44	890	350	25	0	0	8	3
45-59	0	0	–	0	0	0	0
60+	0	0	–	0	0	0	0
All Ages	*890*	*137*	*25*	*0*	*0*	*8*	*1*
Developing Regions							
0-4	0	0	–	0	0	0	0
5-14	150	33	10	2	0	60	13
15-44	11 110	1 176	25	65	7	1 886	200
45-59	385	181	52	1	0	23	11
60+	0	0	–	0	0	0	0
All Ages	*11 645*	*575*	*26*	*68*	*3*	*1 969*	*97*
World							
0-4	0	0	–	0	0	0	0
5-14	150	29	10	2	0	60	11
15-44	12 000	1 001	25	65	5	1 894	158
45-59	385	124	52	1	0	23	7
60+	0	0	–	0	0	0	0
All Ages	*12 535*	*480*	*26*	*68*	*3*	*1 977*	*76*

Table 8 Epidemiological estimates of infertility from maternal sepsis, females, 1990.

Age group (years)	*Incidence*		*Prevalence*		*Avg. age at onset (years)*	*Avg. duration (years)*	*YLDs*	
	Number ('000s)	Rate per100 000	Number ('000s)	Rate per100 000			Number ('000s)	Rate per100 000
Established Market Economies								
0-4	0	0	–	–	–	–	0	0
5-14	0	0	–	–	–	–	0	0
15-44	10	6	150	84	25	15	32	18
45-59	0	0	0	0	–	–	0	0
60+	0	0	0	0	–	–	0	0
All Ages	*10*	*3*	*150*	*37*	*25*	*15*	*32*	*8*
Formerly Socialist Economies of Europe								
0-4	0	0	–	–	–	–	0	0
5-14	0	0	–	–	–	–	0	0
15-44	33	44	491	655	25	15	104	139
45-59	0	0	0	0	–	–	0	0
60+	0	0	0	0	–	–	0	0
All Ages	*33*	*18*	*491*	*272*	*25*	*15*	*104*	*43*
India								
0-4	0	0	–	–	–	–	0	0
5-14	0	0	–	–	–	–	0	0
15-44	228	124	3 387	1 849	25	15	725	396
45-59	0	0	0	0	–	–	0	0
60+	0	0	0	0	–	–	0	0
All Ages	*228*	*56*	*3 387*	*826*	*25*	*15*	*725*	*177*
China								
0-4	0	0	–	–	–	–	0	0
5-14	0	0	–	–	–	–	0	0
15-44	135	48	2 020	711	25	15	430	151
45-59	0	0	0	0	–	–	0	0
60+	0	0	0	0	–	–	0	0
All Ages	*135*	*25*	*2 020*	*368*	*25*	*15*	*430*	*78*
Other Asia and Islands								
0-4	0	0	–	–	–	–	0	0
5-14	0	0	–	–	–	–	0	0
15-44	148	93	2 199	1 377	25	15	471	295
45-59	0	0	0	0	–	–	0	0
60+	0	0	0	0	–	–	0	0
All Ages	*148*	*44*	*2 199*	*647*	*25*	*15*	*471*	*139*
Sub-Saharan Africa								
0-4	0	0	–	–	–	–	0	0
5-14	0	0	–	–	–	–	0	0
15-44	290	273	4 260	4 009	25	15	923	869
45-59	0	0	0	0	–	–	0	0
60+	0	0	0	0	–	–	0	0
All Ages	*290*	*112*	*4 260*	*1651*	*25*	*15*	*923*	*358*

Table 8 *(continued)*

Age group (years)	*Incidence* Number ('000s)	Rate per100 000	*Prevalence* Number ('000s)	Rate per100 000	*Avg. age at onset* (years)	*Avg. duration* (years)	*YLDs* Number ('000s)	Rate per100 000
Latin America and the Caribbean								
0-4	0	0	–	–	–	–	0	0
5-14	0	0	–	–	–	–	0	0
15-44	77	74	1 151	1 106	25	15	245	235
45-59	0	0	0	0	–	–	0	0
60+	0	0	0	0	–	–	0	0
All Ages	*77*	*35*	*1 151*	*517*	*25*	*15*	*245*	*110*
Middle Eastern Crescent								
0-4	0	0	–	–	–	–	0	0
5-14	0	0	–	–	–	–	0	0
15-44	172	160	2 573	2 400	25	15	547	510
45-59	0	0	0	0	–	–	0	0
60+	0	0	0	0	–	–	0	0
All Ages	*172*	*70*	*2 573*	*1043*	*25*	*15*	*547*	*222*
Developed Regions								
0-4	0	0	0	0	–	–	0	0
5-14	0	0	0	0	–	–	0	0
15-44	43	17	641	252	25.00	12.01	136	54
45-59	0	0	0	0	–	–	0	0
60+	0	0	0	0	–	–	0	0
All Ages	*43*	*7*	*641*	*99*	*25.0*	*12.0*	*136*	*21*
Developing Regions								
0-4	0	0	0	0	–	–	0	0
5-14	0	0	0	0	–	–	0	0
15-44	1 050	111	15 590	1 651	25	15	3 341	354
45-59	0	0	0	0	–	–	0	0
60+	0	0	0	0	–	–	0	0
All Ages	*1 050*	*52*	*15 590*	*770*	*25.0*	*15.0*	*3 341*	*165*
World								
0-4	0	0	0	0	–	–	0	0
5-14	0	0	0	0	–	–	0	0
15-44	1 093	91	16 231	1 354	25.00	14.61	3 477	290
45-59	0	0	0	0	–	–	0	0
60+	0	0	0	0	–	–	0	0
All Ages	*1 093*	*42*	*16 231*	*621*	*25.0*	*14.6*	*3 477*	*133*

Table 9 Epidemiological estimates for pelvic inflammatory disease and reproductive tract infections, females, 1990.

Age group (years)	*Incidence* Number ('000s)	Rate per100 000	*Prevalence* Number ('000s)	Rate per100 000	*Avg. age at onset* (years)	*Avg. duration* (years)	*YLDs* Number ('000s)	Rate per100 000
Established Market Economies								
0-4	0	0	0	0.00	–	–	0	0
5-14	1	1	0	0.00	13	0.03	24	48
15-44	104	58	3	1.67	22.1	0.04	30	17
45-59	2	3	0	0.11	52.4	0.02	139	206
60+	1	1	0	0.03	72.4	0.02	242	287
All Ages	*108*	*27*	*3*	*0.76*	*23.2*	*0.03*	*436*	*107*
Formerly Socialist Economies of Europe								
0-4	0	0	0	0.00	–	–	0	0
5-14	1	5	0	0.00	13.0	0.00	68	257
15-44	148	197	5	7.15	22.1	0.04	85	113
45-59	3	10	0	0.23	52.4	0.02	390	1 300
60+	2	5	0	0.00	71.5	0.00	679	1 865
All Ages	*154*	*63*	*5*	*2.24*	*23.2*	*0.04*	*1221*	*503*
India								
0-4	0	0	0	0.00	–	–	0	0
5-14	13	14	0	0.51	13.0	0.04	95	100
15-44	1 032	563	45	24.37	22.1	0.04	119	65
45-59	13	28	0	1.05	52.4	0.04	548	1 190
60+	4	14	0	0.67	70.1	0.05	953	3 293
All Ages	*1 062*	*259*	*46*	*11.17*	*22.5*	*0.04*	*1714*	*418*
China								
0-4	0	0	0	0.00	–	–	0	0
5-14	3	4	0	0.00	13.0	0.00	1 070	1 184
15-44	603	212	22	7.64	22.1	0.04	1 338	471
45-59	8	12	0	0.00	52.4	0.00	6 158	9 562
60+	3	6	0	0.00	70.6	0.00	10 711	20 731
All Ages	*617*	*113*	*22*	*3.95*	*22.6*	*0.04*	*19 278*	*3 515*
Other Asia and Islands								
0-4	0	0	0	0.00	–	–	0	0
5-14	8	10	0	0.39	13.0	0.04	78	97
15-44	669	419	29	18.15	22.1	0.04	97	61
45-59	7	21	0	0.90	52.3	0.04	448	1 277
60+	2	10	0	0.00	70.3	0.00	780	3 440
All Ages	*687*	*202*	*30*	*8.72*	*22.5*	*0.04*	*1403*	*413*
Sub-Saharan Africa								
0-4	0	0	0	0.00	–	–	0	0
5-14	20	29	1	1.41	13.0	0.05	121	173
15-44	1 259	1 185	55	51.84	22.1	0.04	151	142
45-59	13	59	0	2.22	52.2	0.04	697	3 150
60+	4	30	0	0.96	69.7	0.03	1 212	9 518
All Ages	*1 296*	*503*	*57*	*21.97*	*22.4*	*0.04*	*2 181*	*845*

Table 9 *(continued)*

Age group (years)	Incidence		Prevalence		Avg. age at onset (years)	Avg. duration (years)	YLDs	
	Number ('000s)	Rate per100 000	Number ('000s)	Rate per100 000			Number ('000s)	Rate per100 000
Latin America and the Caribbean								
0-4	0	0	0	0.00	–	–	0	0
5-14	4	9	0	0.29	13.0	0.03	72	142
15-44	349	335	13	12.32	22.1	0.04	88	84
45-59	4	17	0	0.63	52.4	0.04	416	1 780
60+	2	9	0	0.00	72.4	0.00	723	4 299
All Ages	*359*	*161*	*13*	*5.89*	*23.2*	*0.04*	*1299*	*583*
Middle Eastern Crescent								
0-4	0	0	0	0.00	–	–	0	0
5-14	11	18	0	0.00	13.0	0.00	412	665
15-44	783	730	28	26.50	22.1	0.04	516	481
45-59	8	37	0	0.00	52.3	0.00	2 372	10 642
60+	3	19	0	0.00	70.4	0.00	4 126	26 708
All Ages	*805*	*326*	*28*	*11.52*	*22.4*	*0.04*	*7 427*	*3 011*
Developed Regions								
0-4	0	0	0	0.00	–	–	0	0
5-14	2	3	0	0.00	13.0	0.0	92	119
15-44	252	99	8	3.29	22.1	0.0	115	45
45-59	5	5	0	0.15	52.4	0.0	530	541
60+	3	3	0	0.02	72.1	0.0	921	761
All Ages	*262*	*40*	*9*	*1.31*	*23.2*	*0.0*	*1658*	*255*
Developing Regions								
0-4	0	0	0	0.00	–	–	0	0
5-14	61	14	2	0.43	13	0	1 849	412
15-44	4 695	497	192	20.29	22	0	2 310	245
45-59	53	25	1	0.67	52	0	10 639	4 989
60+	18	12	0	0.21	70	0	18 504	12 481
All Ages	*4 827*	*238*	*195*	*9.64*	*22.5*	*0.0*	*33 302*	*1 644*
World								
0-4	0	0	0	0.00	–	–	0	0
5-14	63	12	2	0.37	13.0	0.0	1 941	369
15-44	4 947	413	200	16.68	22.1	0.0	2 425	202
45-59	58	19	2	0.51	52.3	0.0	11 168	3 590
60+	21	8	0	0.13	70.7	0.0	19 425	7 216
All Ages	*5 089*	*195*	*204*	*7.80*	*22.5*	*0.0*	*34 960*	*1 338*

Table 10 Epidemiological estimates for maternal sepsis, females, 1990.

Age group (years)	*Incidence* Number ('000s)	Rate per 100 000	*Prevalence* Number ('000s)	Rate per 100 000	*Deaths* Number ('000s)	Rate per 100 000	*YLLs* Number ('000s)	Rate per 100 000	*YLDs* Number ('000s)	Rate per 100 000	*DALYs* Number ('000s)	Rate per 100 000
Established Market Economies												
0-4	0	0		0	0	0	0	0	0	0	0	0
5-14	0	0		0	0	0	0	0	0	0	0	0
15-44	530	296	150	84	0	0	2	1	32	18	34	19
45-59	0	0	0	0	0	0	0	0	0	0	0	0
60+	0	0	0	0	0	0	0	0	0	0	0	0
All Ages	*530*	*130*	*150*	*37*	*0*	*0*	*2*	*0*	*32*	*8*	*34*	*8*
Formerly Socialist Economies of Europe												
0-4	0	0		0	0	0	0	0	0	0	0	0
5-14	0	0		0	0	0	0	0	0	0	0	0
15-44	403	538	491	655	0	0	6	8	104	139	110	147
45-59	0	0	0	0	0	0	0	0	0	0	0	0
60+	0	0	0	0	0	0	0	0	0	0	0	0
All Ages	*403*	*166*	*491*	*202*	*0*	*0*	*6*	*2*	*104*	*43*	*110*	*45*
India												
0-4	0	0		0	0	0	0	0	0	0	0	0
5-14	0	0		0	0	0	0	0	0	0	0	0
15-44	2 809	1 533	3 387	1 848	18	10	523	285	725	396	1 248	681
45-59	84	183	0	0	1	2	9	20	0	0	9	20
60+	0	0	0	0	0	0	0	0	0	0	0	0
All Ages	*2 893*	*705*	*3 387*	*826*	*19*	*5*	*532*	*130*	*725*	*177*	*1 257*	*307*
China												
0-4	0	0		0	0	0	0	0	0	0	0	0
5-14	0	0		0	0	0	0	0	0	0	0	0
15-44	1 644	579	2 020	711	1	0	42	15	430	151	472	166
45-59	95	148	0	0	0	0	1	2	0	0	1	2
60+	0	0	0	0	0	0	0	0	0	0	0	0
All Ages	*1 739*	*317*	*2 020*	*368*	*1*	*0*	*43*	*8*	*430*	*78*	*473*	*86*
Other Asia and Islands												
0-4	0	0		0	0	0	0	0	0	0	0	0
5-14	0	0		0	0	0	0	0	0	0	0	0
15-44	1 820	1 140	2 199	1 378	8	5	234	147	471	295	705	442
45-59	70	199	0	0	0	0	5	14	0	0	5	14
60+	0	0	0	0	0	0	0	0	0	0	0	0
All Ages	*1 890*	*557*	*2 199*	*648*	*8*	*2*	*239*	*70*	*471*	*139*	*710*	*209*
Sub-Saharan Africa												
0-4	0	0		0	0	0	0	0	0	0	0	0
5-14	142	203		0	2	3	60	86	0	0	60	86
15-44	2 808	2 643	4 260	4 009	28	26	823	775	923	869	1 746	1 643
45-59	5	23	0	0	0	0	1	5	0	0	1	5
60+	0	0	0	0	0	0	0	0	0	0	0	0
All Ages	*2 955*	*1 146*	*4 260*	*1 651*	*30*	*12*	*884*	*343*	*923*	*358*	*1 807*	*701*

Table 10 *(continued)*

Age group (years)	Incidence		Prevalence		Deaths		YLLs		YLDs		DALYs	
	Number ('000s)	Rate per100 000	Number ('000s)	Rate per100 000	Number ('000s)	Rate per100 000	Number ('000s)	Rate per100 000	Number ('000s)	Rate per100 000	Number ('000s)	Rate per100 000
Latin America and the Caribbean												
0-4	0	0		0	0	0	0	0	0	0	0	0
5-14	6	12		0	0	0	0	0	0	0	0	0
15-44	949	912	1 151	1 106	2	2	47	45	245	235	292	281
45-59	6	26	0	0	0	0	0	0	0	0	0	0
60+	0	0	0	0	0	0	0	0	0	0	0	0
All Ages	*961*	*432*	*1 151*	*517*	*2*	*1*	*47*	*21*	*245*	*110*	*292*	*131*
Middle Eastern Crescent												
0-4	0	0		0	0	0	0	0	0	0	0	0
5-14	2	3		0	0	0	0	0	0	0	0	0
15-44	2 130	1 987	2 573	2 400	8	7	217	202	547	510	764	713
45-59	125	561	0	0	0	0	7	31	0	0	7	31
60+	0	0	0	0	0	0	0	0	0	0	0	0
All Ages	*2 257*	*915*	*2 573*	*1 043*	*8*	*3*	*224*	*91*	*547*	*222*	*771*	*313*
Developed Regions												
0-4	0	0	0	0	0	0.00	0	0	0	0	0	0
5-14	0	0	0	0	0	0.00	0	0	0	0	0	0
15-44	933	367	641	252	0	0.00	8	3	136	54	144	57
45-59	0	0	0	0	0	0.00	0	0	0	0	0	0
60+	0	0	0	0	0	0.00	0	0	0	0	0	0
All Ages	*933*	*144*	*641*	*99*	*0*	*0.00*	*8*	*1*	*136*	*21*	*144*	*22*
Developing Regions												
0-4	0	0	0	0	0	0.00	0	0	0	0	0	0
5-14	150	33	0	0	2	0.45	60	13	0	0	60	13
15-44	12 160	1 287	15 590	1 651	65	6.88	1 886	200	3 341	354	5 227	553
45-59	385	181	0	0	1	0.47	23	11	0	0	23	11
60+	0	0	0	0	0	0.00	0	0	0	0	0	0
All Ages	*12 695*	*627*	*15 590*	*770*	*68*	*3.36*	*1 969*	*97*	*3 341*	*165*	*5 310*	*262*
World												
0-4	0	0	0	0	0	0.00	0	0	0	0	0	0
5-14	150	29	0	0	2	0.38	60	11	0	0	60	11
15-44	13 093	1 092	16 231	1 354	65	5.42	1 894	158	3 477	290	5 371	448
45-59	385	124	0	0	1	0.32	23	7	0	0	23	7
60+	0	0	0	0	0	0.00	0	0	0	0	0	0
All Ages	*13 628*	*521*	*16 231*	*621*	*68*	*2.60*	*1 977*	*76*	*3 477*	*133*	*5 454*	*209*

nal deaths due to puerperal sepsis (excluding abortion-related sepsis) fell from 25 per cent to 3 per cent in about 30 years (Ministry of Health, Sri Lanka various years).

Such dramatic declines in sepsis-related mortality may be offset by increasing incidence of puerperal infection as a result of iatrogenic factors including increased use of operative interventions such as a caesarean delivery. And the rising prevalence of reproductive tract infections including sexually transmitted diseases and HIV/AIDS, is associate with increasing incidence of postpartum infections. Even where access to health care and to antibiotic therapy is relatively easy, sepsis continues to play a significant role in maternal mortality. In the USA, over the period 1987–1990, sepsis was the cause of death in some 12 per cent of all maternal deaths where the outcome was a stillbirth (Table 3).

Conclusions

Deaths due to sepsis are almost entirely avoidable through a combination of preventive and treatment interventions. The incidence of sepsis can be substantially reduced by ensuring clean delivery for all births whether they take place at home or in an institutional setting and by avoiding certain traditional practices (such as inserting foreign bodies into the vagina during labour or the postpartum period). Other interventions that can help reduce the incidence and case fatality from sepsis include detection and management of sexually transmitted diseases and other reproductive tract infections during pregnancy, prophylactic administration of antibiotics in cases of prolonged rupture of the membranes and timely intervention for prolonged labour. Many controlled trials have demonstrated that prophylactic administration can reduce the incidence of surgical infections (Charles and Larsen 1989).

Experience from developing and industrialized countries alike has shown that sepsis is usually the first cause of death to decline when maternity care becomes accessible.

It has been estimated that by the end of the century 75 per cent of all sepsis deaths could be prevented given the application of interventions to ensure clean delivery for all births (World Health Organization 1994).

Notes

1 The author wishes to express particular thanks to Anne Thompson, Odile Frank and Eve Loftus who contributed to this paper.

2 "Gishiri" cuts result from a traditional operation which involves cutting the anterior vaginal wall. The practice is used in the treatment of a wide variety of gynaecological conditions and is mainly confined to the Hausa people of Nigeria (World Health Organization 1991a).

3 This section on fertility estimates (Table 6 and text) was contributed by Dr Odile Frank, World Health Organization.

References

Adetoro OO, Ebomoyi EW (1991) The prevalence of infertility in a rural Nigerian community. *African journal of medicine and medical science*, 20(1):23–27.

Atrash H et al. (1990) Maternal mortality in the United States, 1979–1986. *Obstetrics and Gynaecology*, 76:1055.

Awan AK et al. (1994) Reproductive morbidity in an urban community in Lahore. *Maternity and Child Welfare Association of Pakistan.*

Bang RA et al. (1989) High prevalence of gynaecological diseases in rural Indian women. *Lancet*, 1(8629):85–88.

Berg CJ, et al. (1996) Pregnancy related mortality in the United States, 1987–1990. *Obstetrics and Gynaecology*; 88:161–7.

Brabin L et al. (1995) Reproductive tract infections and abortion among adolescent girls in rural Nigeria. *Lancet*, 345(8945):300–304.

Cantrelle P and Ferry E (1979) *Approach to natural fertility in contemporary populations.* In: Leridon H and Menken J, eds. Patterns and determinants of natural fertility. Natural fertility: Proceedings of a seminar on natural fertility. Liège, Ordina Editions.

Charles D and Larsen B. (1989) Puerperal sepsis. In: Turnball A & Chamberlain G, eds. *Obstetrics.* Churchill Livingstone.

Demographic and Health Surveys (1993) *Philippines National Safe Motherhood Survey 1993.* Calverton (MD). National Statistics Office and Macro International Inc.

Department of Health and Social Security (1980) Report on Confidential Enquiries into maternal deaths in England and Wales 1973–1975. Her Majesties Stationary Office, London.

Eschenbach DA, Wager GP (1980) Puerperal infections. *Clinical Obstetrics and Gynecology*, 23:1003.

Frank O (1983) *Infertility in sub-Saharan Africa*, Center for Policy Studies Working Paper Number 97. New York: The Population Council.

Frank O (1993) *The demography of fertility and infertility.* In: Campana A, ed. *Reproductive Health.* Rome: Ares-Serono Symposia Publications (Frontiers in Endocrinology Volume 2, pp. 80–91).

Gibbs RS, Weinstein AJ (1976) Puerperal infection in the antibiotic era. *American Journal of Obstetrics & Gynecology*, 124:769.

Gordon A (1795) A treatise on epidemic puerperal fever of Aberdeen, Robinson, London.

Guo Y et al. (1995) Primary caesarean section and its social determinants in Shanghai Municipality. *Journal Of Reproductive Medicine* 4 (Suppl.1):51–63.

Harrison KA, Rossiter CE (1985) Maternal Mortality. *British Journal of Obstetrics & Gynaecology*, 5:100.

Kess EH (1971) Infectious diseases and social change. *Journal of Infectious Diseases* 123:110–114.

Locko-Mafouta et al. (1988) La mortalite maternelle au Congo etude preliminaire. *Medicine d'Afrique Noire*, 35(7):517–518.

MacFarlane A and Mugford M (1984) Birth counts: Statistics of pregnancy and childbirth. Her Majesty's Stationary Office, London.

Murray CJL and Lopez AD (1996a) Estimating causes of death: new methods and global and regional applications for 1990. In: Murray CJL and Lopez AD, eds. *The global burden of disease: a comprehensive assessment of mortality and disability from diseases, injuries, and risk factors in 1990 and projected to 2020.* Cambridge, Harvard University Press.

Murray CJL and Lopez AD (199b) Global and regional descriptive epidemiology of disability: incidence, prevalence, health expectancies and Years lived with Disability. In: Murray CJL and Lopez AD, eds. *The global burden of disease: a comprehensive assessment of mortality and disability from diseases, injuries, and risk factors in 1990 and projected to 2020.* Cambridge, Harvard University Press.

Plummer FA et al. (1987) Postpartum upper genital tract infections in Nairobi, Kenya: epidemiology, etiology, and risk factors. *Journal of Infectious Diseases*, 156:92.

Sachs BP et al. (1988) Hemorrhage, infection, toxemia, and cardiac disease, 1954–1985: causes for the declining role in maternal mortality. *American Journal of Public Health*, 78:671.

Semmelweis P (1861) The etiology, the concept and the prophylaxis. Excerpts cited in 1981, *Reviews of Infectious Disease* 3:808–811.

Semprini AE et al. (1995) The Incidence of complications after caesarean section in 156 HIV positive women, *AIDS* 9(8): 913–17.

Sweet RL, Ledger WJ (1973) Puerperal infectious morbidity. *American Journal of Obstetrics and Gynecology*, 17(8):1093–1100.

World Health Organization (1991a) Maternal Health and Safe Motherhood Programme. *Maternal Mortality: A Global Factbook*. WHO/MCH/MSM/91.3. Geneva.

World Health Organization (1991b) Obstetric fistula: a view of available information WHO/MCH/MSM/91.S.

World Health Organization (1994) The Mother-Baby Package: Implementing safe motherhood in countries. WHO/FHE/MAM/94.11.

World Health Organization (1996) The prevention and mangement of puerperal sepsis. Report of Technical Working Group. WHO/FHE/MSM/95.4.

Weström L and Mard PA (1990) Acute pelvic inflammatory disease (PID). In: Holmes KK et al. (eds.) *Sexually transmitted diseases*, 2nd edition. New York, McGraw Hill.

Weström L (1980) Incidence, prevalence and trends of acute pelvic inflammatory disease and its consequences in industrial countries. *American journal of obstetrics and gynecology*, 138(7):880–892.

Younis N et al. (1993) A community study of gynecological and related morbidities in rural Egypt. *Studies in family planning*, 24(3):175–186.

Chapter 6

Hypertensive Disorders of Pregnancy

Carla AbouZahr
Richard Guidotti

Introduction

The hypertensive disorders of pregnancy represent several distinct entities generally associated with hypertension, proteinuria and, in some cases, convulsions which may result in death. The entities that are responsible for the most serious consequences for mother and fetus are pre-ecalmpsia and eclampsia. Both are characterized by vasospasm, pathologic vascular lesions in multiple organ systems, increased platelet activation and subsequent activation of the coagulation system in the micro-vasculature. The pathogenesis of pre-eclampsia has not been firmly established; however, recent work tends to support the hypothesis that this unique disease of pregnancy is a result of a maternal immunologic maladaptation to fetal and placental tissue leading to a disturbance of trophoblastic invasion of the spiral arteries. The resulting hypoxia and hypoperfusion leads to a complex cascade of bio-chemical events which is expressed in the clinical syndrome known as pre-eclampsia. Eclampsia, a serious sequel of the former, is a central nervous system seizure which often leaves the patient unconscious, and if not treated promptly may lead to death.

Definition and Measurement

Classification of hypertensive disorders of pregnancy

The classification of hypertensive disorders of pregnancy (HDP) is fraught with difficulties due to our limited knowledge of its etiology and lack of conformity on definitions. Two distinct entities of HDP are pregnancy-induced hypertension (PIH) and pre-existing hypertension. Pregnancy-induced hypertension (referred to as gestational hypertension by some authors) occurs after the 20th week of gestation and regresses after the delivery of the infant. Some authors assert that it can exist without other signs or symptoms. Others describe it as being accompanied by proteinuria (in which case it is defined as pre-eclampsia) and/or oedema. PIH consists of a matrix of sub-categories, characterized by severity of hypertension (mild or severe), and timing of onset (antepartum, intrapartum, and puerperium). It may finally result in seizures or convulsions, at which point it is defined as eclampsia. It can cause premature delivery, fetal growth retardation, abruptio placentae, and fetal and maternal death. Pre-existing hypertension, on the other hand, can be detected before 20 weeks of gestation, is a result of non-pregnancy related pathology and is not resolved with the delivery of the baby. Both entities can complicate a pregnancy either independently or jointly.

The classification of HDP as stated by a WHO Study Group (World Health Organization 1987) consists of eight distinct components. These are:

1. Gestational hypertension — hypertension without the development of significant proteinuria (<0.3 g/l),
   a) After 20 weeks of gestation,
   b) During labour and/or within 48 hours of delivery.
2. Unclassified hypertension in pregnancy — hypertension found when blood pressure is recorded for the first time:
   a) After 20 weeks of gestation,
   b) During labour and/or within 48 hours of delivery.
   This type of hypertension should be reclassified as gestational hypertension if blood pressure returns to normal during the postnatal period, although some of these patients may have underlying hypertension caused by renal diseases.
3. Gestational proteinuria — development of significant proteinuria (>= 0.3 g/l):
   a) After 20 weeks of gestation,
   b) During labour and/or within 48 hours of delivery.
4. Pre-eclampsia — development of gestational hypertension and significant proteinuria:
   a) After 20 weeks of gestation,
   b) During labour and/or within 48 hours of delivery.
5. Eclampsia (convulsions):
   a) Antepartum,
   b) Intrapartum,
   c) Postpartum.
6. Underlying hypertension or renal disease (for example, in women who initially have hypertension only during pregnancies, being normotensive between pregnancies, but develop sustained hypertension later in life):
   a) Underlying hypertension,
   b) Underlying renal disease,
   c) Other known causes of hypertension (such as phaeochromocytoma).

7. Pre-existing hypertension or renal hypertension and/or proteinuria in pregnancy (for example, in women known to have disease prior to pregnancy):
   a) Pre-existing hypertension,
   b) Pre-existing renal disease,
   c) Pre-existing other known causes of hypertension.
8. Superimposed pre-eclampsia/eclampsia:
   a) Pre-existing hypertension with superimposed pre-eclampsia or eclampsia (a worsening of hypertension, with an increase in diastolic blood pressure to at least 15 mmHg (2.0 kPa) above non-pregnancy values, accompanied by the development or worsening of proteinuria),
   b) Pre-existing renal disease with superimposed pre-eclampsia or eclampsia.

The terms superimposed pre-eclampsia and eclampsia should be used only when hypertension was known to be present prior to pregnancy, or when hypertension is discovered early in pregnancy (<20 weeks of gestation) and proteinuria develops in late pregnancy.

ICD classification

The Tenth Revision of the International Classification of Diseases groups (ICD-10) hypertensive disorders of pregnancy as follows:

- 010 Oedema, proteinura and hypertensive disorders in pregnancy, childbirth and the puerperium
- 010 Pre-existing hypertension complicating pregnancy, childbirth and the puerperium (pre-existing essential hypertension, hypertensive heart and/or renal disease, and secondary hypertension)
- 011 Pre-existing hypertensive disorder with superimposed proteinuria
- 012 Gestational (pregnancy-induced) oedema and proteinuria without hypertension
- 013 Gestational (pregnancy-induced) hypertension without significant proteinuria (gestational hypertension and mild pre-eclampsia)
- 014 Gestational (pregnancy-induced) hypertension with significant proteinuria (moderate or severe pre-eclampsia)
- 015 Eclampsia (in pregnancy, labour or the puerperium)
- 016 Unspecified maternal hypertension

There are some differences between the ICD-10 classification and that developed by the WHO Study Group. While the study group classified HDP into eight major components and 19 minor components ICD-10 classified this condition into seven major components and 16 minor components. The major difference between these two classifications is that while the ICD-10 includes gestational oedema alone and with proteinuria in the same section entitled oedema, proteinura and hypertensive disorders in pregnancy, childbirth and the puerperium, the WHO Study Group did not include oedema in their classification at all. However it is noteworthy that both agree in leaving oedema out of the definition of pre-eclampsia. Therefore, pre-eclampsia, as noted above, has both gestational hypertension with significant proteinuria in its definition. Eclampsia refers to the convulsions associated with any of the aforementioned conditions.

The main differences between ICD-9 and ICD-10 are that the latter has dropped the term "benign" essential hypertension in favour of "pre-existing" hypertension complicating pregnancy, childbirth and the puerperium. More importantly, oedema has been dropped in the classification of pre-eclampsia, thus agreeing with the conclusions of the WHO Study Group.

Diagnosis of hypertensive disorders, pre-eclampsia and eclampsia

The diagnosis of PIH and eclampsia is based on blood pressure measurements (and their timing during pregnancy), urine testing, and clinical observation of seizures or convulsions. Blood pressure measurements should be taken in a standard manner, taking into account the position of the patient, the condition of the equipment and the size of the pneumatic cuff. Studies have demonstrated enormous observer variability in measuring blood pressures which accounts for some of the poor quality of many epidemiologic studies on HDP (Villar et al. 1989). Furthermore there is no general consensus which Korotkoff phase should be used to estimate diastolic blood pressure. The WHO Study Group recommended phase IV (muffling), while recent studies suggest that phase V (disappearance of sounds) is better.

Nor is there consensus with regard to the definition of pregnancy-induced or gestational hypertension. The two most frequently employed definitions differ in several important respects. The World Health Organization recommends that a diagnosis of hypertension should be made when the diastolic blood pressure persists at or above 90 mmHg for two consecutive readings taken four or more hours apart after a period of rest, or if the diastolic blood pressure is equal to or greater than 110 mmHg on any occasion. The American College of Gynecologists and Obstetriciancs (ACOG) definition includes both the systolic and diastolic blood pressures and defined hypertension in pregnancy as a measurement greater than or equal to 140/90 mmHg on two occasions of at least 6 hours apart. The ACOG definition also includes an increase of 30 mmHg or more in the systolic or an increase of 15 mmHg or more in the diastolic over baseline measurements as valid for the definition of HDP. (Davey and MacGillivray 1988).

Proteinuria is defined as a positive test of >= 0.3 g/24 hours or >= 30 mg/dl (1+dipstick) on two occasions >= 6 hours apart.

Eclampsia comprises the convulsions complicating pregnancy-induced hypertension, in the absence of other neurological explanations (e.g. epilepsy) for the seizures.

Incidence, Mortality and Disability due to hypertensive disorders of pregnancy

There are very few population-based studies on the frequency with which hypertensive disorders occur in pregnancy. There is also little information on the magnitude of the risk of pre-eclampsia developing in a woman with pregnancy-induced hypertension. However, it is known that eclampsia is more common in certain conditions, including:

- low maternal age
- primigravidity
- previous abortions and paternal change
- molar pregnancy;
- where there is a large amount of placental tissue as in twin pregnancy, diabetes and triploidy;
- in obese women;
- where there is a familial tendency;
- where there are geographic and racial differences in incidence (Collins and Wallenberg 1989).

Because uniform diagnostic criteria are not always followed by those who study and report on hypertensive disorders of pregnancy, reported incidence may not be readily comparable between study sites (Davies 1971). Most reports on the epidemiology of the condition have dealt with the occurrence of eclampsia (convulsions). Convulsions or "fits" occurring in pregnancy are fairly easily recognized even without fully trained medical personnel and the condition is likely to be recorded. Therefore, for the purposes of these calculations, attention is focused largely on the incidence, case fatality and long-term morbidities arising from eclampsia.

Incidence of hypertensive disorders of pregnancy

There is no doubt that the incidence of eclampsia can be very much influenced by the availability and quality of antenatal care. Moreover, in parts of the world where care is unavailable or substandard and the incidence of eclampsia is likely to be high, there is usually inadequate recording of births (and maternal deaths) so that it is not possible to determine the number of pregnant women at risk or the incidence and mortality by parity. To add to the difficulty of estimating incidence, most studies have concentrated on data from hospital sources which are, like other aspects of maternal mortality and morbidity, inadequate and biased as sources of incidence and mortality.

Rates of eclampsia reported from different countries at around 0.1 per cent have been reported from around the world (Australia, Canada, France, Germany, Israel, Netherlands, New Zealand, Switzerland, and United Kingdom) from 1950 onwards (MacGillivray 1983). Over the same period much higher rates (10–17 per cent) have been recorded in India, Italy, Korea, and Nigeria. Historically even higher rates have been recorded. However, these are all largely hospital incidence rates which reflect the referral rate of emergencies and standards of antenatal care rather than the true incidence of the condition.

There is evidence from countries which have maintained good clinical records for several decades that the incidence of eclampsia is falling, though the reasons for the decline are not fully understood. Table 1 shows the rate of eclampsia per 100 deliveries and case fatality rates — both of which decreased significantly — in Glasgow Royal Maternity Hospital over a 50-year period (Walker 1992).

Surveys of eclampsia have been undertaken in England and Wales since 1922 and these have continued to show a decline in both incidence and deaths from eclampsia. However, a new national survey of eclampsia was started in 1992 because of continuing concern about the problem and the many unresolved issues relating to the condition and its management. Eclampsia is still a major cause of maternal mortality in the United Kingdom and in a large proportion of eclampsia deaths substandard care has been identified as contributing to the poor outcome.

In order to determine more accurately the epidemiology of hypertensive disorders and eclampsia in different settings, WHO sponsored an inter-regional collaborative study (World Health Organization 1991). This showed considerable variation in the incidence of hypertensive disorders in general and of pre-eclampsia and eclampsia in particular despite the considerable care taken to standardize the definitions and methods used (Table 2). The authors concluded that there are genuine differences in the incidence of hypertensive disorders of pregnancy in the populations studied and that these are not caused by underlying differences in the baseline blood pressure levels in these populations.

Table 3 shows the incidence of eclampsia in selected developing countries. A large scale community study in Jamaica, a country with a high rate of hypertension, recorded an incidence of eclampsia of 0.7 per cent (Thomas et al. 1991). Based on the evidence from the WHO collaborative study and other studies undertaken around the world, an incidence of eclampsia of 0.5 per cent of live births was taken for the developing countries. This is equivalent to around 0.47 per cent of pregnancies. This incidence is high in relation to incidence in most developed countries today where incidence is estimated to be around 0.1 per cent (Duley 1991).

Mortality from hypertensive disorders of pregnancy

Although eclampsia is responsible for the majority of deaths associated with the hypertensive disorders of pregnancy, death can also occur with-

Table 1 Decrease in incidence of, and case fatality from eclampsia at Glasgow Royal Maternity Hospital 1933–82

Period	*Incidence (per 100 000 deliveries)*	*Case fatality (per 100 000 cases)*
1933-42	729	13 700
1943-52	707	12 000
1953-62	235	2 400
1963-72	130	1 300
1973-82	51	0

Source: Walker (1992)

Table 2 Incidence of hypertensive disorders of pregnancy in different settings, 1990

Antenatal Findings	*Burma*	*Thailand*	*China*	*Viet Nam*
Diastolic > 90 mmHg+	7.3% (6.4-8.2%)	20.9% (19.6-22.2%)	33.1% (31.8-34.5%)	5.3% (4.5-5.8%)
Systolic > 140 mmHg+	3.6% (3.0-4.3%	3.4% (2.8-3.9%)	20.0% (18.9-21.1%)	1.6% (1.2-1.9%)
Proteinuria	6.5% (5.6-7.4%)	9.1% (8.2-10.1%)	5.2% (4.6-5.9%)	6.8% 6.1-7.6%
Oedema	6.5% (5.6-7.4%)	8.4% (7.5-9.3%)	37.5% (36.1-38.9%)	2.0% (1.6-2.5%)
Proteinuric Pre-eclampsia	4.4% (3.1-5.8%)	7.5% (6.2-8.8%)	8.3% (7.4-9.2%)	1.5% (0.9-2.1%)
Eclampsia	0.33% (0.13-0.54%)	0.90% (0.59-1.21%)	0.19% (0.07-0.32%)	0.36% (0.19-0.55%)
Clinically diagnosed HDP	5.3% (3.9-6.8%)	1.1% (0.6%-1.7%)	30.9% (29.5-32.3%)	1.2% (0.7-1.7%)

Source: World Health Organization (1991)

out manifested convulsions. Pregnancy-induced hypertension may progressively deteriorate as pregnancy nears term, and result in death due to placental abruption, disseminated intravascular coagulapathy, adult respiratory distress syndrome or cerebral haemorrhage.

Estimates of the proportion of maternal deaths associated with non-convulsive pregnancy-induced hypertension and eclampsia indicate wide intercountry variations. For the purposes of these calculations it has been assumed that two-thirds of all HDP deaths are associated with eclampsia. This is a somewhat arbitrary figure, but appears to be consistent with evidence from different countries as shown in Table 4. Tables 4 and 5 summarize the available country-specific mortality data for hypertensive disorders of pregnancy.

Eclampsia, though uncommon has a high case fatality rate. By contrast, pregnancy-induced hypertension is more common but less likely to result

Table 3 Reported incidence and case fatality rates for eclampsia

Region	*Area*	*Years*	*No. of cases*	*Incidence per 1 000 births*	*Case Fatality Rate (%)*	*Reference*
India						
1985	Calcutta	1976-83	152	–	5.9	Ghose and Das
1990	Pune	1988-89	33	–	6.0	Goyaji and Otiv
Other Asia & Islands						
Bangladesh	Okkalapa	1978-82	–	–	12.0	Tin and Kyow-Myint
Myanmar	Kuala Lumpur	1987-89	109	1.4	6.4	Duley 1991
Thailand	Bangkok	1967-74	298	2.0	4.7	Porapakkham 1979
Sub-Saharan Africa						
Nigeria	Ilorin	1972-87	651	3.8	14.4	Adetoro 1989
	Zaria	1976-79	525	2.3	9.1	Harrison 1985
South Africa	Pietermaritzburg	1985*	**55	4.7	7.0	Moore and Munoz 1985
	Durban	1980	67	0.3	11.9	Moodley and Daya 1994
	Durban	1990	135	0.6	8.9	Moodley and Daya 1994
Zambia	Lusaka	1975-76	79	2.2	16.4	Chatterjee et al. 1978
Zimbabwe	Gwern	1982-84	8	1.6	25	De Muylder 1987
Weighted average					*11.2*	
Latin America & Caribbean						
Colombia	Bogota	1989	83	8.1	4.8	Duley 1991
	Cali	1989	80	7.7	3.8	Duley 1991
Jamaica	National	1986	68	7.2	2.9	Thomas et al. 1991
Weighted average					*3.1*	
Middle Eastern Crescent						
Egypt	Kar el Aini	1981-82	**124	11.9	13.7	Darwish and Sarhan 1983
	Cairo	1973-76	105	6.9	7.6	Mahran 1977
Weighted average					*10.1*	

* Year of publication
** Referral centre, denominator not adjusted.

in death or permanent disability. The case fatality rate varies from region to region as a function of the assumed amount and quality of health care available (Table 3). It is widely believed that the system of regular and frequent monitoring of blood pressure and proteinuria coupled with effective treatment have helped to reduce mortality in many settings. Where these interventions are unavailable, both incidence of eclampsia and case-fatality rates are likely to be high.

Epidemiological data on mortality have been used by the authors to derive a first set of regional mortality estimates. When considered in con-

Table 4 Estimates of the percentage of maternal deaths associated with hypertensive disorders of pregnancy (HDP)

Country	*Number of maternal deaths*	*Number of deaths associated with HDP without convulsions*	*Number of deaths associated with Eclampsia*	*% of HDP deaths associated with eclampsia*
Bahrain	37	5	4	80
Bhutan	44	4	3	75
Brazil	34	8	8	100
Chile	454	49	36	74
Egypt	69	15	8	53
India	7985	730	653	89
Indonesia	50	8	8	100
Iran	125	9	9	100
Israel	27	4	3	75
Jamaica	181	49	37	76
Japan	406	125	50	40
Kuwait	50	11	9	82
Lebanon	45	3	3	100
Malaysia	726	125	70	58
Myanmar	44	5	5	100
Nepal	81	6	6	100
Nigeria	116	18	16	89
Pakistan	545	72	69	96
Qatar	9	5	4	80
Syria	22	2	2	100
Tanzania	224	43	25	58
Thailand	263	35	23	66
Yemen	482	30	29	97

Source: Duley (1992)

junction with mortality estimates proposed by other authors for other diseases and injuries in the Global Burden of Disease Study, the implied level of overall mortality usually exceeded the rate estimated by various demographic methods. In order not to exceed this upper bound for mortality within each age-sex and broad-cause group, an algorithm has been applied by the editors to reduce mortality estimates for specific conditions so that their sum did not exceed this upper bound. The algorithm has been described in more detail in *The Global Burden of Disease* (Murray and Lopez 1996a).

Disabilities due to hypertensive disorders of pregnancy

If little is known about the incidence of and mortality from pre-eclampsia and eclampsia, there is even less knowledge about the extent of seri-

Table 5 Estimates of percentage of deaths and cause-specific mortality for hypertensive disorders of pregnancy (HDP) per 100 000 live births, around 1990

Country or territory	*Deaths due to maternal conditions per 100 000 live births*	*Per cent of maternal deaths due to HDP*	*Deaths from HDP conditions per 100 000 live births*
Established Market Economies			
Japan	15	30	5
India	640	11	70
China	45	10	5
Other Asia And Islands			
Bangladesh	565	15	85
Bhutan	875	9	80
Hong Kong	25	22	5
Indonesia	470	14	65
Malaysia	270	16	45
Myanmar	300	11 †	35
Nepal	245	9	25
Philippines	150	22	35
Singapore	35	21	10
Thailand	90	11	10
Viet Nam	575	4	25
Sub-Saharan Africa			
Botswana *	90	27	25
Burkina Faso *	810	1	10
Cameroon	145	4	10
Chad *	835	21	175
Congo	80	10	10
Ethiopia	645	8	50
Gabon	155	10	15
The Gambia	1130	13	150
Ghana	670	9	60
Guinea *	835	15	125
Guinea-Bissau	790	17 †	135
Ivory Coast	1140	8	90
Kenya	215	3	10
Malawi	260	4	10
Mauritius ‡	95	12	10
Mozambique	370	23	85
Niger	390	18	70
Nigeria	590	12	70
Senegal	795	11 †	90
Sierra Leone	635	12	75
South Africa	115	26	30
Swaziland	95	10	10
Tanzania	270	7	20
Togo	475	7	35
Uganda	345	3	10
Zaire	105	10	10
Zambia	145	21	30
Zimbabwe	140	9	15

Table 5 *(continued)*

Country or territory	*Deaths due to maternal conditions per 100 000 live births*	*Per cent of maternal deaths due to HDP*	*Deaths from HDP conditions per 100 000 live births*
Latin America and the Caribbean			
Argentina	180	10	20
Brazil	110	17	20
Chile	110	10	10
Colombia	295	21	60
Ecuador	165	25	40
Jamaica	80	30	25
Mexico *	360	37	135
Paraguay ‡	470	13	60
Peru	165	17	30
Puerto Rico	40	35	15
Trinidad and Tobago *	30	73	20
Venezuela	125	23	30
Middle Eastern Crescent			
Algeria	140	9	15
Bahrain ‡	35	15	5
Egypt	305	15	45
Israel *	40	15	10
Kuwait	20	22	5
Lebanon *	130	7	10
Morocco	435	7	30
Pakistan	905	13	120
Qatar *	15	55	10
Saudi Arabia	55	3	5
Sudan	515	13	70
Syria	340	11	40
Tunisia	135	12	15
Turkey	105	11	10
Yemen	700	13	90

* Data from one hospital only
† Cause of death data on less than 20 per cent of recorded deaths
‡ Vital registration data only
Source: Duley (1992)

ous morbidity associated with them. As already mentioned, pre-eclampsia affects many vital organ systems. Renal and liver damage, pulmonary oedema, cerebral haemorrhage and retinal detachment may follow eclamptic convulsions. It is not clear to what extent these conditions are temporary and very little long-term follow-up of women who have suffered from eclamptic convulsions has been undertaken. A study in Nigeria found that of 741 eclamptic survivors, 65 (8.8 per cent) had associated complications including acute renal failure (22 women), cerebrovascular haemorrhage (6 women), and acute cardio-pulmonary failure (5 women). Many of these conditions have long-term sequelae. Another 32 women had other acute conditions including haemorrhage, sepsis and ruptured uterus (Odum 1991).

A study in the United States followed a total of 223 women with eclampsia for an average of 7.2 years (Sibai et al. 1992). Twenty of the women (8.9 per cent) developed chronic hypertension following the index pregnancy though they had had no evidence of pre-existing hypertension. Two women (0.9 per cent) had long-term complications — one patient had hypertensive cardiomyopathy and another developed progressive renal failure. Another woman died of cardiovascular complications after 13 years of follow-up though it is not clear that this was related to the eclamptic convulsion. None of the surviving women in this series had evidence of neurologic deficit or seizures. An earlier study had found an association between eclampsia and future development of epilepsy, neurologic deficit and seizures (Sexton 1976). It is assumed that improved management of both pre-eclampsia and eclampsia reduces the impact of long-term complications.

On the basis of this evidence, we have estimated that approximately ten per cent of eclamptic cases developed long-term complications such as chronic hypertension, renal failure or neurological sequelae. Admittedly these are very small numbers and it is difficult to extrapolate from them. On the other hand, the women in the United States study were closely monitored during pregnancy and during subsequent follow-up. Moreover, they received intensive treatment during the eclamptic period. It is reasonable to assume that long-term complications will be more common among women who receive treatment only *in extremis*, as is the case in much of the developing world. The disability estimates for the Global Burden of Disease Study (GBD) take into account only Years Lived with Disability (YLDs) due to neurological sequelae; chronic hypertension and mild renal failure (with the exception of end-stage renal disease) have not been considered to be disabilities *per se*. Based on the limited evidence from follow-up studies, we have assumed that 0.1 per cent of eclampsia cases develop permanent neurological sequelae. It should be noted, however, that women who develop hypertension following an eclamptic episode during pregnancy are more likely to develop serious hypertension during subsequent pregnancies (Sibai et al. 1992).

Table 6 shows the disability weights used in the calculation of Years Lived with Disability (YLDs) and Disability-Adjusted Life Years (DALYs) for the neurological sequelae considered in the Global Burden of Disease Study. As there is no effective treatment for conditions resulting from hypertensive disorders of pregnancy the disability weights used for treated and untreated forms of neurological sequelae are identical. The distribution of episodes of hypertensive disorders, as well as neurological sequelae arising from them, across the seven disability classes used in the GBD are shown in Table 7.

Epidemiological data may be available for incidence, prevalence, case-fatality or mortality. Where data on more than one of these parameters are available, estimates of each of the epidemiological parameters derived from the data may not be internally consistent or consistent with the

Table 6 Disability weights used to calculate the burden of disease from hypertensive disorders of pregnancy, treated and untreated forms.

Condition	*Age (years)* 0-4	5-14	15-44	45-59	60+
Neurological sequelae	—	—	0.388	0.397	0.468

Table 7 Distribution of episodes of hypertensive disorders of pregnancy and neurological sequelae arising from them across the seven classes of disability by age group, females, 1990.*

	Disability class I	II	III	IV	V	VI	VII
Age (years)				**Episodes**			
0-4	0	0	0	0	0	0	0
5-14	0	0	0	0	0	0	0
15-44	0	0	100	0	0	0	0
45-59	0	0	0	0	0	0	0
60+	0	0	0	0	0	0	0
				Neurological sequelae			
0-4	0	0	0	0	0	0	0
5-14	0	0	0	0	0	0	0
15-44	0	8	16	26	18	21	8
45-59	0	8	17	24	18	22	10
60+	0	7	14	19	16	24	20

*For a description of the seven disability classes, see Murray and Lopez (1996b).

adjusted mortality rates described above. To ensure that all epidemiological information concerning a given condition is internally consistent, the editors have undertaken extensive analyses using computer models of the natural history of disease as described in Murray and Lopez (1996b). The incidence, prevalence, and duration estimates have consequently been revised where necessary. In view of these adjustments to the basic epidemiological estimates originally provided for the GBD, the estimates which have undergone the GBD validation process are the joint responsibility of the authors and the editors.

The estimates of number of deaths, Years of Life Lost (YLLs), YLDs and DALYs from episodes of eclampsia and the neurological sequelae are presented in Tables 8–10.

Table 8 Epidemiological estimates for episodes of eclampsia, females, 1990.

Age	*Incidence*		*Avg. age*	*Deaths*		*YLLs*	
group (years)	Number ('000s)	Rate per100 000	at onset (years)	Number ('000s)	Rate per100 000	Number ('000s)	Rate per100 000
Established Market Economies							
0-4	0	0	–	0	0.00	0	0
5-14	0	0	–	0	0.00	0	0
15-44	447	249	30.00	0	0.20	11	6
45-59	0	0	–	0	0.00	0	0
60+	0	0	–	0	0.10	0	0
All Ages	*447*	*110*	*30.00*	*0*	*0.00*	*11*	*3*
Formerly Socialist Economies of Europe							
0-4	0	0	–	0	0.00	0	0
5-14	0	0	–	0	0.00	0	0
15-44	264	352	29.80	0	0.40	9	12
45-59	0	0	52.40	0	0.00	0	0
60+	0	0	–	0	0.00	0	0
All Ages	*264*	*146*	*30.50*	*0*	*0.20*	*9*	*4*
India							
0-4	0	0	–	0	0.00	0	0
5-14	0	0	–	0	0.00	0	0
15-44	1 290	704	29.80	13	5.80	393	214
45-59	42	92	52.40	0	0.80	7	15
60+	0	0	–	0	0.00	0	0
All Ages	*1 332*	*325*	*30.50*	*14*	*2.80*	*400*	*98*
China							
0-4	0	0	–	0	0.00	0	0
5-14	0	0	–	0	0.00	0	0
15-44	1 257	442	29.90	2	0.80	72	25
45-59	79	123	52.40	0	0.20	2	3
60+	0	0	–	0	0.00	0	0
All Ages	*1 336*	*244*	*30.50*	*2*	*0.40*	*74*	*13*
Other Asia and Islands							
0-4	0	0	–	0	0.00	0	0
5-14	0	0	–	0	0.00	0	0
15-44	943	591	29.80	6	3.00	176	110
45-59	39	112	52.20	0	0.50	4	11
60+	0	0	–	0	0.00	0	0
All Ages	*982*	*289*	*30.70*	*6*	*1.60*	*180*	*53*
Sub-Saharan Africa							
0-4	0	0	–	0	0.00	0	0
5-14	71	102	10.00	1	1.30	45	64
15-44	1 259	1 185	29.50	21	14.60	619	583
45-59	3	12	52.20	0	0.20	1	5
60+	0	0	–	0	0.00	0	0
All Ages	*1 333*	*517*	*28.50*	*22*	*6.40*	*665*	*258*

Table 8 *(continued)*

Age group (years)	*Incidence* Number ('000s)	Rate per100 000	*Avg. age at onset* (years)	*Deaths* Number ('000s)	Rate per100 000	*YLLs* Number ('000s)	Rate per100 000
Latin America and the Caribbean							
0-4	0	0	–	0	0.00	0	0
5-14	4	0	10.00	0	0.00	1	2
15-44	623	599	29.80	3	2.40	92	88
45-59	4	17	52.40	0	0.10	0	0
60+	0	0	–	0	0.00	0	0
All Ages	*631*	*284*	*29.80*	*3*	*1.10*	*93*	*42*
Middle Eastern Crescent							
0-4	0	0	–	0	0.00	0	0
5-14	1	0	10.00	0	0.00	0	0
15-44	979	913	29.80	8	5.30	217	202
45-59	63	281	52.30	0	1.50	7	31
60+	0	0	–	0	0.00	0	0
All Ages	*1 043*	*1 043*	*31.10*	*8*	*2.50*	*224*	*91*
Developed Regions							
0-4	0	0	–	0	0.00	0	0
5-14	0	0	–	0	0.00	0	0
15-44	711	280	29.93	0	0.00	20	8
45-59	0	0	–	0	0.00	0	0
60+	0	0	–	0	0.00	0	0
All Ages	*711*	*109*	*29.9*	*0*	*0.00*	*20*	*3*
Developing Regions							
0-4	0	0	–	0	0.00	0	0
5-14	76	17	10	1	0.22	46	10
15-44	6 351	672	30	53	5.61	1 569	166
45-59	230	108	52	0	0.00	21	10
60+	0	0	–	0	0.00	0	0
All Ages	*6 657*	*329*	*30.3*	*54*	*2.67*	*1 636*	*81*
World							
0-4	0	0	–	0	0.00	0	0
5-14	76	14	10.0	1	0.19	46	9
15-44	7 062	589	29.78	53	4.42	1 589	133
45-59	230	74	52.3	0	0.00	21	7
60+	0	0	–	0	0.00	0	0
All Ages	*7 368*	*282*	*30.3*	*54*	*2.07*	*1 656*	*63*

Table 9 Epidemiological estimates for neurological sequelae arising from hypertensive disorders of pregnancy, females, 1990.

Age group (years)	*Incidence* Number ('000s)	*Incidence* Rate per100 000	*Prevalence* Number ('000s)	*Prevalence* Rate per100 000	*Avg. age* at onset (years)	*Avg.* duration (years)	*YLDs* Number ('000s)	*YLDs* Rate per100 000
Established Market Economies								
0-4	0	0.00	0	0.00	–	–	0	0
5-14	0	0.00	0	0.00	–	–	0	0
15-44	0	0.10	4	2.10	30.00	50.00	3	2
45-59	0	0.00	3	4.20	–	–	0	0
60+	0	0.00	3	4.20	–	–	0	0
All Ages	*0*	*0*	*10*	*2.5*	*30.00*	*50.00*	*3*	*1*
Formerly Socialist Economies of Europe								
0-4	0	0.00	0	0.00	–	–	0	0
5-14	0	0.00	0	0.00	–	–	0	0
15-44	0	0.20	2	3.00	29.90	46.80	2	3
45-59	0	0.00	2	6.00	–	–	0	0
60+	0	0.00	2	6.00	–	–	0	0
All Ages	*0*	*0.1*	*6*	*3.4*	*29.90*	*46.80*	*2*	*1*
India								
0-4	0	0.00	0	0.00	–	–	0	0
5-14	0	0.00	0	0.00	–	–	0	0
15-44	1	0.70	19	10.50	29.80	41.70	14	8
45-59	0	0.00	10	21.30	–	–	0	0
60+	0	0.00	6	21.30	–	–	0	0
All Ages	*1*	*0.3*	*35*	*8.6*	*29.80*	*41.70*	*14*	*3*
China								
0-4	0	0.00	0	0.00	–	–	0	0
5-14	0	0.00	0	0.00	–	–	0	0
15-44	1	0.50	19	6.80	29.90	44.20	15	5
45-59	0	0.00	9	13.70	–	–	0	0
60+	0	0.00	7	13.70	–	–	0	0
All Ages	*1*	*0.2*	*35*	*6.4*	*29.90*	*44.20*	*15*	*3*
Other Asia and Islands								
0-4	0	0.00	0	0.00	–	–	0	0
5-14	0	0.00	0	0.00	–	–	0	0
15-44	1	0.60	13	8.30	29.80	41.40	10	6
45-59	0	0.00	6	16.90	–	–	0	0
60+	0	0.00	4	16.90	–	–	0	0
All Ages	*1*	*0.3*	*23*	*6.8*	*29.80*	*41.40*	*10*	*3*
Sub-Saharan Africa								
0-4	0	0.00	0	0.00	–	–	0	0
5-14	0	0.00	0	0.00	–	–	0	0
15-44	1	1.20	19	17.70	29.50	37.20	14	13
45-59	0	0.00	8	36.70	–	–	0	0
60+	0	0.00	5	36.70	–	–	0	0
All Ages	*1*	*0.5*	*32*	*12.3*	*29.50*	*37.20*	*14*	*5*

Table 9 *(continued)*

Age group (years)	*Incidence* Number ('000s)	Rate per100 000	*Prevalence* Number ('000s)	Rate per100 000	*Avg. age at onset* (years)	*Avg. duration* (years)	*YLDs* Number ('000s)	Rate per100 000
Latin America and the Caribbean								
0-4	0	0.00	0	0.00	–	–	0	0
5-14	0	0.00	0	0.00	–	–	0	0
15-44	1	0.60	9	8.60	29.80	42.60	7	7
45-59	0	0.00	4	17.30	–	–	0	0
60+	0	0.00	3	17.30	–	–	0	0
All Ages	*1*	*0.3*	*16*	*7.1*	*29.80*	*42.60*	*7*	*3*
Middle Eastern Crescent								
0-4	0	0.00	0	0.00	–	–	0	0
5-14	0	0.00	0	0.00	–	–	0	0
15-44	1	0.90	15	13.90	29.80	42.60	11	10
45-59	0	0.00	6	28.00	–	–	0	0
60+	0	0.00	4	28.00	–	–	0	0
All Ages	*1*	*0.4*	*25*	*10.3*	*29.80*	*42.60*	*11*	*4*
Developed Regions								
0-4	0	0.00	0	0.00	–	–	0	0
5-14	0	0.00	0	0.00	–	–	0	0
15-44	0	0.00	6	2.36	–	–	5	2
45-59	0	0.00	5	5.11	–	–	0	0
60+	0	0.00	5	4.13	–	–	0	0
All Ages	*0*	*0.00*	*16*	*2.46*	–	–	*5*	*1*
Developing Regions								
0-4	0	0.00	0	0.00	–	–	0	0
5-14	0	0.00	0	0.00	–	–	0	0
15-44	6	0.64	94	9.95	30	42	71	8
45-59	0	0.00	43	20.16	–	–	0	0
60+	0	0.00	29	19.56	–	–	0	0
All Ages	*6*	*0.30*	*166*	*8.20*	*29.8*	*41.6*	*71*	*4*
World								
0-4	0	0.00	0	0.00	–	–	0	0
5-14	0	0.00	0	0.00	–	–	0	0
15-44	6	0.50	100	8.34	29.8	41.6	76	6
45-59	0	0.00	48	15.43	–	–	0	0
60+	0	0.00	34	12.63	–	–	0	0
All Ages	*6*	*0.23*	*182*	*6.96*	*29.8*	*41.6*	*76*	*3*

Table 10 Epidemiological estimates for hypertensive disorders of pregnancy, females, 1990.

Age group (years)	Incidence		Prevalence		Deaths		YLLs		YLDs		DALYs	
	Number ('000s)	Rate per100 000	Number ('000s)	Rate per100 000	Number ('000s)	Rate per100 000	Number ('000s)	Rate per100 000	Number ('000s)	Rate per100 000	Number ('000s)	Rate per100 000
Established Market Economies												
0-4	0	0	0	0.00	0	0.00	0	0	0	0	0	0
5-14	0	0	0	0.00	0	0.00	0	0	0	0	0	0
15-44	447	249	4	2.23	0	0.00	11	6	3	2	14	8
45-59	0	0	3	4.42	0	0.00	0	0	0	0	0	0
60+	0	0	3	3.55	0	0.00	0	0	0	0	0	0
All Ages	*447*	*110*	*10*	*2.46*	*0*	*0.00*	*11*	*3*	*3*	*1*	*14*	*3*
Formerly Socialist Economies of Europe												
0-4	0	0	0	0.00	0	0.00	0	0	0	0	0	0
5-14	0	0	0	0.00	0	0.00	0	0	0	0	0	0
15-44	264	352	2	2.67	0	0.00	9	12	2	3	11	15
45-59	0	0	2	6.67	0	0.00	0	0	0	0	0	0
60+	0	0	2	5.50	0	0.00	0	0	0	0	0	0
All Ages	*264*	*109*	*6*	*2.47*	*0*	*0.00*	*9*	*4*	*2*	*1*	*11*	*5*
India												
0-4	0	0	0	0.00	0	0.00	0	0	0	0	0	0
5-14	0	0	0	0.00	0	0.00	0	0	0	0	0	0
15-44	1 291	705	19	10.37	13	7.09	393	214	14	8	407	222
45-59	42	91	10	21.74	0	0.00	7	15	0	0	7	15
60+	0	0	6	20.74	0	0.00	0	0	0	0	0	0
All Ages	*1 333*	*325*	*35*	*8.53*	*13*	*3.17*	*400*	*98*	*14*	*3*	*414*	*101*
China												
0-4	0	0	0	0.00	0	0.00	0	0	0	0	0	0
5-14	0	0	0	0.00	0	0.00	0	0	0	0	0	0
15-44	1 258	443	19	6.69	2	0.70	72	25	15	5	87	31
45-59	79	123	9	13.97	0	0.00	2	3	0	0	2	3
60+	0	0	7	13.55	0	0.00	0	0	0	0	0	0
All Ages	*1 337*	*244*	*35*	*6.38*	*2*	*0.36*	*74*	*13*	*15*	*3*	*89*	*16*
Other Asia and Islands												
0-4	0	0	0	0.00	0	0.00	0	0	0	0	0	0
5-14	0	0	0	0.00	0	0.00	0	0	0	0	0	0
15-44	944	591	13	8.14	6	3.76	176	110	10	6	186	117
45-59	39	111	6	17.10	0	0.00	4	11	0	0	4	11
60+	0	0	4	17.65	0	0.00	0	0	0	0	0	0
All Ages	*983*	*289*	*23*	*6.77*	*6*	*1.77*	*180*	*53*	*10*	*3*	*190*	*56*
Sub-Saharan Africa												
0-4	0	0	0	0.00	0	0.00	0	0	0	0	0	0
5-14	71	102	0	0.00	1	1.43	45	64	0	0	45	64
15-44	1 260	1 186	19	17.88	21	19.76	619	583	14	13	633	596
45-59	3	14	8	36.17	0	0.00	1	5	0	0	1	5
60+	0	0	5	39.28	0	0.00	0	0	0	0	0	0
All Ages	*1 334*	*517*	*32*	*12.41*	*22*	*8.53*	*665*	*258*	*14*	*5*	*679*	*263*

Table 10 *(continued)*

Age group (years)	Incidence		Prevalence		Deaths		YLLs*		YLDs*		DALYs*	
	Number ('000s)	Rate per100 000	Number ('000s)	Rate per100 000	Number ('000s)	Rate per100 000	Number ('000s)	Rate per100 000	Number ('000s)	Rate per100 000	Number ('000s)	Rate per100 000
Latin America and the Caribbean												
0-4	0	0	0	0.00	0	0.00	0	0	0	0	0	0
5-14	4	8	0	0.00	0	0.00	1	2	0	0	1	2
15-44	624	600	9	8.65	3	2.88	92	88	7	7	99	95
45-59	4	17	4	17.13	0	0.00	0	0	0	0	0	0
60+	0	0	3	17.83	0	0.00	0	0	0	0	0	0
All Ages	*632*	*284*	*16*	*7.19*	*3*	*1.35*	*93*	*42*	*7*	*3*	*100*	*45*
Middle Eastern Crescent												
0-4	0	0	0	0.00	0	0.00	0	0	0	0	0	0
5-14	1	2	0	0.00	0	0.00	0	0	0	0	0	0
15-44	980	914	15	13.99	8	7.46	217	202	11	10	228	213
45-59	63	283	6	26.92	0	0.00	7	31	0	0	7	31
60+	0	0	4	25.89	0	0.00	0	0	0	0	0	0
All Ages	*1 044*	*423*	*25*	*10.13*	*8*	*3.24*	*224*	*91*	*11*	*4*	*235*	*95*
Developed Regions												
0-4	0	0	0	0.00	0	0.00	0	0	0	0	0	0
5-14	0	0	0	0.00	0	0.00	0	0	0	0	0	0
15-44	711	280	6	2.36	0	0.00	20	8	5	2	25	10
45-59	0	0	5	5.11	0	0.00	0	0	0	0	0	0
60+	0	0	5	4.13	0	0.00	0	0	0	0	0	0
All Ages	*711*	*109*	*16*	*2.46*	*0*	*0.00*	*20*	*3*	*5*	*1*	*25*	*4*
Developing Regions												
0-4	0	0	0	0.00	0	0.00	0	0	0	0	0	0
5-14	76	17	0	0.00	1	0.22	46	10	0	0	46	10
15-44	6 357	673	94	9.95	53	5.61	1 569	166	71	8	1 640	174
45-59	230	108	43	20.16	0	0.00	21	10	0	0	21	10
60+	0	0	29	19.56	0	0.00	0	0	0	0	0	0
All Ages	*6 663*	*329*	*166*	*8.20*	*54*	*2.67*	*1 636*	*81*	*71*	*4*	*1 707*	*84*
World												
0-4	0	0	0	0.00	0	0.00	0	0	0	0	0	0
5-14	76	14	0	0.00	1	0.19	46	9	0	0	46	9
15-44	7 068	590	100	8.34	53	4.42	1589	133	76	6	1 665	139
45-59	230	74	48	15.43	0	0.00	21	7	0	0	21	7
60+	0	0	34	12.63	0	0.00	0	0	0	0	0	0
All Ages	*7 374*	*282*	*182*	*6.96*	*54*	*2.07*	*1656*	*63*	*76*	*3*	*1 732*	*66*

Impact of Interventions on the Burden

Management of eclampsia requires timely intervention such as anti-convulsant treatment and/or expedited delivery of the infant. Poor access to facilities that can provide these services will greatly decrease a woman's chance of survival. Treatment of eclampsia may require special care to address its complex pathophysiology; for example, hepatic involvement could lead to the HELLP syndrome with concurrent haemolysis, elevated liver enzymes and low platelet counts. In one study of 254 eclamptic cases (Sibai 1990), this condition was reported as a complication in 9.8 per cent of cases. In the same study, other complications included placental abruption (9.8 per cent), and disseminated intravascualr coagulophathy (5.1 per cent). Eclampsia may also be complicated by cerebral pathology leading to cerebral haemorrhage and oedema resembling that of hypertensive encephalopathy, pulmonary oedema including adult respiratory distress syndrome, renal cortical necrosis, and hepatic rupture. About two thirds of women dying from eclampsia have specific lesions in the liver and various grades of infarction including complete infarction. However, cerebral pathology, particularly cerebral haemorrhage, is usually the most significant cause of death (Redman 1992).

The hypertensive disorders of pregnancy pose a dilemma for the health care provider for the following reasons. Women often attend antenatal care late in pregnancy precluding the possibility of taking a "baseline' blood pressure measurement. An abnormal reading should be reconfirmed within 4–6 hours, a practice that is not always possible. Therefore, in these situations it is difficult to predict which women will develop pre-eclampsia. Moreover, in most developing country settings, women are unable or unwilling to follow the kind of antenatal care regimen common in the industrialized world with regular visits and close monitoring of blood pressure and proteinuria at each visit. The presence of significant proteinuria with hypertension greatly increases the risk of developing eclampsia, however in most developing country settings, urine is not tested.

It has now been established that the drug of choice in the treatment of eclamptic convulsions is magnesium sulphate (The Eclampsia Trial Collaborative Group 1995). However, it is not always available in a form suitable for administration to eclamptic women. In order to promote its wider availability, WHO has included magnesium sulphate (and its antidote) in the WHO List of Essential Drugs. It is hoped that this will help to ensure increased availability of the drug around the world. The administration of magnesium sulphate and the general care of women with eclamptic convulsions require health care providers with relatively advanced midwifery skills. Further research is needed as to the feasibility of providing treatment with magnesium sulphate at lower levels of the health care system where providers may have only a minimum of training and where back-up and supportive supervision are often lacking. Further research is also needed as to the role and effectiveness of magnesium sulphate in the management of pre-eclampsia and the prevention of eclamptic convulsions.

Conclusions

Hypertensive disorders of pregnancy continue to represent a major cause of maternal mortality even where access to care is assured. In developed countries they account for 10–15 per cent of maternal deaths and the proportion is considerably higher in many developing areas. As with haemorrhage, mortality from eclampsia and hypertensive disorders is relatively slow to decline as overall maternal mortality falls because it too depends on the availability of highly qualified professional health care.

This is well illustrated by the case of Sweden, a country which now has an extremely low maternal mortality ratio (around 4 deaths per 100 000 live births), where the decline in eclampsia deaths was not only due to a decline in the incidence but also to a reduction in the case fatality rate from 14 per cent in 1950–55 to 3 per cent in 1971–80 (Hogberg 1985).

Adequate antenatal monitoring and timely referral for signs and symptoms of eclampsia could result in a 65 per cent reduction of mortality due to eclampsia by the year 2000 (World Health Organization 1994).

Much about the epidemiology and etiology of hypertensive disorders is still unclear and even though treatment of eclampsia is now clearly defined, prevention strategies are still subject to debate. For reasons that are not well understood, the incidence of eclampsia appears to have been falling steadily in developed countries over the past three decades. There is insufficient evidence to be able to draw any conclusions about changing patterns of incidence in the developing world. However, in much of the developing world, eclampsia remains a major source of maternal death and one of the slowest to decline. Although improved case management of convulsions will help to accelerate the decline, continued attention to prevention strategies and to early detection and prevention of eclamptic convulsions is essential.

References

Adetoro OO (1989) A sixteen year survey of maternal mortality associated with eclampsia in Ilorin, Nigeria. *International Journal of Gynecology and Obstetrics*, 30:117–121.

Chatterjee TK, Hickey MU, Chikamta MD (1978) A review of 79 cases of eclampsia at the University Teaching Hospital, Lusaka. *Medical Journal of Zambia*, 12:77–80.

Collins R and Wallenburg HCS (1989) Pharmacological prevention and treatment of hypertensive disorders of pregnancy. In: Chalmers I. et al. (eds). *Effective care in pregnancy and childbirth*. Oxford University Press.

Coyaji KJ, Otiv SR (1990) Single high dose of intravenous phenytoin sodium for the treatment of eclampsia. *Acta Obstetrica Gynaecologica Scandinavia*, 69:115–118.

Darwish N, Sarhan D (1983) Maternal mortality in cases of pregnancy toxaemia in Kasr el-Aini hospital: a two year experience. In: Fayao M, Abdulla M. (eds). *Medical Education in the Field of Primary Maternal Child Health Care. Proceedings of International Conference, Cairo, Egypt. Dec 5–7th 1983.*

Davey DA, MacGillivray I (1988) The classification and definition of the hypertensive disorders of pregnancy. *American Journal of Obstetrics and Gynecology*, 158:892–8.

Davies AM (1971) Geographical epidemiology of the toxaemias of pregnancy. *Israeli Journal of Medical Science*, 7(6).

De Muylder X (1987) Maternity services in a general hospital. Part 1: Obstetrical data. *Central African Journal of Medicine*, 32:240–243.

Duley L (1991) *Maternal mortality and eclampsia: An assessment of levels and possible interventions.* Report prepared for the Maternal Health and Safe Motherhood Research Programme of the World Health Organization.

Duley L (1992) Maternal mortality associated with hypertensive disorders of pregnancy in Africa, Asia, Latin America and the Caribbean. *British Journal of Obstetrics and Gynaecology*, 99:547–553.

Ghose N, Das B (1985) Treatment of eclampsia. *Journal of the Indian Medical Association.* 83(9):299–302.

Harrison KA (1985 suppl. 5) Child bearing, health and social priorities. A survey of 22,774 consecutive births in Zaria, Northern Nigeria. *British Journal of Obstetrics and Gynaecology.*

Heuberger J *Diazepam and magnesium sulphate in the management of eclampsia.* (Personal communication).

Hogberg U (1985) *Maternal mortality in Sweden.* Umea University, Umea.

MacGillivray I (1983) *Pre-Eclampsia. The Hypertensive Disease of Pregnancy.* W.B. Saunders Company Ltd, London, Philadelphia, Toronto.

Mahran M (1977) *The extent of the problem of eclampsia and pre-eclampsia in arab countries.* WHO Document MCH/77.5.

Moodley J, Daya P (1994) Eclampsia: a continuing problem in developing countries. *International Journal of Gynaecology and Obstetrics*, 44(1):9–14.

Moore PJ, Munoz AP (1985) Eclampsia in the black population of the Natal midlands. *South African Medical Journal*, 67:597–599.

Murray CJL and Lopez AD (1996a) Estimating causes of death: new methods and global and regional applications for 1990. In: Murray CJL and Lopez AD, eds. *The global burden of disease: a comprehensive assessment of mortality and disability from diseases, injuries, and risk factors in 1990 and projected to 2020.* Cambridge, Harvard University Press.

Murray CJL and Lopez AD (199b) Global and regional descriptive epidemiology of disability: incidence, prevalence, health expectancies and Years lived with Disability. In: Murray CJL and Lopez AD, eds. *The global burden of disease: a comprehensive assessment of mortality and disability from diseases, injuries, and risk factors in 1990 and projected to 2020.* Cambridge, Harvard University Press.

Odum CU (1991) Eclampsia: An analysis of 845 cases treated in the Lagos University Teaching Hospital, Nigeria over a 20-Year period. *Journal of Obstetrics and Gynaecology of East and Central Africa*, 9:16.

Porapakkham S (1979) An epidemiologic study of eclampsia. *Obstetrics and Gynaecology*, 54:26–30.

Redman CWG (1992) Pathophysiology of pre-eclampsia and eclampsia — Why is it dangerous? In: *Royal College of Obstetricians and Gynaecologists Maternal mortality — The Way forward*, London, RCOG.

Sexton JA (1976) Epilepsy as a sequal of obstetrical complications. *Journal of the Kenya Medical Association*, 74:595–601.

Sibai BM (1990) Eclampsia VI. Maternal — perinatal outcome in 254 consecutive cases. *American Journal of Obstetrics and Gynecology*, 162:777.

Sibai BM et al. (1992) Pregnancy outcome after eclampsia and long-term prognosis. *American Journal of Obstetrics and Gynaecology*, 166:1757–1763.

The Eclampsia Trial Collaborative Group (1995) Which anticonvulsant for women with eclampsia? Evidence from the Collaborative Eclampsia Trial. *Lancet* 345:1455-1463

Thomas P et al. (1991) *Pre-eclampsia, Eclampsia and Maternal Mortality in Jamaica.* Report of a study.

Tin U, Kyaw-Myint TO, eds. *Report of the perinatal mortality and low birth weight sutdy project – Burma* WHO SEARO Inter-Country Collaborative Project. Rangoon Department of Medical Education, Ministry of Health.

Villar J et al. (1989) The measurement of blood pressure during pregnancy. *American Journal of Obstetrics and Gynecology*, 161:1019–1024.

Walker JJ (1992) What can current management offer? In: *Royal College of Obstetricians and Gynaecologists Maternal Mortality- The Way Forward*, London, RCOG.

World Health Organization (1975) *International Statistical Classification of Diseases. Ninth Revision.* Geneva, World Health Organization.

World Health Organization (1987) *The Hypertensive Disorders of Pregnancy: Report of a WHO Study Group.* Technical Report Series, No. 758, Geneva.

World Health Organization (1991) *Hypertensive disorders of pregnancy: Report of a WHO/MCH Interregional Collaborative Study.* WHO/MCH/91.4. Geneva.

World Health Organization (1992) *International Statistical Classification of Diseases and Related Health Problems. Tenth Revision.* Geneva, World Health Organization.

World Health Organization. Maternal Health and Safe Motherhood Programme (1994) *The Mother-Baby Package. Implementing Safe Motherhood in Countries.* Geneva.

Chapter 7

Prolonged and Obstructed labour

Carla AbouZahr

Introduction

Prolonged and obstructed labour are more common in humans than in other primates because the birth canal of a woman is not straight and wide as in other primates, but varies in width. The baby's head, which is large compared with the rest of the body, has to turn and flex as it negotiates the birth canal (Rosenberg 1992). The unique aspects of the mechanism of birth in humans are the following:

- the transverse or oblique position of the fetal head as it enters the maternal pelvic inlet;
- the rotation and flexion of the fetal head as it traverses the birth canal; and
- the emergence of the fetal head from the birth canal in an occiput-anterior position.

In humans, the infant cranium is actually longer than the anterior-posterior dimensions of the pelvic inlet, requiring the head to rotate and flex in order to pass through. Evolution has resulted in a variety of compensatory mechanisms for dealing with the resulting difficulties in childbirth. For example, in the mother increased levels of the hormone relaxin cause a relaxation of the ligaments at the sacroiliac articulations and the pubic symphysis. This increased joint mobility adds a certain amount to the dimensions of pelvic inlet. Also, during labour, the fetal skull bones are subjected to compressive forces arising during maternal uterine contractions. Because the sutures of the fetal cranial bones are not fused, movement can occur between the individual bones. The resultant alteration in shape or moulding may account for a reduction in fetal cranial diameter of 5–10 mm. Although fetal cranial moulding is an important adaptive response to a tight fit in the birth canal, excessive moulding is disadvantageous as it may cause cerebral trauma, mental retardation and cerebral palsy.

This tight fit between the human pelvis and the fetal head is one reason why prolonged labour is a relatively common complication of delivery. The adaptive mechanisms may be insufficient to prevent damage to mother, infant or both. A slight disproportion between the size of the fetal head and the space in the bony birth canal (cephalo-pelvic disproportion) is commonly a result of physical immaturity or stunting in the mother or distortion of her pelvis through disease or malnutrition. Obstructed labour may also be caused by an abnormal position of the fetus when the mother goes into labour.

Prolonged labour due to cephalopelvic disproportion may result in obstructed labour, maternal dehydration, ruptured uterus and obstetric fistulae (and also, but less directly, in postpartum haemorrhage and neonatal infection). In the infant, prolonged obstructed labour may cause asphyxia, brain damage and death. Obstructed labour, with or without ruptured uterus, features among the five major causes of maternal death in almost every developing country, although its relative importance varies from region to region. Abnormally prolonged labour and its effects are important contributors to maternal (and perinatal) mortality and morbidity worldwide.

Definition and Measurement

The classification of obstructed labour has not changed significantly through the different revisions of the International Classification of Diseases. In the Tenth Revision of the ICD, obstructed labour is assigned to three major categories:

O64 Obstructed labour due to malposition and malpresentation of fetus
O65 Obstructed labour due to maternal pelvic abnormality
O66 Other obstructed labour

In addition, two other related codes are:

O62 Abnormalities of forces of labour
O63 Long labour

The Ninth Revision of the International Classification of Diseases classified prolonged and obstructed labour under the general heading of "Complications occurring mainly in the course of labour and delivery" (660–669). The primary category is:

660 Obstructed labour

Other causes associated with prolonged labour may be categorized under:

661 Abnormality of forces of labour
662 Long labour
663 Umbilical cord complications
664 Trauma to perineum and vulva during delivery
665 Other obstetrical trauma.

According to the Eighth Revision, the categories referring to obstructed labour are listed under the general category Delivery (650–662) and include the following:

657 Delivery complicated by prolonged labour of other origin includes delivery complicated by obstructed labour NOS, retarded birth NOS, rigid cervix uteri, prolonged labour of other origin.
658 Delivery with laceration of perineum, without mention of other laceration
659 Delivery with rupture of uterus
660 Delivery with other obstetrical trauma

Etiology of obstructed labour

Labour is said to be obstructed when there is no advance of presenting part despite strong uterine contractions. (Bennett and Brown 1995). The causes of obstructed labour include:

Cephalopelvic disproportion — the fetus may be large in relation to maternal size, such as the fetus of a diabetic woman, or the pelvis may be contracted; contracted pelvis is more common when malnutrition is prevalent.

Deep transverse arrest — this is a common outcome of occipitoposterior position.

Fetal abnormalities — includes hydrocephalic fetus

Locked twins — this is a rare cause of obstruction

Malpresentations — vaginal delivery is impossible in cases of shoulder or brow presentation or persistent mentoposterior position

Pelvic tumors — in rare instances, cervical fibriods, an ovarian tumour or a tumour of the bony pelvis may prevent the head from entering the pelvis.

If obstruction cannot be overcome by manipulation or instrumental delivery, caesarean delivery is needed. Neglected obstructed labour is a major cause of both maternal and newborn morbidity and may result in death for one or both. Maternal complications include intrauterine infections following prolonged rupture of the membranes, trauma to the bladder due to pressure from the fetal head or damage during delivery, and ruptured uterus with consequent haemorrhage, shock and even death. The fetus may suffer intra-uterine asphyxia leading to still birth or permanent brain damage. Intracranial haemorrhage may be caused by asphyxia or trauma sustained during an instrumental delivery. Ascending infection may cause neonatal pneumonia which may also result from meconium aspiration.

As a general rule, cephalopelvic disproportion is most likely to be detected at first birth. However, disproportion in parous women also occurs and presents a different problem than in nulliparae. A past history of uneventful delivery may falsely reassure the birth attendant as well as the woman herself. However, in a subsequent labour, the fetus may be bigger, or the presentation may be abnormal. Because the tempo of labour is more rapid in a parous woman and uterine action in the presence of disproportion is likely to be vigorously reactive, uterine rupture is an ever-present possibility. The risk of uterine rupture is magnified if oxytocin augmentation is used.

In parts of the world where malnutrition, disease and early marriage are common, obstructed labour is primarily due to cephalo-pelvic disproportion and would be classified under categories of the ICD-10. The women most at risk are the very young and women of small stature. Rupture of the uterus is rare in first pregnancies but is a common consequence of obstructed labour among women who have borne many children. In countries where cephalo-pelvic disproportion is less prevalent, prolonged and obstructed labour is more likely to be due to either malpresentation of the fetus (ICD-10 O64) or to inefficient uterine contractions (ICD-10 O62).

Diagnosis of obstructed labour

Disproportion or obstructed labour is detected when labour is prolonged and cannot be successfully resolved except through operative intervention. In order to detect prolonged labour it is necessary to define precisely the onset of labour, and to determine an appropriate rate of cervical dilation during the active phase. A normal cervical dilation pattern is shown in Figure 1 below (Friedman 1955).

The definition of the presence of prolonged or obstructed labour is based on the following principles:

- the active phase of labour commences at 3cm cervical dilation with cervical effacement *and* regular uterine contractions;
- during active labour, the rate of cervical dilatation should not be slower than 1 cm/hour;
- a lag time of 4 hours between a slowing of labour and the need for intervention is unlikely to compromise the fetus or the mother and, if respected, avoids unnecessary interventions.

In fact, in many developing countries where most deliveries take place at home in the presence only of the immediate family or a traditional birth attendant, labour lasting for several days is relatively common (Kelly 1991). Although many local traditions include the exhortation "never let the sun set twice on the same labour" and information, education and communication campaigns such as "Facts-for-Life" recommend seeking medical assistance "when labour has gone on for too long (more than 12 hours)" the fact remains that for many women in developing countries the physical, economic, emotional and cultural obstacles to seeking care in cases of prolonged labour are overwhelming (Thaddeus et al. 1990).

Figure 1 Normal cervical dilation pattern during labour

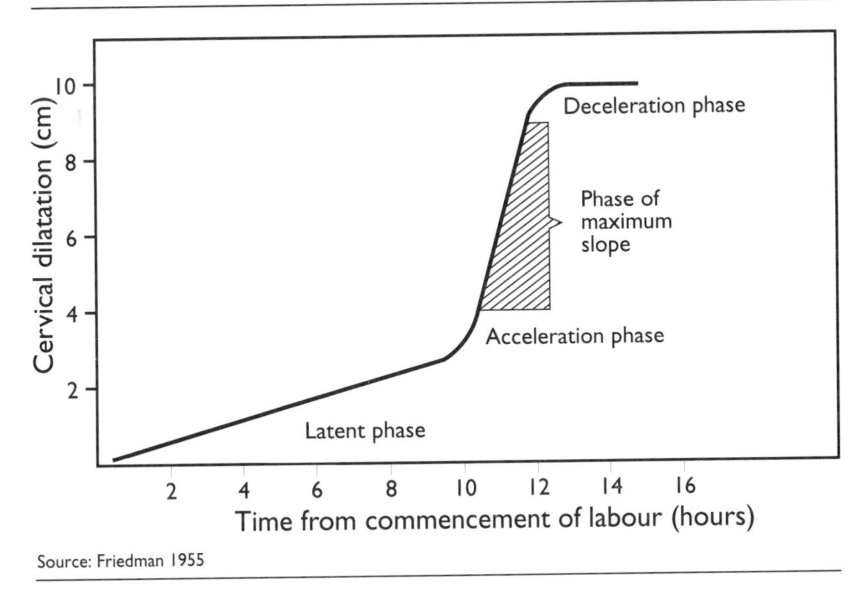

Source: Friedman 1955

Incidence, mortality and disability due to obstructed labour

Incidence of obstructed labour

Information on the incidence of, and mortality from prolonged or obstructed labour is incomplete and patchy. In part this is because when a woman dies as a result of obstructed labour the death is often classified under the final cause of death which may be sepsis, ruptured uterus or haemorrhage rather than ascribed to the underlying cause, that is cephalopelvic disproportion or abnormal presentation.

Any case of prolonged labour will normally require some form of obstetric intervention if it is to be brought to a successful outcome. Cephalopelvic disproportion or abnormal fetal position will require instrumental or caesarean delivery. It is, therefore, possible to use the rate of operative delivery — caesarean, forceps, and vacuum extraction—as a proxy indicator of the incidence of obstructed labour.

This is very approximate, however. Rates of instrumental delivery vary from country to country and from one institution to another within the same country. Even among the developed countries where such data are relatively easier to obtain than in developing areas, there are marked international variations in almost every aspect of delivery: the rates of total operative delivery, the relative proportions of instrumental, vaginal and caesarean delivery, and the rates of change in all these over time (Lomas and Enkin 1989).

Alongside the widely divergent rates of operative delivery, there are also differences in the reasons for operative interventions. There are many indications for instrumental delivery including, for example, fetal distress, eclampsia, and cord complications such as prolapse. The availability of such indication-specific data is limited in the case of caesarean delivery and non-existent in the case of instrumental vaginal delivery. A review of all available information found that previous caesarean section and breech presentation were the only important indications for which there were reliable and comparative data (Lomas and Enkin 1989). It proved impossible to reconcile differences in the use of the term dystocia (difficult labour), which in some cases included cephalo-pelvic disproportion and prolonged labour while in others it included the former only (see Table 1). However, an analysis of all hospital births in the Canadian Province of Ontario permits an analysis of the percentage of deliveries in which a diagnosis of caesarean section for dystocia was made. The diagnosis of dystocia varied from a low of 4.1 per cent to a high of 14 per cent (see Table 2).

Bearing in mind all these caveats, for the purposes of these calculations it has been assumed that the incidence of dystocia varies between the narrow range from 3 to 6 per cent. The lower figure is assumed to apply

Table 1 Rates of operative instrumental intervention in selected developed countries around 1980

Country	*(a) Caesarean*	*(b) Forceps*	*(c) Vacuum*	*(b+c) Instrum.*	*(a+b+c) total op.*
Canada 1980	16.5	17.8	0.5	18.3	34.4
USA 1980	16.5	18.4	0.5	18.9	35.4
England & Wales 1980	8.8	12.5	21.3	33.8	42.6
Sweden 1979	12.0	0.3	6.8	7.1	19.1
Scotland 1979	10.7	13.0	0.3	13.3	24.0
Denmark 1979	10.7	0.7	8.6	9.3	20.0
Norway 1979	8.3	3.2	3.4	6.6	14.9
France 1981	10.7	n.a.	n.a.	n.a.	n.a.
Finland 1979	11.9	0.3	3.4	3.7	15.6
Czechoslovakia 1981	4.0	1.3	1.0	2.3	6.3

Sources:

Canada — Statistics Canada. Institutional care statistics (Dr Nair). Data are for fiscal year 1980-81. Adjustments for under-reporting in the province of Quebec were not made for this year and result in an underestimate of the caesarean section rate for Canada of about 1.5 percentage points

England and Wales - Macfarlane and Mugford (1984)

Sweden, Scotland, Denmark, Norway, Czechoslovakia — Bergsjø et al. (1983).

Switzerland — Federal Office of Statistics (Dr Paccaud), Switzerland

USA — National Center for Health Statistics (Dr Placek): National hospital discharge survey for caesarean section rates and for instrumental vaginal delivery.

Adapted from: Lomas J, Enkin M. (1989).

Table 2 Deliveries diagnosed as caesarean section for dystocia, Ontario, Canada, 1982

	Percentage of all births with this diagnosis							
Hospital type	*Teaching Hospitals*				*Community Hospitals*			
	1	2	3	4	1	2	3	4
Dystocia	4.1	11.2	8.9	13.6	7.2	12.4	11.3	14.0

Adapted from: Lomas J, Enkin M. (1989).

in more developed areas and those where early marriage and childhood malnutrition especially among girls is not widespread. The higher figure is applied to Africa, the Middle East and South West Asia and India. When weighted by numbers of live births in each region, the global incidence of obstructed labour is estimated as 5.1 per cent of all live births (live births used as a proxy for deliveries).

We have been unable to find comparable data on the specific incidence of cephalo-pelvic disproportion and obstructed labour. Based on historical evidence from developed countries it has been asserted that obstructed labour due to cephalo-pelvic disproportion or abnormal lie occurs in only 1 and 2 per cent of all deliveries (Van Lerberghe and De Brouwere 1997). Rates of caesarean delivery in developing country settings, on the other hand, are generally considerably higher, even when efforts are made to avoid unnecessary operative interventions. A WHO study in three developing countries (Indonesia, Malaysia and Thailand) during which the partograph was introduced for the monitoring of labour and the early detection of abnormal progress, found that rates of caesarean delivery among "normal" women (those without serious complications or high risk already on admission) were reduced from 5.2 to 3.7 per cent — still well above the threshold (World Health Organization 1993). A report from Nigeria examined rates of disproportion among healthy women and among women attending as emergencies (Harrison 1997). The rate of disproportion was 2.4 per cent for healthy women who had booked for hospital deliveries. Among women identified prenatally as having signs and symptoms of complications, the rate of disproportion was 8 per cent and for the emergency admissions it was 13.9 per cent. Very high rates of disproportion such as these may be a reflection of special circumstances in parts of West Africa where cephalo-pelvic disproportion is known to be higher than elsewhere in part due to the shape of the female pelvis in certain ethnic groups.

Mortality from obstructed labour

Although measures of incidence of obstructed labour are rare, more information is available on maternal mortality due to prolonged or obstructed labour. However, such data must also be treated with caution because in many instances the cause of death is classified under another

Table 3 Per cent of maternal deaths due to obstructed labour and/or ruptured uterus for countries reporting either as a cause of death

*Country**	*No. of studies*	*Total maternal deaths*	*No. of studies reporting RUU** and/or OBL*** as cause of death*	*Total deaths in the studies reporting RUU** and/or OBL****	*% of deaths due to RUU** and/or OBL****
Africa					
Algeria	3	383	2[a]	177	18.6
Benin	2	319	2[a]	319	16.6
Burkina Faso	1	384	1[c]	384	25.3
Ivory Coast	3	297	1[a]	181	16.6
Egypt	9	1 541	7[a]	949	11.5
Ethiopia	5	446	4[b]	429	11.4
Ghana	2	447	2[b]	447	14.3
Guinea	1	212	1[a]	212	7.1
Kenya	3	284	3[a]	284	10.6
Malawi	4	420	4[b]	420	18.8
Morocco	2	214	2[a]	214	15.4
Niger	2	330	2[a]	330	27.3
Nigeria	18	2 570	18[b]	2 570	35.1
Senegal	1	152	1[a]	152	7.2
Sierra Leone	2	134	2[b]	134	17.9
South Africa	3	936	2[a]	855	7.0
Sudan	8	565	4[b]	262	15.3
Togo	2	251	1[a]	41	17.1
Tunisia	5	363	5[a]	363	15.1
Uganda	3	1 048	3[b]	1 048	18.6
Tanzania	12	1 514	11[b]	1 506	13.1
Zambia	4	376	4	376	11.4
Latin America					
Brazil	6	750	2	68[a]	5.9
Chile	4	744	1	45[a]	2.2
Colombia	7	3 372	3	367[a]	2.4
Honduras	1	381	1	381[c]	4.2
Jamaica	3	269	1	193[b]	2.6
Peru	2	706	1	168[a]	3.6
Venezuela	3	423	2	132[a]	11.4
Asia					
Bangladesh	5	563	4	515[b]	7.6
China	9	8 613	5	964[b]	2.7
India	15	7 841	14	7 826[b]	8.1
Indonesia	4	479	1	26[a]	7.7
Iraq	2	125	2	125[a]	4.8
Pakistan	6	680	6	680[a]	7.6
Philippines	3	3 613	1	306[a]	5.9
Sri Lanka	3	2 421	1	1 839[b]	2.4
Thailand	3	478	3	478[b]	4.6
Oceania					
Fiji	1	164	1	164[a]	4.3
Papua New Guinea	3	1 341	3	1 341[b]	10.9

* Countries reporting causes for at least 100 maternal deaths
** Ruptured uterus
*** Obstructed labour

a Reported ruptured uterus only
b Reported both obstructed labour and ruptured uterus
c Reported obstructed labour only

Source: Abstracted from: World Health Organization. (1991).

heading including sepsis, ruptured uterus or haemorrhage, all of which could be secondary complications of obstructed labour.

Table 3 provides country estimates for both obstructed labour and ruptured uterus as a cause of maternal death. The countries included in this table are only those reporting 100 maternal deaths or more, and listing either obstructed labour or ruptured uterus as a cause of death. We have further categorized each country as reporting only ruptured uterus, reporting only obstructed labour or reporting both.

Epidemiological data on mortality have been used by the author to derive a first set of regional mortality estimates. When considered in conjunction with mortality estimates proposed by other authors for other diseases

Table 4 Disability weights used to calculate the burden from obstructed labour, treated and untreated form.

Condition	*0-4*	*5-14*	*15-44*	*45-59*	*60+*
Stress incontinence	0	0	0.025	0.025	0.033
Rectovaginal fistula	0	0	0.43	0	0

Table 5 Distribution of episodes of obstructed labour and cases of stress incontinence and rectovaginal fistula resulting from obstructed labour across the seven classes of disability by age group, females, 1990.

	Disability class						
	I	**II**	**III**	**IV**	**V**	**VI**	**VII**
Age (years)				**Episodes**			
0-4	0	0	0	0	0	0	0
5-14	0	0	0	0	0	0	0
15-44	0	0	100	0	0	0	0
45-59	0	0	0	0	0	0	0
60+	0	0	0	0	0	0	0
				Stress incontinence			
0-4	0	0	0	0	0	0	0
5-14	0	0	0	0	0	0	0
15-44	61	27	0	0	0	0	0
45-59	61	27	0	0	0	0	0
60+	49	37	1	0	0	0	0
				Rectovaginal fistula			
0-4	0	0	0	0	0	0	0
5-14	0	0	0	0	0	0	0
15-44	0	0	0	0	100	0	0
45-59	0	0	0	0	0	0	0
60+	0	0	0	0	0	0	0

Source: Murray and Lopez 1996b

and injuries in the GBD study, the implied level of overall mortality usually exceeded the rate estimated by various demographic methods. In order not to exceed this upper bound for mortality within each age-sex and broad-cause group, an algorithm has been applied by the editors to reduce mortality estimates for specific conditions so that their sum did not exceed this upper bound. The algorithm has been described in more detail in *The Global Burden of Disease* (Murray and Lopez 1996a).

Following the analysis of the percentage of maternal mortality due to obstructed labour, regional estimates were derived ranging from less than 1 per cent to 10 per cent, with a global average of 7.5 per cent of direct maternal deaths. This amounts to some 34 000 maternal deaths annually due to obstructed labour.

Disability following obstructed labour

Table 4 shows the disability weights used in the calculation of Years Lived with Disability (YLDs) and Disability-Adjusted Life Years (DALYs) for two major sequelae of obstructed labour, rectovaginal fistula and stress incontinence. As there is no effective treatment for conditions resulting from obstructed labour, the disability weights used for treated and untreated forms of stress incontinence and rectovaginal fistula are identical. The estimated distribution of obstructed labour episodes, as well as cases of stress incontinence and rectovaginal fistula, across the seven disability classes used in the Global Burden of Disease Study are shown in Table 5.

By far the most severe and distressing long-term condition following obstructed labour is obstetric fistula — a hole which forms in the vaginal wall communicating into the bladder (vesico-vaginal fistula) or the rectum (recto-vaginal fistula) or both. In developing countries, fistulae are commonly the result of prolonged obstructed labour and follow pressure necrosis caused by impaction of the presenting part during difficult labour. It is the duration of impaction without relief rather than the magnitude of the pressure which determines the degree of tissue necrosis. The fistula site depends greatly on the degree of cervical effacement and dilatation, and the level at which the presenting part impacts (Zacharin 1988).

In some settings fistulae result from traditional practices; certain birth canal damage predisposes to prolonged labour and development of fistulae, especially female genital mutilation and inserting caustics into the postpartum vagina. The immediate consequences of such damage are urinary incontinence, faecal incontinence if the rectum is affected, and excoriation of the vulva from the constantly leaking urine and faeces. Secondary amenorrhoea is a frequently associated problem. Women who have survived prolonged obstructed labour may also suffer from local nerve damage which results in difficulty in walking, including drop foot.

The true incidence of obstetric fistula is very difficult to determine because it is a result of poor or absent obstetric care associated with a range of social conditions such as lack of health services, early marriage, seclusion of women and socio-economic deprivation. Most reports on the incidence of the problem are based on hospital records and are reported by the surgeons who operated on the women. Their primary concern is the degree of successful repair rather than the incidence of the problem. Such reports do provide an indication of the existence of the problem in particular areas but do not furnish adequate data as to incidence or prevalence. In general, cases are reported as a proportion of admissions or gynaecological admissions or as a proportion of hospital deliveries. Moreover, such reports indicate only those cases which reach a hospital setting for treatment. Since most fistula sufferers are treated as outcasts, divorced by their husbands and live in isolation (Murphy 1981) they are unlikely to come to the attention of researchers unless special efforts are made to locate them.

Only patchy information is available from countries where fistulae are known to occur. In one area of Nigeria, for example, at hospitals serving a population of some 15 million which could expect some 600 000 births annually, surgeons estimate a need for 1500 fistula repairs each year to cope with new cases and backlog. Reports estimate the prevalence of fistulae in sub-Saharan Africa to be 1.5 to 2.0 million women, with 50 000 to 100 000 new cases occurring each year (Waldijk 1994). A study of 203 cases of prolonged labour in India found the incidence of vulval haematoma to be 2.9 per cent (6 cases), of vesico-vaginal fistula to be 3.9 per cent (8 cases) and of obstetric palsies to be 2.4 per cent (5 cases). (Randhowa et al. 1991) The overall incidence of prolonged labour was 4.4 per cent, of which one-third (31.9 per cent) were emergency admissions. It has been estimated that incidence of fistulae probably ranges between 50 and 80 per 100,000 births. In calculating the regional estimates of the number of new cases annually, the higher figure has been applied for Africa, Middle East/South West Asia and India and a lower figure of 30 per 100 000 births used for Latin America and China. This gives a world average incidence of 1.1 per cent of cases of obstructed labour, a figure considerably lower than the 3.9 per cent reported from India, above.

Women with prolonged and/or obstructed labour are more likely to also develop complications related to sepsis particularly if there is premature or prolonged rupture of the membranes.

Another complication frequently associated with obstructed labour, particularly in women who have had several children already, is uterine rupture. When the membranes rupture and the amniotic fluid drains away, the thick, muscular upper body of the uterus retracts, forcing the fetus down into the increasingly thin, overstretched lower segment of the uterus. If contractions continue uterine rupture of the lower segment becomes a dangerous possibility. Rupture of the uterus may be complete, in which case bleeding will occur within the peritoneum, or incomplete, in which case bleeding will occur behind the viscreal peritneum. Rupture of the uterus causes haemorrhage and shock and without treatment is rapidly fatal.

Obstructed labour is one of the most important causes of fetal death and disability. If labour is allowed to continue the fetus dies because of reduced oxygen availability and severe ketosis. The dead fetus becomes macerated and may trigger the onset of disseminated intravascular coagulation (DIC) resulting in maternal haemorrhage, shock and death.

As well as the immediate consequences of poorly managed obstructed labour such as fistulae, prolonged obstructed labour can cause less severe, though chronic, disabilitites, even in areas where obstetric interventions are available. Perineal trauma due to the manipulations used in managing prolonged and obstructed labour is common and can cause discomfort to a degree that can dominate the experience of early motherhood and may result in significant disability during the months and years that follow.

Although there is debate about the extent to which stress incontinence is caused or aggravated by vaginal delivery, it is generally agreed that such sequelae are particularly likely to occur where delivery has been prolonged or difficult. Prolonged labour is more likely to result in injury to the pelvic floor muscles and ligaments or to their nerve supply or to the interconnecting fascia. This in turn may cause uterine or vaginal wall prolapse or stress incontinence. It has long been thought that episiotomy prevents perineal overstretching during delivery and thereby prevents genital prolapse and urinary incontinence, though the evidence remains inconclusive (Sleep et al. 1989).

The evidence indicates that even in developed countries with high standards of obstetric care, around 6 per cent of first-time mothers and 10 per cent of multiparous mothers had stress incontinence at their six weeks postnatal check-up. Other studies have found that both urinary and faecal incontinence result from damage to the nerves of the pelvic floor muscles (MacArthur et al. 1997). In calculating the burden of disability caused by prolonged and obstructed labour, it has been assumed that almost all will result in either stress incontinence in the short term or prolapse in the longer term. This is equivalent to 4.9 per cent of all births — a relatively conservative estimate.

Uterovaginal prolapse causes much local discomfort and also affects the passing of urine and other bodily functions. The affected woman is sometimes unable to control her bladder and may leak urine when coughing or sneezing (stress incontinence). Alternatively, the prolapsed uterus may partially block urination. There may be constipation and low backache as well as pain on intercourse. The cervix, if displaced permanently outside the introitus, ulcerates, bleeds and becomes infected, exuding a foul-smelling discharge. Many women with prolapse are still young and the presence of prolapse affects subsequent pregnancies, increasing the risk of both spontaneous abortion and premature labour. A survey in nine countries found that the percentage of women with uterovaginal prolapse ranged from 2 per cent to as high as 28 per cent. Higher parity and older women are most likely to be affected (Omran and Stanley 1978). Community-based studies have found between one-third and two-thirds of women with prolapse in Lahare, Pakistan; Istanbul, Turkey; and Giza, Egypt (Omran and Stanley 1981, Younis et al. 1993).

Depending on the condition under study, epidemiological data may be available for incidence, prevalence, case-fatality or mortality. Where data on more than one of these parameters are available, estimates of each of the epidemiological parameters derived from the data may not be internally consistent or consistent with the adjusted mortality rates described above. To ensure that all epidemiological information concerning a given condition is internally consistent, the editors have undertaken extensive analyses using computer models of the natural history of disease described in Murray and Lopez (1996b). The incidence, prevalence, and duration estimates have consequently been revised where necessary. In view of these adjustments to the basic epidemiological estimates originally provided for the Global Burden of Disease Study, the data which have undergone the GBD validation process are the joint responsibility of the authors and the editors.

The estimates of number of deaths, Years of Life Lost (YLLs), Years Lived with Disability adjusted for severity of the disability (YLDs) and Disability-Adjusted Life Years (DALYs) from obstructed labour episodes, stress incontinence and rectovaginal fistula are presented in Tables 6–9.

Impact of interventions on the burden

Obstructed labour is particularly common among the poor in developing areas of the world. Where environmental hygiene is inadequate and malnutrition and infectious diseases in childhood endemic, growth in stature of girls may be stunted (Harrison 1985). Where girls suffer discrimination in terms of food allocation and health care, such stunting may be particularly commonplace. The risks to women during labour and delivery are considerably higher in such circumstances and are further greatly aggravated by early marriage and childbearing before girls are fully grown. Prevention strategies to reduce the incidence of obstructed labour must, therefore, include attention to the nutrition of adolescent girls, delayed childbearing and special attention to the nutritional needs of women both preconceptually and throughout pregnancy.

Although short maternal stature is associated with higher incidence of obstructed labour, maternal height alone is a poor predictor of obstructed labour; both sensitivity and specificity low (World Health Organization 1995). The indicator performs better for the prediction of adverse pregnancy outcomes when combined with age and when the cut-off value for height is based on reference values determined locally rather than according to standardized criteria (Dujardin 1993). It is not the actual height as such that is important, but the deviation from the norm in the reference population. WHO does not recommend routine risk screening of pregnant women on the basis of height alone (Rooney 1992). However, in settings where women live far from health care facilities and where obstructed

Table 6 Epidemiological estimates for episodes of obstructed labour, females, 1990.

Age group (years)	*Incidence* Number ('000s)	Rate per100 000	*Avg. age at onset* (years)	*Deaths* Number ('000s)	Rate per100 000	*YLLs* Number ('000s)	Rate per100 000
Established Market Economies							
0-4	0	0	–	0	0.00	0	0
5-14	0	0	–	0	0.00	0	0
15-44	312	174	19.00	0	0.00	0	0
45-59	0	0	–	0	0.00	0	0
60+	0	0	–	0	0.00	0	0
All Ages	*312*	*77*	*19.00*	*0*	*0*	*0*	*0*
Formerly Socialist Economies of Europe							
0-4	0	0	–	0	0.00	0	0
5-14	0	0	–	0	0.00	0	0
15-44	212	283	19.00	0	0.00	0	0
45-59	0	0	–	0	0.00	0	0
60+	0	0	–	0	0.00	0	0
All Ages	*212*	*117*	*19.00*	*0*	*0*	*0*	*0*
India							
0-4	0	0	–	0	0.00	0	0
5-14	0	0	–	0	0.00	0	0
15-44	1 549	845	19.00	9	4.90	263	144
45-59	51	110	52.40	0	0.60	5	11
60+	0	0	–	0	0.00	0	0
All Ages	*1 600*	*390*	*20.10*	*9*	*2.2*	*268*	*65*
China							
0-4	0	0	–	0	0.00	0	0
5-14	0	0	–	0	0.00	0	0
15-44	1 005	354	19.00	0	0.10	13	5
45-59	63	98	52.4	0	0.00	0	0
60+	0	0	–	0	0.00	0	0
All Ages	*1 068*	*195*	*21.00*	*0*	*0.1*	*13*	*2*
Other Asia and Islands							
0-4	0	0	–	0	0.00	0	0
5-14	0	0	–	0	0.00	0	0
15-44	1 046	655	19.00	4	2.50	117	73
45-59	44	124	52.20	0	0.50	3	9
60+	0	0	–	0	0.00	0	0
All Ages	*1 090*	*321*	*20.30*	*4*	*1.2*	*120*	*35*
Sub-Saharan Africa							
0-4	0	0	–	0	0.00	0	0
5-14	85	122	10.00	1	1.10	30	43
15-44	1 511	1 422	19.00	14	13.30	413	389
45-59	3	15	52.20	0	0.10	0	0
60+	0	0	–	0	0.00	0	0
All Ages	*1 600*	*620*	*18.60*	*15*	*5.8*	*443*	*172*

Table 6 *(continued)*

Age group (years)	*Incidence* Number ('000s)	Rate per100 000	*Avg. age at onset* (years)	*Deaths* Number ('000s)	Rate per100 000	*YLLs* Number ('000s)	Rate per100 000
Latin America and the Caribbean							
0-4	0	0	–	0	0.00	0	0
5-14	4	7	10.00	0	0.00	0	0
15-44	498	478	19.00	2	1.50	48	45
45-59	3	14	52.40	0	0.00	0	0
60+	0	0	19.20	0	0.70	0	0
All Ages	*505*	*227*	*19.20*	*2*	*0.7*	*48*	*21*
Middle Eastern Crescent							
0-4	0	0	–	0	0.00	0	0
5-14	1	2	10.00	0	0.00	0	0
15-44	1 175	1 096	19.00	4	3.50	109	102
45-59	75	337	52.30	0	1.10	4	18
60+	0	0	–	0	0.00	0	0
All Ages	*1 252*	*507*	*21.00*	*2*	*0*	*113*	*46*
Developed Regions							
0-4	0	0	–	0	0	0	0
5-14	0	0	–	0	0	0	0
15-44	524	206	19.00	0	0	0	0
45-59	0	0	–	0	0	0	0
60+	0	0	–	0	0	0	0
All Ages	*524*	*81*	*19.0*	*0*	*0*	*0*	*0*
Developing Regions							
0-4	0	0		0	0	0	0
5-14	90	20	10	1	0	30	7
15-44	6 784	718	19	33	3	962	102
45-59	239	112	52	0	0	12	6
60+	0	0	–	0	0	0	0
All Ages	*7 113*	*351*	*19.5*	*34*	*2*	*1 004*	*50*
World							
0-4	0	0	–	0	0	0	0
5-14	90	17	10.0	1	0	30	6
15-44	7 308	610	19.00	33	3	962	80
45-59	239	77	38.5	0	0	12	4
60+	0	0	–	0	0	0	0
All Ages	*7 637*	*292*	*19.5*	*34*	*1*	*1 004*	*38*

Table 7 Epidemiological estimates for stress incontinence resulting from obstructed labour, females, 1990.

Age group (years)	Incidence		Prevalence		Avg. age at onset (years)	Avg. duration (years)	YLDs•	
	Number ('000s)	Rate per100 000	Number ('000s)	Rate per100 000			Number ('000s)	Rate per100 000
Established Market Economies								
0-4	0	0	–	–	–	–	0	0
5-14	0	0	–	–	–	–	0	0
15-44	312	174	4 715	2 631	29.80	50.10	230	129
45-59	0	0	3 541	5 223	–	–	0	0
60+	0	0	4 417	5 223	–	–	0	0
All Ages	*312*	*77*	*12 673*	*3 111*	*29.80*	*50.10*	*230*	*57*
Formerly Socialist Economies of Europe								
0-4	0	0	–	–	–	–	0	0
5-14	0	0	–	–	–	–	0	0
15-44	212	283	3 217	4 292	29.70	47.00	155	206
45-59	0	0	2 546	8 484	–	–	0	0
60+	0	0	3 088	8 484	–	–	0	0
All Ages	*212*	*117*	*8 850*	*4 892*	*29.70*	*47.00*	*155*	*64*
India								
0-4	0	0	–	–	–	–	0	0
5-14	0	0	–	–	–	–	0	0
15-44	1 528	834	23 639	12 901	29.10	42.40	1 095	598
45-59	0	0	11 485	24 966	–	–	0	0
60+	0	0	7 221	24 966	–	–	0	0
All Ages	*1 528*	*373*	*42 346*	*10 325*	*29.10*	*42.40*	*1 095*	*267*
China								
0-4	0	0	0	0	–	–	0	0
5-14	0	0	0	0	–	–	0	0
15-44	746	263	11 284	3 972	29.70	44.40	536	189
45-59	0	0	5 073	7 877	–	–	0	0
60+	0	0	4 070	7 877	–	–	0	0
All Ages	*746*	*136*	*20 427*	*3 724*	*29.70*	*44.40*	*536*	*98*
Other Asia and Islands								
0-4	0	0	–	–	–	–	0	0
5-14	0	0	–	–	–	–	0	0
15-44	1 026	643	0	0	29.30	41.90	731	458
45-59	0	0	6 757	19 257	–	–	0	0
60+	0	0	4 364	19 257	–	–	0	0
All Ages	*1 026*	*302*	*26 826*	*7 900*	*29.30*	*41.90*	*731*	*215*
Sub-Saharan Africa								
0-4	0	0	–	–	–	–	0	0
5-14	0	0	0	0	–	–	0	0
15-44	1 491	1 403	23 422	22 043	28.40	38.20	1 047	985
45-59	0	0	9 229	41 727	–	–	0	0
60+	0	0	5 312	41 727	–	–	0	0
All Ages	*1 491*	*578*	*37 963*	*14 717*	*28.50*	*38.20*	*1 047*	*406*

Table 7 *(continued)*

Age group (years)	Incidence		Prevalence		Avg. age at onset (years)	Avg. duration (years)	YLDs*	
	Number ('000s)	Rate per100 000	Number ('000s)	Rate per100 000			Number ('000s)	Rate per100 000
Latin America and the Caribbean								
0-4	0	0	0	0	–	–	0	0
5-14	0	0	0	0	–	–	0	0
15-44	486	467	7 403	7 113	29.50	45.00	352	338
45-59	0	0	3 269	13 999	–	–	0	0
60+	0	0	2 355	13 999	–	–	0	0
All Ages	*486*	*218*	*13 028*	*5 850*	*29.50*	*45.00*	*352*	*158*
Middle Eastern Crescent								
0-4	0	0	0	0	–	–	0	0
5-14	0	0	0	0	–	–	0	0
15-44	1 159	1 081	18 324	17 092	29.00	43.50	838	782
45-59	0	0	7 217	32 374	–	–	0	0
60+	*0*	*0*	*5 002*	*32 374*	–	–	*0*	*0*
All Ages	*1 159*	*470*	*30 543*	*12 381*	*29.00*	*43.50*	*838*	*340*
Developed Regions								
0-4	0	0	0	0	–	–	0	0
5-14	0	0	0	0	–	–	0	0
15-44	524	206	7 932	3 121	29.76	43.02	385	151
45-59	0	0	6 087	6 224	–	–	0	0
60+	0	0	7 505	6 205	–	–	0	0
All Ages	*524*	*81*	*21 524*	*3 311*	*29.8*	*43.0*	*385*	*59*
Developing Regions								
0-4	0	0	0	0	–	–	0	0
5-14	0	0	0	0	–	–	0	0
15-44	6 436	681	84 072	8 901	29	42	4 599	487
45-59	0	0	43 030	20 177	–	–	0	0
60+	0	0	28 324	19 105	–	–	0	0
All Ages	*6 436*	*318*	*155 426*	*7 673*	*29.1*	*42.0*	*4 599*	*227*
World								
0-4	0	0	0	0	–	–	0	0
5-14	0	0	0	0	–	–	0	0
15-44	6 960	581	92 004	7 676	29.10	42.22	4 984	416
45-59	0	0	49 117	15 790	–	–	0	0
60+	0	0	35 829	13 309	–	–	0	0
All Ages	*6 960*	*266*	*176 950*	*6 770*	*29.1*	*42.2*	*4 984*	*191*

Table 8 Epidemiological estimates for rectovaginal fistula resulting from obstructed labour, females, 1990.

Age group (years)	Incidence Number ('000s)	Incidence Rate per100 000	Prevalence Number ('000s)	Prevalence Rate per100 000	Avg. age at onset (years)	Avg. duration (years)	YLDs Number ('000s)	YLDs Rate per100 000
Established Market Economies								
0-4	0	0.00	0	0.00	–	–	0	0
5-14	0	0.00	0	0.00	–	–	0	0
15-44	0	0.00	0	0.00	–	–	0	0
45-59	0	0.00	0	0.00	–	–	0	0
60+	0	0.00	0	0.00	–	–	0	0
All Ages	*0*	*0.00*	*0*	*0.00*	–	–	*0*	*0*
Formerly Socialist Economies of Europe								
0-4	0	0.00	0	0.00	–	–	0	0
5-14	0	0.00	0	0.00	–	–	0	0
15-44	0	0.00	0	0.00	–	–	0	0
45-59	0	0.00	0	0.00	–	–	0	0
60+	0	0.00	0	0.00	–	–	0	0
All Ages	*0*	*0.00*	*0*	*0.00*	–	–	*0*	*0*
India								
0-4	0	0.00	0	0.00	–	–	0	0
5-14	0	0.00	0	0.00	–	–	0	0
15-44	21	11.50	139	76.00	19.00	12.40	141	77
45-59	0	0.00	34	74.00	–	–	0	0
60+	0	0.00	21	74.00	–	–	0	0
All Ages	*21*	*5.1*	*194*	*47*	*19.00*	*12.40*	*141*	*34*
China								
0-4	0	0.00	0	0.00	–	–	0	0
5-14	0	0.00	0	0.00	–	–	0	0
15-44	8	2.80	27	9.40	19.00	6.20	29	10
45-59	0	0.00	5	8.20	–	–	0	0
60+	0	0.00	4	8.20	–	–	0	0
All Ages	*8*	*1.5*	*36*	*6.6*	*19.00*	*6.20*	*29*	*5*
Other Asia and Islands								
0-4	0	0.00	0	0.00	–	–	0	0
5-14	0	0.00	0	0.00	–	–	0	0
15-44	13	8.00	58	36.00	19.00	8.00	59	37
45-59	0	0.00	12	33.00	–	–	0	0
60+	0	0.00	7	33.00	–	–	0	0
All Ages	*13*	*3.8*	*77*	*23*	*19.00*	*8.00*	*59*	*18*
Sub-Saharan Africa								
0-4	0	0.00	0	0.00	–	–	0	0
5-14	0	0.00	0	0.00	–	–	0	0
15-44	20	18.80	196	184.00	19.00	17.40	174	164
45-59	0	0.00	42	190.00	–	–	0	0
60+	0	0.00	24	190.00	–	–	0	0
All Ages	*20*	*7.7*	*262*	*102*	*19.00*	*17.40*	*174*	*68*

Table 8 *(continued)*

Age group (years)	Incidence		Prevalence		Avg. age at onset (years)	Avg. duration (years)	YLDs	
	Number ('000s)	Rate per100 000	Number ('000s)	Rate per100 000			Number ('000s)	Rate per100 000
Latin America and the Caribbean								
0-4	0	0.00	0	0.00	–	–	0	0
5-14	0	0.00	0	0.00	–	–	0	0
15-44	4	3.80	13	12.70	19.00	6.10	15	14
45-59	0	0.00	3	11.00	–	–	0	0
60+	0	0.00	2	11.00	–	–	0	0
All Ages	*4*	*1.8*	*18*	*7.9*	*19.00*	*6.10*	*15*	*7*
Middle Eastern Crescent								
0-4	0	0.00	0	0.00	–	–	0	0
5-14	0	0.00	0	0.00	–	–	0	0
15-44	16	14.90	52	48.00	19.00	5.80	55	51
45-59	0	0.00	9	41.00	–	–	0	0
60+	0	0.00	6	41.00	–	–	0	0
All Ages	*16*	*6.5*	*67*	*27*	*19.00*	*5.80*	*55*	*22*
Developed Regions								
0-4	0	0.00	0	0.00	–	–	0	0
5-14	0	0.00	0	0.00	–	–	0	0
15-44	0	0.00	0	0.00	–	–	0	0
45-59	0	0.00	0	0.00	–	–	0	0
60+	0	0.00	0	0.00	–	–	0	0
All Ages	*0*	*0.00*	*0*	*0.00*	–	–	*0*	*0*
Developing Regions								
0-4	0	0.00	0	0.00	–	–	0	0
5-14	0	0.00	0	0.00	–	–	0	0
15-44	82	8.68	485	51.35	19	11	474	50
45-59	0	0.00	105	49.24	–	–	0	0
60+	0	0.00	64	43.17	–	–	0	0
All Ages	*82*	*4.05*	*654*	*32.29*	*19.0*	*10.7*	*474*	*23*
World								
0-4	0	0.00	0	0.00	–	–	0	0
5-14	0	0.00	0	0.00	–	–	0	0
15-44	82	6.84	485	40.46	19.0	10.7	474	40
45-59	0	0.00	105	33.75	–	–	0	0
60+	0	0.00	64	23.77	–	–	0	0
All Ages	*82*	*3.14*	*654*	*25.02*	*19.0*	*10.7*	*474*	*18*

Table 9 Summary table of epidemiological estimates for obstructed labour, females, 1990.

Age group (years)	*Incidence*		*Prevalence*		*Deaths*		*YLLs*		*YLDs*		*DALYs*	
	Number ('000s)	Rate per100 000	Number ('000s)	Rate per100 000	Number ('000s)	Rate per100 000	Number ('000s)	Rate per100 000	Number ('000s)	Rate per100 000	Number ('000s)	Rate per100 000
Established Market Economies												
0-4	0	0	0	0	0	0	0	0	0	0	0	0
5-14	0	0	0	0	0	0	0	0	0	0	0	0
15-44	312	0	4 715	0.03	0	0	0	0	230	129	230	129
45-59	0	0	3 541	0.05	0	0	0	0	0	0	0	0
60+	0	0	4 417	0.05	0	0	0	0	0	0	0	0
All Ages	*312*	*0*	*12 673*	*0.03*	*0*	*0*	*0*	*0*	*230*	*57*	*230*	*57*
Formerly Socialist Economies of Europe												
0-4	0	0	0	0	0	0	0	0	0	0	0	0
5-14	0	0	0	0	0	0	0	0	0	0	0	0
15-44	212	0	3 217	0.04	0	0	0	0	155	206	155	206
45-59	0	0	2 546	0.08	0	0	0	0	0	0	0	0
60+	0	0	3 088	0.08	0	0	0	0	0	0	0	0
All Ages	*212*	*0*	*8 851*	*0.04*	*0*	*0*	*0*	*0*	*155*	*64*	*155*	*64*
India												
0-4	0	0	0	0	0	0	0	0	0	0	0	0
5-14	0	0	0	0	0	0	0	0	0	0	0	0
15-44	1 549	0.01	23 778	0.13	9	0	263	0	1 236	675	1 499	818
45-59	0	0	11 519	0.25	0	0	5	0	0	0	5	11
60+	0	0	7 242	0.25	0	0	0	0	0	0	0	0
All Ages	*1 549*	*0*	*42 539*	*0.1*	*9*	*0*	*268*	*0*	*1 236*	*301*	*1 504*	*367*
China												
0-4	0	0	0	0	0	0	0	0	0	0	0	0
5-14	0	0	0	0	0	0	0	0	0	0	0	0
15-44	754	0	11 311	0.04	0	0	13	0	566	199	579	204
45-59	0	0	5 078	0.08	0	0	0	0	0	0	0	0
60+	0	0	4 074	0.08	0	0	0	0	0	0	0	0
All Ages	*754*	*0*	*20 463*	*0.04*	*0*	*0*	*13*	*0*	*566*	*103*	*579*	*105*
Other Asia and Islands												
0-4	0	0	0	0	0	0	0	0	0	0	0	0
5-14	0	0	0	0	0	0	0	0	0	0	0	0
15-44	1039	0.01	58	0	4	0	117	0	790	495	907	569
45-59	0	0	6 769	0.19	0	0	3	0	0	0	3	9
60+	0	0	4 371	0.19	0	0	0	0	0	0	0	0
All Ages	*1 039*	*0*	*11 198*	*0.03*	*4*	*0*	*120*	*0*	*790*	*233*	*910*	*268*
Sub-Saharan Africa												
0-4	0	0	0	0	0	0	0	0	0	0	0	0
5-14	0	0	0	0	1	0	30	0	0	0	30	43
15-44	1 511	0.01	23 618	0.22	14	0	413	0	1 221	1 149	1 634	1 538
45-59	0	0	9 271	0.42	0	0	0	0	0	0	0	0
60+	0	0	5 336	0.42	0	0	0	0	0	0	0	0
All Ages	*1 511*	*0.01*	*38 225*	*0.15*	*15*	*0*	*443*	*0*	*1 221*	*473*	*1 664*	*645*

Table 9 *(continued)*

Age group (years)	Incidence Number ('000s)	Incidence Rate per100 000	Prevalence Number ('000s)	Prevalence Rate per100 000	Deaths Number ('000s)	Deaths Rate per100 000	YLLs Number ('000s)	YLLs Rate per100 000	YLDs Number ('000s)	YLDs Rate per100 000	DALYs Number ('000s)	DALYs Rate per100 000
Latin America and the Caribbean												
0-4	0	0	0	0	0	0	0	0	0	0	0	0
5-14	0	0	0	0	0	0	0	0	0	0	0	0
15-44	490	0	7 416	0.07	2	0	47	0	366	352	414	398
45-59	0	0	3 272	0.14	0	0	0	0	0	0	0	0
60+	0	0	2 357	0.14	0	0	0	0	0	0	0	0
All Ages	*490*	*0*	*13 045*	*0.06*	*2*	*0*	*47*	*0*	*366*	*164*	*414*	*186*
Middle Eastern Crescent												
0-4	0	0	0	0	0	0	0	0	0	0	0	0
5-14	0	0	0	0	0	0	0	0	0	0	0	0
15-44	1 175	0.01	18 376	0.17	4	0	109	0	893	833	1 002	935
45-59	0	0	7 226	0.32	0	0	4	0	0	0	4	18
60+	0	0	5 008	0.32	0	0	0	0	0	0	0	0
All Ages	*1 175*	*0*	*30 610*	*0.12*	*4*	*0*	*113*	*0*	*893*	*362*	*1 006*	*408*
Developed Regions												
0-4	0	0	0	0	0	0	0	0	0	0	0	0
5-14	0	0	0	0	0	0	0	0	0	0	0	0
15-44	524	206.17	7 932	3 120.89	0	0	0	0	385	151	385	151
45-59	0	0	6 087	6 223.61	0	0	0	0	0	0	0	0
60+	0	0	7 505	6 204.58	0	0	0	0	0	0	0	0
All Ages	*524*	*80.61*	*21 524*	*3 311.15*	*0*	*0*	*0*	*0*	*385*	*59*	*385*	*59*
Developing Regions												
0-4	0	0	0	0	0	0	0	0	0	0	0	0
5-14	0	0	0	0	1	0.22	30	7	0	0	30	7
15-44	6 518	690.11	84 557	8 952.72	33	3.49	962	102	5 072	537	6 035	639
45-59	0	0	43 135	20 226.29	0	0	12	6	0	0	12	6
60+	0	0	28 388	19 147.96	0	0	0	0	0	0	0	0
All Ages	*6 518*	*321.8*	*156 080*	*7 705.76*	*34*	*1.68*	*1 004*	*50*	*5 072*	*250*	*6 077*	*300*
World												
0-4	0	0	0	0	0	0	0	0	0	0	0	0
5-14	0	0	0	0	1	0.19	30	6	0	0	30	6
15-44	7 042	587.5	92 489	7 716.15	33	2.75	962	80	5 457	455	6 420	536
45-59	0	0	49 222	15 823.6	0	0	12	4	0	0	12	4
60+	0	0	35 893	13 332.47	0	0	0	0	0	0	0	0
All Ages	*7 042*	*269.42*	*177 604*	*6 795.07*	*34*	*1.3*	*1 004*	*38*	*5 457*	*209*	*6 462*	*247*

labour is common, women deemed to be at particular risk can be advised to await delivery in a maternity waiting home located near a first referral level hospital (World Health Organization 1997). This is one way of ensuring that if problems arise, women can be referred to a higher level of care in a timely manner.

Mortality due to obstructed labour can be greatly reduced through early detection of the problem and referral to a facility where operative delivery is an option. The use of the partograph permits early detection of abnormal progress and prevention of prolonged labour and would eliminate the risk of obstructed labour and significantly reduced the incidence of associated conditions such as uterine rupture, postpartum haemorrhage and sepsis (World Health Organization 1993). Although caesarean delivery will be needed for many cases of obstructed labour , alternative delivery techniques such as forceps, venoutse and symphisiotomy may be feasible in certain circumstances and settings and may be easier to provide where skills in surgery and anaesthesia are unavailable. Ensuring widespread accessibility of skilled health care workers able to perform operative interventions may require innovative approaches given the extremes shortages of practitioners, especially in rural areas. Experiences with training nurses, midwives and paramedical personnel in the techniques of emergency caesarean delivery have shown that outcomes in such cases can be at least as good as for interventions performed by highly trained doctors (White et al. 1987).

Community information and mobilization is an essential component of efforts to reduce maternal mortality due to obstructed labour. All too often, women and their families wait for many hours and even days before seeking assistance from the health care system during which time the woman can become dehydrated, infected and ruptured uterus can occur (Thaddeus and Maine 1994). It is under circumstances such as these that obstetric fistulae are common.

Conclusions

Preventing deaths from obstructed labour requires professional expertise and relatively sophisticated facilities. Antenatal care has a vital role to play in informing women and communities about signs and symptoms of obstructed labour and the need for early referral. The incidence of the condition also declines as a result of socioeconomic development such as raising the age at marriage, eliminating discrimination against female children and combating poverty.

Deaths from obstructed labour are now extremely rare in industrialized countries though they may occur following a caesarean delivery (such post-caesarean deaths have not been included in this analysis). The major barriers to effective care for prolonged/obstructed labour are poor transport and communication infrastructures and failure of the woman and/or her family to seek assistance in a timely manner when labour has gone on for too long. The World Health Organization estimates that a combination of information, education and communication to alert communities to the dangers of prolonged and obstructed labour, together with improved access to referral facilities, could lead to a reduction in deaths due to obstructed labour of 80 per cent by the year 2000 (World Health Organization 1994).

REFERENCES

Bennet VR and Brown LK (1995) Myles textbook for midwives. Churchill Livingstone.

Dujardin B et al. (1987) How accurate is maternal height measurement in Africa? *International Journal of Gynaecology and Obstetrics*, 41(2):139–145.

Friedman EA (1955) Primigravid labour. A graphicostatistical analysis. *Obstetrics and Gynecology*, 6(6):567–589.

Harrison K (1985) Childbearing, health and social priorities: A survey of 22, 774 consecutive hospital births in Zoria, Northern Nigeria. *British Journal of Obstetrics and Gynecology*. 92 (suppl 5):1–119

Harrison K (1997) Maternal mortality in Nigeria: The real issues. *African Journal of Reproductive Health*. 1(1):7–13

Kelly J (1991) *Epidemiological study of vesico-vaginal fistula in Ethiopia* (Unpublished project report).

Lomas J, Enkin M (1989) Variations in operative delivery. In: Chalmers I, Enkin M, Keirse M (eds.) *Effective care in pregnancy and childbirth*. Oxford University Press.

MacArthur C et al. (1997) Faecal incontinence after childbirth. *British Journal of Obstetrics and Gynecology*. 104:46–50.

Murray CJL and Lopez AD (1996a) Estimating causes of death: new methods and global and regional applications for 1990. In: Murray CJL and Lopez AD, eds. *The global burden of disease: a comprehensive assessment of mortality and disability from diseases, injuries, and risk factors in 1990 and projected to 2020.* Cambridge, Harvard University Press.

Murray CJL and Lopez AD (1996b) *The Global Burden of Disease: a comprehensive assessment of mortality and disability from diseases, injuries, and risk factors in 1990 and projected to 2020.* Cambridge, Harvard University Press.

Murphy M (1981) Social consequences of vesico-vaginal fistula in Northern Nigeria. *Journal of Biosocial Science*, 13.

Omran AR, Stanley CC (1976 & 1978) *Family Formation Patterns and Health.* Vols. I and II. World Health Organization, Geneva.

Randhowa I et al. (1991) A study of prolonged labour. *Journal of the Indian Medical Association.*, 89:6.

Rooney C. *Antenatal Care and Maternal Health: How effective is it?* World Health Organization, WHO/MSM/92.4.

Rosenberg K (1992) The evolution of modern human childbirth. *Yearbook of Physical Anthropology,* 35:89–124.

Sleep J, Roberts J, Chalmers I (1989) Care during the second stage of labour. In: Chalmers I, Enkin M, Keirse M (eds.) *Effective Care in Pregnancy and Childbirth.* Oxford University Press.

Thaddeus S, Maine D (1994) *Too far to walk: Maternal mortality in context. Social Science and Medicine.* 38(8):1091–1110.

Waldijk K (March–June 1994) Surgeons show success in early fistula repairs. *Safe Motherhood newsletter*, Issue 14.

White SM et al. (1987) Emergency obstetric surgery performed by nurses in Zaire. *Lancet.* 2:612–613.

World Health Organization (1993) *Preventing prolonged labour: a practical guide.* The pathograph WHO/FHE/msm/93.8 WHO, Geneva, Switzerland.

World Health Organization (1994) Maternal Health and Safe Motherhood Programme. *Obstetric fistulae: a review of available information.* WHO/MCH/MSM/91.5.

World Health Organization (1994) Maternal Health and Safe Motherhood Programme. *The Mother-Baby Package. Implementing Safe Motherhood in Countries.* World Health Organization, Geneva.

World Health Organization (1995) A WHO collaborative study of maternal anthropometry and pregnancy outcomes. *Bulleting of WHO* 73(suppl).

World Health Organization (1997) *Maternity waiting homes: A review of experiences.* WHO/RHT.msm.96.21 WHO, Geneva, Switzerland.

Younis N et al. (1994) *Learning about the gynecological health of women.* Policy Series in Reproductive Health 1002, Giza, Egypt. The Population Council.

Zacharin RF (1988) *Obstetric Fistula.* Springer-Verlag, Wien, New York.

Chapter 8

Unsafe Abortion and Ectopic Pregnancy

Carla AbouZahr
Elizabeth Åhman

Introduction

Pregnancy with abortive outcome covers a variety of conditions arising during early pregnancy including both conditions such as hydatidiform mole and ectopic pregnancy as well as spontaneous and induced abortion. In general, the term abortion is usually used to denote induced abortion — a deliberate procedure to terminate an established pregnancy — and spontaneous abortion is called miscarriage. In medical parlance, on the other hand, the term abortion is used to describe both types of pregnancy termination.

There are important differences in the dimensions and nature of deaths and disabilities resulting from different kinds of abortion. Ectopic pregnancy is a serious complication which can result in maternal death. The pregnancy is situated outside the normal nidation site within the uterine cavity, usually in the fallopian tube. Pregnancies implanted in the fallopian tubes almost invariably cause tubal rupture and present a threat to the health or life of the woman. Hydatidiform mole is the term applied to a gross malformation of the trophoblast in which the chorionic villi proliferate and become avascular and the fetus, deprived of oxygen and nutrition dies and becomes absorbed. The condition may develop into malignant choriocarcinoma which can be fatal to the woman if left untreated.

Spontaneous abortion occurring early in pregnancy is seldom fatal even in the absence of medical treatment. Induced abortion can be one of the safest of all medical procedures when carried out in appropriate medical settings by qualified and skilled health personnel. On the other hand, induced abortion by unskilled providers in settings where standards of hygiene are inadequate results in a major burden of suffering and death around the world.

Given the lack of epidemiological information about incidence and mortality from ectopic pregnancy or hydatidiform mole, and the relatively small health risks associated with spontaneous and safely induced abortion, this chapter focuses on deaths and disabilities due to unsafe abortion, which represent a major portion of the global burden of reproductive ill-health.

ICD Classification

The ICD-10 classification has a main grouping under the title "Pregnancy with abortive outcome" (O00–O08) which consists of the following categories:

- O00 Ectopic pregnancy
  - O00.0 Abdominal pregnancy (excluding delivery of viable fetus in abdominal pregnancy and maternal care associated with it)
  - O00.1 Tubal pregnancy: fallopian pregnancy, rupture of fallopian tube due to pregnancy and tubal abortion
  - O00.2 Ovarian pregnancy
  - O00.8 Other ectopic pregnancy: cervical, cornual, intraligamentous, mural
  - O00.9 Ectopic pregnancy, unspecified
- O01 Hydatidiform mole
  - O01.0 Classical hydatidiform mole
  - O01.1 Incomplete and partial hydatidiform mole
  - O01.9 Hydatidiform mole, unspecified; trophoblastic disease and vesicular mole
- O02 Other abnormal products of conception
  - O02.0 Blighted ovum and non-hydatidiform mole
  - O02.1 Missed abortion (early fetal death with retention of dead fetus)
  - O02.2 Other specified abnormal products of conception
  - O02.9 Abnormal product of conception, unspecified
- O03 Spontaneous abortion
- O04 Medical abortion
- O05 Other abortion
- O06 Unspecified abortion

Categories O03–O06 include the following subcategores:

- .0 Incomplete, complicated by genital tract and pelvic infection
- .1 Incomplete, complicated by delayed or excessive haemorrhage
- .2 Incomplete, complicated by embolism
- .3 Incomplete, with other or unspecified complications
- .4 Incomplete, without complications
- .5 Complete or unspecified, complicated by genital tract and pelvic infection

.6 Complete or unspecified, complicated by delayed or excessive haemorrhage
.7 Complete or unspecified, complicated by embolism
.8 Complete or unspecified, with other or unspecified complications
.9 Complete or unspecified, without complications

O07 Failed attempted abortion
O07.0 Failed medical abortion, complicated by genital tract and pelvic infection
O07.1 Failed medical abortion, complicated by delayed or excessive haemorrhage
O07.2 Failed medical abortion, complicated by embolism
O07.3 Failed medical abortion, with other or unspecified complications
O07.4 Failed medical abortion, without complications
O07.5 Other and unspecified failed attempted abortion, complicated by genital tract and pelvic infection
O07.6 Other and unspecified failed attempted abortion, complicated by delayed or excessive haemorrhage
O07.7 Other and unspecified failed attempted abortion, complicated by embolism
O07.8 Other and unspecified failed attempted abortion, with other or unspecified complications
O07.9 Other and unspecified failed attempted abortion, without complications

O08 Complications following abortion and ectopic and molar pregnancy (primarily intended for morbidity coding) and comprising:
O08.0 Genital tract and pelvic infection following abortion and ectopic and molar pregnancy
O08.1 Delayed or excessive haemorrhage following abortion and ectopic and molar pregnancy
O08.2 Embolism following abortion and ectopic and molar pregnancy
O08.3 Shock following abortion and ectopic and molar pregnancy
O08.4 Renal failure following abortion and ectopic and molar pregnancy
O08.5 Metabolic disorders following abortion and ectopic and molar pregnancy
O08.6 Damage to pelvic organs and tissues following abortion and ectopic and molar pregnancy
O08.7 Other venous complications following abortion and ectopic and molar pregnancy
O08.8 Other complications following abortion and ectopic and molar pregnancy

O08.9 Complications following abortion and ectopic and molar pregnancy, unspecified

Ectopic pregnancy

Definition and measurement

Ectopic pregnancy occurs when the fertilized ovum implants outside the uterine cavity, usually in the fallopian tubes, hence the term tubal pregnancy. Occasionally the implantation site may be the abdominal cavity or the cervical canal but such cases are rare (Turner 1989). In the initial stages of the pregnancy, the woman experiences the usual signs and symptoms of pregnancy, including enlargement of the uterus under the influence of pregnancy hormones. If the ovum is implanted in the fallopian tube, the woman is likely to experience abdominal pain as the tube becomes distended. There may be some vaginal bleeding, though the condition is uterine in origin and signifies endometrial degeneration (Sweet 1997). If the site of implantation is the narrow proximal end of the tube, tubal rupture is likely to occur between the fifth and seventh weeks of pregnancy. If the site of implantation is the wider ampullary section, the gestation may continue until the tenth week. When the tube ruptures, there will be severe intra-peritoneal haemorrhage accompanied by acute abdominal pain. Ruptured tubal pregnancy is an acute medical emergency requiring rapid intervention.

Diagnosis of ectopic pregnancy is difficult, as the clinical picture may appear similar to pelvic inflammatory disease or threatened abortion. Classic symptomatology includes a short history of acute abdominal pain, amenorrhoea, and vaginal bleeding. The availability of ultrasound and hormonal assays has greatly facilitated diagnosis in developed countries, though they remain the exception in developing country institutions.

The etiology of ectopic pregnancy is poorly understood, though certain high risk factors have been identified. These factors include a history of pelvic inflammatory disease, a previous ectopic pregnancy, or past tubal surgery, particularly for tubes damaged by pelvic inflammatory disease (Turner 1989). Other identified risk factors include older age, low parity, hormonal stimulation of ovulation, salpingitis (especially chlamydial), and iatrogenic factors such as *in-vitro* fertilization (Sweet 1997). Intrauterine contraceptive devices and the progestogen-only pill have also been implicated in the etiology of ectopic pregnancies; however, the evidence is equivocal at best and generally weak, with the exception of the progestogen-loaded intrauterine device (Turner 1989). Ectopic pregnancy appears to be peculiar to the human species, perhaps because pelvic inflammatory disease is also confined to humans, and also perhaps because of the particularly invasive properties of human tophoblast (Turner 1989).

Table 1 Incidence of ectopic pregnancy, selected studies.

Country	*Year of study*	*Incidence*	*Denominator*	*Source*
Jamaica	1954-61	1:28	Births	Douglas (1963)
USA	1970-78	1:108	Reported pregnancies	Rubin et al. (1983)
USA	1980	1:150-200	Conceptions	Benson (1980)
United Kingdom	1980	1:175	Live and stillbirths	Macafee (1982)
United Kingdom	1980-84	1:99	Deliveries	Pillai (1984)

Incidence of ectopic pregnancy

There is wide variation in the reported incidence of ectopic pregnancy. A frequently quoted figure from Jamaica is one ectopic pregnancy for every 28 births; this figure has changed little since it was first quoted in 1963 (Douglas 1963; Turner 1989). However, there is wide variation both in quoted incidence and in ways of presenting the results rendering global or regional generalizations unsure (Table 1).

Unfortunately, there are no comparable data sets for other developing countries. Rates are thought to be particularly high in Africa, probably because of the high prevalence of sexually transmitted diseases and pelvic inflammatory disease. However, because diagnosis of the condition is difficult, many cases in the developing world probably go unreported. Incidence varies both between countries, geographical areas, and between ethnic groups within countries. In the United States, average incidence of ectopic pregnancy over the period 1970–87 was 9.7 per 1000 pregnancies for white women, compared with 14.2 for women of other races (including blacks).

There is evidence of a rising trend in the incidence of ecctopic pregnancy in industrialized countries. In the United States, the reported incidence per 1000 reported pregnancies increased from 4.5 to 17 over the period 1970–88 (Figure 1) (Wilcox and Marks 1995).

Mortality from ectopic pregnancy

Little is known about the natural history of ectopic pregnancy if left untreated. It may resolve spontaneously, or it may cause death due to catastrophic intra peritoneal haemorrhage. An early study of conservative approaches to treatment found that one-third of cases resolved without surgery (Lund, 1955). As deaths from other obstetric causes are brought under control, ectopic pregnancy accounts for a rising proportion of maternal deaths. In the United Kingdom, it accounts for some 10 per cent of all maternal deaths (Department of Health and Social Security, 1986). In the United States, ectopic pregnancy accounted for 13 per cent of maternal deaths over the period 1979–96 (Wilcox and Marks 1995). In the overwhelming majority of cases, death resulted from haemorrhage (Table 2).

Figure 1 Cases of ectopic pregnancy per 1000 reported pregnancies, United States, 1970–1988

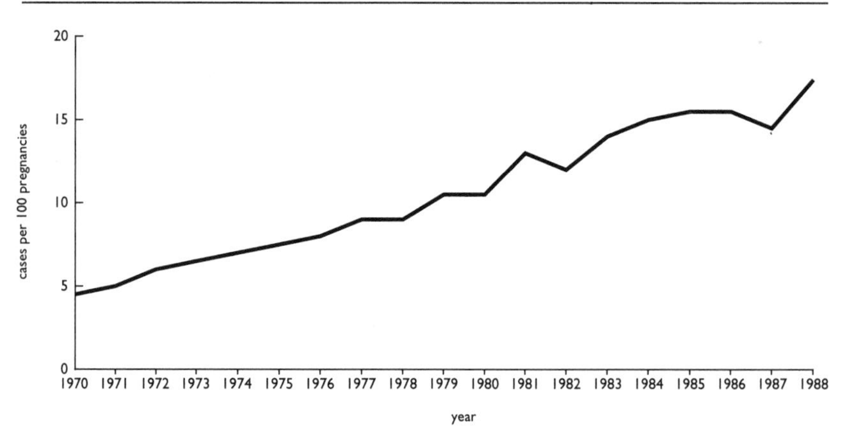

Source: Wilcox and Marks (1995).

Global estimates of mortality due to ectopic pregnancy have not been attempted in these calculations because so little is known about the incidence of the condition or associated mortality. However, for the three regions with relatively good vital reporting of deaths associated with ectopic pregnancy (Established Market Economies, Formerly Socialist Economies of Europe, and Latin America and the Caribbean), such deaths are included in the primary tabulations on abortion. For the rest of the world, estimates of mortality due to ectopic pregnancy are included in the overall chapter on maternal mortality, but excluded from the primary tabulations on abortion which cover only deaths and disabilities associated with unsafe abortion. Disabilities associated with ectopic pregnancy

Table 2 Causes of maternal deaths due to ectopic pregancy, United States, 1979–86

Cause of death	*Per cent of ectopic deaths*
Haemorrhage	89
Pulmonary embolism	3
Pregnancy-induced hypertension	<1
Infection	2
Anaesthesia complications	1
Other	5
Total deaths due to ectopic pregnancy	*100 (n=343)*

Source: Wilcox and Marks (1995)

have been counted in the primary tabulations with sexually transmitted diseases.

Hydatidiform mole and choriocarcinoma

Hydatidiform mole is a condition occurring as a result of degeneration of the chorionic villi at an early stage of the pregnancy. Choriocarcinoma is a malignant disease of trophoblastic tissue. A World Health technical report describes the following histopathological entities:
Hydatidiform mole: consists of two distinct entities, partial and complete, neither of which generally has any serious sequelae.
Partial hydatidiform mole: consists of an abnormal conceptus with an embryo or fetus that tends to die early.
Complete hydatidiform mole: consists of an abnormal conceptus without an embryo or fetus.
Invasive mole: consists of a tumor or tumor-like process invading the myometrium and may metastasize, though it does not exhibit the progression of a true cancer and may regress spontaneously. It can, however, result in death.
Gestational choriocarcinoma: a carcinoma arising from the trophoblastic epithlelium that may arise from conceptions that give rise to a live birth, an abortion, an ectopic pregnancy, or a hydatidiform mole. It appears to follow some 3 per cent of the latter (Sweet 1997). In the absence of treatment, this condition is rapidly fatal.
Placental site trophoblastic tumor: a tumor that arises from the trophoblast of the placental bed (World Health Organization 1983).

Given the paucity of data on the incidence of and mortality from hydatidiform mole, we have not included any estimates in the current calculations of the Global Burden of Disease Study (Murray and Lopez 1996a).

Spontaneous abortion

Of all clinically diagnosed pregnancies, between 15 per cent and 20 per cent end in spontaneous abortion (World Health Organization 1970). Of these abortions, approximately 80 per cent take place before 13 weeks (Jeffcoate 1975). Though these figures refer to clinically diagnosed pregnancies, it is likely that rates of pregnancy wastage are much higher.

Spontaneous abortions early in pregnancy are almost always preceded by the death of the embryo, unlike those later in pregnancy. In first trimester abortions, fetal death may be associated with abnormalities of the ovum itself, immunological factors, abnormalities in the reproductive tract or systemic disease in the woman (Turnbull 1989). Whereas first trimester spontaneous abortions are often associated with chromosomal abnormalities, second trimester abortions are usually associated with factors such as cervical incompetence, abnormalities of the uterine body, and infections such as *listeria monocytogenes*.

Other factors that can result in spontaneous abortion include maternal disease, particularly those associated with high fever, but also conditions such as diabetes, thyroid disease, renal disease, and hypertensive disorders (Sweet 1997). Other causes of spontaneous abortion include environmental factors such as radiation, drugs, and severe stress.

Spontaneous abortions seldom present severe complications and are rarely fatal. However, the psychological effects can be significant, and some women may become clinically depressed. The intensity of the reaction appears to be greater in women with no living children, in those who have had abortions previously, and in those whose abortion occurred during the second trimester, rather than early in pregnancy.

No attempt has been made to quantify death or disability resulting from spontaneous abortion in the Global Burden of Disease Study. The overwhelming majority of deaths and disabilities due to pregnancies with abortive outcome are caused by complications arising from unsafe abortions, such as when induced abortion is carried out by unskilled practitioners or in settings where minimal conditions of hygiene cannot be assured.

Unsafe abortion

Millions of women every year have an unwanted pregnancy. Some unwanted pregnancies are carried to term, others end in an induced abortion. An estimated 26 to 31 million legal abortions were performed in 1987 (Henshaw and Morrow 1990). Millions of abortions, however, were performed outside the legal system, often by unskilled providers.

Induced abortion is restricted by law in many countries. In others, pregnancy termination is legal on broad medical and social grounds. Sometimes, even where induced abortion is legal, services may be insufficient to meet demand or are inadequately distributed. Alternatively, women may be unaware of their availability. Despite restrictive laws and lack of adequate services, women continue to seek to terminate unwanted pregnancies.

Women who resort to unauthorized facilities and/or unskilled providers put their health and lives at risk. Restrictive legislation is associated with high rates of unsafe abortion. It is, however, the number of maternal deaths, not abortions, that is most affected by legal codes (Jacobson 1990). In the case of Romania, for example, the number of abortion-related deaths increased sharply after November 1966 when the government tightened a previously liberal abortion law (Figure 2). The figure rose from 20 per 100 000 live births in 1965 to almost 100 in 1974 and 150 in 1983 (Royston and Armstrong 1989). Abortions were legalized again in December 1989 and, by the end of 1990, maternal deaths caused by abortions dropped to around 60 per 100 000 live births.

The World Health Organization is particularly concerned with the public health aspects of abortion. As early as 1967, the World Health Assembly passed Resolution WHA20.41 which stated that "abortions .... constitute a serious public health problem in many countries ..."

Evidence from Demographic and Health Surveys carried out in some 40 developing countries shows that a large number of women want no more children or want to space births (Westoff 1991). For example, between 16 per cent and 49 per cent of women in sub-Saharan Africa said that they wanted no more children, and between 40 per cent and 77 per cent of women either wanted no more children or wanted to space births. In Latin America the figures are higher, being 55–72 per cent and 74–85 per cent respectively.

Studies also show that many *married* women in developing countries often do not have access to the contraception they require (Westoff and Ochoa 1991) to space their children or limit family size. The situation is even worse for unmarried women, particularly adolescents, who rarely have access to reproductive information and counselling, and frequently are excluded from contraceptive services.

Where contraception is unavailable or inaccessible there will inevitably be large numbers of unwanted pregnancies. These will also arise following contraceptive failure. Women may resort to unsafe abortion to terminate such pregnancies. Despite the paucity of data, inevitable in the

Figure 2 Effects of the introduction of anti-abortion law in 1966 and the legalization of abortion in 1989, Romania

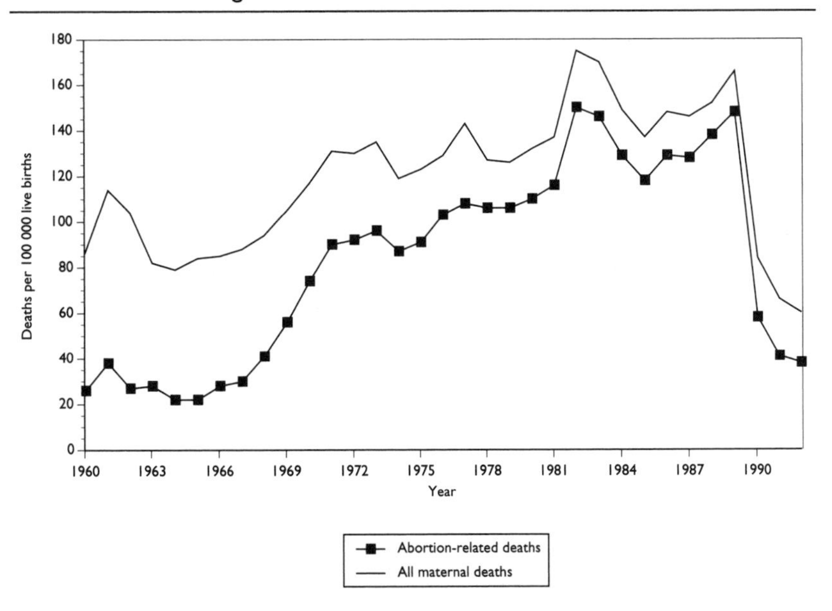

context of a procedure that most women wish to keep secret even when it is legal, it has been clear for many years that unsafe abortion is a public health problem of considerable magnitude. In some countries, up to 80 per cent or more of all abortion cases admitted to hospitals may have been induced. While a spontaneous or an uncomplicated abortion may require up to 3 days of hospitalization, complicated cases may require a stay 5 times longer.

The treatment of abortion complications in hospitals uses a disproportionate share of resources, including hospital beds, blood supply, medication, as well as access to operating theatres, anaesthesia and medical specialists. Thus unsafe abortion and its consequences places great clinical, material and financial demands on the scarce hospital resources of many developing countries (Figa-Talamanca et al. 1986, Fortney 1981, Tshibangu 1984). Up to 50 per cent of the resources of some hospitals are often used to treat patients admitted for complications of unsafe abortions (Genasci 1986). This undoubtedly compromises other maternity services.

Definition and measurement of unsafe abortion

Unsafe abortion is defined by the World Health Organization as a procedure for terminating an unwanted pregnancy either by persons lacking the necessary skills or in an environment lacking the minimal medical standards or both (World Health Organization 1992). Complications of unsafe abortion account for a substantial proportion of all maternal deaths around the world. In developing countries with high levels of maternal mortality, the risk of death following complications of unsafe abortion may be 100 to 500 times higher than that following an abortion performed under these conditions. In developed countries where abortions are performed professionally under safe conditions, induced abortion can be a relatively safe procedure. In the United States, for example, the death rate for induced abortion is now 0.6 per 100 000 procedures, making it safer than an injection of penicillin (Gold 1990).

For the purpose of the WHO database and tabulations (World Health Organization 1994), unsafe abortion has been defined as an "abortion not provided through approved facilities and/or persons". What constitutes "approved facilities and/or persons" will vary according to the legal and medical standards of each country. The definition does not take into consideration differences in quality, services available or the other substantial differences between health systems. Unsafe abortions are characterized by the lack or inadequacy of skills of the provider, hazardous techniques and unsanitary facilities (World Health Organization 1992).

ICD Classification

The ICD-9 has separate codes for spontaneous, legally and illegally induced abortion as follows:

634 Spontaneous abortion (complete and incomplete)
635 Legally induced abortion (legal and therapeutic)

636 Illegally induced abortion (criminal and illegal)
637 Unspecified abortion (complete, incomplete and retained products of conception following abortion not classifiable elsewhere)
638 Failed attempted abortion

The Tenth revision of the ICD does not distinguish between legal and illegal abortion but retains separate codes for spontaneous abortion, medical abortion and others as follows:

O03 Spontaneous abortion
O04 Medical abortion
O05 Other abortion
O08 Unspecified abortion

Reports of maternal deaths due to abortion-related complications may separately distinguish abortion and ectopic pregnancy but rarely make explicit reference to the type of abortion responsible for the maternal deaths analysed. In countries where induced abortion is not permitted by law, it has been assumed that the majority of abortion-related maternal deaths were due to unsafe abortions. In a number of cases, there appears to be under-reporting of abortion deaths by health care providers because of the stigma attached for both the patient and provider (Chukudebulu and Ozaumba 1988).

For the estimation of mortality due to abortion in the Global Burden of Disease Study the analysis focused on mortality and disability from unsafe abortion. The disability from ectopic preganncy has been counted in the primary tabulations with sexually transmitted diseases but mortality from ectopic pregnancy is included in the estimates presented in the overview chapter of maternal mortality (Chapter 3 in this volume).

Etiology of unsafe abortion

Unsafe abortion is a neglected problem of health care in developing countries and a serious concern to women during their reproductive lives. Contrary to common belief, most women seeking abortion are married or live in stable unions and already have several children (Ampofo et al. 1993). They use abortion to limit family size, or space births (Bulut et al. 1993) They may resort to abortion in the event of contraceptive failure or the lack of access to modern contraception. A recent study in the United States of almost 10 000 women who had abortions found that more than half had been using a contraceptive during the month they became pregnant; the proportion whose pregnancy was attributed to condom failure was 32 per cent (Henshaw and Kost 1996). However, in all parts of the world, particularly in urban areas, an increasing proportion of those having abortions are unmarried adolescents; in some urban centres, they represent the majority of all abortion seekers.

Unsafe abortions may be induced by the woman herself, by non-medical persons or by health workers in unhygienic conditions. Such abortions may be induced by insertion of a solid object (usually root, twig or catheter) into the uterus, an improperly performed dilatation and curettage procedure, ingestion of harmful substances, or exertion of external force. The mortality and morbidity risks of induced abortion depend on the facilities and skill of the abortion provider, the method used and certain characteristics of the woman herself, such as her general health, presence of reproductive tract infections (RTI) or sexually transmitted disease (STD), age, parity, and the stage of her pregnancy. The risks involved also depend on the availability and the utilization of treatment facilities once complications have occurred.

Measurement of unsafe abortion

Data on unsafe abortion are scarce and inevitably unreliable because of legal and ethical/moral constraints which hinder data collection. Underreporting and misreporting are common because women may be reluctant to admit to an induced abortion especially when it is illegal.

Few studies have achieved higher than 75 per cent accuracy of reporting and in some cases only a quarter of abortions known to have been performed have been admitted to by respondents (Jones and Forrest 1992, Van der Tak 1974, Wilcox and Horney 1984). In a rare follow-up study of 118 women admitting only to spontaneous abortion in Merida, Mexico in 1979, 77 per cent later admitted that the abortion had been induced (Canto de Cetina et al. 1985).

Hospital admissions for abortion complications are often used as an indicator of the problem of unsafe abortion. Hospital records show the number of women admitted for abortion complications and the number of subsequent deaths in a given period. This is particularly useful when information on births and maternal deaths is also available for the same period of time. Assuming that spontaneous abortions are relatively constant in a given population, and that they are unlikely to cause sepsis and death, the excess may be considered to be the result of unsafe abortion.

Hospital records rarely differentiate between induced and spontaneous abortions. When they do, induced abortions invariably are under-reported. A WHO protocol has been developed to assist researchers to distinguish between induced, probably induced and possibly induced abortions in hospital studies.

Between 10 per cent and 50 per cent of unsafe abortion cases will need medical attention (Armijo and Monreal 1965, Morris 1979). However, not all women seek health care when complications arise. Their decision to seek help depends on the accessibility (geographic and financial) of the health service and social attitudes, as well as the attitudes of health centre staff. Admissions data are, therefore, only indicative of a small proportion of the total number. On admission, women are reluctant to admit the true nature of the abortion and usually insist it is spontaneous.

Community surveys attempt to collect data on incidence by interviewing a random sample of women of reproductive age in the community. The success of this approach depends on factors such as the legal status of abortion and on the skill of the interviewers. These studies are vulnerable to under-reporting of induced abortions, coupled with over-reporting of spontaneous abortions. Indirect methods such as the Random Response Technique (RRT) (Abernathy et al. 1970) have been used in community studies to establish the proportion of women ever resorting to induced abortion. Prospective community studies follow women in a community and record the pregnancy outcomes.

Abortion providers' surveys are rare but, when available, may be used to estimate the incidence of abortion. These studies tend to report higher rates than other research methods, but may be the least biased method.

Mortality studies are often used in developing countries where vital registration systems are poor or nonexistent. Many deaths, particularly in rural areas, are not registered at all. When a death is reported, the cause is frequently not known, not indicated or deliberately concealed. An abortion may not be mentioned in order to protect the family and all references to pregnancy may be avoided, particularly in the case of unmarried women. Case findings, using a variety of sources of information, may actually be the most successful form of mortality studies. These studies usually begin by identifying all deaths of women of reproductive age, and then go on to determine the cause of death (Royston 1989). No single source of information is likely to yield all of the deaths. The sisterhood method (Graham et al. 1989) for estimating maternal deaths has also been used to identify deaths from abortion (Chiphangwi 1992).

Mortality and Disability Due to Unsafe Abortion

Incidence

Because of the difficulties surrounding the measurement of unsafe abortion, estimates of its incidence and mortality are imprecise. The approach used varies according to the information available for the particular area. Estimates were made for each country with a population of one million or more, from which sub-region, region and world totals were derived.

For the estimates of the numbers of unsafe abortions, the starting point was usually information about the ratio of abortion (both induced and spontaneous) treated in hospitals to deliveries in the same hospitals. The information came from individual hospital studies, or in a few cases, from national statistics on some or all of the country's hospitals. Differences between countries in the propensity to utilize hospitals for pregnancy-related conditions were thus taken into account to the extent that they apply equally to treatment of abortion complications and deliveries.

The abortion/birth ratio was adjusted by subtracting 0.034 to account for spontaneous abortions, following the procedure suggested by Singh and Wulf (1993). The fraction subtracted corresponds to the expected number of miscarriages at 13 to 22 weeks gestation. It was assumed that these would necessitate hospital treatment whilst women in developing countries having miscarriages prior to 13 weeks would rarely turn to hospitals.

The ratio was further adjusted on the assumption that half or more of induced abortions are accomplished without complications requiring hospitalization, and that abortion ratios are lower in rural than in urban areas. These adjustments took into account the existing abortion law (*de jure*) and its interpretation (*de facto*), information on the providers of unsafe abortions, and cultural and rural/urban differences. Careful consideration was given to total fertility rates, contraceptive prevalence, and the proportion of deliveries that take place in hospitals or other health care facilities.

To arrive at the estimated number of induced abortions, the adjusted ratio was applied to the number of births which, in turn, was calculated from the 1990 population and birth rate estimates. A few countries for which no data on the abortion ratio were available were assumed to have the same ratio as other countries in the region or as other countries having similar fertility and development indicators, and abortion laws.

The global estimate of the incidence of unsafe abortion suggests that worldwide some 20 million unsafe abortions take place each year. This represents almost one in ten pregnancies, or a ratio of one unsafe abortion to seven births. Nearly 90 per cent of unsafe abortions take place in the developing world. Despite liberalization of abortion laws in several countries during the 1980s and some improvement in service provision, many women still resort to abortions outside of approved facilities or with unskilled providers.

Mortality

According to the conditions in which the unsafe abortions are performed and the methods used, both of which are related to the legal status of abortion, a variety of severe complications may occur. Complications such as sepsis, haemorrhage, genital and abdominal trauma, perforated uterus or poisoning from abortifacient medicines can lead to death if left untreated. Death may also result from secondary complications such as gas gangrene and acute renal failure. Typical complications from illegally induced abortion are illustrated by a study of 840 patients in Ibadan, Nigeria, in 1989: sepsis (86 per cent), haemorrhage (35 per cent), uterine perforation (16 per cent), lower genital tract injury (10 per cent), renal failure (0.4 per cent), coma (0.4 per cent), embolism (0.2 per cent), and death (7 per cent) (Adewole 1992). Another study of 230 illegally induced septic abortions in Ibadan reported an even more extensive list of complications (see Table 3) (Konje et al. 1992).

To estimate the number of maternal deaths resulting from unsafe abortions, the starting point was information on abortion deaths as a percentage of all maternal deaths. For many countries, this information also came from individual hospital studies (see Table 4). However, where such in-

Table 3 Complications in patients with sepsis after induced abortion.

Complication	*No.*	*(%)*
Pelvic peritonitis	94	40.9
Generalized peritonitis	63	27.4
Pelvic abscess	60	26.1
Jaundice	28	12.2
Septicaemia	29	12.6
Uterine perforation	24	10.4
Maternal death[a]	19	8.3
Abdominopelvic abscess	15	6.5
Cervical laceration	10	4.3
Psychiatric disorders	8	3.5
Acute renal failure	7	3.0
Post fornix perforation	6	2.6
Septic shock	4	1.7
DIC[b]	3	1.3
Heart failure	3	1.3
Hepatorenal failure	3	1.3
Small bowel injury	3	1.3
Gynetresia	2	0.9

(a) Causes of mortality: septicaemic shock; acute renal failure; haemorrhage from perforation; DIC; choriocarcinoma; hepatorenal failure; cardiopulmonary failure after repair of burst abdomen.

(b) DIC, disseminated intravascular coagulation

Source: Konje (1992).

formation was available from community studies it was used in preference to that derived from hospital data. After the results of individual studies were combined and adjustment for rural/urban differences made, the percentage of abortion deaths to total maternal deaths in each country was weighted by the estimated number of births to arrive at regional estimates of the proportion of maternal mortality caused by abortion-related complications. These were then applied to the estimated number of maternal deaths in the region (World Health Organization 1991) to arrive at regional and world totals.

The estimates of the incidence of unsafe abortion and resulting maternal mortality necessarily have a high degree of uncertainty and may well be too low. They reflect the epidemiological judgement of experts but should be viewed as "best guesses" based on the information currently available.

On the basis of the assumptions and methodology described above and bearing in mind the large degree of uncertainty due to the incompleteness of the original data sources, it would appear that approximately one in eight maternal deaths occur each year as a result of complications following unsafe abortions and ectopic pregnancy. These estimates inevitably

Table 4 Mortality from unsafe aborion in selected countries, by region

Region/country	Year	Deaths from unsafe abortion per 100 000 live births	Deaths from unsafe abortion %of all maternal deaths
Established Market Economies			
Canada	1984	–	9
Finland	1970–79	0.8	9.8
Germany	1977	–	8.5
Portugal	1987	–	40
Spain	1985	–	45
United Kingdom	1974	–	4.9
USA	1987	–	18
Formerly Socialist Economies of Europe			
Albania	1994	8.4	20.6
Armenia	1988	3	9.1
Azerbaijan	1988	2	7.5
Belarus	1988	6	25
Estonia	1988	–	0
Kazakhstan	1988	9	17.7
Kurgyzstan	1988	5	9.7
Latvia	1988	7	25
Lithuania	1990	6	25
Romania	1992	38	63.3
Russian Federation	1991	22	42
Tajukistan	1988	2	3.4
Turkmenistan	1988	5	14.2
Ukaine	1988	10	27.1
Uzbekistan	1988	2	4.8
India	1991	–	20
Other Asia and Islands			
Bangladesh	1991	–	20.7
Fiji	1969–76	17	13.8
Mauritius	1989	5	25
Mongolia	1993	16	6.5
Myanmar	1990	–	40
Papua New Guinea	1984–86	46	6.6
Philippines	1987	10	9.9
Singapore	1985–87	–	30
Sub-Saharan Africa			
Angola	1987	69	7.4
Botswana	1982–86	7	10.6
Ethiopia	1986	14	54
Guinea-Bissau	1989–90	51	5.6
Madagascar	1987–91	–	22–40
Nigeria	1993	–	40–50
Senegal	1988	25	8.5
South Africa	1980–82	4	4.9
Tanzania	1983–84	45	16.5
Uganda	1994	180	33

Table 4 *(continued)*

Region/country	Year	Deaths from unsafe abortion per 100 000 live births	%of all maternal deaths
Latin America and the Caribbean			
Argentina	1990	17	32.9
Bolivia	1988	77	15.2
Brazil	1986	6	13.2
Chile	1991	13	37
Colombia	1986	18	10.3
Costa Rica	1988	1	6.7
Cuba	1988	9	21.8
Dominican Republic	1988	–	17
Ecuador	1988	8	7.3
El Salvador	1984	5	7.1
Guatemala	1987	–	11.5
Guyana	1984	62	30.8
Haiti	1987–89	41	11.9
Honduras	1989–90	19	8.7
Jamaica	1986–87	6	4.8
Mexico	1987–89	28	6.4
Nicaragua	1979	13	9.5
Panama	1988	–	11
Paraguay	1899	30	13.6
Peru	1985	–	16.1
Suriname	1985	10	14.2
Trinidad and Tobago	1986	55	51.7
Uruguay	1988	2	5
Venezuela	1987	10	19.4
Middle Eastern Crescent			
Bahrain	1977–86	2	5.4
Egypt	1992–93	7	4.1
Kuwait	1973–77	2	5.3

Source: World Health Organization (1993)

have a large margin of error; the numbers could be as low as 50 000 or as high as 100 000.

The calculations indicate that, in 1990, the mortality risk associated with unsafe abortion and ectopic pregnancy is at least 15 times higher in developing areas than in industrialised areas and in some regions it may be as much as 40–50 times higher. However, even in developed areas, the risk of death from unsafe abortion is substantially higher than in cases when abortion is legal.

There are large differences in the incidence of, and mortality from, abortion between regions. In most developing regions there are 20 or more unsafe abortions per 1000 women of reproductive age. In Latin America and the Caribbean, the rate is even higher. Every year there are 40 unsafe abortions per 1000 women of reproductive age, representing more than

abortions per 1000 women of reproductive age, representing more than one unsafe abortion for every three births. Abortion mortality represents nearly a quarter of all maternal deaths.

Although induced abortion is legal in the countries of the Formerly Socialist Economies of Europe, problems of confidentiality and quality of care result in reliance on unsafe abortion, with abortion related deaths accounting for almost 25 per cent of maternal deaths. In less developed regions, abortion-related deaths account for 8–13 per cent of all maternal deaths, a relatively low percentage because of overall high maternal mortality.

Epidemiological data on mortality have been used by the authors to derive a first set of regional mortality estimates. When considered in conjunction with mortality estimates proposed by other authors for other diseases and injuries in the GBD Study, the implied level of overall mortality usually exceeded the rate estimated by various demographic methods. In order not to exceed this upper bound for mortality within each age-sex and broad-cause group, an algorithm has been applied by the editors to reduce mortality estimates for specific conditions so that their sum did not exceed this upper bound. The algorithm has been described in more detail in *The Global Burden of Disease* (Murray and Lopez 1996a).

Disability

The consequences of an unsafe abortion can be permanent disability. In a hospital study in Durban, South Africa (1983–84), 42 of 647 patients with septic abortion underwent laparotomy. A hysterectomy was necessary in 35 patients, 18 of whom were primigravid. Eight patients were under the age of 20 at the time of hysterectomy (Richards et al. 1985). However, long-term consequences of abortion may include chronic pelvic pain, pelvic inflammatory disease, tubal occlusion and secondary infertility. High incidence of ectopic pregnancy and premature delivery, and increased risks of spontaneous abortion in subsequent pregnancies are other possible consequences of poorly performed abortions. For example, in prospective European studies it has been demonstrated that women harbouring sexually transmitted disease infections are at increased risk of an ascending postabortal infection: 22 per cent to 38 per cent of chlamydia-infected women developed pelvic infection after legal abortion, compared with from 2 per cent to 10 per cent of women without chlamydia (Giertz et al. 1987, Moller et al. 1982, Osser and Persson 1984, Westergaard 1982). Other studies show that the risk of infertility, for example, increases with each episode of salpingitis (Robertson and Ward 1988, Westrom 1980). Extrapolations from these and other studies indicate that about 20 to 30 per cent of unsafe abortions may lead to reproductive tract infections of which between 20 per cent and 40 per cent lead to pelvic inflammatory disease (PID) and infertility.

The likelihood that an infection will develop subsequent to an induced abortion will depend on the abortion method, who induced it, the environment where it took place and the general health status of the abortion seeker. It will also depend on access to health facilities as well as health-seeking behaviour should complications occur. It is estimated that between 20 and 30 per cent of unsafe abortion procedures result in reproductive tract infections. The upper range was used in regions with high incidence of unsafe abortion using methods that may introduce infectious agents and/ or with poor availability of hospital and medical care, i.e. sub-Saharan Africa and India. A lower estimate of 15 per cent was used in the regions where abortions are induced in "safer" circumstances and abortion seekers may receive skilled care in case of an infection. Depending on external factors, in particular the accessibility and use of health services, between 20 and 40 per cent of such reproductive tract infections are estimated to develop into bilateral tubal occlusion and infertility.

The outcome of these calculations is displayed in Chapter 2 in this volume; the total number of cases of reproductive tract infections and infertility is high in sub-Saharan Africa, India and large parts of Asia as well as in Latin America where many cases occur despite relatively good health facilities, because of the large number of unsafe abortions taking place in the region. Further description of the long-term sequelae of post-abortion infection is given in Chapter 5 in this volume, on Puerperal Sepsis and Other Puerperal Infections (AbouZahr 1996).

Depending on the condition under study, epidemiological data may be available for incidence, prevalence, case-fatality or mortality. Where data on more than one of these parameters are available, estimates of each of the epidemiological parameters derived from the data may not be internally consistent or consistent with the adjusted mortality rates described above. To ensure that all epidemiological information concerning a given condition is internally consistent, the editors have undertaken extensive analyses using computer models of the natural history of disease described in Murray and Lopez (1996b). The incidence, prevalence, and duration estimates have consequently been revised where necessary. In view of these adjustments to the basic epidemiological estimates originally provided for the Global Burden of Disease Study, the data which have undergone the GBD validation process are the joint responsibility of the authors and the editors.

The estimates of number of deaths, Years of Life Lost (YLLs), YLDs and DALYs from abortion episodes and infertility following abortion are presented in Tables 5–7. All episodes of abortion and all cases of subsequent infertility were classified as a class III disability and assigned a disability weight of 0.18; as there is no effective treatment, the disability weight was the same for treated and untreated forms of infertility.

Table 5 Epidemiological estimates for episodes of unsafe abortions, females, 1990.

Age group (years)	*Incidence* Number ('000s)	Rate per100 000	*Avg. age at onset* (years)	*Deaths* Number ('000s)	Rate per100 000	*YLLs* Number ('000s)	Rate per100 000
Established Market Economies							
0-4	0	0	–	0	0	0	0
5-14	0	0	–	0	0	0	0
15-44	123	69	30.00	0	0.10	3	2
45-59	3	4	52.40	0	0.00	0	0
60+	0	0	–	0	0.00	0	0
All Ages	*126*	*31*	*30.40*	*0*	*0.00*	*3*	*1*
Formerly Socialist Economies of Europe							
0-4	0	0	–	0	0	0	0
5-14	0	0	–	0	0	0	0
15-44	1 948	2 599	29.90	1	1.40	29	39
45-59	10	33	52.40	0	0.00	0	0
60+	0	0	–	0	0.00	0	0
All Ages	*1 958*	*565*	*30.00*	*1*	*0.30*	*29*	*12*
India							
0-4	0	0	–	0	0	0	0
5-14	0	0	–	0	0	0	0
15-44	4 152	2 268	29.60	16	9.00	486	265
45-59	136	295	52.40	1	1.20	8	17
60+	0	0	–	0	0.00	0	0
All Ages	*4 292*	*1 047*	*30.30*	*17*	*4.20*	*494*	*120*
China							
0-4	0	0	–	0	0.00	0	0
5-14	0	0	–	0	0.00	0	0
15-44	8	3	–	2	0.80	74	26
45-59	0	0	–	0	0.20	2	3
60+	0	0	–	0	0.00	0	0
All Ages	*8*	*2*	–	*3*	*0.50*	*76*	*14*
Other Asia and Islands							
0-4	0	0	–	0	0.00	0	0
5-14	0	0	–	0	0.00	0	0
15-44	3 402	2 131	29.70	7	4.20	195	122
45-59	142	404	52.20	0	0.80	4	11
60+	0	0	–	0	0.00	0	0
All Ages	*3 544*	*1 044*	*30.60*	*7*	*2.00*	*199*	*59*
Sub-Saharan Africa							
0-4	0	0	–	0	0.00	0	0
5-14	194	277	10.00	1	1.90	51	73
15-44	3 424	3 222	29.20	24	22.40	696	655
45-59	7	34	52.20	0	0.20	1	5
60+	0	0	–	0	0.00	0	0
All Ages	*3 625*	*1 405*	*28.20*	*25*	*9.80*	*748*	*290*

Table 5 *(continued)*

Age group (years)	Incidence Number ('000s)	Incidence Rate per100 000	Avg. age at onset (years)	Deaths Number ('000s)	Deaths Rate per100 000	YLLs Number ('000s)	YLLs Rate per100 000
Latin America and the Caribbean							
0-4	0	0	–	0	0.00	0	0
5-14	33	66	10.00	0	0.10	1	2
15-44	4 655	4 472	29.70	4	4.10	130	125
45-59	30	131	52.40	0	0.10	0	0
60+	0	0	29.70	4	2.00	0	0
All Ages	*4 719*	*2 119*	*29.70*	*4*	*2.00*	*131*	*59*
Middle Eastern Crescent							
0-4	0	0	–	0	0	0	0
5-14	3	4	10.00	0	0.00	0	0
15-44	2 190	2 043	29.80	4	3.50	109	102
45-59	140	629	52.30	0	1.10	4	18
60+	0	0	–	0	0.00	0	0
All Ages	*23 333*	*946*	*31.10*	*4*	*1.60*	*113*	*46*
Developed Regions							
0-4	0	0	-	0	0	0	0
5-14	0	0	-	0	0	0	0
15-44	2 071	815	29.91	1	0	32	13
45-59	13	13	52.40	0	0	0	0
60+	0	0	-	0	0	0	0
All Ages	*2 084*	*321*	*30.0*	*1*	*0*	*32*	*5*
Developing Regions							
0-4	0	0	-	0	0	0	0
5-14	230	51	10	1	0	52	12
15-44	17 831	1 888	30	57	6	1 690	179
45-59	455	213	52	1	0	19	9
60+	0	0	-	4	3	0	0
All Ages	*18 516*	*914*	*29.9*	*63*	*3*	*1 761*	*87*
World							
0-4	0	0	-	0	0	0	0
5-14	230	44	10.0	1	0	52	10
15-44	19 902	1 660	29.6	58	5	1 722	144
45-59	468	150	52.3	1	0	19	6
60+	0	0	-	4	1	0	0
All Ages	*20 600*	*788*	*29.9*	*64*	*2*	*1 793*	*69*

Table 6 Epidemiological estimates of infertility arising from unsafe abortion, 1990, Females.

Age group (years)	Incidence Number ('000s)	Incidence Rate per100 000	Prevalence Number ('000s)	Prevalence Rate per100 000	Avg. age at onset (years)	Avg. duration (years)	YLDs Number ('000s)	YLDs Rate per100 000
Established Market Economies								
0-4	0	0.00	0	0	–	–	0	0
5-14	0	0.00	0	0	–	–	0	0
15-44	4	2.20	60	34	25.00	15.00	12 722	7 099
45-59	0	0.00	0	0	–	–	0	0
60+	0	0.00	0	0	–	–	0	0
All Ages	*4*	*1.00*	*60*	*15*	*25.00*	*15.00*	*12 722*	*3 123*
Formerly Socialist Economies of Europe								
0-4	0	0.00	0	0	–	–	0	0
5-14	0	0.00	0	0	–	–	0	0
15-44	57	76.00	860	1 147	25.00	15.00	182 445	243 393
45-59	0	0.00	0	0	–	–	0	0
60+	0	0.00	0	0	–	–	0	0
All Ages	*57*	*32.00*	*860*	*475*	*25.00*	*15.00*	*182 445*	*75 161*
India								
0-4	0	0.00	0	0	–	–	0	0
5-14	0	0.00	0	0	–	–	0	0
15-44	479	262.00	7 192	3 925	25.00	15.00	1 525 746	832 640
45-59	0	0.00	0	0	–	–	0	0
60+	0	0.00	0	0	–	–	0	0
All Ages	*479*	*117*	*7 192*	*1 754*	*25.00*	*15.00*	*1 525 746*	*372 031*
China								
0-4	0	0.00	0	0	–	–	0	0
5-14	0	0.00	0	0	–	–	0	0
15-44	0	0.00	0	0	–	–	0	0
45-59	0	0.00	0	0	–	–	0	0
60+	0	0.00	0	0	–	–	0	0
All Ages	*0*	*0.00*	*0*	*0*	–	–	*0*	*0*
Other Asia and Islands								
0-4	0	0.00	0	0	–	–	0	0
5-14	0	0.00	0	0	–	–	0	0
15-44	252	158.00	3 779	2 368	25.00	15.00	801 705	502 287
45-59	0	0.00	0	0	–	–	0	0
60+	0	0.00	0	0	–	–	0	0
All Ages	*252*	*74*	*3 779*	*1 113*	*25.00*	*15.00*	*801 705*	*236 096*
Sub-Saharan Africa								
0-4	0	0.00	0	0	–	–	0	0
5-14	0	0.00	0	0	–	–	0	0
15-44	389	366.00	5 833	5 489	25.00	15.00	1 237 371	1 164 508
45-59	0	0.00	0	0	–	–	0	0
60+	0	0.00	0	0	–	–	0	0
All Ages	*389*	*151*	*5 833*	*2 261*	*25.00*	*15.00*	*1 237 371*	*479 690*

Table 6 *(continued)*

Age group (years)	Incidence		Prevalence		Avg. age at onset (years)	Avg. duration (years)	YLDs	
	Number ('000s)	Rate per100 000	Number ('000s)	Rate per100 000			Number ('000s)	Rate per100 000
Latin America and the Caribbean								
0-4	0	0.00	0	0	–	–	0	0
5-14	0	0.00	0	0	–	–	0	0
15-44	137	132.00	2 059	1 978	25.00	15.00	436 722	419 582
45-59	0	0.00	0	0	–	–	0	0
60+	0	0.00	0	0	–	–	0	0
All Ages	*137*	*62*	*2 059*	*924*	*25.00*	*15.00*	*436 722*	*196 117*
Middle Eastern Crescent								
0-4	0	0.00	0	0	–	–	0	0
5-14	0	0.00	0	0	–	–	0	0
15-44	107	100.00	1 611	1 502	25.00	15.00	341 675	318 694
45-59	0	0.00	0	0	–	–	0	0
60+	0	0.00	0	0	–	–	0	0
All Ages	*107*	*44*	*1 611*	*653*	*25.00*	*15.00*	*341 675*	*138 506*
Developed Regions								
0-4	0	0.00	0	0	-	-	0	0
5-14	0	0.00	0	0	-	-	0	0
15-44	61	24.00	920	362	25.00	11.44	195 167	76 790
45-59	0	0.00	0	0	-	-	0	0
60+	0	0.00	0	0	-	-	0	0
All Ages	*61*	*9.38*	*920*	*142*	*25.0*	*11.4*	*195 167*	*30 024*
Developing Regions								
0-4	0	0.00	0	0	-	-	0	0
5-14	0	0.00	0	0	-	-	0	0
15-44	1 364	144.42	20 474	2 168	25	15	4 343 219	459 851
45-59	0	0.00	0	0	-	-	0	0
60+	0	0.00	0	0	-	-	0	0
All Ages	*1 364*	*67.34*	*20 474*	*1 011*	*25.0*	*15.0*	*4 343 219*	*214 427*
World								
0-4	0	0.00	0	0	-	-	0	0
5-14	0	0.00	0	0	-	-	0	0
15-44	1 425	118.88	21 394	1 785	25.0	14.5	4 538 386	378 627
45-59	0	0.00	0	0	-	-	0	0
60+	0	0.00	0	0	-	-	0	0
All Ages	*1 425*	*54.52*	*21 394*	*819*	*25.0*	*14.5*	*4 538 386*	*173 637*

Table 7 Epidemiological Estimates for unsafe abortion, females, 1990.

Age group (years)	*Incidence*		*Prevalence*		*Deaths*		*YLLs*		*YLDs*		*DALYs*	
	Number ('000s)	Rate per100 000	Number ('000s)	Rate per100 000	Number ('000s)	Rate per100 000	Number ('000s)	Rate per100 000	Number ('000s)	Rate per100 000	Number ('000s)	Rate per100 000
Established Market Economies												
0-4	0	0.00	0	0.00		0.00	0	0.00	0	0.00	0	0.00
5-14	0	0.00	0	0.00		0.00	0	0.00	0	0.00	0	0.00
15-44	4	0.00	60	0.00	0	0.00	3	0.00	12 722	0.07	12 725	0.07
45-59	0	0.00	0	0.00	0	0.00	0	0.00	0	0.00	0	0.00
60+	0	0.00	0	0.00	0	0.00	0	0.00	0	0.00	0	0.00
All Ages	*4*	*0.00*	*60*	*0.00*	*0*	*0.00*	*3*	*0.00*	*12 722*	*0.03*	*12 725*	*0.03*
Formerly Socialist Economies												
0-4	0	0.00	0	0.00		0.00	0	0.00	0	0.00	0	0.00
5-14	0	0.00	0	0.00		0.00	0	0.00	0	0.00	0	0.00
15-44	57	0.00	860	0.01	1	0.00	29	0.00	182 445	2.43	182 474	2.43
45-59	0	0.00	0	0.00	0	0.00	0	0.00	0	0.00	0	0.00
60+	0	0.00	0	0.00	0	0.00	0	0.00	0	0.00	0	0.00
All Ages	*57*	*0.00*	*860*	*0.00*	*1*	*0.00*	*29*	*0.00*	*182 445*	*0.75*	*182 474*	*0.75*
India												
0-4	0	0.00	0	0.00		0.00	0	0.00	0	0.00	0	0.00
5-14	0	0.00	0	0.00		0.00	0	0.00	0	0.00	0	0.00
15-44	479	0.00	7 192	0.04	16	0.00	486	0.00	1 525 746	8.33	1 526 232	8.33
45-59	0	0.00	0	0.00	1	0.00	8	0.00	0	0.00	8	0.00
60+	0	0.00	0	0.00	0	0.00	0	0.00	0	0.00	0	0.00
All Ages	*479*	*0.00*	*7 192*	*0.02*	*17*	*0.00*	*494*	*0.00*	*1 525 746*	*3.72*	*1 526 240*	*3.72*
China												
0-4	0	0.00	0	0.00	0	0.00	0	0.00	0	0.00	0	0.00
5-14	0	0.00	0	0.00	0	0.00	0	0.00	0	0.00	0	0.00
15-44	0	0.00	0	0.00	2	0.00	74	0.00	0	0.00	74	0.00
45-59	0	0.00	0	0.00	0	0.00	2	0.00	0	0.00	2	0.00
60+	0	0.00	0	0.00	0	0.00	0	0.00	0	0.00	0	0.00
All Ages	*0*	*0.00*	*0*	*0.00*	2	*0.00*	*76*	*0.00*	*0*	*0.00*	76	*0.00*
Other Asia and Islands												
0-4	0	0.00	0	0.00	0	0.00	0	0.00	0	0.00	0	0.00
5-14	0	0.00	0	0.00	0	0.00	0	0.00	0	0.00	0	0.00
15-44	252	0.00	3 779	0.02	7	0.00	195	0.00	801 705	5.02	801 900	5.02
45-59	0	0.00	0	0.00	0	0.00	4	0.00	0	0.00	4	0.00
60+	0	0.00	0	0.00	0	0.00	0	0.00	0	0.00	0	0.00
All Ages	252	*0.00*	*3 779*	*0.01*	*7*	*0.00*	*199*	*0.00*	*801 705*	2.36	*801 904*	2.36
Sub-Saharan Africa												
0-4	0	0.00	0	0.00	0	0.00	0	0.00	0	0.00	0	0.00
5-14	0	0.00	0	0.00	1	0.00	51	0.00	0	0.00	51	0.00
15-44	389	0.00	5 833	0.05	24	0.00	696	0.01	1 237 371	11.65	1 238 067	11.65
45-59	0	0.00	0	0.00	0	0.00	1	0.00	0	0.00	1	0.00
60+	0	0.00	0	0.00	0	0.00	0	0.00	0	0.00	0	0.00
All Ages	*389*	*0.00*	*5 833*	*0.02*	*25*	*0.00*	*748*	*0.00*	*1 237 371*	*4.80*	*1 238 119*	*4.80*

Table 7 *(continued)*

Age group (years)	*Incidence*		*Prevalence*		*Deaths*		*YLLs*		*YLDs*		*DALYs*	
	Number ('000s)	Rate per100 000	Number ('000s)	Rate per100 000	Number ('000s)	Rate per100 000	Number ('000s)	Rate per100 000	Number ('000s)	Rate per100 000	Number ('000s)	Rate per100 000
Latin America and the Caribbean												
0-4	0	0.00	0	0.00	0	0.00	0	0.00	0	0.00	0	0.00
5-14	0	0.00	0	0.00	0	0.00	1	0.00	0	0.00	1	0.00
15-44	137	0.00	2 059	0.02	4	0.00	130	0.00	436 722	4.20	436 852	4.20
45-59	0	0.00	0	0.00	0	0.00	0	0.00	0	0.00	0	0.00
60+	0	0.00	0	0.00	4	0.00	0	0.00	0	0.00	0	0.00
All Ages	*137*	*0.00*	*2 059*	*0.01*	*8*	*0.00*	*131*	*0.00*	*436 722*	*1.96*	*436 853*	*1.96*
Middle Eastern Crescent												
0-4	0	0.00	0	0.00		0.00	0	0.00	0	0.00	0	0.00
5-14	0	0.00	0	0.00	0	0.00	0	0.00	0	0.00	0	0.00
15-44	107	0.00	1 611	0.02	4	0.00	109	0.00	341 675	3.19	341 784	3.19
45-59	0	0.00	0	0.00	0	0.00	4	0.00	0	0.00	4	0.00
60+	0	0.00	0	0.00	0	0.00	0	0.00	0	0.00	0	0.00
All Ages	*107*	*0.00*	*1 611*	*0.01*	*4*	*0.00*	*113*	*0.00*	*341 675*	*1.39*	*341 788*	*1.39*
Developed Regions												
0-4	0	0.00	0	0.00	0	0.00	0	0	0	0	0	0
5-14	0	0.00	0	0.00	0	0.00	0	0	0	0	0	0
15-44	61	24.00	920	361.98	1	0.39	32	13	195 167	76 790	195 199	76 802
45-59	0	0.00	0	0.00	0	0.00	0	0	0	0	0	0
60+	0	0.00	0	0.00	0	0.00	0	0	0	0	0	0
All Ages	*61*	*9.38*	*920*	*141.53*	*1*	*0.15*	*32*	*5*	*195 167*	*30 024*	*195 199*	*30 028*
Developing Regions												
0-4	0	0.00	0	0.00	0	0.00	0	0	0	0	0	0
5-14	0	0.00	0	0.00	1	0.22	52	12	0	0	52	12
15-44	1 364	144.42	20 474	2 167.74	57	6.04	1 690	179	4 343 219	459 851	4 344 909	460 030
45-59	0	0.00	0	0.00	1	0.47	19	9	0	0	19	9
60+	0	0.00	0	0.00	4	2.70	0	0	0	0	0	0
All Ages	*1 364*	*67.34*	*20 474*	*1 010.81*	*63*	*3.11*	*1 761*	*87*	*4 343 219*	*214 427*	*4 344 980*	*214 514*
World												
0-4	0	0.00	0	0.00	0	0.00	0	0	0	0	0	0
5-14	0	0.00	0	0.00	1	0.19	52	10	0	0	52	10
15-44	1 425	118.88	2 1394	1 784.85	58	4.84	1 722	144	4 538 386	378 627	4 540 108	378 771
45-59	0	0.00	0	0.00	1	0.32	19	6	0	0	19	6
60+	0	0.00	0	0.00	4	1.49	0	0	0	0	0	0
All Ages	*1 425*	*54.52*	*2 1394*	*818.53*	*64*	*2.45*	*1 793*	*69*	*4 538 386*	*173 637*	*4 540 179*	*173 706*

Impact of interventions on the burden

Maternal deaths from unsafe abortion are particularly tragic because this complication is almost entirely preventable. Access to family planning information and services helps to avoid unwanted pregnancies and thus recourse to unsafe abortion. Access implies more than simply physical proximity; it involves paying particular attention to the barriers that prevent women from reaching services and obtaining the method of contraception that is most stable and appropriated for them. Barriers include the economic and opportunity costs for women; social and cultural constraints; lack of privacy and confidentiality; provider attitudes; fear and shame.

Even when access to high quality family planning services is available, unwanted pregnancies will continue to occur, including among women who were using a method of contraception at the time of conception (Henshaw and Kost 1996). Methods fail for a variety of reasons including factors related to the method and factors related to the user. Whatever the reasons for the failure, health services need to be available to provide sympathetic and compassionate counseling for the woman and advice and information on the options available to her.

The legal status of abortion is a key determinant of access to safe abortion. However, even where safe abortion is legally available, unsafe abortions continue to occur (Bulut et al. 1993). Women continue to resort to unsafe abortions because safe services are inaccessible to them due to distance, financial costs, lack of confidentiality, provider attitudes and poor quality of care (McLaurin et al. 1990). In general, where abortions are against the law, women will obtain them anyway – the better off women usually safely and poor women suffering the consequences of poorly performed procedures. Adolescents are particularly vulnerable to unsafe abortion (Mpangile et al. 1992). Lack of knowledge about their bodies, about pregnancy and about when and where to seek help and shortage of resources, mean that they often seek car too late or they turn to unqualified practitioners.

Where legal termination of pregnancy is not available, much can be done to prevent abortion-related mortality by prompt and high quality treatment for complications (World Health Organization 1994). Treatment for uncomplicated early incomplete abortion is surgical: the retained products of conception are removed, bleeding stops and infection is then unlikely. Prophylactic antibiotic therapy should be considered even if there are no signs of infections. Treatment of complicated incomplete abortion requires high dosage of intravenous antibiotics, in some cases blood transfusion; total hysterectomy may be necessary in some cases (World Health Organization 1995).

Recently available technologies have rendered the treatment of incomplete abortion both relatively simple and safe. Manual vacuum aspiration (MVA) of retained products is both simpler and safer than the traditional dilatation and curettage. MVA can also be used to induce abortion; it is cost-effective and can be performed at the peripheral level. More recently still, drug induced abortion has been successfully introduced into a variety of settings as diverse as India, Viet Nam, China, France and the United Kingdom.

Conclusions

This chapter has focused entirely on deaths and morbidities due to unsafe abortion. It does not cover ectopic pregnancy, molar pregnancy or spontaneous abortion. Spontaneous abortion is unlikely to result in the death of the mother though this can happen, especially when the abortion occurs late in pregnancy and/or the condition is treated inappropriately.

Unsafe abortion is both widespread and a major cause of maternal death in developing countries. Neither access to safe procedures nor its illegal status seem to deter women from having abortions to terminate an unwanted pregnancy. Unlike many other causes of maternal deaths, unsafe abortion is almost entirely preventable. Access for all individuals and couples to information and services for family planning, together with management of abortion-related complications could result in the reduction of abortion-related mortality by 80 per cent by the year 2000.

References

Abernathy J, Greenberg B, Horvitz D (1970) Estimates of induced abortion in urban North Carolina. *Demography*, 7(1):19–29.

AbouZahr C (1996) Puerperal infections. In: Murray CJL and Lopez AD, eds. *Health Dimensions of Sex and Reproduction: the global burden of sexually transmitted diseases, HIV, maternal conditions, perinatal disorders, and congenital anomalies.* Cambridge, Harvard University Press.

Adewole IF (1992) Trends in postabortal mortality and morbidity in Ibadan, Nigeria. *International journal of gynecology and obstetrics*, 38(1):115–118.

Ampofo DA et al. (1993). *Contraceptives cause infertility. Determinants of decision-making factors in women with knowledge of contraception who resort to induced abortion.* Accra, University of Ghana Medical School.

Armijo R, Monreal T (1965) Epidemiology of provoked abortion in Santiago, Chile. In: Muramatsu M, Harper PA, eds. *Population dynamics: International Action and Training Programmes*. Baltimore, Johns Hopkins Press.

Benson RC (1980) Ectopic pregnancy. In: *Handbook of obstetrics and gynecology.* Lange, California, p.248.

Bulut A et al. (1993) *Abortion services in two public sector hospitals in Istanbul, Turkey: how well do they meet women's needs?* Istanbul, University of Istanbul.

Canto de Cetina TE et al. (1985) Aborto incompleto: caracteristicas de las pacientes tratadas en el Hospital O'Horan de Merida, Yucatan. [Incomplete abortion: characteristics of patients treated in the O'Horan de Merida Hospital, Yucatan.] *Salud Publica de Mexico*, 27(6):507–513.

Chiphangwi JD et al. (1992) Maternal Mortality in the Thyolo district of Southern Malawi. *East African Medical Journal*, 69(12):675–679.

Chukudebulu WO and Ozaumba BC (1988) Maternal mortality in Anambra State of Nigeria. *International Journal of Gynecology and Obstretrics* 27:171–176.

Department of Health and Social Security (1986) *Confidential enquiries into maternal deaths in England and Wales 1979–81*. HMSO, London.

Douglas CP (1963) Tubal ectopic pregnancy. *British Medical Journal,* 838–841.

Figa-Talamanca I et al. (1986) Illegal abortion: an attempt to assess its costs to the health services and its incidence in the community. *International Journal of Health Services*,16(3):375–389.

Fortney JA (1981) The use of hospital resources to treat incomplete abortions: examples from Latin America. *Public Health Reports*, 96(6):574–579.

Genasci L (1986) Brazil to launch national programme. *People*, 13(3):25.

Giertz G et al. (1987) A prospective study of Chlamydia trachomatis infection following legal abortion. *Acta obstetricia et gynaecologica*, 66:107–109.

Gold RB (1990) *Abortion and women's health. A turning point for America?* New York and Washington DC, The Alan Guttmacher Institute.

Graham W et al. (1989) Estimating maternal mortality: the sisterhood method. *Studies in Family Planning*, 20(3):125–135.

Henshaw SK and Kost K (1996) Abortion patients in 1994–95; characteristics and contraceptive use. *Family planning perspectives* 28(4):140–147/158.

Henshaw SK and Morrow E (1990 suppl.) *Induced abortion. A world review*. New York, The Alan Guttmacher Institute.

Jacobson JL (1990) The global politics of abortion. *Worldwatch Paper*.

Jeffcoate N (1975) *Principles of gynaecology*, 3rd edition. Butterworth, London.

Jones EF, Forrest JD (1992) Under-reporting of abortion in surveys of U.S. women: 1976 to 1988. *Demography*, 29(1):113–126.

Konje JC et al. (1992) Health and economic consequences of septic induced abortion. *International journal of gynecology and obstetrics*, 37(3):193–197.

Lund JJ (1955) Early ectopic pregnancy. Comments on conservative treatment. *Journal of obstetrics and gynaecology of the British Empire* 62:70–76.

Macafee CAJ (1982) Diagnoses not to be missed: ectopic pregnancy. *British Journal of Hospital Medicine* 9:246–248.

McLaurin KE (1990) *Health systems' role in abortion care: the need for a proactive approach. Issues in abortion care*. IPAS. Carborro.

Moller BR et al. (1982) Pelvic infection after elective abortion associated with Chlamydia trachomatis. *Obstetrics and Gynecology*, 66:107–109.

Morris L et al. (1979) Contraceptive use and demographic trends in El Salvador. *Studies in Family Planning*, 10(2):43–52.

Mpangile GS et al. (1992) *Factors associated with induced abortion in public hospitals in Dar es Salaam, Tanzania*. Dar es Salaam, Tanzania Family Planning Association.

Murray CJL and Lopez AD (1996a) Estimating causes of death: new methods and global and regional applications for 1990. In: Murray CJL and Lopez AD, eds. *The global burden of disease: a comprehensive assessment of mortality and disability from diseases, injuries, and risk factors in 1990 and projected to 2020*. Cambridge, Harvard University Press.

Murray CJL and Lopez AD (1996b) Global and regional descriptive epidemiology of disability: incidence, prevalence, health expectancies and Years lived with Disability. In: Murray CJL and Lopez AD, eds. *The global burden of disease: a comprehensive assessment of mortality and disability from diseases, injuries, and risk factors in 1990 and projected to 2020*. Cambridge, Harvard University Press.

Osser S, Persson K (1984) Postabortal pelvic infection associated with Chlamydia trachomatis and the influence of humoral immunity. *American Journal of Obstetrics and Gynecology*, 150(6):699–703.

Pillai (1984) Current trends in ectopic pregnancy (unpublished). Quoted in: Turner G (1989) Ectopic pregnancy. In: Turnbull A and Chamberlain G, eds. *Obstetrics*, Churchill Livingstone.

Richards A et al. (1985) The incidence of major abdominal surgery after septic abortion — an indicator of complications due to illegal abortion. *South African Medical Journal*, 68:799–800.

Robertson JN, Ward ME (1988) Gonococcal and chlamydial infection in infertility and ectopic pregnancy. *Contemporary Review in Obstetrics and Gynaecology*, 1(9):60–66.

Rowley J, Berkley S (1996) Sexually transmitted diseases. In: Murray CJL and Lopez AD, eds. *Health Dimensions of Sex and Reproduction: the global burden of sexually transmitted diseases, HIV, maternal conditions, perinatal disorders, and congenital anomalies*. Cambridge, Harvard University Press.

Royston E (1989) Methodological Issues in Abortion Research. *Proceedings of a seminar presented under the Population Council's Robert H. Ebert Program on Critical Issues in Reproductive Health, in collaboration with International Projects Assistance Services and the World Health Organization*. New York.

Royston E, Armstrong S (1989) *Preventing maternal deaths*. Geneva, World Health Organization.

Rubin GL et al. (1983) ectopic pregnancy in the United States: 1970–1978. *Journal of the American Medical Association* 249:1725–1729.

Singh S, Wulf D (1993) *Estimates of induced abortion levels in Brazil, Chile, Colombia*. New York, The Alan Guttmacher Institute.

Sweet B, ed. (1997) *Mayes' midwifery: A textbook for midwives*. 12th edition. Bailliere Tindall, London.

The Tbilisi Declaration. "*From abortion to contraception*", 10–13 October 1990.

Tshibangu K et al. (1984) Avortement clandestin, problème de santé publique a Kinshasa. [Clandestine Abortion, a public health issue in Kishasa.] *Journal de Gynecologie, Obstetrique et Biologie de la Reproduction*, 13(7):759–763.

Turnbull A (1989) Spontaneous abortion. In: Turnbull A and Chamberlain G, eds. *Obstetrics*, Churchill Livingstone.

Turner G (1989) Ectopic pregnancy. In: Turnbull A and Chamberlain G, eds. *Obstetrics*, Churchill Livingstone.

Van der Tak J (1974) *Abortion, fertility and changing legislation: an international review*. Lexington, Lexington Books.

Westergaard L et al. (1982) Significance of cervical chlamydia trachomatis infection in postabortal pelvic inflammatory disease. *Obstetrics & Gynecology*, 60(3):322–325.

Westoff CF (1991) *Demographic and Health Surveys. Reproductive preferences: a comparative view. Comparative studies 3*. Columbia, MD, Institute for Resource Development/Macro Systems, Inc.

Westoff CF, Ochoa LH (1991) *Demographic and Health Surveys. Unmet need and the demand for family planning. Comparative studies 5*. Columbia MD, Institute for Resource Development/Macro International, Inc.

Weström L (1980) Incidence, prevalence and trends of acute pelvic inflammatory disease and its consequences in industrialised countries. *American Journal of Obstetrics and Gynecology*, 138(7) :880–892.

Wilcox AJ, Horney LF (1984) Accuracy of spontaneous abortion recall. *American Journal of Epidemiology*, 120(5):727–733.

Wilcox LS and Marks JS (1995) *From data to action: CDC's public health surveillance for women, infants and children*. US Department of Health and Human Services, Centers for Disease Control and Prevention, Atlanta, USA.

World Health Organization (1970) Spontaneous and induced abortion. *Technical report series* no.41, Geneva.

World Health Organization (1974). *Abortion: A Tabulation on the Frequency and Mortality of Unsafe Abortion. 2nd edition*. WHO/FHE/MSM/93.13. Geneva, 1994.

World Health Organization (1983) Gestational trophoblastic diseases. Technical report series 692, Geneva.

World Health Organization (1991) *Essential elements of obstetric care at first referral level*. Geneva, Switzerland.

World Health Organization (1991) Maternal Health and Safe Motherhood Programme. *Maternal mortality ratios and rates. A tabulation of available information*. Third edition. WHO/MCH/MSM/91.6. Geneva.

World Health Organization (1992) Maternal Health and Safe Motherhood Programme. *The prevention and management of unsafe abortion. Report of a Technical Working Group*, Geneva, 12–15 April 1992, WHO/MSM/92.5.

World Health Organization (1992) *The prevention and management of unsafe abortion. Report of a Technical Working Group*. WHO/MSM/92.5, Geneva.

World Health Organization (1993) *Abortion: a tabulation of available data on the frequency and mortality of unsafe abortion*. 2nd edition. WHO/FHE/MSM/93.13

Chapter 9

HIV AND AIDS

DANIEL LOW-BEER, RAND STONEBURNER,
THIERRY MERTENS, ANTHONY BURTON, SETH BERKLEY

INTRODUCTION

If the global burden of disease had been assessed for 1980, a decade earlier than for the present volume, HIV would not have been featured. It is an epidemic which has emerged during the last quarter of the twentieth century, accumulating an estimated 20.5 million HIV infections by 1996, and has become a leading cause of mortality in certain areas (Mulder et al. 1994, Lindan et al. 1992, Wagner et al. 1993, Selik et al. 1993). AIDS cases have been reported in 192 countries, and although it imposes a truly global burden, HIV is concentrated in less developed countries in young adults often central to economic, social and family activity.

The rapid emergence of HIV as a pandemic has come to characterize the continued modern burden of infectious disease which occurs alongside advances in medical treatment, hygiene and health indicators. This characterization of AIDS draws from ancient fears of infectious disease epidemics but also of new emerging viruses which are able to survive in the inter-connected modern world. Its identification in 1981 is often contrasted with the formal eradication of smallpox in 1979[1] and the hopes of, for example, William McNeil the medical historian who, ironically unaware of HIV, wrote in 1983 "One of the things that separates us .. from other ages ... is the disappearance of epidemic disease as a serious factor in human life" (McNeil 1983).

What is the scale of the impact of HIV on loss of life, and its position relative to other diseases which burden humanity? What priorities do HIV interventions assume in the range of demands on public health decision makers?

Perhaps it is worth recalling Bailey's classic justification of epidemiology in terms of the burden of disease "The fearful toll of human life and happiness exacted through the ages by widespread disease and pestilence affords a spectacle that is both fascinating and repellent. A recital of the astronomical number of casualties ... makes the consequences of all past wars seem almost trivial in comparison ... The total load of human misery and suffering from communicable disease in the world today is incalculable" (Bailey 1957). The DALY method is an attempt to calculate just that, and provide "a framework for objectively identifying epidemiological priorities" (Murray et al. 1994).

The chapter is organized into six sections and a conclusion, as follows.

1. A brief introduction, which presents the various disease terms associated with AIDS, its global distribution, methods of transmission, and components of its disease burden.
2. The definitions of disease states in relation to the natural history of HIV, and the choice of the appropriate disease measure for the Global Burden of Disease study, in this case HIV incidence.
3. The review of empirical databases for disease estimation by region.
4. The method of disease estimation, presentation of all parameters used, and HIV incidence results by region, age and sex; their use with mortality and morbidity weights to calculate total loss of life due to HIV.
5. Important considerations for the 1990 HIV DALY calculation including: relating the 1990 point measure to changing HIV incidence over a period, the build-up of prevalence which accompanies HIV incidence, and disease interactions particularly with sexually transmitted diseases (STDs) and tuberculosis.
6. Some reflections on the burden of HIV measured in DALYs.

The burden of HIV is calculated based on estimates of HIV incidence by region, sex and age group. As HIV incidence could not be estimated directly, estimates of HIV prevalence by region were used and WHO's *Epimodel* was applied to convert this to HIV incidence for 1990. From this source of HIV incidence, the subsequent stream of disability was divided into two stages, a chronic and a final AIDS stage, followed by mortality after a median incubation interval. These were weighted and cumulated to calculate total years of life lost. Thus for the disease calculations three types of inputs were required from this chapter:

1. The natural history of HIV by region and for adults and children, including the duration of the chronic and AIDS stages, and the median time to mortality.
2. HIV prevalence by region. The date of onset of the epidemic and position on the epidemic curve for WHO's *Epimodel*, to calculate HIV incidence. The distribution of HIV incidence by sex and for five age groups, for each region.
3. Information on the disabling sequelae of HIV, their duration and descriptions of their severity.

If the reader wishes to pass quickly through the chapter the results are presented in Tables 12–13, and all the parameters used in the estimation process shown in Table 7. Despite limits to the availability and quality of data on HIV and AIDS, considerable validation of the 1990 estimates produced for the GBD enables us to be relatively confident in our results for most regions. However the HIV epidemic evolves rapidly, and for

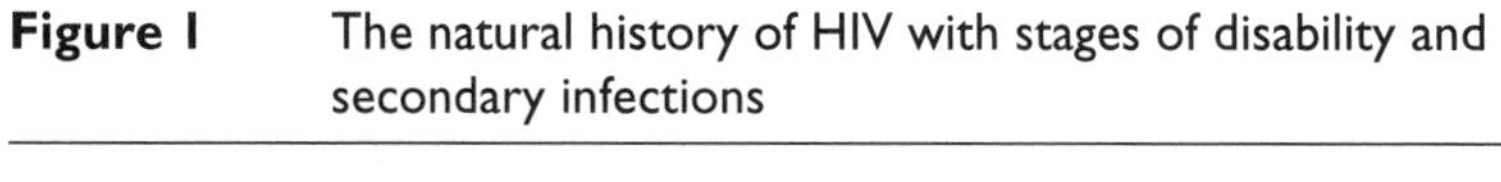

Figure 1 The natural history of HIV with stages of disability and secondary infections

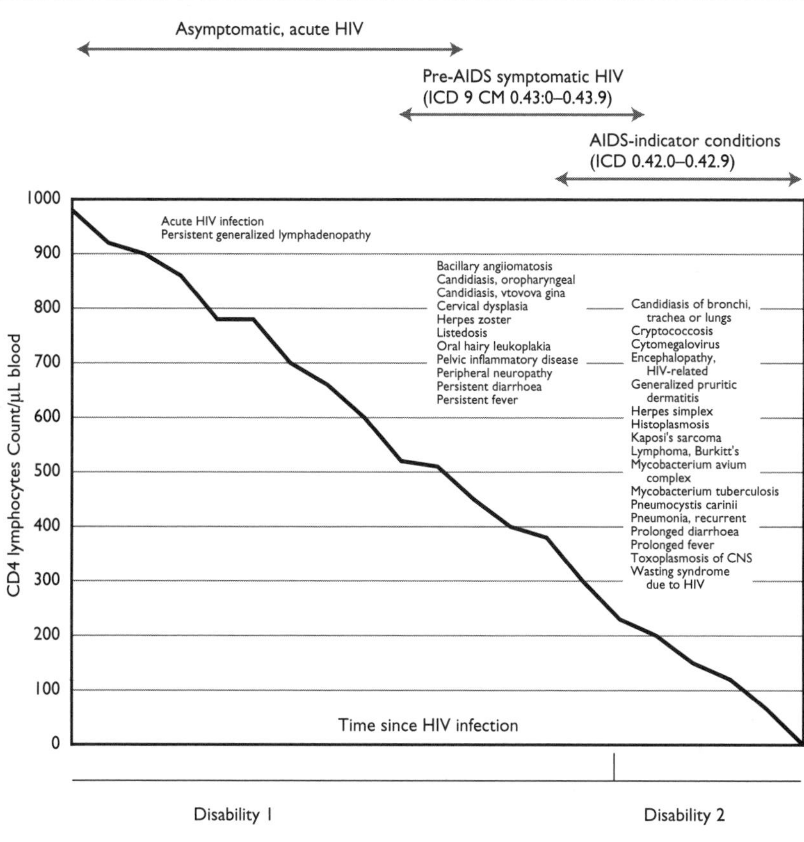

example in India and China its development since 1990 has been particularly unclear, requiring a concerted surveillance programme. Although the disease estimates are the result of an immense effort from many data sources and areas of expertise, the parameters and methods used in estimation and modelling are all presented, so that the results may be reproduced in the appropriate public health contexts.

GENERAL CHARACTERISTICS OF HIV TRANSMISSION

The epidemic of HIV has given rise to a number of disease terms including AIDS, ARC and the considerable list of secondary diseases associated with it. Firstly it is important to understand how these disease states are connected in relation to the incubation period of HIV and stages of morbidity and mortality (see Figure 1).

Human immunodeficiency virus (HIV)[2] is the viral infection resulting in a progressive immunodeficiency of the host, marked by numerous secondary diseases and cancers, the most severe of which define the clinical syndrome known as Acquired Immunodeficiency Syndrome (AIDS). AIDS occurs on average 7-10 years after infection with HIV (Hendriks et al. 1993), and is thought to be 100 per cent fatal, mortality occurring usually within 1 to 2 years. Disability associated with HIV is concentrated in the later periods of disease, with episodes of opportunistic diseases and cancers, the most common of which include tuberculosis (Perriens et al. 1991) pneumocystis carinii pneumonia, chronic diarrhoea with enteritis, HIV wasting syndrome and Kaposi's sarcoma (Lucas et al. 1991). Figure 1 characterizes the natural history of HIV in the host. It shows the progressive immunodeficiency marked by a decline in CD4 counts *(y axis)* and the emergence of secondary diseases. This is classified into two stages of disability, one chronic, the second defined as AIDS, followed by mortality, which form the basis of the disability states used for calculating DALYs.

In response to the spread of HIV, extraordinary progress has been made in the identification of the causative viral agent known as HIV, its methods of transmission, its interaction with its host to produce morbidity and mortality, and the implementation of programmes for disease prevention and care (World Health Organization 1993). The majority of HIV transmission world-wide occurs through sexual intercourse, though HIV is also transmitted with varying efficiency by contact with infected blood, intravenous drug use (IDU), and from mother to child before or after birth or during the postpartum period through breast feeding. There is considerable variation between regions in the relative importance of risk behaviours, with IDU and male to male sexual transmission playing a greater role in the Established Market Economies than in other regions, and some variation in the incubation period and secondary diseases. Knowledge of the transmission and course of the disease has provided a basis for interventions, focused on the prevention of initial infection and care at later stages of disease, but has not led to a curative ability to help the larger numbers with prevalent HIV infection.

This global spread contrasts with the geographical diversity in epidemic conditions, with the burden heavily concentrated in certain populations where HIV prevalence levels can reach 30 per cent (Lindan et al. 1992, De Cock et al. 1990), and may account for over 50 per cent of estimated adult mortality (Mulder et al. 1994, Lindan et al. 1992, Wagner et al. 1993). Other areas exhibit lower stable HIV prevalence, but epidemic growth in infections can be very rapid: for example in Thailand HIV prevalence increased from 1.9 per cent to 8 per cent in Chaing Mai from 1990 to 1993 (Brown et al. 1994).

THE BURDEN OF HIV

Direct impact of HIV on mortality and morbidity

Longitudinal cohorts or repeat sampling studies, for example in Uganda, the United States and Amsterdam, have been the major source for documenting the impact of HIV on mortality and disability. Mulder et al. (1994) estimated that HIV accounted for 47 per cent and 53 per cent of adult mortality in males and females respectively, and 23 per cent in children, in a cohort in Masaka, Uganda, where adult HIV prevalence was 8.2 per cent. The highest mortality rate ratios were found at ages 14-44 years, with a maximum excess mortality at ages 25-34 years. Other epidemiological studies have found HIV-1 attributable mortality in adults of 15 per cent in Abidjan (De Cock et al. 1990), 20-24 per cent in Kinshasa (Ryder et al. 1990) and 90 per cent in childbearing women aged 25-34 in Kigali, Rwanda (Lindan et al. 1992).

Secondary impacts of HIV

The secondary or indirect impacts involve the burden which extends beyond the individual with disease, including the burden on the community of care, loss of labour, orphanhood and demographic and social changes. HIV is also shown to be a major cause of infant mortality in several regions (Hira et al. 1989, Ryder et al. 1989), and its impact on family structure and orphanhood has been documented (Barnett and Blaikie 1992). The concept of the multiple "downstream" impacts of HIV infection on household, family and community structures, labour and farming practices and regional development was also pursued by Barnett and Blaikie (1992). The timescale before a demographic impact will be observed has been estimated at several decades (Anderson et al. 1991), and there has been little consensus as to the scale (World Health Organization 1991). Changes in population structure consistent with the impact of AIDS have been noted in selected areas, but even in a study of one of the first African districts to be affected by HIV, a positive rate of population increase of 17.6 per 1000 population was maintained (Sewankambo et al. 1994).

Economic analysis of the impact of AIDS has ranged from simulations of its possible effects on GNP (Rowley et al. 1990), specific labour sources (Nkowane, 1988), to food production and consumption systems (Abel et al. 1988; Gillespie 1989). The importance of the concept of indirect costs (*"the value of the time lost to the sick person and to his family, friends and employer, because of illness and/or death"*, Over et al. 1989) as compared to direct costs (*"the cost of treatment and health care services")* has been stressed, with their ratio estimated as 4:1 in Puerto Rico (Alameda-Lozada and Gonzalez-Martinez 1989) and 16:1 in Tanzania (Over et al. 1988). Nevertheless, recent econometric studies have failed to demonstrate an impact on macro-economic performance (Bloom and Mahal 1997).

The impact of HIV has also been compared to other diseases, with Over et al. (1988, 1989) estimating that in Zaire and Tanzania only the most lethal diseases of early childhood caused more loss of life than HIV infection.

Definition and Measurement

The definitions used for AIDS, HIV and the staging sequences including the associated ICD disabling sequelae are described below with methods of their measurement including modelling approaches.

Disease states and the natural history of HIV infection

HIV-1 directly infects host CD4+ T lymphocytes resulting in the loss of important immune co-ordinating functions, and leading to progressive impairment of the host immune response, and ultimately irreversible immunodeficiency. HIV integrates into the CD4+ T lymphocyte genome[4] and over many years results in a continuous decline from approximately 900 CD4+ T cells/ml of blood (Kaslow and Francis 1989) to less than 200/ml at end-stage disease. This eventually results in the inability to respond to a host of viral, bacterial, fungal and parasitic infections, some of which are latent infections reactivated by immunosuppression (Redfield and Burke 1988).

Natural history studies of HIV infection have documented the occurrence of a broad spectrum of disease states ranging from asymptomatic to life-threatening severe immunodeficiency manifested by the occurrence of serious opportunistic infections and cancer (WHO 1994; Baltimore and Feinberg 1989). The risk and severity of these opportunistic illnesses increases as the number of CD4+ lymphocytes decline.

HIV is a relatively new disease, having first been described 15 years ago. A definitive test for HIV was not available until a decade ago. Except for unique episodes such as single contaminated blood transfusions or needlestick injuries, it is difficult to be sure of the exact date of infection. Prospective cohort studies give approximate dates of seroconversion (seroconversion sometime between the two examinations) but have only been underway for the last decade for a disease that has a median incubation period of almost that long. Fortunately, a few cohort studies with serum banked for other purposes (for example Hepatitis B vaccination) were underway at the time HIV/AIDS appeared allowing a retrospective analysis of date of onset of infections in its members.

The difficulties in studying the natural history of infection mean that the course of disease beyond 12-15 years is unknown. In addition, recent studies of natural history may be biased by an increased AIDS-free time due to use of inhibitors of reverse transcriptase and the use of prophylaxis against pneumocystis carinii or tuberculosis (Graham et al. 1991). Hence, current cohorts in the Established Market Economies (EME) may not provide accurate data on natural history; historic data, although with limited follow-up, may be more accurate in predicting the natural history of infection in the absence of treatment. Most of the information available on the natural history of infection comes from studies done in the EME. It is unknown how much of this information will be pertinent for less developed country settings.

Natural History in Adults

Established Market Economies

There have been a number of attempts to create staging systems for clinical disease with the purpose of standardizing studies of the clinical course of infection. The two most common systems are the Walter-Reed staging system (Redfield et al. 1986) and the CDC system (CDC 1986) revised in 1993 (CDC 1993). These systems require sophisticated laboratory or diagnostic facilities and are therefore not very useful for developing countries. The WHO convened a meeting in 1989 and published their own classification system in 1990 which can be used in most settings (WHO 1990). (Table 1)

A recent study of intravenous drug users validated this clinical staging system and demonstrated a progression rate to AIDS within three years of 6.5 per cent for those in clinical stage I, 10.4 per cent in stage II and 17.1 per cent for those in stage III (Aylward et al. 1994). There is a wide distribution of progression times and some individuals may pass directly from early clinical stages to AIDS.

Conceptually, the process of HIV infection can be divided into three stages: early or acute phase which lasts for a few weeks and is characterized by a mild and short flu like illness; a middle, or chronic phase lasting many years and characterized by long periods of no symptoms punctuated by periods of mild illness; and a final phase lasting months to years characterized by opportunistic infections and resulting in death (Baltimore and Feinberg 1989). In terms of disability the significant phases are the chronic and final AIDS phases.

Acute Phase

The acute phase (WHO phase I) relates to acute HIV viremia and causes a symptomatic illness in 50-90 per cent of persons (Tindall et al. 1988). This illness is described as a mononucleosis-like syndrome and may include fever, muscle and joint aches, headaches, diarrhoea, sore throat, swollen lymph nodes and a generalized rash. In addition, various neurological

Table 1 WHO Staging System

Stage	*Category*	*Physical Activity*	*Example of Symptoms/diseases*
I	Asymptomatic	normal activity, (asymptomatic)	none
II	Early Disease	normal activity, (symptomatic)	minor weight loss, minor skin conditions
III	Intermediate Disease	Bed-bound < 50% of the day	weight loss > 10% body weight, tuberculosis, thrush
IV	Late Disease	Bed-bound > 50% of the day	AIDS-defining illness

manifestations have been reported. This illness lasts for a few weeks and can easily be confused with a myriad of other febrile illnesses including viral syndromes and malaria.

Chronic Phase

The chronic phase (WHO phase II & III) lasts for years. During this period, virus replication occurs and there is slow destruction of the immune system. Recent studies have suggested an average loss of 60 CD4+ cells/ μL of blood per year after the initial infection. This would lead to a laboratory-based prediction of AIDS (CD4+ < 200) to occur in 10-11 years, similar to that found in current studies (see below). The reason for this gradual loss of CD4+ over time is still not known (Levy 1993). Although it is clear that most persons who are HIV infected will have progressive disease and go on to develop AIDS, it is not known if all persons will eventually develop AIDS. A small number of individuals remain asymptomatic with normal or only mildly reduced immunological markers 8-15 years after infection (Buchbinder et al. 1994). While the natural history in these non-progressors, representing 8 per cent of the infected population is not clear, the vast majority of infected individuals progress to clinical illness.

Most studies have shown few cases of AIDS in the first couple of years after seroconversion (Lifson et al. 1988), but then a steady increase in cases with about 50 per cent having developed AIDS by 10 years (Rutherford et al. 1990). In fact a large number of studies suggests that in the absence of treatment the median time for progression to AIDS is 7–10 years (Hendricks 1993, Moss and Bacchetti 1989, Rutheford et al. 1990). The appearance of AIDS deaths relating to this median incubation period may be well approximated by a Weibull distribution (Hendricks 1993, Taylor et al. 1990, Brookmeyer and Damians 1989), with an elongation function to represent the extended outlier survival of certain individuals for up to twenty years (Hendricks 1993). The following table lists the median time from progression to AIDS in a collection of studies. (Table 2)

Table 2 Estimates of median time from HIV infection to progression to AIDS

Parametric analysis of 84 men in SFCC* cohort	7.8 years
Non-parametric analysis of 513 men in SFCC cohort	9.8 years
SFGH** cohort	9.0 years
US transfusion data	7.3 years
Hershey haemophilia cohort	8.3 years

Source: Moss AR, and Bacchetti P 1989

*San Francisco Clinic Control

**San Francisco General Hospital

In addition to AIDS, persons in the chronic phase may develop bothersome chronic illnesses that are not necessarily life threatening. These conditions such as severe weight loss, chronic diarrhoea, recurrent bacterial infections, oral candidiasis with difficulty swallowing and eating etc., often result in time spent under therapy, at limited activity or complete bed rest.

Final Phase

The final phase (WHO stage IV) is manifest by the occurrence of serious, life-threatening opportunistic infections. In the EME countries, some progress has been made extending life during this period. This generally requires expensive therapies and diagnostic equipment, out of reach of most people living in developing counties. Regardless of location, much of the time in this stage is spent either bed-ridden or in in-patient health care facilities, and is the major source of HIV-related disability.

Other factors influencing the rate of progression to AIDS

There may also be differences in the rate of progression to AIDS based upon mode of transmission, gender and age. Initially it was suggested that those infected with a higher viral inoculum such as those infected through IDU or transfusion may progress faster than those infected sexually. Recent data have suggested this is not true once controlling for other factors such as age (Von Overbeck et al. 1993). Gender has also been suggested as an important factor with females progressing at a faster rate than males. Recent data, however, suggests that there is no difference and that previous reported differences were due to gender specific differences in diagnosis (Von Overbeck et al. 1993; Till et al. 1993). Age has clearly been shown to be a modifier. Adults infected at an older age progress to AIDS at a faster rate than those infected at a younger age (Carre et al. 1994; Rosenberg et al. 1994). In fact, with each ten year increase in age at seroconversion, there was a 1.3-1.6 fold increase in rate of progression.

Developing Countries

Information on disease progression is even more limited in developing countries. Widespread testing was not available until recently and cohorts are more difficult to establish and follow. A few cohorts have been established and followed for five years in Africa and for two to three years in Thailand. In most other regions, these sort of studies are only now just getting underway. The limited data that exists from sub-Saharan Africa and Thailand, however, suggests a faster progression than in EME from HIV infection to AIDS. This may relate to the higher exposure to infectious diseases in general with continuous stimulation of the immune system. Nutrition may also play a role.

There has been a longterm study of prostitutes of lower socio-economic status from the Pumwani area of Nairobi, Kenya, underway since 1985 (Nagelkerke et al. 1990). This population is transient and is followed up irregularly. Despite these shortcomings, it is the African cohort with the longest follow-up. Using a Markov model, the authors demonstrated a much shorter progression to lymphadenopathy and AIDS than is found in EME studies. They report a mean time of 34.2 months to symptomatic disease and 44.6 months to AIDS (Anzala et al. 1991).

A well conducted prospective community study in Masaka district in Uganda demonstrated a one-year mortality rate of 10.3 per cent which compares to an annual progression rate of 5-6 per cent for cohorts in the EME (Mulder et al. 1994). More recent follow up suggests a higher rate of 12.4 per cent per annum (Mulder et al. 1993), supporting the assumption that those HIV infected persons living in Africa (and probably other developing countries) have a faster progression to AIDS. Not all studies support this. A study in ambulatory HIV infected women in Rwanda demonstrated a very low two-year mortality of 7 per cent for those with HIV infection and a 21 per cent two-year mortality in those meeting the criteria for AIDS (Lindan et al. 1992).

There are no good data on the clinical course of patients with WHO stage III and IV disease in developing countries. In Africa, where the best data are available, HIV infection creates enormous morbidity. In a number of studies, more than 80 per cent of those admitted to a hospital with HIV disease had lost > 10 per cent of their body weight, 90 per cent had severe weakness and >40 per cent had chronic diarrhoea (Colebunders and Latif 1991). Over 40 per cent of those with HIV wasting were found to have disseminated tuberculosis at autopsy (Lucas et al. 1994). In addition, due to the lack of effective therapy, those who develop AIDS tend to die quickly often with the first episode of an opportunistic infection (Colebunders and Latif 1991). Thus, not only is the time from HIV infection to AIDS shorter in Africa, but probably so is the time from AIDS to death. Data are not yet available from other areas in the developing world; however, progression is also likely to be accelerated as is the time from AIDS to death. Owing to this lack of data, we have used a shorter but conservative progression time for Africa, as well as other developing countries, in estimating the burden of disease.

Natural History in Children

Difficulties in distinguishing diagnosis of infection in newborns from later passive carriage of maternal antibody renders neonatal studies particularly difficult to undertake in developing countries. The incubation period from HIV infection to death in children infected perinatally is believed to be shorter than in adults and substantially shorter in developing countries (Ryder et al 1989; Turner et al 1995).

Established Market Economies

Studies in EME have shown the period of progression from infection to AIDS to be shorter in children than in adults (Lepage et al. 1993). Over 80 per cent of untreated perinatally infected infants will have symptoms of HIV infection by 18-24 months (Pizzo et al. 1995). In the European Collaborative study, 90 per cent had symptoms early in the first year of life, but not all of these children were continuously symptomatic (European Collaborative Study 1994). Many children improved during the second and third year of life. Early studies suggested a median incubation time of 12-18 months. Longer follow-up has shown a bimodal distribution of progression with better survival of infected children than previously suspected. For example the Italian register for HIV infection in children has shown a cumulative survival of 49.5 per cent at nine years (Tova et al. 1992). In that cohort, the mortality rate was 8.9 per cent in the first year of life and then stabilized at 3.5 per cent per year. In the European study, 23 per cent developed AIDS in the first year of life and 39 per cent within four years. Furthermore in the European study 48 per cent of children were still alive 2 years after their AIDS diagnosis, demonstrating the improved survival in the EME countries.

The median incubation period for children may consist of two progression rates, 15-25 per cent of infected infants suffering severe immunodeficiency in the first year, and the remaining 75 to 85 per cent progressing at a slower rate of 11-12 per cent annually (Gibb and Wara 1994). Analysis of over 90 per cent of all child AIDS cases diagnosed in Europe also suggested a bimodal rate, a sub group progressing to AIDS at a median age estimated at 5 months with 20 per cent of children developing AIDS by age 1, and an overall median incubation period of 4.4 years and 74 per cent diagnosed with AIDS by age 8 (Downs et al. 1995).

Similar to adults, there may be differences in incubation and survival based upon mode of transmission and other variables. In the CDC AIDS register, the estimated incubation period for paediatric transmitted AIDS including transmission via transfusion (3.5 years median) was longer than for vertically transmitted cases (1.75 median) (Jones et al. 1992). However following AIDS diagnosis, survival was similar in both groups (approximately 14 months).

A community based surveillance study in California showed somewhat different findings (Rederick et al. 1994). They also found that those with vertical infection had an earlier onset of symptoms — the median symptom-free survival time was 6.4 months for perinatally-acquired versus 17.8 months for transfusion-acquired infection. But unlike the results from analysis of the CDC registry, they found survival differences as well — 75 per cent of children infected perinatally survived 44 months compared to 71 months for children infected by transfusion. Other studies have not shown these differences in incubation period and survival times. At the present time, no firm conclusions can be drawn.

Developing countries

In a study in Rwanda, most HIV infected children presented with symptoms in the first two years of life (Lepage et al. 1993). Similar to AIDS in adults, the mortality in developing countries is substantially higher. In Kigali, Rwanda, mortality at 24 months of age was 19 per cent in a cohort that had regular follow-up and received much better medical care than the norm (Lepage et al. 1993).

Definition and Measurement

The stream of disease emanating from the progressive deterioration of immune function following infection, shown in Figure 1, introduces the potential points of measurement of HIV. Accurate estimates require precise, consistently interpretable and specific definitions of disease states. This section describes the types of HIV disease data and their definitions, together with modelling approaches which can link them, given a knowledge of the incubation period.

AIDS case definitions for surveillance purposes

A case definition for AIDS in adults was first developed in the United States by the Centers for Disease Control and Prevention (CDC) for surveillance purposes soon after the recognition of this new disease in 1981 (CDC 1982). AIDS was defined, rather narrowly in retrospect, at a time when the causative viral agent HIV had not yet been identified, as the occurrence of numerous rare disease manifestations common to this new entity of clinical immunodeficiency "predictive of a defect of cell-mediated immunity, occurring in a person with no known cause for diminished resistance to that disease" (CDC 1982). Subsequent modifications increased the sensitivity of the original AIDS definition, including a recognition of the broader clinical spectrum of severe HIV disease and the wider use of diagnostic tests for HIV infection and immune suppression.

The 1987 CDC/WHO AIDS surveillance case definition included 23 AIDS indicator conditions, some of which require HIV serological confirmation, and encompassed both adult and paediatric AIDS. The CDC recently introduced an expanded version of the 1987 CDC/WHO definition adding serologically confirmed HIV infection together with immunological criteria indicative of severe immunosuppression (CD4+ lymphocyte counts of <200µl), and recurrent pneumonia, pulmonary tuberculosis or invasive cervical cancer. This latter case definition is used solely in the United States and a modified version without the use of immunological criteria has been introduced in Western Europe. These definitions have been widely used in the EME countries and some LAC countries. AIDS cases in persons under 13 years of age are defined by the 1987 CDC/WHO paediatric surveillance case definition in most developed countries, which, with a few exceptions, is similar to that in adults.

The problems with a "gold standard" AIDS definition, represented by the CDC definition, have led to a number of surveillance definitions relative to specific epidemiological and diagnostic conditions. AIDS case surveillance definitions for developing countries were designed for surveillance purposes in the absence of sophisticated diagnostic facilities, to be "simple, universally applicable and usable by all health service personnel" (World Health Organization 1985).

The provisional WHO clinical definition for AIDS (the "Bangui" definition) was developed in 1985[5] on the basis of the identification of a restricted combination of at least two major and one minor sign of AIDS, including chronic diarrhoea, prolonged fever, recurrent herpes zoster, or other signs such as Kaposi's sarcoma and cryptococcal meningitis, regarded as sufficient AIDS diagnostic criteria. Although the definition was simple and widely used in sub-saharan Africa (SSA), low sensitivity and specificity (World Health Organization 1994) particularly with respect to tuberculosis, one of the most common HIV-related opportunistic infections in Africa, necessitated further modifications. However it is still useful in geographic areas where diagnostic capabilities are limited, and shows significant increases in identifying AIDS cases which previously did not meet the CDC definition (Deschamps 1988).

Table 3 Case definitions of AIDS surveillance by WHO

WHO Case Definition for Aids Surveillance		Expanded WHO Case Definition for Aids Surveillance
2 major and 1 minor sign from		*HIV antibody test positive and one or more of following*
Major sign	**Minor sign**	
weight loss >= 10%	persistent cough for more than 1 month[1,2]	>= 10% body weight loss of cachexia, with diarrhoea or fever, or both, intermittent or constant, for at least 1 month, not known to be due to condition unrelated to HIV.
chronic diarrhoea for more than 1 month	generalized pruritic dermatitis	cryptococcal meningitis
prolonged fever for more than 1 month (intermittent or constant)	history of herpes zoster[2]	pulmonary or extra-pulmonary tuberculosis
	oropharyngeal candidiasis	Kaposi sarcoma
	chronic progressive or disseminated herpes simplex	neurological impairment sufficient to prevent independent daily activities, not known to be due to non-HIV condition.
	generalized lymphadenopathy	candidiasis of the oesophagus (may be presumptively diagnosed on basis of oral candidiasis with dysphagia)
		clinically diagnosed life-threatening or recurrent episodes of pneumonia, with or without etiological confirmation
		invasive cervical cancer

Notes: 1. For patients with tuberculosis, persistent cough for more than 1 month should not be considered as a sign

2. Change from "Bangui definition"

Since 1993, WHO recommends two case definitions for AIDS surveillance "for use in adults and adolescents in countries with generally limited clinical and laboratory diagnostic capabilities" shown in Table 3: the WHO case definition, a modified version of the "Bangui" definition, and the recently developed Expanded WHO case definition for AIDS surveillance (WHO 1994). The Expanded WHO AIDS surveillance case definition requires HIV serological testing and includes a broader spectrum of clinical disease manifestations. Although it requires more sophisticated diagnostic capabilities it should prove more sensitive and specific than the "Bangui" definition.

The Pan American Health Organisation (Caracas) AIDS surveillance definition was developed in 1989 for countries in Central and South America, requires a positive HIV serological test and depends upon a point scoring schema for 14 different manifestations of HIV disease including tuberculosis. The development of AIDS surveillance definitions and of HIV test and status definitions through time is shown in Figure 2.

The accuracy of AIDS case surveillance data may be influenced somewhat by the sensitivity and specificity of particular AIDS surveillance case definitions. However under-recognition of AIDS cases by the healthcare system and the completeness and timeliness of reporting of identified AIDS cases by the surveillance system are more important. In industrialized countries about 80 per cent of AIDS cases are reported, while in areas of sub-Saharan Africa, perhaps only 10–20 per cent of AIDS cases are ever reported (Mertens et al. 1995). Nevertheless if adjusted for delays in, and under-reporting, AIDS cases can represent an important sample of individuals at the stage of HIV disease associated with greatest morbidity and mortality.

HIV Mortality — Vital registration

Since HIV-1 infection is a fatal illness, vital registration systems with reasonably accurate cause-specific reporting of mortality can be a useful data source. However the accuracy both of reporting mortality and diagnosing HIV as a cause of death vary widely. Even in the United States, reported deaths may underestimate current HIV related mortality by 15-35 per cent in young men and 20-45 per cent in young women (Selik et al. 1993). Nevertheless, with adjustment for bias, the analysis of mortality statistics even in less developed areas has been central to estimating the mortality of HIV.

The International Classification of Disease 9th Revision (ICD-9) codes used to designate manifestations of HIV infection aims to allow classification and comparability of information on disease mortality and morbidity reported to WHO. The classification of HIV has been periodically revised as knowledge has improved rapidly. HIV was originally included as an addendum to the 1975 ICD-9-CM (clinical modification) grouped with other immunity disorders. In 1983[6], the pre-existing code (ICD-9 No. 279.1) was adopted for HIV/AIDS and used through to 1986. During 1986

Figure 2 Surveillance definitions of AIDS and of HIV test and status

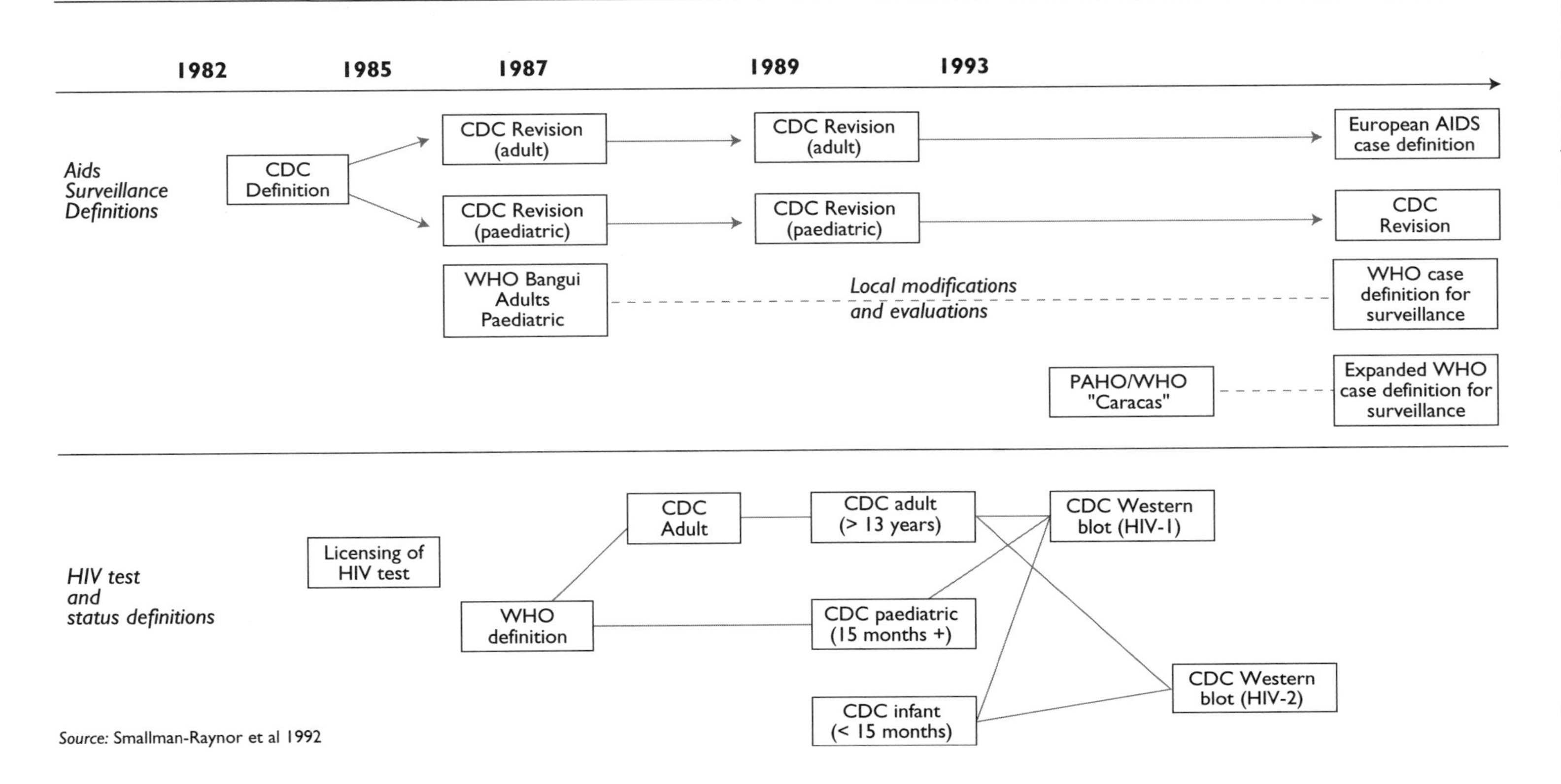

Source: Smallman-Raynor et al 1992

and 1987 there were two official addenda to the ICD-9 CM which introduced a detailed set of codes (*042–*044) for classifying and coding HIV infection (CDC 1987). The ICD-10th Revision classifies HIV disease into 5 categories designated as B20-B24 and it has been recommended that this should come into effect as from 1 January 1993 (World Health Organization 1992).

HIV mortality data has been used in several studies (De Cock et al. 1990; Selik et al. 1993) and represents the end and most critical stage of morbidity and mortality for the disease burden. However its systematic use for estimation of regional totals for HIV is limited, due to the bias and quality of the records, difficulties in diagnosing HIV as the cause of death, and the number of mortality records which need to be analysed to locate those related to HIV.

HIV prevalence and incidence

Knowledge of the magnitude and trends of HIV incidence and resulting HIV prevalence are, in principle, the most important data from which to monitor the epidemic, estimate the HIV disease burden and assess the impacts of interventions. They allow the impact of present day activities to prevent infections to be related to the future burdens of morbidity and mortality, if an incubation period is assumed.

Tests to detect HIV viral antibodies in blood samples have been available since 1984-5, and the tests used for HIV surveillance at present are the enzyme-linked immunosorbent assay (ELISA) and the more specific Western blot (WB) assay which detects antibodies to specific HIV proteins. General methods for evaluating diagnostic tests are available elsewhere (Fletcher et al. 1988) and have been applied to HIV (Schwartz et al. 1988).

Two important measures of the accuracy of a test are its sensitivity, the probability that the test is positive among individuals with HIV, and specificity, the probability that the test will be negative among individuals without HIV. Of further concern for HIV is the "window" interval following infection of up to six months, where HIV antibody levels may be too low to be identified by tests. Initially reactive ELISA tests should be repeated twice to improve specificity, or be confirmed with a Western blot test.

In lieu of evaluating HIV prevalence by random samples of general populations, which can prove costly, and may often provide risk-biased estimates as the populations at risk are not randomly distributed in the general population, HIV prevalence data can be obtained by sequential cross-sectional sero-surveys of HIV prevalence in sentinel sub-populations at particular high risk (homosexual males, injecting drug users, attendees of sexually transmitted disease clinics) or who reflect to some extent infection in the general population (pregnant women, newborns, military recruits).

Prevalence data from sentinel studies may suffer from a number of biases related to the methods of selecting the population, including sample size, laboratory methods for testing, the period of testing, and generalizability to the larger population. In addition, since HIV incidence may change over time, it is unknown what stage of disease progression HIV prevalent infections represent. With reasonably accurate estimates of the size of subpopulations, sentinel HIV prevalence rates can be useful in making estimates of population prevalence. Methods for measuring HIV prevalence, HIV incidence and AIDS, and the cohorts and reporting routes involved, are shown in Figure 3.

Measuring HIV incidence suffers from many of the methodological constraints of HIV prevalence. Major limitations of these data from cohort studies are generalizability to the larger population, and the large samples required to identify significant numbers of new infections. The features of epidemic expansion, saturation and geographic diversity make the measure of HIV incidence a "moving target". Thus a direct measure of incidence generalizable to larger populations is difficult to achieve, and is more easily estimated using models which produce incidence scenarios which can then be subjected to validation. It is therefore often necessary to combine empirical data with a modelling approach to produce consistent epidemiological estimates.

Modelling approaches

Due to limited epidemiological data, difficulties in measuring underlying HIV incidence, and the need to understand disease trends both before data were available and into the future, a number of modelling approaches have been used. The many techniques used may be simplified into three major approaches.

Firstly, extrapolation methods use a mathematical function and fitting procedures to extend available data on any one disease measure into the future (Curran et al. 1985, Karon et al. 1988). They assume that past trends will continue into the future, and are limited by their dependence on defined mathematical functions (Gail and Rosenberg 1992) and the lack of an empirical basis for application to HIV incidence. Extrapolation has therefore generally been applied to AIDS cases for short term forecasts of up to 3 years with some success, but it has been suggested that their use in recent years is severely limited by signs of saturation in some risk groups (Hethcote and Van Ark 1992).

The second group of methods, including backcalculation, exploit additional knowledge of the incubation period and progression rates linking HIV incidence, HIV prevalence and AIDS. AIDS incidence data as the endpoint of infection is regarded as the sum of progressors from a series of earlier annual HIV incidence. AIDS cases in year t_j are therefore the sum up to time t_j of the product of HIV incidence at time t_i and the probability of developing AIDS, t_j-t_i years after infection. AIDS cases can therefore be distributed backwards along an assumed incubation distribution to reconstruct earlier incidence rates. These in turn are projected forward to provide quantitative estimates of the size of the epidemic, and short term

Figure 3 Methods for measuring HIV incidence and prevalence

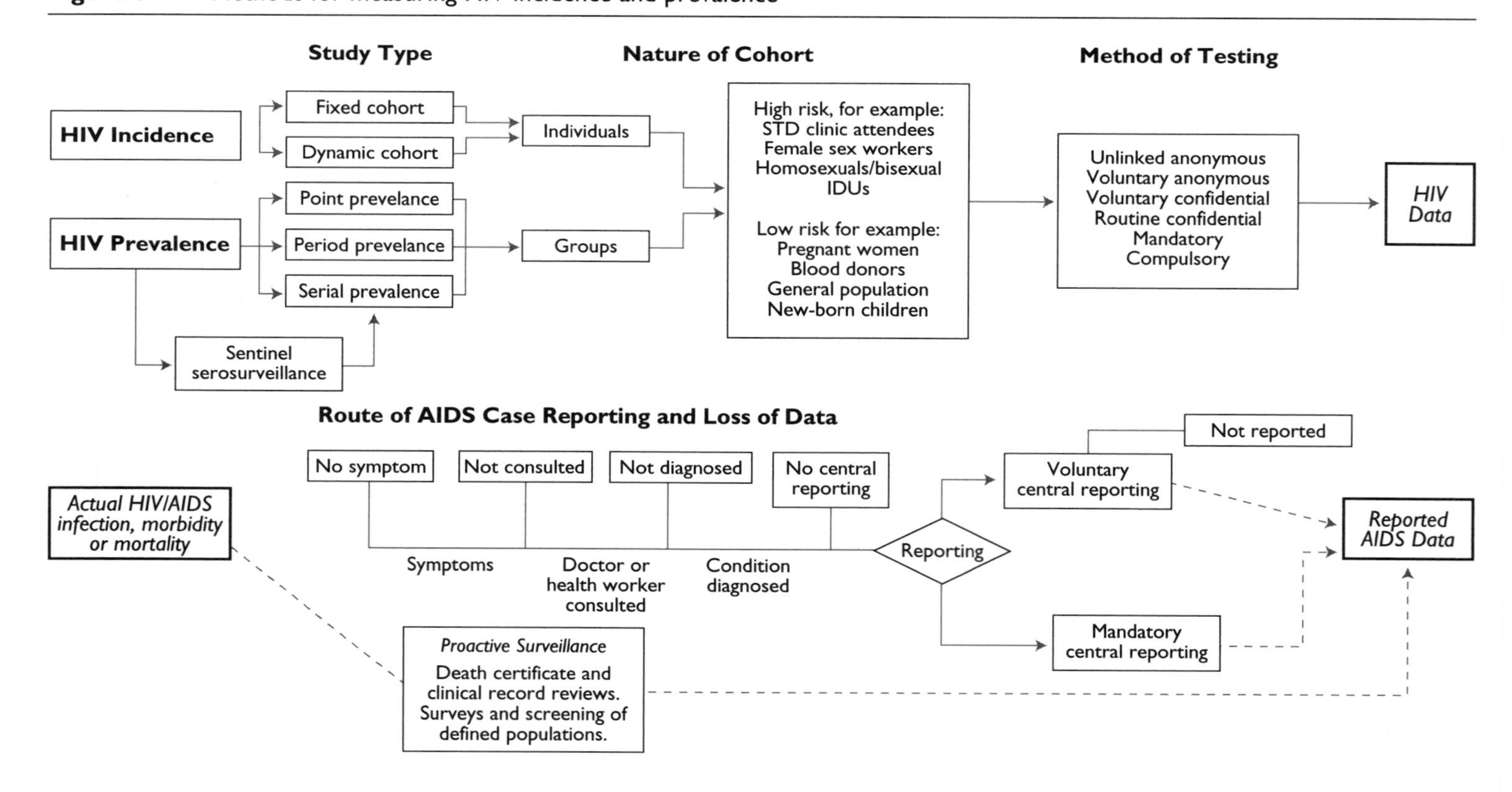

projections into the future. These methods have proved widely useful for quantitative estimates, but estimates of recent HIV incidence are imprecise because they are not yet reflected in AIDS cases, and additional assumptions of the shape of the incidence curve are usually required to prevent implausible oscillations in estimates (Brookmeyer, Gail 1994). The method is also very sensitive to the median length and distribution used for the incubation period (Brookmeyer and Damiano 1989, Hyman and Stanley 1988).

The third group of methods apply principles of epidemic theory including the mixing dynamics between susceptibles and infectives to generate underlying HIV incidence patterns. They require estimates of the magnitude and distribution of risk behaviours, probabilities of contact and transmission, an incubation period distribution, and an estimate of the initial number of HIV infections. They have illustrated several features of the epidemic, including the influence of partner rates (Anderson 1989), assortative and disassortative mixing (whether the individuals in a group are more likely to mix with others from the same or from different groups, respectively) (Gupta et al.. 1989), possible periods of infectiousness related to viral load (Anderson 1988, Seitz 1994), and the concept of reproductive threshold levels above which an epidemic will be sustained (Anderson, May, 1991). While they have provided considerable qualitative insight into the HIV epidemic (Anderson 1991; Auvert et al. 1990; Seitz and Mueller 1994; Way and Stanecki 1991), there is minimal consensus on the basic shape of the infection curve and therefore on a basis for quantitative estimates. A useful review of the diversity of their approaches and estimates is provided by a WHO publication on estimating the demographic impact of the HIV epidemic (WHO, 1991).

REVIEW OF EMPIRICAL DATABASES BY REGION

The interpretation of data collected from the AIDS epidemic is not straightforward. Understanding of the disease process, surveillance and the underlying disease incidence have all evolved rapidly over the history of the epidemic. The development of a diagnostic test for HIV in 1984, the onset of disease reporting for example in East Africa in 1987, and the changing AIDS definitions, for example the revision of the CDC AIDS definition in 1992, have an impact on HIV statistics which are inseparable from the disease trends. There are problems with delayed and under-reporting, but paradoxically in regions like SSA where underreporting is high, AIDS surveillance and HIV prevalence studies may provide the most reliable samples of HIV infection for disease estimation. With a grasp of definitional and reporting problems, and the relation between incidence, prevalence and AIDS during an epidemic, HIV and AIDS data may provide a better basis for calculating the global disease burden than data on most other diseases.

We have made estimates of HIV incidence for 1990 by region, sex and age group; as HIV incidence data by region are incomplete estimates have been made indirectly using WHO's *Epimodel*. The empirical data used are therefore:

1. HIV prevalence studies usually providing rates for sub-groups in a country, for example urban/rural, IDU or pregnant women attending antenatal clinics.
2. Further estimates of the population size of these sub-populations, the date of onset of the epidemic in a region, and the shape of, and present position on the epidemic curve provided by *Epimodel*.
3. Data on the sex and age distribution of AIDS cases and HIV prevalence, as the basis for estimating the age and sex distribution of HIV incidence.
4. HIV prevalence and AIDS cases databases are cross-compared and used in the validation of estimates.

Examples of data sources on HIV and AIDS

Initially we introduce examples of data on AIDS and HIV prevalence available from the regions and selected countries, before discussing the systematic choice of data sources for HIV estimation in a subsequent section. Data quality by region is discussed in the regional descriptions, and examples of the data are given in Tables 4 and 5 and Figures 4, 5 and 6.

AIDS case data used comes from the global AIDS surveillance system established by WHO and National AIDS Control Programmes. This system provides data for 192 countries with estimated reporting completeness from 80 per cent in EME, 30 per cent in LAC, to 10 per cent in SSA (Mertens et al. 1994). The sex ratios and age distributions of reported AIDS cases for selected countries are used to estimate the distributions of HIV incidence by age and sex with which they are consistent. The distribution of AIDS cases by risk group, shown in Figure 5, gives an idea of the regional characteristics of the epidemic, and into which major groups HIV prevalence should be disaggregated for the estimation process.

For regions for which we undertake estimates directly we use HIV prevalence studies; in 1990, 444 good quality studies, peer reviewed and with a full description of methodology were recorded (U.S. Bureau of the Census). In addition the LAC region and most countries in the EME produce their own direct estimates using their own expertise. Table 4 shows HIV prevalence for all reviewed studies in 1989-90 for Tanzania, Brazil and India by different sub-populations together with ranges, mean and medians. The number of scientifically reviewed studies for urban and rural areas in 14 countries from all regions is shown in Table 5. In contrast to the estimated low completeness of AIDS case reporting, countries in SSA have some of the largest number of HIV prevalence studies, though the relative lack of rural studies may be most critical in this region. As shown in Table 6 Asia has only more recently collected HIV prevalence data, with a limited time-series, as HIV becomes a priority.

Figure 4 HIV prevalence and incidence and AIDS incidence, by region

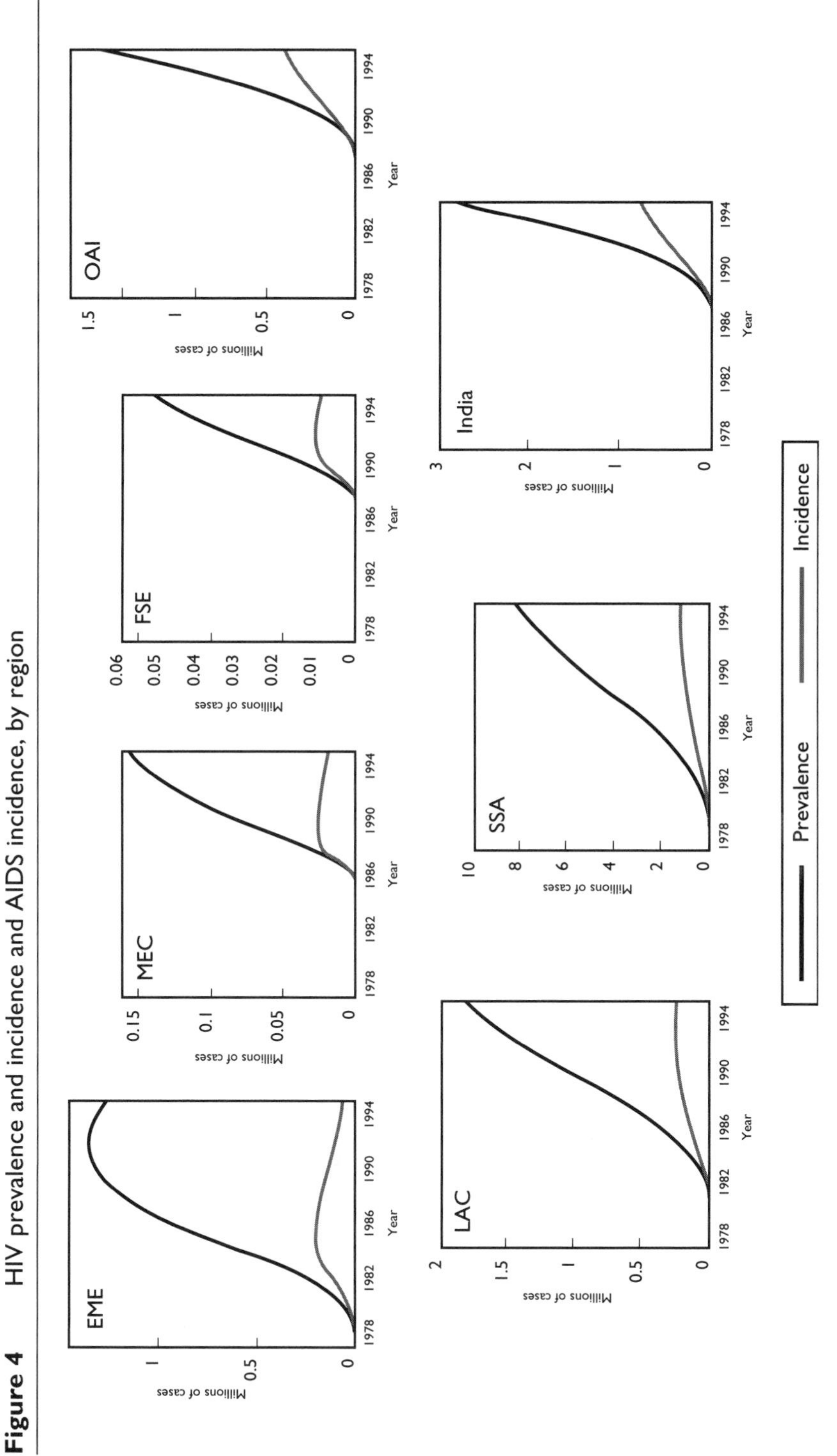

Figure 5 Distribution of AIDS cases by risk group for selected countries

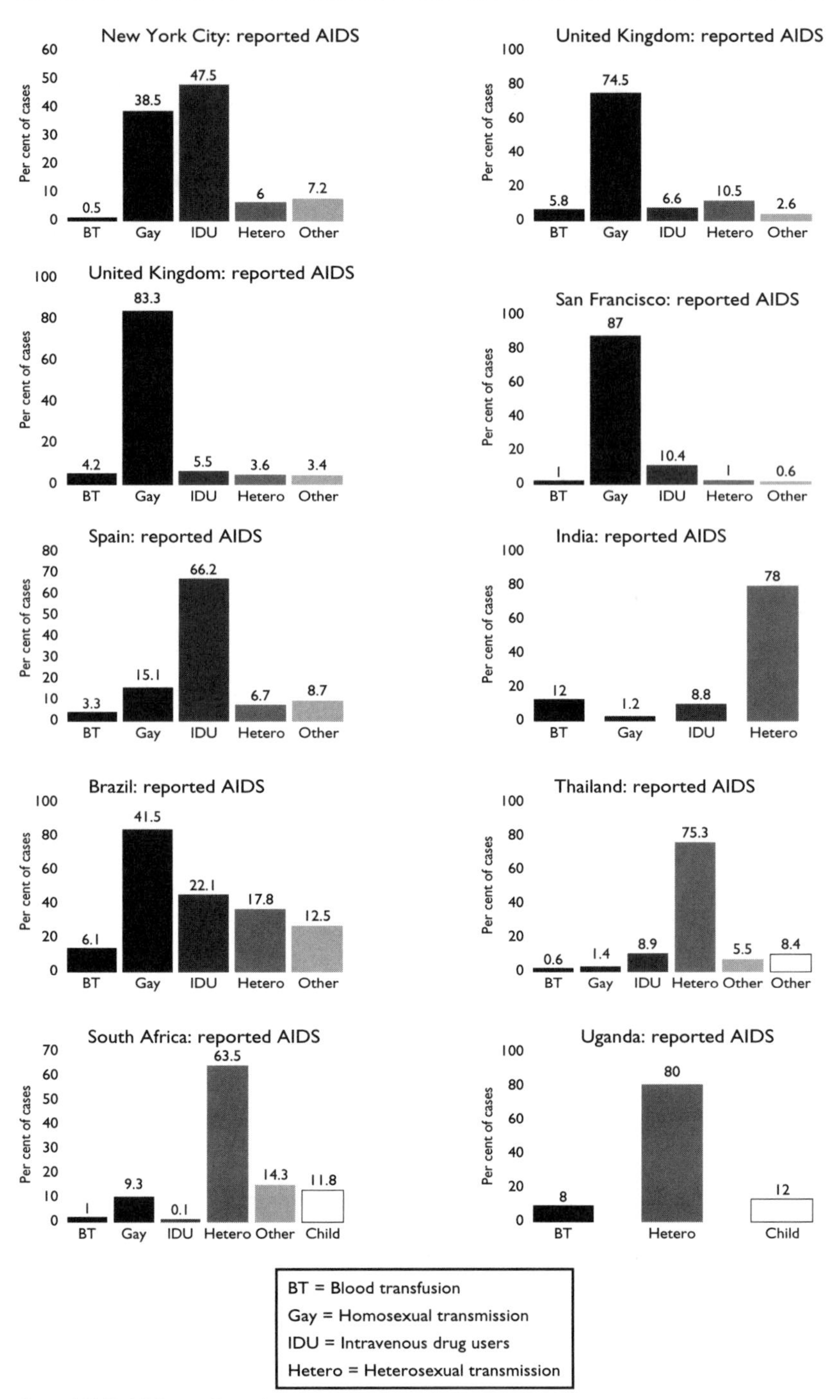

Source: WHO AIDS surveillance data

Figure 6 The age distribution of reported AIDS cases by sex for selected countries

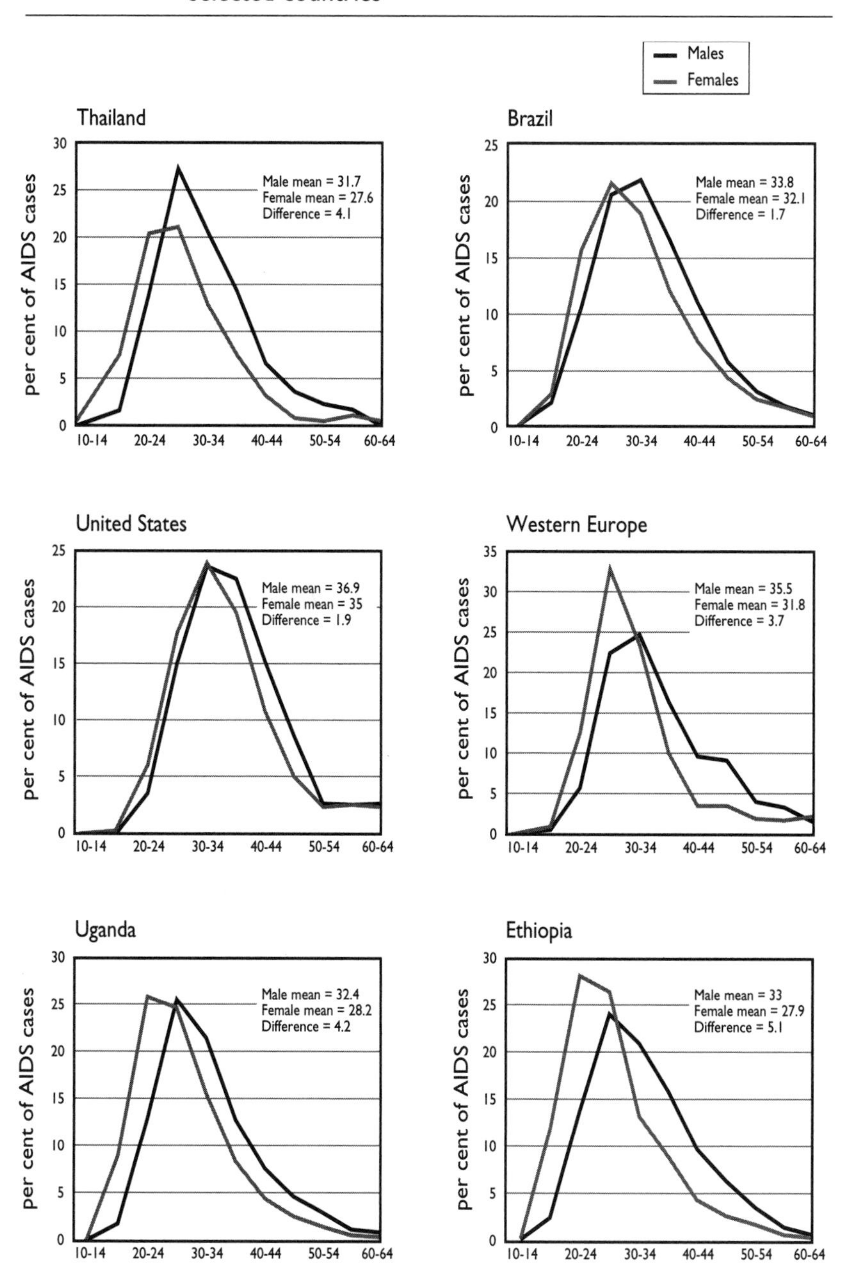

Source: AIDS cases reported to National AIDS programmes.
Note: Means are based on the mid-age of five year age groups. The median with continuous data would be more representative and give a younger average.

Table 4 Prevalence of HIV in selected countries

	Urban high risk	*Urban*	*Rural*	*Gay/Bisexual*
Tanzania				
No. Studies	40	35	51	
Mean	29.07	13.28	5.66	
Median	27.00	11.80	3.90	
Range	{0.3-75}	{0.7-27}	{0.1-17.4}	
Std. Deviation	17.17	5.78	4.86	
Brazil				
No. Studies	67	33	3	13
Mean	15.93	15.92	0.60	0.48
Median	12.00	8.80	0.20	0.30
Range	{0-42}	{0-80}	{0-3.7}	{0.23-0.9}
Std. Deviation	14.87	18.66	0.90	0.37
India				
No. Studies	36	10	11	
Mean	9.06	0.08	0.26	
Median	2.53	0.02	0.05	
Range	{0-54}	{0-0.25}	{0-1.1}	
Std. Deviation	14.44	0.10	0.40	

Despite the large range in HIV prevalence rates in different groups within the three countries, the difference in HIV prevalence patterns in 1990 is apparent (see Table 4). HIV prevalence in Tanzania is at least 4 per cent in all groups although there is a clear gradient among them, with a median of 27 per cent in high risk urban, 12 per cent in general urban, and 4 per cent in general rural, while in Brazil and India HIV prevalence

Table 5 Number of HIV prevalence studies

Country	*Urban*	*Rural*
Uganda	63	33
Zambia	28	10
Haiti	24	9
Kenya	56	3
Ethiopia	31	0
Argentina	36	0
South Africa	60	5
Morocco	15	0
China	1	2
Pakistan	10	0
Australia	25	0
Jamaica	5	0
Columbia	10	0
Botswana	1	2

Source: WHO country files, US Bureau of the Census

Table 6 Completeness of AIDS case reporting

Region	*HIV surveys 1990–1994*	*Reported AIDS cases*	*Estimated AIDS cases*	*% Reporting Completeness*
Africa	554	442735	4100000	~ 10%
LAC	54	146223	500000	30%
Asia	83	28630	300000	<10%
N.America	NA	501310	550000	~ 90%
Europe	NA	154103	220000	~ 70%

Source: WHO country files

is much more concentrated in urban high risk groups. There are considerable data on HIV, but the changing incidence pattern, and the problems of monitoring certain groups for example general male populations, are compounded by the large areas where HIV prevalence studies are sparse. For example, 3 studies are reported in China in 1990 in Tables 5. Due to the availability of empirical data and the stage of the epidemic we are most confident of our estimates for EME and SSA, have medium confidence for LAC, OAI and FSE, and low confidence for MEC, India and China.

How is this available data used to calculate the disease estimates for the global burden study? The first estimates required are of the number of HIV prevalent infections by region, and the following section presents the data sources used and the methods of estimation and forecasting.

DATA SOURCES FOR ESTIMATION OF HIV LEVELS

Having provided examples of the data available for regions, we now look at how they are systematically used in estimation. As the estimation process is primarily based on the proportion of HIV positive tests, WHO draws on a variety of sources of information additional to AIDS case surveillance, such as HIV seroprevalence studies and the estimated size of various population groups (Mertens et al. 1994). The following data sources are systematically considered for estimation of HIV prevalence:

Published studies. The US Bureau of the Census maintains a database of HIV prevalence data which appear in the scientific literature, the press, and international conferences. The completeness of the database is limited by the time taken for the results of studies to appear in the literature, the omission of methodological details from certain abstracts, and because data from routine surveillance activities, blood screening programmes, and service statistics rarely appear in the published literature. The HIV prevalence rates are also biased as studies in high risk groups, for example STD clinic attendees, are over represented, and any simple mathematical measure for example mean or medians would be misleading.

Blood banking systems. In most countries, blood donated for transfusion is screened for HIV as well as other pathogens. While HIV prevalence levels from such screening may not reflect levels in the general population due to donor selection, they provide important trends in HIV prevalence in that population. The large number of individuals tested over a few months in many blood banks' screening programmes improves the confidence interval on the estimated seroprevalence level. However systematic bias, for example the exclusion of those who are HIV positive or with risk behaviours, can make this seroprevalence level unrepresentative.

Routine surveillance activities: Many countries have implemented HIV surveillance activities. These activities may consist of sero-surveys in which individuals are selected on a random or voluntary basis, reports of identified HIV-positive individuals, and sentinel surveillance systems to monitor HIV trends in selected populations. For methodological and ethical considerations, WHO recommends that sentinel populations be selected where blood is already being drawn for other reasons, and that an unlinked anonymous testing method be used over a period of two to three months (WHO 1991). Common sentinel populations are STD clinic attendees and women attending antenatal clinics, although some groups are difficult to contact, for example males representative of the general population.

Research activities: A variety of research activities may involve testing individuals for serological evidence of HIV. One-time cross-sectional studies and cohort studies have been undertaken in many parts of the world. Preliminary reports of these are abstracted on a regular basis.

Institutional requirements: In some areas, HIV testing has been practised for non-public health purposes for example in visa applicants, military recruits, and job applicants, and the results communicated to WHO.

When reviewing findings from HIV prevalence studies for estimation purposes, there are several important considerations. The time interval for which blood samples were drawn is used to ascertain whether the HIV prevalence rate is a point estimate (over a few months) or a period estimate (over a period of more than 6 months). Geographical location is also important, so that for example estimates of urban/rural-specific rates of infection are usually made. When available, information on age and sex-specific HIV levels is taken into account to describe the local patterns of HIV transmission.

Estimates may be biased depending on the enrolment method used. Unlinked anonymous testing of blood drawn for other purposes minimises bias due to differential participation, while the results of voluntary and mandatory testing will usually be affected by participation bias. The representativeness of the sample is also influenced by the sampling method used, such as random, consecutive, or convenience sampling. Finally, the sample size influences the precision of the HIV prevalence estimate.

WHO augments the US Bureau of the Census data base with data from country files (Mertens et al. 1995). A total of about 1500 data points with sufficient methodological, geographic and demographic information have served as the basis of WHO global and regional estimates for the period 1990–1993.

AIDS cases reported to WHO

AIDS cases have been officially reported to WHO headqaters from Member States via WHO's regional offices. The usefulness of reported AIDS cases for estimation is limited by varying completeness of AIDS surveillance, and limited capacities in many countries to diagnose patients with conditions which satisfy one of the commonly used AIDS surveillance definitions. Although essential for monitoring the magnitude and course of the epidemic, for estimation purposes WHO uses reported AIDS cases mostly to validate current estimates of HIV infection and to estimate patterns of HIV incidence by age and sex.

Estimation of national/regional HIV prevalence

Most HIV prevalence studies represent levels of HIV infection in different segments of the population and are therefore not representative of the country. Nonetheless, it is possible to estimate national prevalence of seropositive individuals from such data, if they are interpreted in their own context, and if the entire population is stratified into mutually exclusive and exhaustive subpopulations, and the prevalence rate in each subpopulation estimated from a variety of surveys of that subpopulation (Brookmeyer and Gail 1994). Such estimates are subject to uncertainty due to selection bias, variability in observed prevalence rates from one sample to the next, and difficulties in estimating the size of subpopulations. Our estimation procedure for country-specific prevalent infections is described in five basic stages, and illustrated in Figures 7 and 8:

1. Subpopulations in which there was evidence of HIV infection were identified. This was achieved by reviewing all data available regardless of their quality.
2. Prevalence studies were reviewed for their methodological qualities according to the criteria described previously, including sampling method, point/period estimate, scientific review process, HIV test type, representativeness of sample, and studies with a predetermined threshold sample size were selected.
3. Using all remaining seroprevalence data points to provide upper and lower bounds, a conservative estimate (usually lower than the median value of all prevalence levels) was selected for each subpopulation – in accordance with the WHO approach (Chin and Lwanga 1991) – taking into account seroprevalence trends over the past two years.
4. The best available information was used to estimate the size of the subpopulation.
5. Finally, the estimated prevalence rates were applied to the estimated subpopulations' sizes and totalled to provide an estimate of prevalent infections for the country.

Once a provisional country-specific estimate was obtained, reported and estimated AIDS cases were compared with the numbers that were expected from estimated past and present HIV levels, using WHO's cur-

Figure 7 Estimation procedure for HIV infection

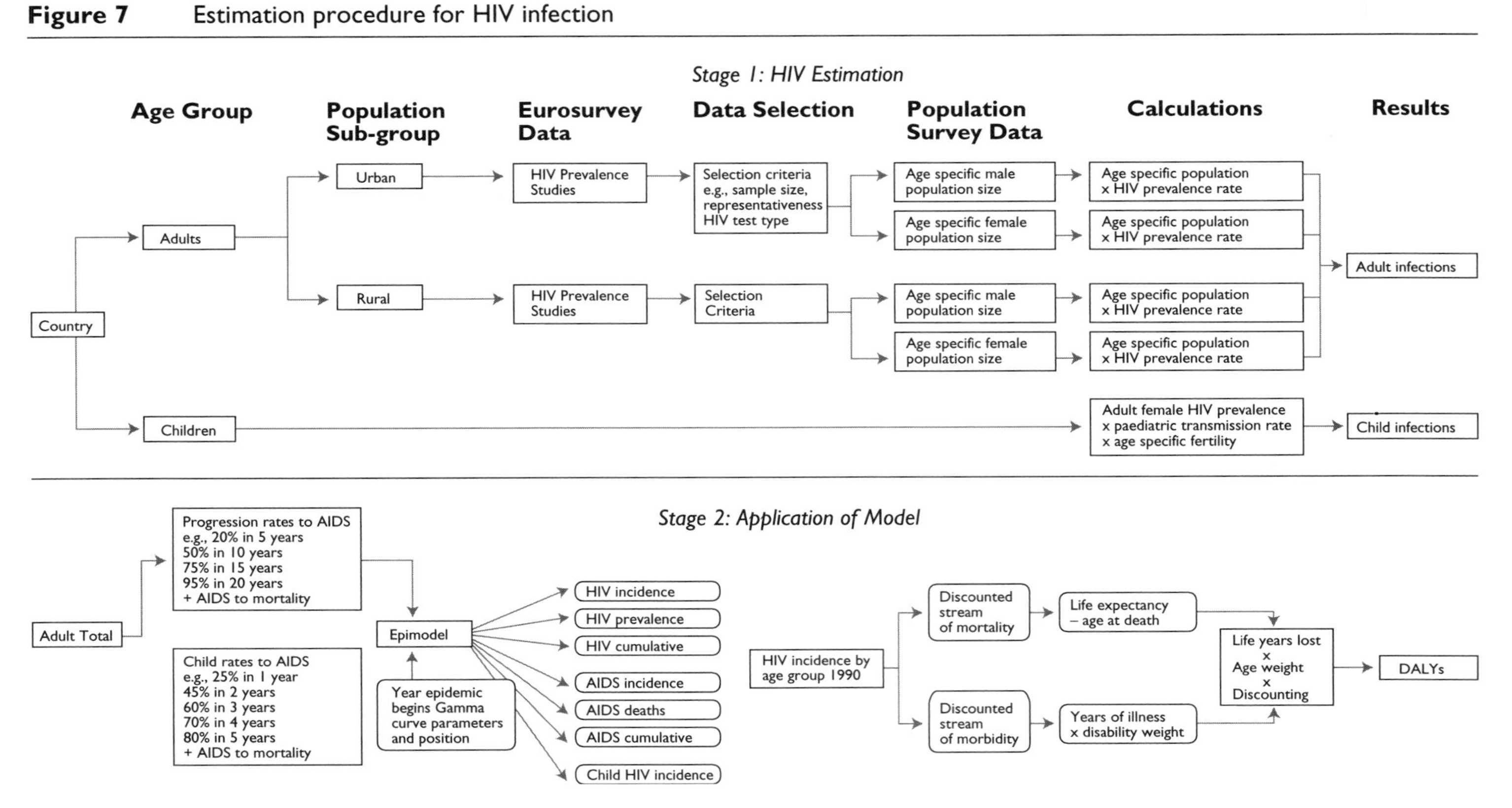

rent model (described below), and the estimate was adjusted accordingly. All estimates were discussed with each country's national UNAIDS programme.

Estimates of perinatally acquired HIV infections were calculated as the product of the estimated number of HIV-infected women and age-specific fertility rates for the region, together with an average HIV infection transmission rate of 30 per cent from an infected woman to her offspring (Chin and Lwanga 1991). Thus if there were 1000 HIV prevalent women aged 20-25 with an annual fertility rate of 200 births per 1000 women, then the number of HIV positive children born in this group would be:

$$\text{\# of HIV}^{+}\text{ women x Fertility rate x Transmission rate}$$

$$1000 \times (200/1000) \times 0.3 = 60$$

This figure was aggregated across all female ages and those HIV positive children who had survived from earlier years are included.

There were some exceptions to the use of these procedures. For industrialized countries, HIV estimates developed by national experts and National UNAIDS programmes were generally used. For Latin America, including the Caribbean, the US Bureau of Census and the UNAIDS database were used together with estimates made by UNAIDS experts.

FORECASTING AIDS CASES AND HIV INFECTIONS

On the basis of estimates of regional HIV prevalence and trends in 1993, WHO uses a mathematical model to generate estimates of AIDS cases and HIV infections since the beginning of the epidemic. The model, illustrated in Figure 8, combines: a point-prevalence for HIV; progression rates from HIV to AIDS and from AIDS to death; a gamma curve value and position on the epidemic curve (see below); and the year of epidemic onset. It projects HIV incidence, prevalance, AIDS and mortality into the future for a period selected by the user. Figure 8 shows the application of the model for two values of gamma.

The model currently used by WHO has been described by Chin and Lwanga (1991). The initial input for this model is a regional estimate of HIV prevalence and the model then distributes past cumulative HIV incidence along a gamma distribution from the present year backward to the time at which extensive spread of HIV infection is estimated to have begun. The gamma curve representing cumulative HIV infections stems from classical epidemiological theory and the use of deterministic models to attempt forecasts of the future course of epidemics (Bailey 1957). Such a curve is characteristic of a single source epidemic with person to person transmission (Bailey 1957, Chin and Lwanga 1991). Further inputs to define the epidemic curve include:

1. *The onset year of extensive spread of HIV infections* — defined as at least 1 per cent HIV seroprevalence in groups with high risk behaviours, or the reporting of a substantial rise in AIDS cases. It is not when the first AIDS case was reported.

Figure 8 A country level example of HIV prevalence estimation and application of a model to estimate HIV incidence for Botswana

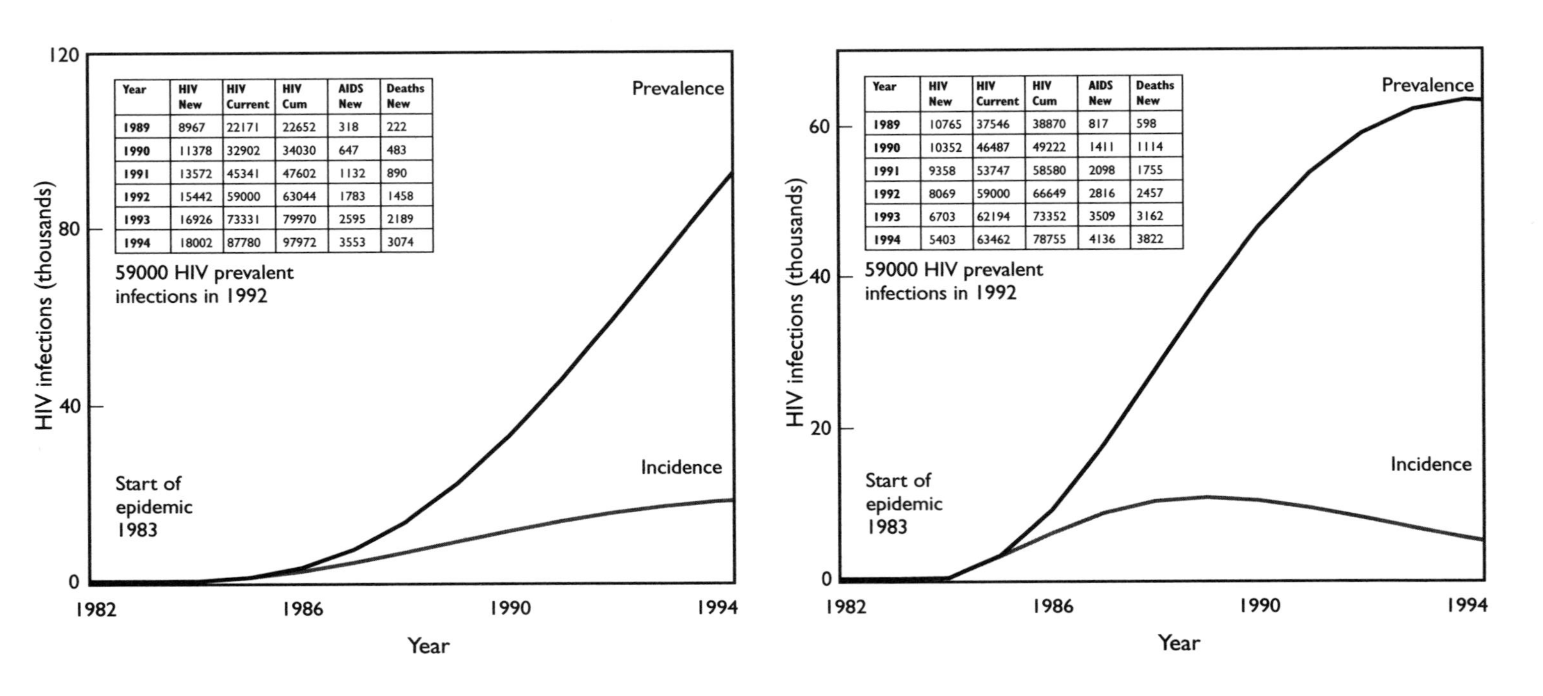

Year	HIV New	HIV Current	HIV Cum	AIDS New	Deaths New
1989	8967	22171	22652	318	222
1990	11378	32902	34030	647	483
1991	13572	45341	47602	1132	890
1992	15442	59000	63044	1783	1458
1993	16926	73331	79970	2595	2189
1994	18002	87780	97972	3553	3074

Year	HIV New	HIV Current	HIV Cum	AIDS New	Deaths New
1989	10765	37546	38870	817	598
1990	10352	46487	49222	1411	1114
1991	9358	53747	58580	2098	1755
1992	8069	59000	66649	2816	2457
1993	6703	62194	73352	3509	3162
1994	5403	63462	78755	4136	3822

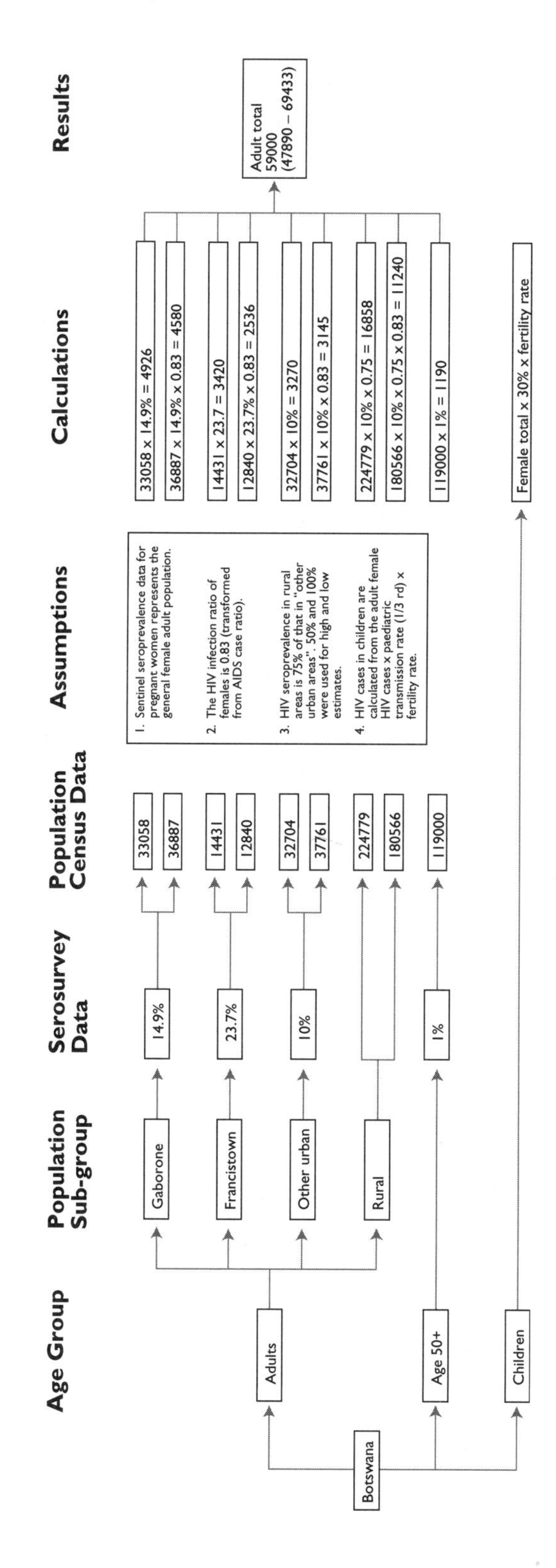

Figure 8 *(continued)*

2. *Position and shape of the HIV epidemic curve* — The fundamental assumption in the model is that cumulative HIV infections follow a sigmoid curve, skewed with a long right tail, defined by the gamma function:

$$Y_t = t^{(p-1)}e^{-t}/(p-1)!$$

describing Y_t (HIV incidence) at time t since the onset of widespread infection. Parameter p defines the steepness of the HIV epidemic curve, and is referred to in this chapter as the "gamma value". The "position" of the reference year on the gamma curve is also defined (effectively scaling and proportional to t), suggesting whether HIV incidence is increasing, at its peak value, or decreasing (as the position value increases).

An incubation distribution from infection to AIDS and a survival time from AIDS to death are applied to each annual cohort of incident HIV infections. Further details of the epidemiological basis for this model and its numerous applications for projecting AIDS and HIV infections have been published elsewhere (Chin and Lwanga 1991).

The key parameter is the position, which is best thought of in terms of when HIV incidence may peak in the region; whether the reference year (1990 for this study) is before, at the maximum or on the extended downslope of the gamma curve. Figure 9 shows the 1990 estimate at different positions, using a gamma value of 3 and 5 and an onset of spread in 1980, and the resulting curves of HIV prevalence and HIV incidence. It should be stressed that *EPIMODEL* works best for short term forecasts as it is based on present trends, and is not inconsistent for a new fit for extrapolation to be provided when new data emerge.

While we have considerable data for HIV estimation over the period 1990-94 for this study, the future trends of the epidemic are uncertain and subject to much debate. WHO has estimated there may be 30–40 million cumulative HIV infections by the year 2000 (Mertens et al. 1995), while Mann et al. (1992) estimate 30–120 million. WHO projections are based on current HIV prevalence studies and trends, and therefore may be seen as conservative, as new developments, for example HIV prevalence studies showing considerable spread in China (or declines elsewhere), are included only when evidence emerges. When such data are forthcoming, the trajectory should be adjusted if necessary, which is why the method is restricted to 3–5 year projections based on present estimates.

Despite uncertainties of forecasting the HIV epidemic, for this study we are more confident of the short term trajectory of the epidemic from the 1990 estimates. This is based on:

1. The regional characteristics of the epidemic, transmission patterns, and sentinel data, presented in the following section.
2. A review of HIV and AIDS data at the country level for 1994, providing country by country and regional estimates. These were compared

Figure 9 Estimated HIV incidence and prevalence in 1990 for different positions and gamma values.

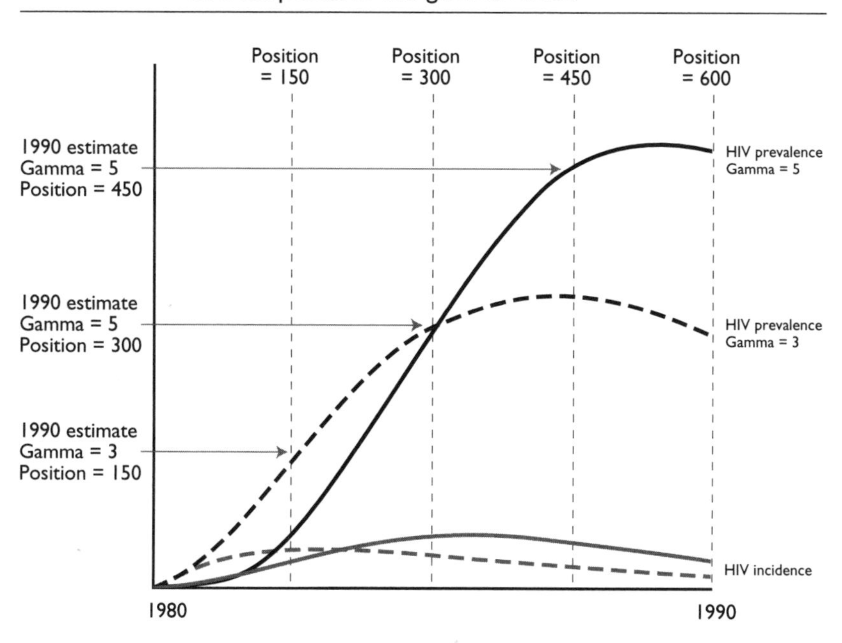

to what the 1990 estimate and the parameters used in the study would forecast for 1994, to validate the short-term trend.

The trajectory used for the 1990-94 trend was based on the parameters presented in this chapter, and assumed HIV incidence had peaked in the mid-1980s for the EME, was increasing past the 1990 estimate until at least the mid-1990s in SSA and LAC, and was increasing most steeply in Asia and would not peak there before 2000.

Gender and age distributions of HIV incidence are estimated by simple extrapolation from reported AIDS cases and HIV prevalence by age and sex, using the median incubation period, the stage of the epidemic, and knowledge of transmission characteristics. HIV incidence by age may be similar to the distribution of AIDS cases in the first years of an epidemic, thereafter becoming progressively different until HIV incidence is, on average, a mean incubation period younger (this varies in younger age groups, and if the age distribution of HIV incidence changes rapidly). Female to male ratios of HIV incidence are also approximated from HIV prevalence and AIDS data, and tend to fall into three patterns:

1. High HIV prevalence in pregnant women (5 per cent), and mainly heterosexual transmission in the general population (women 50 per cent of HIV incidence).

2. Medium HIV prevalence in pregnant women (1-3 per cent), and heterosexual transmission but related to high risk sexual behaviour e.g. sex workers and clients (women 15-35 per cent of HIV incidence).
3. High HIV prevalence in IDUs and homosexuals, HIV prevalence in pregnant women < 1 per cent (women 10-20 per cent of HIV incidence).

Combinations of and transitions between the above transmission types in a region result in intermediary ratios of female:male HIV incidence. As above, this proportion is multiplied by the estimated annual births to women infected with HIV, and a separate shorter incubation distribution is applied to each annual cohort of incident child HIV infections.

Major uncertainties for these projections include the accuracy of the prevalence estimates, the timing and level at which HIV incidence peaks, the shape of the incidence curve in populations with different demographic and geographic characteristics, the rate at which children and adults ultimately develop AIDS and die, and how this progression rate may change over time as a result of factors related to the host, viral agent, or medical interventions.

The model provides estimates of HIV incidence by region for 1990 presented in Table 7, used as the disease basis of the DALY burden calculations. The parameters in the estimation process include: an HIV prevalence estimate for a year; the regional date of onset of rapid growth in HIV infections; the gamma value and position on the epidemic curve; the age and sex distribution of HIV incidence. These parameters used for the GBD estimates are presented in Table 7, so that the process can be systematically reproduced by readers for their region using the mathematical model *Epimodel* which can be obtained from the U.N. Programme on AIDS. The basis for the choice of these parameters comes from the regional characteristics of the epidemic as described below.

Regional characteristics of the HIV epidemic

Despite its global extent with 192 countries having reported AIDS cases, the AIDS epidemic has developed distinctive characteristics in the different cultures through which it has spread. This section describes the infection patterns, transmission characteristics, and sex and age distributions for each region.

From these regional characteristics, the following parameters for estimation are derived which are discussed in the text: the estimate of epidemic onset; the position and gamma value of the epidemic curve; and the age and sex distribution of HIV incidence. For the interpretation of the DALY burdens based on HIV incidence, the number of prevalent infections which accompany HIV incidence are highlighted, together with the quality of AIDS and HIV reporting.

Table 7 GBD Estimation exercise

Regions	Year of Index estimate	Index Estimate of HIV prevalence for 15 and above	Gamma value	Position	Start Year	% female HIV incidence	% age 0-14	% age 15-44	% age 45-59
N. America	1990	800 000	5	538	1978	17.5	2	90	7
Europe	1990	425 000	3	345	1982	17.3	2	90	7
SSA	1990	5 000 000	5	271	1978	50	11	86	2.7
LAC	1990	1 000 000	5	261	1980	22.5	2	92.5	5
India	1992	1 009 000	5	180	1987	35	1	94	4
China	1990	2 780	3	152	1989	12.7	0.5	94	5
OAI	1992	500 000	5	180	1987	35	0.8	94	4
FSE	1991	20 000	3	190	1988	12.7	0.3	91	8
MEC	1991	95 000	3	230	1986	15	1	91	8

Regions	1990 HIV prevalence for all ages	1990 HIV incidence for all ages	Source
N. America	851 058	79 215	National Estimates
Europe	452 125	59 192	Regional Estimate
SSA	5 465 241	1 071 215	WHO Estimate
LAC	1 014 364	228 042	PAHO/WHO
India	262 383	178 781	WHO Estimate
China	2 790	2 791	WHO Estimate
OAI	126 007	89 442	WHO Estimate
FSE	11 866	7 952	WHO Estimate
MEC	75 034	25 072	WHO Estimate

Sub-Saharan Africa

Infection patterns and data quality

Sub-Saharan Africa accounts for the majority of both cumulative and prevalent estimated world-wide HIV infections, with 11.5 million and over 8.5 million respectively. It has some of the earliest evidence of HIV infection from the 1970s and before (Nzilambi et al. 1988, Getchell et al. 1987), with epidemic spread estimated to occur from 1978 in this study (N'Galy and Ryder 1988; Morvan et al. 1989, Piot et al. 1984). The diagnosis and reporting of AIDS are of limited completeness, and the 442 735 AIDS cases reported by end 1995, represent only around 10 per cent of the over 4 million AIDS cases estimated by WHO. In contrast there is frequently a wealth of HIV seroprevalence studies, with for example 2087 recorded for 1990-4 with 554 of these peer reviewed and of high scientific standard (U.S. Bureau of the census). The region had a population of 510 million in 1990 and a total health expenditure of 22 US$ per capita (even this figure is very skewed by South Africa), presenting the highest burden of HIV but with low health-related resources to deal with it. (Murray et al. 1994) Due to the limited diagnostic and surveillance capabilities of much of the region, the Bangui AIDS surveillance definition, described earlier, was applied.

Heterosexual transmission accounts for over 80 per cent of HIV infections, resulting in high rates of HIV prevalence reported in the general population, pregnant women and blood donors (Kapiga et al. 1992; Asiimwe et al. 1992; Ladner et al. 1992; De Cock et al. 1990). Other transmission modes include contact with infected blood particularly due to contamination of blood supplies and reuse of injection equipment, and infection from mother to child. HIV prevalence is highest in East and Central Africa, accounting for 60 per cent of HIV infections, though HIV prevalence rates among pregnant women were at similar high levels of 10-20 per cent (Diallo et al. 1992, Adjorlolo 1992) in parts of West Africa, namely Cote d'Ivoire.

Position on the epidemic curve

The GBD estimates that HIV incidence increases past the 1990 estimate at least until the mid 1990s, and a gamma value of 5 and early position of 271 (compared to 538 for North America with the same year of onset) are used. Considerable HIV incidence is associated with the HIV prevalence estimate in 1990, with a ratio of 1:5.5. These parameters appear to have some validity for the trend between the two HIV prevalence estimates for 1990 and 1994 (see Table 7). Beyond this period there is much uncertainty, and the major question is the potential scale of the expanding HIV epidemics in West and South Africa. The forecasting methods used for the 1990 estimate should not be extended more than 3-5 years, but prevalent HIV infections may increase to greater than 9 million by the year 2000 (Mertens et al. 1995), if HIV incidence already at a high level peaks in the mid-1990s. This may occur due to:

1. High rates of HIV prevalence which have already occurred in East and Central Africa, and there are indications of stability in some rural and urban areas of Uganda, Burundi (Sokal et al. 1993), Tanzania (Kigadye et al. 1993) and Zaire (Magazani et al. 1993). Sokal et al. (1993) suggested HIV prevalence may have been stable in Bujumbara, Burundi since 1986, also showing geographical stability between districts. HIV prevalence may also have been stable since 1986 in Kinshasa, Zaire (N'Galy and Ryder 1988). This can be associated with high incidence (Batter et al. 1994), and a continued risk to youth as 46 per cent of the population are under the age of 15 (Stoneburner et al. 1995). Wawer et al. (1994) for example noted a decline in HIV prevalence in a rural, population based, open cohort in Uganda 1990-92, but adult HIV incidence remained stable at 2.1 per 100 person years. A decline in HIV prevalence in Masaka, Uganda was also shown by Mulder et al. (1995), HIV incidence declining in males aged 13-24 but remaining relatively stable overall at 7/1000 person years. Substantial declines in HIV prevalence in ante-natal clinic (ANC) attendees in Kampala, Uganda from 29.1 per cent in 1989 to 16.2 per cent in 1993 have recently been reported with the declining trend unrelated to changes in fertility and continuing to 1995 (Bagenda et al. 1995). Other evidence may suggest a

decline in HIV incidence in restricted urban and rural areas (Mertens et al. 1995; Kegeya-Kayondo et al. 1994), though trends in rural areas are difficult to monitor.

2. Expansion of the epidemic to West and South Africa is occurring, particularly to Nigeria with a population of about 100 million and South Africa with some 40 million. There is evidence of rising HIV prevalence in Nigeria, with 2.1 per cent reported among pregnant women (Harry et al. 1994), and 5.8 per cent in one State, though several rural States remain below 1 per cent (Asagba et al. 1992). Data aggregated from antenatal clinics in the Republic of South Africa suggested an HIV prevalence of 2.4 per cent among pregnant women (Mertens et al. 1995). More recent increases in HIV prevalence from 4.5 per cent to 8 per cent in urban ANC from 1992-94 have been recorded, with rural ANC more stable at 3 per cent (Wilkinson 1994). Surrounding countries already had high HIV prevalence in pregnant women by 1990-93, for example 15-30 per cent in urban areas of Botswana (Namboze 1993), and 18 per cent in Harare, Zimbabwe by 1990 (Mahomed et al. 1991). Although Nigeria and South Africa have a population twice those of the countries with already severe epidemics, HIV prevalences recorded in pregnant women remain 3-5 times lower. Notable exceptions include Cote d'Ivoire, Botswana, and Zimbabwe which had reached high HIV prevalence levels by 1992 (U.S. Bureau of the Census).

The longer term infection patterns remain uncertain and depend on two major questions: will evidence of stability and possibly decline in HIV prevalence in limited areas in the worst epidemics be confirmed more generally, and will HIV prevalence in the general population in Nigeria and South Africa continue to rise to 5-10 per cent? The epidemic in SSA is very tightly balanced between these two trends, and WHO projects the high incidence of HIV will continue and maybe increase until the mid to late 1990s (Mertens et al. 1995).

Sex and age distributions

Uganda and Zambia form a distinct grouping compared to Brazil, Europe, USA and Thailand, in that females constitute around 50 per cent of all reported AIDS cases (51 per cent in Zambia and 55 per cent in Uganda in 1993). Some studies have suggested female infections may exceed males in certain areas (Berkley et al. 1990; Barongo et al. 1992; Mathiot et al. 1990). The age distribution of AIDS cases is also young with a marked lag of almost five years between male and younger females cases (see Figure 6). The high levels of infection among young females leads to considerable perinatal transmission, resulting in around 1 million cumulative child infections. Eighty-six per cent of all HIV incidence is estimated to occur in the 15-44 age group, while a smaller proportion than in other regions occurs in the 45-59 age group. SSA is estimated to have the highest proportion of HIV incidence of all regions in the 0-14 year age group of 11 per cent. The HIV epidemic in SSA therefore has the youngest age distribution, with an even ratio of males to females, and suggestions that youth has an increasing relative risk as the epidemic matures (Stoneburner et al. 1996).

Latin America and Caribbean

Infection patterns and data quality

Latin America and the Caribbean is estimated to account for over 2 million cumulative and over 1.8 million prevalent HIV infections by the end of 1995. They represent a very heterogeneous epidemic, associated with restricted risk behaviours in many countries, but in some countries, for example in much of the Caribbean, also showing the capability for widespread heterosexual spread. HIV infections have been reported since the 1970s, and extensive spread is estimated to have occurred from 1980 (Pradinaud et al. 1989). The diagnosis and reporting of AIDS cases are of intermediate quality, and the 146223 reported AIDS cases represent 30 per cent of what is estimated to be more than 410000 cases. AIDS case data are supplemented by 884 HIV reported seroprevalence studies from 1990-4, with 54 of these peer review and meeting high scientific standards (U.S. Bureau of the Census 1995). The region had a population of 444 million in 1990, and an average health expenditure per capita of $98, and in keeping with its intermediate diagnostic capabilities a special Caracas AIDS surveillance definition was developed, described earlier.

Transmission characteristics of epidemics in the region are heterogeneous, with two major patterns. In Latin America, the majority of infections have been among homosexual or bisexual men with considerable infections also among injecting drug users. However heterosexual transmission has increased for example in Brazil from 7.5 per cent of reported AIDS cases in 1987 to 26 per cent in 1993-4. HIV prevalence rates in antenatal clinic attendees in Brazil were 0.5 per cent in Sao Paulo State, 0.3 per cent in Rio de Janeiro (Rodrigues 1994). Figure 4 shows the much lower HIV prevalence results among pregnant women, blood donors or the working population compared to high risk groups for 1990. However there are signs that a more widely distributed epidemic in the general population occur: for example in Honduras in pregnant women HIV prevalence reached 2-4 per cent in some cities in 1991-2 (Ministry of Health 1994), and contacts between risk groups and the general population exist through which transmission could occur. Brazil accounts for almost 50 per cent of the whole region's reported AIDS cases, with Mexico reporting over 20 000 cases and Argentina around 5 000.

The second transmission pattern covers most of the Caribbean, with heterosexual transmission predominating for over a decade. HIV prevalence rates among pregnant women are reported at 3.6 per cent in the Bahamas, 1.2 per cent in the Dominican republic, and 7.5 per cent in urban and 5.5 per cent in rural areas of Haiti (Bernard et al. 1994). These countries contribute much lower total AIDS case to the regional total because of their smaller populations, but have some of the highest reported AIDS case rates per 100 000 population in the world.

Position on the epidemic curve

For LAC, HIV incidence is estimated to be increasing past the 1990 estimate, at least until the mid-1990s, and a gamma value of 5 and position of 261 are used. In 1990 the ratio of HIV incidence to HIV prevalence was high, 1:5. Widespread heterosexual transmission has been found in a number of countries in the Caribbean and at a lower rate in Honduras of 2-4 per cent (U.S. Bureau of the Census). However sentinel surveillance in the most populous countries, for example Brazil and Argentina, has identified HIV prevalence in pregnant women, but generally at less than 1 per cent (U.S. Bureau of the Census; Rodrigues et al. 1994). In some areas of Brazil, increased IDU use may lead to heterosexual transmission: for example HIV prevalence in pregnant women in Itajai, southern Brazil, was 2.2 per cent, and there was substantial HIV prevalence in attendees of STD clinics (see Table 8). However the major question is whether heterosexual spread in Brazil and the other larger South American countries will emerge, following evidence in the Caribbean, Honduras and Guyana. The table shows HIV prevalence studies in South America, suggesting at present there remains a large difference between HIV prevalence rates in high risk groups in Brazil, Argentina and Mexico (and pregnant women in the Caribbean and Honduras) compared to sentinel groups representing the general population.

When a 1994 estimate is projected from the parameters and the 1990 estimate, there is evidence that the LAC estimate and trajectory is overestimated compared to the 1994 country calculations. Because of the heterogeneous transmission characteristics and the uncertain heterosexual element, we have used the 1990 estimate of one million infections for the GBD study.

Sex and age distributions

The age distribution of HIV incidence in LAC countries is estimated to be similar but slightly younger than that in North America and Europe, with 85 per cent of HIV incidence in the 15-44 year age group. The age distribution of AIDS cases in Brazil (see Figure 6) shows an extended distribution into the older age groups 40-59, reflecting the contribution of cases in homosexuals/ bisexuals. The proportion of HIV incidence in females was estimated at 22.5 per cent in 1990, and their proportion of reported AIDS cases in Brazil provides some supporting evidence, reaching 21.5 per cent by 1993. The female proportion of reported AIDS cases in Brazil shows a steady increase from 1985 to 1993. This possibly reflects the increasing proportion of injecting drug users, their partners and heterosexual spread, but remains much more similar to Europe and North America than the more widespread heterosexually transmitted epidemics.

Table 8 HIV prevalence in South American countries

Country	Year	Group	HIV Prevalence	Reference
Brazil				
	1994	Atenatal clinic attendees (ANC), Rio de Janeiro	0.3%	Rodrigues et al. 1994
	1994	ANC, Sao Paulo	0.5%	Rodrigues et al. 1994
	1994	ANC, Itajai	2.2%	Rodrigues et al. 1994
	1993	STD clinics, North	5.2%	Brazil NAP 1995
	1993	STD clinics, South	4.5%	Brazil NAP 1995
	1993	STD clinics, Central	2.9%	Brazil NAP 1995
	1993	STD clinics, North East	10.4%	Brazil NAP 1995
Argentina				
	1992	Blood donors, urban	0.2%	Fay et al 1992
	1992	Sex workers	2%	Fay et al 1992
	1992	Military recruits	0.4%	Avolio et al 1993
Mexico				
	1992	Blood donors, urban	0.1%	Herrera et al 1992
	1991	ANC	0.1%	Valdespino et al 1992
Guyana				
	1993	Sex workers	25%	Guyana Min. Health
	1992	ANC	6.9%	Guyana Min. Health
Honduras				
	1992	ANC	2-4%	U.S. Bureau of the Census

Established Market Economies

Infection patterns and data quality

The established market economies include North America, Western Europe, Australia, Japan and New Zealand and account for over 1.9 million cumulative and 1.3 million prevalent estimated HIV infections. There is sporadic early evidence of CDC-defined AIDS cases with serological evidence of HIV infection in St. Louis, USA in 1968 and Norway in 1976 (Smallman-Raynor et al. 1992), but extensive spread is estimated to occur only from 1978 (Gottlieb et al. 1981; Auerbach et al. 1984). Most EME countries have well developed AIDS surveillance systems established since the early to mid-1980s, and over 650000 AIDS cases have been reported, representing almost 85 per cent of the WHO estimate of 760000 AIDS cases. HIV prevalence studies are routinely carried out though many of these do not appear in the published literature, and sentinel populations have to be carefully chosen for the number of positive HIV infections identified to be statistically significant. EME constituted a population of 798 million in 1990, the quality of HIV and AIDS data reflecting a developed health structure, with health expenditure per capita of US$1869.

However there are problems identifying low levels of HIV infection in the general population, which would require large sample sizes for example to measure HIV incidence directly. HIV prevalence is estimated at below 1 per cent in the general population, but despite sophisticated health surveillance it may be as difficult to monitor as for example in SSA.

The majority of HIV infections are associated with IDU and homosexual populations, but there is an increasing proportion of heterosexually transmitted infections (Holmes et al. 1990; Prevots et al. 1994). Over 80 per cent of reported cumulative AIDS cases in the EME countries are associated with IDU or homosexuality, but one-third of new HIV infections in some Spanish cities have been shown to be transmitted heterosexually (Mertens et al. 1995). HIV prevalence among women in London attending antenatal clinics, an approximate reflection of the general adult population, were 1-5 per 1000 and in the United States 1.7 per 1000 (WHO-EC Collaborating Centre 1994; Peterson et al. 1994). The relative increase of heterosexual transmission is partly due to a decline in incidence among homosexuals (Lemp et al. 1994), but also due to the build-up of the number infected with HIV, which can increase exposure and further transmission.

The major heterogeneity among EME epidemics is the relative proportion of AIDS cases among IDU and homosexuals. This is apparent between the East and West coast of the United States, where 87 per cent of AIDS cases occur in homosexuals in San Francisco, while IDU is the major transmission characteristic in New York. Similarly in Europe the United Kingdom has reported 6.6 per cent of AIDS cases among IDU, compared to 63 per cent in Spain (Rebagliato et al. 1995). These differences have implications for the lower rates of heterosexual transmission. Of particular concern are increases in heterosexual transmission associated with IDU and crack use (Edlin et al. 1994), particularly among women. Furthermore while HIV incidence among homosexuals may be slowing, the relative importance of IDU has increased, for example from 16 to 44 per cent of recent reported AIDS cases in Western Europe since 1985, and from 17 to 25 per cent in the United States.

AIDS has become a leading cause of mortality in younger adults in countries throughout EME as mentioned previously, and is the leading cause of death in the United States in adults aged 25-44. HIV transmission has also occurred through infected blood and blood products, associated with very high transmission efficiency, and accounts for over 5 per cent of cumulative AIDS cases in some European countries (although after the widespread implementation of HIV screening of blood and blood products it has contributed almost no recent infections).

Position on the epidemic curve

For the EME, HIV incidence is estimated to have peaked before the 1990 estimate, declining slowly on the long right tail of the gamma function (Chin, Lwanga 1991), and a gamma of 5 and position of 538 were used for North America and 3 and 345 for Europe. There was therefore a lower HIV incidence: HIV prevalence ratio in 1990, of 25:1 for North America and 15:1 for Western Europe.

Evidence for this trajectory include the early rapid rise in HIV incidence in homosexuals and IDUs from 1980-86 (Lemp et al. 1994; Mertens et al. 1995), followed by some declines among homosexuals in the number of AIDS cases (CDC 1991; Morris, Dean 1994), HIV seroprevalence (Winkelstein 1987), and other markers of risk, for example rectal gonorrhoea (Johnson and Gill 1989). Some longitudinal studies also reported HIV incidence peaked in the mid-1980s (Kingsley et al. 1991; Van Griensven et al. 1989). Over 500 000 tests from STD clinics across the United States suggested declines in HIV prevalence among gay and bisexual men, and among heterosexual men and women in Whites, with stability in African-Americans and heterosexual IDUs, from 1988-1992 (Weinstock et al. 1995). By 1991 the European Centre for the Epidemiological Monitoring of AIDS (1994) also noticed "signs of levelling off in the incidence of AIDS among IDUs" which had already occurred in homosexuals. The results of backcalculation exercises on AIDS incidence data also suggest similar HIV incidence trends (Brookmeyer and Gail 1994), and many surveys have documented substantial behaviour change in homosexuals over the last decade (CDC 1991; Morris, Dean 1994). Substantial declines have also been noted in HIV incidence among IDUs in some cities (WHO-EC Collaborating Centre 1994; Robert et al. 1990), though trends are less consistent (Edlin et al. 1994). These quantitative trends may be associated with qualitative changes in transmission patterns, and increases at lower levels of infection to heterosexuals (Mertens et al. 1995).

The major question is whether this decline in HIV risk will be passed on to younger generations, and some behavioural studies have observed a relapse to unsafe sex in young gay men (Adib et al. 1991; Osmond 1993). Increases in the median number of sex partners, sex episodes and unprotected oral and anal intercourse were observed in a cohort of gays aged 18-24 in New York (Dean and Meyer 1995). Continued high HIV incidence in young homosexual men in London in contrast to substantial declines in those aged over 30 was also observed (Miller et al. 1995). Results of backcalculation on AIDS data also suggest a decline in the median age at HIV infection from 30 to 25 (Rosenberg et al. 1994), and birth cohort analysis showed diffusion of infection to younger birth cohorts in New York (Stoneburner et al. 1993). Secondly will HIV prevalence levels in IDUs in the United States maintain high levels (Friedman et al. 1994; Mertens et al. 1995), and become increasingly associated with heterosexual transmission particularly to females? (Edlin et al. 1994). While the estimated trajectory around the 1990 estimate can be viewed with confidence, the future trajectory is more uncertain.

Sex and age distributions

A majority (80-85 per cen)t of reported AIDS cases occur in men, though women appear to have a higher proportion of cases transmitted heterosexually. The age distributions vary, due to the younger age of AIDS cases among IDU compared to homosexuals, though both Western Europe and the United States show an extended age distribution into older ages over 40 years old (see Figure 6). The increased risk of heterosexual transmission among women is partly due to the link between IDU and sex for money or drugs, but largely because the majority of people already infected are men. Among homosexuals there is some evidence of declining HIV incidence in groups exposed to HIV for 10 years, despite continued infection levels in younger age groups, either due to behaviour change not being sustained in this age group or because it is at younger ages that susceptibles not already infected move into HIV risk. Overall the sex and age distributions closely reflect transmission characteristics, with cases in homosexuals being slightly older, and males predominating in HIV transmission among homosexuals and IDU.

India, China, Other Asia and Islands

Infection patterns and data quality

Asia (India, China, and OAI) represents the largest concentration of HIV infection outside SSA, with over 4.5 million cumulative and over 4 million prevalent HIV infections. Over 90 per cent of these are concentrated in South and South East Asia. The onset of HIV epidemics in the region is estimated for this study as 1987 (Un-eklabh et al. 1988, Kitayaporn et al. 1993, Indian Council of Medical Research 1988), and is considerably later than other regions. In Thailand HIV prevalence was first measured at 1 per cent among IDUs in Bangkok clinics in 1987 (Unedklabh and Phutiprawn 1988), and in India it was first identified in sex workers in Madras and nearby cities in 1986 (Simoes et al. 1987), in blood donors in 1987 (John et al. 1989) and in IDUs in Manipur state in 1989 (Pavri 1990). In some of the more populous countries, for example China, it is not clear whether the onset of epidemic growth has emerged yet (Zhang et al. 1993). The potential for very rapid growth in HIV prevalence, for example in Rayong, Thailand from 0-10 per cent among pregnant women between 1990 and 1993 (Brown et al. 1994), the size of the region's population of 2.7 billion, and the early stage of the epidemic, has made Asia a major focus for concern and prevention.

Many countries have not yet or have only recently established AIDS case surveillance, and the 28 630 reported AIDS cases represent under 10 per cent of the over 300 000 AIDS cases estimated by WHO. HIV prevalence studies are particularly important to measure changes in the early stages of the epidemic, but while there were 83 peer reviewed HIV studies in South Asia for the period 1990-4, large populations are not well covered; for example, only 2 rural and 1 urban studies were recorded for China in 1990 (Table 4).

For the global burden of disease study the region is subdivided into India, China and 'Other Asia and islands'. Despite Thailand representing the most severe epidemic, India's population size means it contributes the most HIV infections. Overall the development of the epidemic in China and India has been particularly unclear, and countries in Other Asia and Islands show the potential for widespread infection in the region. The trajectory of HIV prevalence can change rapidly, and constitutes much of the uncertainty in global estimates and forecasts.

The major concern has been the predominance of heterosexual transmission in the region, accounting for 75 per cent of reported AIDS cases in Thailand and India. This may be connected to specific transmission characteristics, namely contact with sex workers, though HIV prevalence in pregnant women in Thailand also reached 1.7 per cent by 1994 (Mertens et al. 1995). Consequently HIV infection in children is also important, accounting for 8.4 per cent of reported AIDS cases in Thailand, and is likely to increase as the epidemic evolves.

IDU present a serious transmission risk, with 35 per cent HIV prevalence in IDU in Thailand and 38 per cent in India (Brown et al. 1994; Jain et al. 1994), though the limited size of the population of drug users results in them contributing under 10 per cent to total AIDS cases. The high HIV prevalences in urban high risk groups in India, sex workers, IDUs and STD clinics, are in contrast to much lower prevalences in the general population (see Figure 5). Longitudinal studies in south India provide evidence of increasing HIV prevalence, from 1 to 8.5 per cent in STD patients in Madras (1986-9 to 1991-2), and sentinel surveillance in March 1994 has established HIV prevalence rates among pregnant women of 2.5 per cent in Bombay, 0.7 per cent in Pune, and 0.8 per cent in Rajasthan (Bushaur et al. 1995; Mertens et al. 1995). In Malaysia 80 per cent of HIV infections are among IDUs, though in Viet Nam and Cambodia HIV is also spreading heterosexually, with for example HIV prevalence in blood donors (representing the general population) increasing to 3.5 per cent in Phnom Penh by 1994. There are therefore countries throughout the region with increasing HIV prevalence, and the point 1990 DALY estimate in this chapter should be interpreted in the context of these period trends.

Position on the epidemic curve

All the Asian epidemics are assumed to be at an early position on the HIV epidemic curve, with rapidly increasing HIV incidence past the 1990 estimate until at least the year 2000. A gamma value of 5 and position of 180 are used for "Other Asia and Islands" and for India, and a gamma value of 3 and position of 152 for China due to its slower rate of epidemic growth (gamma of 3) and later onset in 1989. There is therefore very high HIV incidence associated with the HIV prevalence estimate in 1990, with a ratio of under 1:3. This increasing trend in HIV incidence fits the 1990-4 pattern and 1994 estimate satisfactorily (see Table 7). Forecasts beyond

3-5 years are very uncertain until better data on India and China are forthcoming.

The spread of HIV infection in the region has occurred in a number of lagged waves which have yet to be completed — within countries where Brown et al. (1994) describe infection in Thailand rising in IDU then sex workers, then clients of sex workers, then wives and girlfriends of clients, and then to paediatric infection; and between countries with a lagged increase in HIV prevalence among blood donors between Thailand, Viet Nam and Cambodia. The major uncertainty is whether and to what levels this pattern will continue given the extensive heterosexual spread to India and China.

Figure 10 shows that HIV has spread to alarmingly high levels in sex workers and STD clinic attendees in some Indian cities, increasing rapidly through 1990. Table 9 summarizes HIV prevalence data, suggesting low levels of heterosexual transmission in the general population in India and China at present, but increasing trends in Indian cities with 2.5 per cent prevalence among pregnant women in Bombay. Recent evidence suggested 45 per cent HIV prevalence in sex workers and 21 per cent in males attending STD clinics in Pune, India, but also 13 per cent in monogamous, married women attending the STD clinics, providing some evidence of spread to other risk groups (Rodrigues et al. 1995). In China there has been an increase in reported STDs in recent years but these still remain at very low rates, and high HIV prevalence in IDUs in Yunnin province contiguous with south east Asia have been reported (Zhang 1991, Mertens et al. 1994). Reported data from large samples in China suggested very low HIV prevalence even in sex workers and STD patients, although the data generally refer to 1990-92. There is therefore much uncertainty as to the future trends in China and India, but evidence of increasing HIV prevalence in sex workers and more recently among pregnant women in India suggests that the assumption of a rapidly increasing trend around the 1990 estimate may not be unreasonable.

The second important question is whether signs of the success of interventions in defined groups in Thailand can be repeated and affect the trajectory of the epidemic. The Thai HIV-control programme established in 1989 has been associated with a reported increase in the use of condoms in commercial sex from 14 to 94 per cent (1989-93), and a decline in the cases of the five major STDs in men reported to public STD clinics by 79 per cent (Hanenberg et al. 1994). A modest decline in STDs treated by quinolones began from 1986, and the opening of new clinics, some outside the public sector, may affect STD trends (see Chapter 1 in this volume). Recently a decline in HIV incidence has been measured among sex workers (Sawanpanyalert et al. 1994), and from 3.4 to 0.87 per 100 person-years among army conscripts in Northern Thailand (Khanboonruang et al. 1994).

The association of declining HIV prevalence with public health interventions requires evaluation (Mastro and Limpakarnjanarat 1995), and

Figure 10 HIV prevalence in India, 1986–93

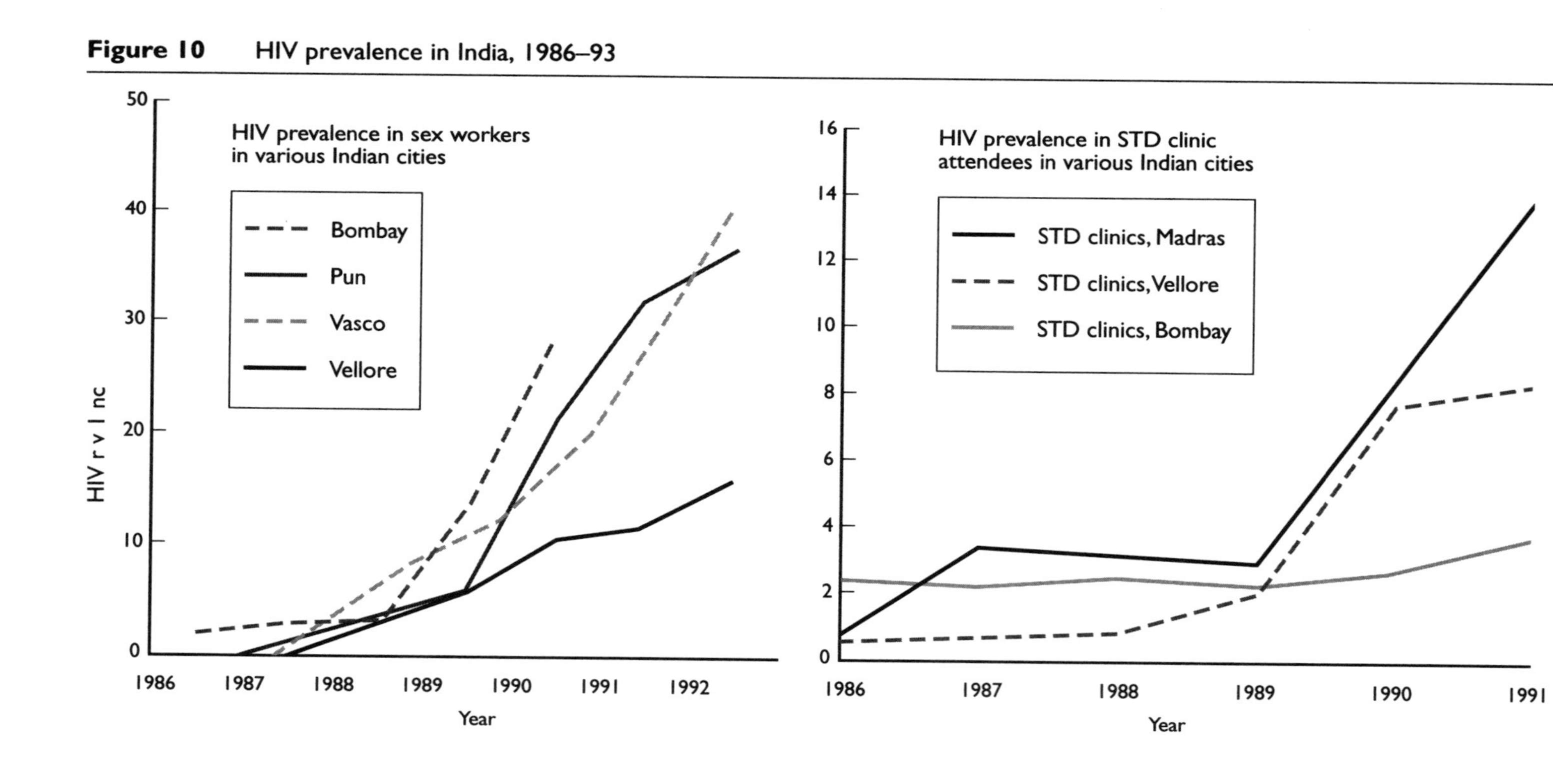

Source: Jain et al 1994

Table 9 HIV prevalence in India and China

Country		*Year*	*Group*	*HIV Prevalence*	*Reference*
India					
	Bombay	1987–88	Sex workers	1.1%	Bhave et al. 1992
		1992	Sex workers	41.2%	Bhave et al. 1992
		1986–92	ANC	1%	Joshi et al. 1992
		1994	ANC	2.5%	Mertens et al. 1995
	Rajasthan	1994	ANC	0.8%	Mertens et al. 1995
	Pune	1994	ANC	0.7%	Mertens et al. 1995
	Gujurat	1992	Blood donors	0.1%	Mertens et al. 1995
	Madras	1991–92	Blood donors	0.35%	Ravinathan et al. 1992
	New Delhi	1992	Blood donors	0.2%	Nanu et al. 1992
	Manipur	1991–92	ANC	0.2%	Ibotomba and Brajachand 1992
China					
	Sichuan	1992	High risk	0.04%	Zhang et al. 1993
	Sichuan	1992	Sex workers	0%	Zhang et al. 1993
	Longchuan	1992	IDU	45%	Zhang et al. 1993
	Ruili county	1989–90	IDU	23%	Zhang 1991
		1990	Blood donors	0%	Zeng 1992
		1990	Sex workers and STD patients	0%	Zeng 1992
		1990	Homosexuals	1%	Zeng 1992

Note: ANC = ante-natal clinic patients

some studies have suggested low rates of consistent condom use among commercial sex workers (Morris et al. 1995). Perhaps the most compelling evidence is the recently reported declines in HIV prevalence in army entry recruits aged 21 by 25 per cent nationwide, in all regions with declines evident in both rural and urban areas, and at all educational levels (Mason et al. 1995). HIV prevalence among these young cohorts aged 21 is a good indicator of recent HIV incidence since the onset of public health interventions.

HIV incidence among IDUs in Bangkok began to decline by 1991-92 (Kitayaporn et al. 1993), but HIV prevalence among pregnant women has increased throughout the country to a mean of 1.7 per cent in mid-1994, although there are signs of stability in several regions from mid-1993 (Brown et al. 1994). The speed of these changes has surprised many, but their impact on national or sub-continental trends is unclear, and until further data are available HIV incidence in all three GBD regions in Asia is assumed to be rapidly increasing from 1990 beyond 2000.

The potential for rapid heterosexual spread in South Asia has been demonstrated in Thailand despite some evidence that HIV incidence has peaked (Brown et al. 1994). The future trajectory of the HIV epidemic for Asia as well as globally depends on whether and to what level the waves of heterosexual transmission in Asia will continue to some of the most populous countries in the world including China, India, Indonesia and Bangladesh. For the GBD estimate, however, and for the trajectory around the 1990 estimate which can be assumed to be rising rapidly, these uncertainties are less important.

Sex and age distributions

Due to the predominance of heterosexual transmission, it was estimated for the GBD study that 35 per cent of HIV incidence occurs among females in India and Other Asia and Islands (see Table 7). However distinct transmission patterns related to a restricted number of sex workers and a larger number of male clients may mean the proportion of female infections is lower. Fifteen per cent of reported AIDS cases in Thailand in 1994 were among females (see Figure 5) clustering at similar levels obserevd in Europe and the United States. However if the waves of infection continue from sex worker clients to their wives and girlfriends, the proportion of HIV incidence in females could increase, with AIDS cases following later. In China, evidence of HIV infection is predominantly among male IDU, and only 12.7 per cent of incidence in 1990 is estimated to occur among females, though direct data are lacking. The age distribution of AIDS cases in Thailand is young, with a peak in females in the 20-24 and 25-29 year age groups with males five years older, similar to the curves for Uganda and Ethiopia. The three regions comprising Asia are estimated to have the highest proportion of HIV incidence of all regions in the 15-44 age group (94 per cent). This is partly because child cases do not yet constitute more than 1 per cent of HIV incidence, though they will certainly increase. For example, as Figure 5 shows, 8.4 per cent of reported AIDS cases in Thailand occur in children.

Formerly Socialist Economies of Europe (FSE)

Countries in this region account for 50 000 cumulative and around 50 000 prevalent HIV infections. The reporting of HIV and AIDS was scant before the social and political changes of the late 1980s, though routes of HIV transmission were apparent in retrospect, including the tragic nosocomial hospital-based transmission of HIV to children in Elista (former USSR) and Romania, which dominated reported HIV and AIDS case totals up to 1990 (Rudin et al. 1990). The onset of the HIV epidemic for this study is estimated to be late compared to other regions, starting in 1988 (Medvedev 1990). There has been rapid growth in estimated HIV infections from 10652 in 1990 to 20000 in 1991 to 50000 in 1995, but these still remain at a low level compared to other regions. High HIV prevalence rates appear concentrated in groups with risk behaviours. For example, 46 per cent of all cases were reported in IDUs in Poland in 1993 (Stark and Wirth 1994). This study therefore uses a low estimate of 12.7 per cent of HIV incidence among females in 1990. This, together with the early stage of the epidemic, results in a comparatively low HIV incidence estimate of 0.3 per cent among children, despite the publicised cases in Romania.

For the GBD estimates it has been assumed that HIV prevalence in 1990 was at low levels but is increasing at a modest rate (gamma = 3) from the 1990 estimate, and is at an early stage on the epidemic curve with a position of 190. This is based on data shown below suggesting firstly that HIV prevalence is at low levels in the general population, and secondly that there may have been some modest increases following the political changes of the early 1990s. These social and political changes have made it difficult to maintain the continuity of disease surveillance, though for some diseases surveillance was of a high standard (Baroyan et al. 1977). HIV spread could change rapidly, but a number of widespread disease studies have confirmed low levels of infection in the general populations. Despite problems of selection bias, the largest HIV survey to date involving several million HIV tests carried out in the Russian Federation in 1992, identified less than 100 positive tests.

HIV prevalence among STD clinic attendees was less than 0.1 per cent in studies from 1991-93 in the Czech Republic, Bulgaria, Azerbaijan, Lithuania, the Slovak Republic and the Ukraine (WHO-EC Collaborating Centre 1994). The cumulative reported AIDS case rates in 1994 are an order of magnitude lower than in Western Europe, except in Romania which has similar levels to Sweden (WHO-EC Collaborating Centre, 1994). AIDS case rates should be treated with caution due to the lower rates of reporting in Eastern compared to Western Europe, and as they do not reflect the most recent trends of HIV incidence.

From this low rate there are some indications of increases: for example HIV prevalence by mass screening in 1993 in St. Petersberg was double that of the previous five years largely due to heterosexual transmission (Kozlov et al. 1994), and rates of syphilis and gonorrhoea have been increasing in the Russian Federation since 1990 (Chaika 1993; Mertens et al. 1995). A major uncertainty is whether the social and political turmoil and increased international mobility will lead to increased HIV infection, but there is only evidence at present for modest increases at rates considerably lower than Western Europe.

Middle Eastern Crescent (MEC)

The countries of the Middle Eastern Crescent region account for over 200000 cumulative and 150000 prevalent HIV infections. For the GBD study we estimated the onset of epidemic spread from 1986. There is evidence of low levels of HIV infection at this date, for example 0.49 per cent among IDUs in Egypt in 1986-7 (Woody et al. 1988), 3.8 per cent among homosexuals in Morocco (Benslimane et al. 1987), and 1.9 per cent among sex workers in Tunisia (Giraldo et al. 1988). Surveillance data are not available for many countries in the region. The estimate of 200 000

Table 10 Distribution of HIV incidence by sex, age and region, 1990

Sex Distribution Of HIV Incidence			*Age Distribution Of HIV Incidence (%)*				
			Age group Years				
Region	Female %	Evidence	0-4	5–14	15–44	45–59	60+
EME	18	Majority of infection in risk groups. Female % AIDS cases 15–20%.	2.00	0	89.21	8.05	0.72
FSE	12.5	Majority of infection in risk groups similar to Europe.	0	0	87.50	12.50	0.00
IND	35	High HIV prevalence in sex workers and STD clinics. Low but increasing levels in pregnant women.	1	0	94.1	3.78	1.12
CHN	12.7	Infection associated with IDU.	0	0	100	0.00	0.00
OAI	35	Infection associated with sex workersand their clients, HIV prevalence in pregnant women increasing to1–4%.	0	0	95.51	3.37	1.12
SSA	50	General population heterosexual transmission. Female % HIV prevalence and AIDS cases 50–60%.	10.63	0.56	85.82	2.71	0.28
LAC	23	Majority of infection in risk groups, with some heterosexual epidemics, female % AIDS cases increasing, 8–23%.	1.75	0	92.54	5.26	0.44
MEC	16	Little information, but HIV prevalence in risk groups.	1	0	91	8.00	0.00

HIV infections is uncertain, particularly as only 1039 AIDS cases have been reported. Despite problems of AIDS surveillance, a considerable number of reviewed HIV prevalence studies have been recorded, 40 from 1990–4 for North Africa (U.S. Bureau of the Census). Most of these are from four countries, Egypt, Tunisia, Morocco and Sudan.

HIV prevalence is, as expected, concentrated in groups with high risk behaviours: for example 1.2 per cent was reported among STD patients in 1991 in Morocco (Rihad et al. 1992), 4 per cent among truck drivers in Sudan (Ahmed and Kheir 1990), and 1.8 per cent among sex workers in Tunisia (Giraldo et al. 1988). For the GBD study, we estimated that 15 per cent of 1990 HIV incidence was in women, with 91 per cent of HIV incidence concentrated at ages 15–44 and 8 per cent extending into age groups 45–59. The GBD study assumes a relatively late position of 230 (considering the date of onset of 1986) on the epidemic curve, but HIV incidence is increasing modestly past the 1990 estimate (gamma of 3). This was based on the low levels of HIV infection in the general population, concentrated in risk groups, but with the potential for HIV transmission as exhibited in neighbouring countries. Most HIV prevalence studies in the general population show very low HIV prevalence, for example 0.01 per cent among blood donors in Morocco (El Alaqui et al. 1993), 0.08 per cent in Sudan (Ahmed and Kheir 1990), and no infection among 1030 ANC attendees in Tunisia (Ben Salem et al. 1993). However bordering countries show substantial HIV prevalence. For example, in Niamey, Niger prevalence was 1.3 per cent in pregnant women, 3.4 per cent in truck drivers and 15.4 per cent in STD patients (Hassane et al. 1993). A major question is whether HIV infection from the severe epidemics in nearby countries will spread to MEC, and why this has not already happened. The HIV epidemic has a low priority in many of these countries, and it is difficult to validate the 1990 estimate or provide forecasts without additional surveillance data.

Estimation of DALYs due to HIV

Summary of the method to estimate HIV incidence

The focus of this chapter has been to draw together data and information on the HIV epidemic to provide as accurate estimates of HIV incidence for 1990 as possible. Estimates of HIV incidence are then followed along the incubation period to establish patterns of morbidity and mortality. This estimation process is in Figure 8 illustrated based on calculations completed by the Botswana national AIDS control programme.

Parameters used for HIV estimation

All the inputs required for the global burden of disease estimates are presented in Table 7. They consist of the HIV prevalence estimates, the parameters used in the forecasting model, and how resulting HIV incidence is distributed by age and sex. The beginning year of the epidemic is based on evidence of the onset of significant HIV spread discussed in the previous regional descriptions. The regions divide into two groupings, firstly those with evidence of HIV spread already apparent when an AIDS surveillance definition was introduced in 1982 and an HIV test was developed in 1984, and further supported by the retrospective testing of stored blood (Nzilambi et al. 1988). Epidemic onset in North America and SSA is estimated to date around the late 1970s (Nzilambi et al., 1988; N'Galy and Ryder 1988; Morvan et al. 1989), and in LAC and Europe to the early 1980s (Pradinaud et al. 1989), with for example no evidence of infection in European blood product recipients prior to 1981. These epidemics have later positions on the gamma curve than in other regions, particularly the United States and Europe (538 and 345), though LAC and SSA have positions of 261 and 271 as HIV incidence is estimated to peak later.

Secondly, there are those epidemics with later onset or without signs of growth at present, the most significant being India and OAI with estimated onset in 1987 and still at early positions of 180 on the gamma curve.

These have a higher gamma value of 5 than the less quickly developing epidemics of the FSE, MEC and China which have a gamma value of 3. The evidence for these choices has been discussed previously, but includes the rapid rise in HIV prevalence reported in Thailand and Viet Nam (Brown et al. 94), and lower levels of HIV prevalence reported in the general populations in China, the Russian Federation, Tunisia and Morocco (Zeng 1992, Ben Salem et al. 1993). Although the estimation of HIV prevalence cannot be reduced to a systematic measure, for example the mean of HIV prevalence studies for the region, once a regional HIV prevalence is established all parameters are provided to allow the reproduction of the global burden of disease results.

Epidemiological data on mortality have been used by the authors to derive a first set of regional mortality estimates. When considered in conjunction with mortality estimates proposed by other authors for other diseases and injuries in the GBD study, the implied level of overall mortality usually exceeded the rate estimated by various demographic methods. In order not to exceed this upper bound for mortality within each age-sex and broad-cause group, an algorithm has been applied by the editors to reduce mortality estimates for specific conditions so that their sum did not exceed this upper bound. The algorithm has been described in more detail in *The Global Burden of Disease* (Murray and Lopez 1996).

Depending on the condition under study, epidemiological data may be available for incidence, prevalence, case-fatality or mortality. Where data on more than one of these parameters are available, estimates of each of the epidemiological parameters derived from the data may not be internally consistent or consistent with the adjusted mortality rates described above. To ensure that all epidemiological information concerning a given condition is internally consistent, the editors have undertaken extensive analyses using computer models of the natural history of disease described in Murray and Lopez (1996). The incidence, prevalence, and duration estimates have consequently been revised where necessary. In view of these adjustments to the basic epidemiological estimates originally provided for the Global Burden of Disease Study, the data presented in the following tables which have undergone the GBD validation process are the joint responsibility of the authors and the editors.

The majority of HIV incidence in all the regions occurs in the 15-44 year age group. The proportion in the 0-14 year age group depends largely on the female prevalence level and the maturity of the epidemic. HIV incidence in the 45-59 year age group results from the older mean age of the general population for example in North America, Europe and FSE, and infection in homosexuals who have an older mean age at infection. The proportion of HIV incidence in females is highest in epidemics with heterosexual transmission, being 50 per cent in SSA, and 35 per cent in India and OAI. Evidence for the estimates in these latter two regions include: over 75 per cent of AIDS cases in India and Thailand result from heterosexual transmission, though this may be linked to contact with sex workers. Conversely, only 15 per cent of reported AIDS cases occur among females in Thailand. The proportions of AIDS cases in females in Uganda, Zambia, Europe, the United States and Brazil for 1994 are also consistent with the 1990 HIV incidence ratios for their regions. However the steady increase in cases among females in some countries and the lag between HIV incidence and AIDS cases should be appreciated.

Validation of Estimates

Finally although the choice of inputs are supported by regional characteristics and individual studies, continual validation of projections against empirical data and estimates is essential. As a projection model is used for HIV prevalence, incidence and AIDS, the 1990 estimates can be validated against HIV prevalence for any nearby year. Such a validation exercise for the SSA regional estimate is shown in Table 7, which represents the majority of HIV infections worldwide. This involved reviewing all HIV prevalence studies and population estimates for countries with significant HIV infection for 1992, and producing HIV estimates by urban and rural regions country by country. These were then aggregated resulting in a 1992 regional estimate of 6,819,392 prevalent infections. This was within 7 per cent of the 1992 projections of 6,381,822, based on the 1990 regional estimates and parameters.

Formally to verify the GBD 1990 estimates and short term trend, projections for 1994 were produced and compared to a country estimation process for 1994. HIV prevalence studies were reviewed by country, and country by country estimates were produced. These were aggregated to provide 1994 regional estimates. Estimates for 1994 were also projected from *Epimodel* based on the 1990 estimates and epidemic curves used for the GBD study.

The exercise suggested that overall the estimates and parameters used for the GBD exercise were consistent with HIV prevalence estimates based on available data for 1994. For LAC, the GBD estimate and trend appears to overestimate 1994 HIV prevalence, and it may be underestimated in Africa. Divergence of the forecasts from the 1990 estimates is expected after 3-5 years, and the higher 1994 estimates for SSA are particularly sensitive to the extent that we have assumed thatsentinel surveillance in pregnant women in South Africa and Nigeria represent the general popu-

Table 11 Disability weights for HIV and AIDS, for treated and untreated individuals, by sex and age group

	Age group (years)				
	0–4	5–14	15–44	45–59	60+
HIV cases	0.123	0.123	0.136	0.136	0.136
AIDS	0.505	0.505	0.505	0.505	0.505

lation. The estimate for SSA for 1990 is less affected by these countries, and the second validation exercise for SSA for 1992 (Table 7) suggested the GBD estimates and trajectory.

Given the many limitations, there are some regions where we are less confident in our estimates. We are most confident in estimates for North America, Europe and SSA, have medium confidence for LAC, Other Asia and FSE and low confidence for MEC, India and China. Of estimates with low confidence, India is the most significant uncertainty, representing 11 per cent of total estimated 1990 HIV incidence. For 1990, regions for which we have lower confidence may not contribute a substantial proportion of total HIV incidence, but their importance has been growing quickly with time. Overall the regions with high confidence accounted for 67 per cent of HIV incidence in 1990, regions with medium confidence 20 per cent, and regions with low confidence 13 per cent. The regions with low confidence in the estimates may have represented 32 per cent of estimated HIV incidence by 1995, and improved surveillance of HIV will be required particularly in India and China.

Tables of results of disease estimation

Table 11 shows the disability weights by sex and age group for treated and untreated chronic HIV infection and AIDS which were used to calculate DALYs by region for HIV in the Global Burden of Disease (Murray and Lopez 1996).

Tables 12–13 present all the basic disease estimates required for the global burden study. Briefly these are:

1. HIV incidence by region, sex and age.
2. The average age at onset of HIV infection.
3. The duration of the two stages of chronic and AIDS-related morbidity.
4. The percentage developing a disability at each stage.
5. The mortality rate by the end of the disease process, which for HIV in this study is 100 per cent.

Further considerations in calculating the burden of HIV

Uncertainty still surrounds the current and future course and impact of the epidemic, although there may be more surveillance data on HIV prevalence and AIDS cases than for most other diseases. Nevertheless, the HIV epidemic may be particularly difficult to calculate due to:

1. The indirect causation of morbidity and mortality through secondary diseases
2. The epidemic pattern of changing HIV incidence
3. The asymptomatic nature of the majority of HIV infections

4. The rapid and long lasting build up of HIV prevalence after HIV incidence
5. The series of secondary impacts which an infection creates epidemiologically, and in the economic and social structure of communities

Epidemic and endemic patterns of disease incidence

HIV infections have increased from zero to 15-16 million in 15 years, and HIV incidence rates vary considerably geographically and over time: in some regions incidence may have peaked and declined slightly, for example in the United States and Europe, while it is in an early stage of rapid growth in HIV incidence in other regions, for example in Asia. If underlying HIV incidence is changing over a period, how do DALYs in 1990 represent the public health priority of HIV? How does this compare to endemic diseases which may have more stable disease incidence? The two diagrams in Figure 11 compare one million infections distributed according to a stable, disease incidence and for a theoretical HIV incidence curve. The table illustrates disease incidence and point DALY values A, B, C comparing them to the average period values. It also shows the estimated future loss of life from a point HIV prevalence. For an epidemic and endemic disease with the same overall incidence, what do we learn from the DALYs at points A, B and C and how do they relate to the period value A-C ?

If successive estimates where taken at time A and C the burden of the epidemic disease would be evaluated to be smaller than that of endemic disease and vice-versa at point B. Important considerations occur on the upslope, where DALYs at point A would give little warning of the importance of interventions to prevent rapidly increasing incidence. The public health priority to prevent the burden of HIV may be greatest from years two to five, where its DALY value is lowest. Similarly on the downslope, the importance of the epidemic disease may be overestimated.

The table shows that a point value for a stable, endemic disease gives a good measure of the period experience from A-C, but this is not captured for an epidemic disease at A, B or C. The prevalence burden of HIV, related closely to the mortality it causes, increases throughout the period, and peaks beyond C, when DALYs are once again low. An important consideration for HIV is to project DALYs over the course when the epidemic is evolving. This is particularly significant as HIV prevalence can change rapidly, for example in Thailand it increased from 0 per cent to 10.53 per cent over the period 1990-93 in antenatal clinics in Rayong and from 1.9 per cent to 8 per cent in Chiang Mai (Brown et al. 1994), and in blood donors in Gonder, Ethiopia from 3.85 per cent to 16 per cent from 1989 to 1993. Furthermore direct empirical measurement of changes in HIV incidence are usually unavailable, and public health responses can be misguided if they rely solely on point measures of HIV infection or DALYs.

Table 12 Epidemiological estimates for HIV cases, 1990, *males*

Age group (years)	*Incidence* Number ('000s)	Rate per100 000	*Prevalence* Number ('000s)	Rate per100 000	*Avg. age at onset* (years)	*Avg. duration* (years)	*Deaths* Number ('000s)	Rate per100 000	*YLDs* Number ('000s)	Rate per100 000
	Established Market Economies									
0-4	1	4.60	3	10.10	0.0	4.0	0	0.00	1	2
5-14	0	0.20	0	0.50	13.0	10.0	0	0.00	0	1
15-44	102	55.70	1 012	550.10	30.0	10.0	0	0.00	243	132
45-59	9	13.60	89	134.10	52.0	10.0	0	0.00	20	30
60+	1	1.30	8	12.80	68.0	10.0	0	0.00	2	3
All Ages	*114*	*29.1*	*1 112*	*284.7*	*31.7*	*9.9*	*0*	*0*	*265*	*68*
	Formerly Socialist Economies of Europe									
0-4	0	0.20	1	3.60	0.0	2.0	0	0.00	0	0
5-14	0	0.00	0	0.40	13.0	7.0	0	0.00	0	0
15-44	6	8.20	9	11.20	30.0	7.0	0	0.00	8	10
45-59	1	2.00	1	2.80	52.0	7.0	0	0.00	0	2
60+	0	0.20	0	0.30	68.0	7.0	0	0.00	0	0
All Ages	*7*	*4.2*	*10*	*6*	*31.9*	*7.0*	*0*	*0*	*9*	*5*
	India									
0-4	0	0.80	1	0.80	0.0	2.0	0	0.00	0	0
5-14	0	0.20	0	0.30	13.0	7.0	0	0.00	0	0
15-44	108	53.80	183	91.40	30.0	7.0	0	0.00	135	67
45-59	6	12.20	10	20.60	52.0	7.0	0	0.00	5	11
60+	2	5.80	3	9.90	68.0	7.0	0	0.00	1	3
All Ages	*116*	*26.4*	*197*	*44.8*	*31.5*	*7.0*	*0*	*0*	*141*	*32*
	China									
0-4	0	0.00	0	0.00	0.0	2.0	0	0.00	0	0
5-14	0	0.00	0	0.00	13.0	7.0	0	0.00	0	0
15-44	2	0.70	2	0.70	30.0	7.0	0	0.00	3	1
45-59	0	0.20	0	0.20	52.0	7.0	0	0.00	0	0
60+	0	0.10	0	0.10	68.0	7.0	0	0.00	0	0
All Ages	*2*	*0.4*	*2*	*0.4*	*31.6*	*7.0*	*0*	*0*	*3*	*1*
	Other Asia and Islands									
0-4	0	0.60	0	0.60	0.0	2.0	0	0.00	0	0
5-14	0	0.10	0	0.10	13.0	7.0	0	0.00	0	0
15-44	54	33.60	78	48.50	30.0	7.0	0	0.00	68	42
45-59	3	8.50	4	12.20	52.0	7.0	0	0.00	2	7
60+	1	4.30	1	6.20	68.0	7.0	0	0.00	1	3
All Ages	*58*	*16.9*	*84*	*24.4*	*31.5*	*7.0*	*0*	*0*	*71*	*21*
	Sub-Saharan Africa									
0-4	57	119.70	114	240.00	0.0	2.0	0	0.00	5	11
5-14	1	1.40	7	10.00	13.0	7.0	0	0.00	3	5
15-44	460	442.90	2 401	2 314.00	30.0	7.0	0	0.00	644	621
45-59	16	77.80	157	771.00	52.0	7.0	0	0.00	18	90
60+	2	22.58	52	497.00	68.0	7.0	0	0.00	3	26
All Ages	*536*	*212.3*	*2 731*	*1082*	*27.7*	*6.5*	*0*	*0*	*674*	*267*

Table 12 (continued)

Age group (years)	Incidence		Prevalence		Avg. age at onset (years)	Avg. duration (years)	Deaths		YLDs	
	Number ('000s)	Rate per100 000	Number ('000s)	Rate per100 000			Number ('000s)	Rate per100 000	Number ('000s)	Rate per100 000
	Latin America and the Caribbean									
0-4	2	7.00	4	12.60	0.0	2.0	0	0.00	0	1
5-14	0	0.30	0	0.70	13.0	7.0	0	0.00	0	0
15-44	164	157.60	761	730.20	30.0	7.0	0	0.00	224	215
45-59	9	39.00	40	180.50	52.0	7.0	0	0.00	9	40
60+	0	2.40	2	11.30	68.0	7.0	0	0.00	1	5
All Ages	*176*	*79.2*	*807*	*364.2*	*30.8*	*6.9*	*0*	*0*	*234*	*106*
	Middle Eastern Crescent									
0-4	0	0.30	0	0.40	0.0	2.0	0	0.00	0	0
5-14	0	0.00	0	0.00	13.0	7.0	0	0.00	0	0
15-44	19	17.10	59	51.90	30.0	7.0	0	0.00	25	22
45-59	2	7.60	5	23.20	52.0	7.0	0	0.00	2	7
60+	0	0.90	0	3.30	68.0	7.0	0	0.00	0	1
All Ages	*21*	*8.4*	*65*	*25.3*	*31.8*	*7.0*	*0*	*0*	*27*	*10*
	Developed Regions									
0-4	1	2.49	4	9.96	0.0	3.3	0	0.0	1	2
5-14	0	0.00	0	0.00			0	0.0	0	0
15-44	108	41.48	1 021	392.18	30.0	9.6	0	0.0	251	96
45-59	10	10.74	90	96.66	52.0	8.8	0	0.0	20	22
60+	1	1.23	8	9.81	68.0	8.3	0	0.0	2	2
All Ages	*120*	*21.59*	*1 123*	*202.05*	*31.9*	*9.5*	*0*	*0.0*	*274*	*49*
	Developing Regions									
0-4	59	23.37	119	47.14	0	2	0	0.0	6	2
5-14	1	0.22	7	1.57	13	7	0	0.0	4	1
15-44	807	86.09	3 484	371.65	30	7	0	0.0	1 098	117
45-59	36	11.95	216	71.69	52	7	0	0.0	36	12
60+	5	3.44	58	39.90	68	7	0	0.0	5	3
All Ages	*908*	*48.39*	*3 884*	*207.01*	*29.1*	*6.7*	*0*	*0.0*	*1 149*	*61*
	World									
0-4	60	18.67	123	38.28	0.0	2.0	0	0.0	6	2
5-14	1	0.18	7	1.27	13.0	7.0	0	0.0	4	1
15-44	915	73.20	4 505	360.42	30.0	7.9	0	0.0	1 349	108
45-59	46	14.73	306	97.96	52.0	7.9	0	0.0	56	18
60+	6	2.74	66	30.16	68.0	7.4	0	0.0	7	3
All Ages	*1 028*	*38.74*	*5 007*	*188.68*	*29.4*	*7.5*	*0*	*0.0*	*1 423*	*54*

Table 12 Epidemiological estimates for HIV cases, 1990, *females*

Age group (years)	*Incidence* Number ('000s)	Rate per 100 000	*Prevalence* Number ('000s)	Rate per 100 000	*Avg. age at onset* (years)	*Avg. duration* (years)	*Deaths* Number ('000s)	Rate per 100 000	*YLDs* Number ('000s)	Rate per 100 000
	Established Market Economies									
0-4	1	4.80	3	10.70	0.0	4.0	0	0.00	1	2
5-14	0	0.20	0	0.80	13.0	10.0	0	0.00	0	1
15-44	22	12.50	178	99.10	30.0	10.0	0	0.00	49	27
45-59	1	1.70	10	15.30	52.0	10.0	0	0.00	2	3
60+	0	0.10	0	0.40	68.0	10.0	0	0.00	0	0
All Ages	*25*	*6.1*	*191*	*47*	*29.6*	*9.7*	*0*	*0*	*52*	*13*
	Formerly Socialist Economies of Europe									
0-4	0	0.20	1	3.80	0.0	2.0	0	0.00	0	0
5-14	0	0.00	0	0.40	13.0	7.0	0	0.00	0	0
15-44	1	1.30	1	1.70	30.0	7.0	0	0.00	1	2
45-59	0	0.20	0	0.20	52.0	7.0	0	0.00	0	0
60+	0	0.00	0	0.00	68.0	7.0	0	0.00	0	0
All Ages	*1*	*0.6*	*2*	*1.1*	*30.3*	*6.9*	*0*	*0*	*1*	*1*
	India									
0-4	0	0.80	1	0.90	0.0	2.0	0	0.00	0	0
5-14	0	0.30	0	0.40	13.0	7.0	0	0.00	0	0
15-44	61	33.30	64	34.70	30.0	7.0	0	0.00	76	42
45-59	1	1.40	1	2.10	52.0	7.0	0	0.00	1	1
60+	0	1.10	0	1.10	68.0	7.0	0	0.00	0	1
All Ages	*63*	*15.3*	*66*	*16*	*30.1*	*7.0*	*0*	*0*	*77*	*19*
	China									
0-4	0	0.00	0	0.00	0.0	2.0	0	0.00	0	0
5-14	0	0.00	0	0.00	13.0	7.0	0	0.00	0	0
15-44	0	0.10	0	0.10	3.0	7.0	0	0.00	0	0
45-59	0	0.00	0	0.00	52.0	7.0	0	0.00	0	0
60+	0	0.00	0	0.00	68.0	7.0	0	0.00	0	0
All Ages	*3*	*0.1*	*3*	*0.1*	*30.0*	*7.0*	*0*	*0*	*0*	*0*
	Other Asia and Islands									
0-4	0	0.60	0	0.70	0.0	2.0	0	0.00	0	0
5-14	0	0.20	0	0.20	13.0	7.0	0	0.00	0	0
15-44	31	19.10	41	25.80	30.0	7.0	0	0.00	38	24
45-59	0	0.90	0	1.20	52.0	7.0	0	0.00	0	1
60+	0	0.70	0	0.90	68.0	7.0	0	0.00	0	0
All Ages	*31*	*9.2*	*42*	*12.4*	*30.1*	*7.0*	*0*	*0*	*39*	*11*
	Sub-Saharan Africa									
0-4	57	120.90	114	243.00	0.0	2.0	0	0.00	5	12
5-14	5	6.90	11	15.00	13.0	7.0	0	0.00	7	10
15-44	460	432.50	2 432	2 289.00	30.0	7.0	0	0.00	647	609
45-59	13	60.60	130	590.00	52.0	7.0	0	0.00	15	67
60+	1	7.50	47	369.00	68.0	7.0	0	0.00	1	10
All Ages	*536*	*207.6*	*2 735*	*1 060*	*27.3*	*6.5*	*0*	*0*	*676*	*262*

Table 12 (continued)

Age group (years)	Incidence Number ('000s)	Incidence Rate per100 000	Prevalence Number ('000s)	Prevalence Rate per100 000	Avg. age at onset (years)	Avg. duration (years)	Deaths Number ('000s)	Deaths Rate per100 000	YLDs Number ('000s)	YLDs Rate per100 000
	Latin America and the Caribbean									
0-4	2	7.30	4	13.10	0.0	2.0	0	0.00	0	1
5-14	0	0.50	0	0.90	13.0	7.0	0	0.00	0	1
15-44	47	44.80	193	185.40	30.0	7.0	0	0.00	62	60
45-59	3	12.90	8	34.80	52.0	7.0	0	0.00	3	12
60+	1	3.00	2	12.10	68.0	7.0	0	0.00	0	2
All Ages	*52*	*23.5*	*207*	*93*	*30.4*	*6.8*	*0*	*0*	*66*	*30*
	Middle Eastern Crescent									
0-4	0	0.30	0	0.40	0.0	2.0	0	0.00	0	0
5-14	0	0.00	0	0.00	13.0	7.0	0	0.00	0	0
15-44	3	3.10	9	8.80	30.0	7.0	0	0.00	4	4
45-59	0	0.90	1	2.50	52.0	7.0	0	0.00	0	1
60+	0	0.00	0	0.10	68.0	7.0	0	0.00	0	0
All Ages	*4*	*1.5*	*10*	*4.1*	*30.3*	*7.0*	*0*	*0*	*4*	*2*
	Developed Regions									
0-4	1	2.62	4	10.47	0.0	3.3	0	0.0	1	2
5-14	0	0.00	0	0.00			0	0.0	0	0
15-44	23	9.05	179	70.43	30.0	9.7	0	0.0	50	20
45-59	1	1.02	10	10.22	52.0	8.3	0	0.0	2	2
60+	0	0.00	0	0.00			0	0.0	0	0
All Ages	*25*	*3.85*	*193*	*29.69*	*29.7*	*9.4*	*0*	*0.0*	*54*	*8*
	Developing Regions									
0-4	59	21.77	119	43.90	0	2	0	0.0	6	2
5-14	5	1.11	11	2.45	13	7	0	0.0	8	2
15-44	602	63.74	2 739	290.00	30	7	0	0.0	829	88
45-59	17	7.97	140	65.65	52	7	0	0.0	19	9
60+	2	1.35	49	33.05	68	7	0	0.0	2	1
All Ages	*685*	*33.82*	*3 058*	*150.98*	*27.9*	*6.6*	*0*	*0.0*	*863*	*43*
	World									
0-4	60	19.40	123	39.77	0.0	2.0	0	0.0	6	2
5-14	5	0.95	11	2.09	13.0	7.0	0	0.0	8	2
15-44	625	52.14	2 918	243.44	30.0	7.3	0	0.0	879	73
45-59	18	5.79	150	48.22	52.0	7.2	0	0.0	21	7
60+	2	0.74	49	18.20	68.0	7.0	0	0.0	2	1
All Ages	*710*	*27.16*	*3 251*	*124.38*	*28.0*	*6.9*	*0*	*0.0*	*917*	*35*

Table 13 Epidemiological Estimates for HIV-AIDS, 1990, *males*

Age group (years)	Incidence Number ('000s)	Incidence Rate per 100 000	Prevalence Number ('000s)	Prevalence Rate per 100 000	Avg. age at onset (years)	Avg. duration (years)	Deaths Number ('000s)	Deaths Rate per 100 000	DALYs Number ('000s)	DALYs Rate per 100 000
	Established Market Economies									
0-4	1	3.00	1	4.60	2.5	2.0	0.0	2	13	52
5-14	0	0.20	0	0.30	10.0	2.0	0.0	0	3	6
15-44	51	27.50	82	44.30	35.0	2.0	25.0	14	156	87
45-59	10	15.10	16	24.40	57.0	2.0	9.0	13	16	24
60+	2	3.10	3	5.00	73.0	2.0	2.0	3	3	4
All Ages	*63*	*16.3*	*102*	*26.1*	*39.2*	*2.0*	*36.0*	*9*	*191*	*47*
	Formerly Socialist Economies of Europe									
0-4	0	2.50	0	2.80	1.5	0.5	0.0	2	10	76
5-14	0	0.20	0	0.20	10.0	1.0	0.0	0	2	8
15-44	0	0.30	0	0.30	33.5	1.0	0.0	0	3	4
45-59	0	0.10	0	0.10	55.5	1.0	0.0	0	0	0
60+	0	0.00	0	0.10	71.5	1.0	0.0	0	0	0
All Ages	*1*	*0.4*	*1*	*0.4*	*16.1*	*0.7*	*1.0*	*0*	*16*	*7*
	India									
0-4	0	0.20	0	0.20	1.5	0.5	0.0	0	5	9
5-14	0	0.00	0	0.00	10.0	1.0	0.0	0	1	1
15-44	0	0.20	0	0.20	33.5	10.0	0.0	0	77	42
45-59	0	0.10	0	0.10	55.5	1.0	0.0	0	1	2
60+	0	0.00	0	0.00	71.5	1.0	0.0	0	0	0
All Ages	*1*	*0.1*	*1*	*0.1*	*27.6*	*0.9*	*0.0*	*0*	*83*	*20*
	China									
0-4	0	0.00	0	0.00			0.0	0	0	0
5-14	0	0.00	0	0.00			0.0	0	0	0
15-44	0	0.00	0	0.00	33.5	1.0	0.0	0	0	0
45-59	0	0.00	0	0.00			0.0	0	0	0
60+	0	0.00	0	0.00			0.0	0	0	0
All Ages	*0*	*0*	*0*	*0*	*33.5*	*1.0*	*0.0*	*0*	*0*	*0*
	Other Asia and Islands									
0-4	0	0.20	0	0.20	1.5	0.5	0.0	0	3	7
5-14	0	0.00	0	0.00	10.0	1.0	0.0	0	1	1
15-44	0	0.00	0	0.00	33.5	1.0	0.0	0	39	24
45-59	0	0.00	0	0.00	55.5	1.0	0.0	0	0	0
60+	0	0.00	0	0.00			0.0	0	0	0
All Ages	*0*	*0*	*0*	*0*	*14.4*	*0.7*	*0.0*	*0*	*42*	*12*
	Sub-Saharan Africa									
0-4	34	71.60	35	74.40	1.5	0.5	32.0	67	1 037	2 205
5-14	4	5.40	4	5.60	10.0	1.0	4.0	6	176	252
15-44	97	93.00	133	128.50	33.5	1.0	64.0	62	3 126	2 942
45-59	9	45.90	13	63.40	55.5	1.0	8.0	42	110	497
60+	4	36.50	5	50.50	71.5	1.0	4.0	33	17	134
All Ages	*147*	*58.5*	*191*	*75.6*	*28.0*	*0.9*	*112.0*	*45*	*4 467*	*1 732*

Table 13 (continued)

Age group (years)	Incidence Number ('000s)	Incidence Rate per100 000	Prevalence Number ('000s)	Prevalence Rate per100 000	Avg. age at onset (years)	Avg. duration (years)	Deaths Number ('000s)	Deaths Rate per100 000	DALYs Number ('000s)	DALYs Rate per100 000
	Latin America and the Caribbean									
0-4	1	3.80	1	3.90	1.5	0.5	1.0	4	34	123
5-14	0	0.20	0	0.20	10.0	1.0	0.0	0	4	8
15-44	25	24.40	34	33.00	33.5	1.0	19.0	18	186	179
45-59	3	13.50	4	18.20	55.5	1.0	3.0	12	8	34
60+	1	10.50	2	14.20	71.5	1.0	1.0	9	2	12
All Ages	*31*	*14.1*	*42*	*18.8*	*36.3*	*1.0*	*23.0*	*11*	*233*	*105*
	Middle Eastern Crescent									
0-4	0	0.10	0	0.10	1.5	0.5	0.0	0	2	5
5-14	0	0.00	0	0.00	10.0	1.0	0.0	0	0	0
15-44	1	0.60	1	0.70	33.5	1.0	0.0	0	6	6
45-59	0	0.60	0	0.70	55.5	1.0	0.0	0	0	0
60+	0	0.20	0	0.20	71.5	1.0	0.0	0	0	0
All Ages	*1*	*0.4*	*1*	*0.4*	*36.2*	*1.0*	*0.0*	*0*	*7*	*3*
	Developed Regions									
0-4	1	2.49	1	2.49	2.5	0.6	0	0	23	60
5-14	0	0.00	0	0.00		0.0	0	0	5	6
15-44	51	19.59	82	31.50	35.0	2.0	25	10	159	63
45-59	10	10.74	16	17.18	57.0	2.0	9	10	16	16
60+	2	2.45	3	3.68	73.0	2.0	2	2	3	2
All Ages	*64*	*11.51*	*102*	*18.35*	*39.1*	*2.0*	*36*	*6*	*206*	*32*
	Developing Regions									
0-4	35	13.86	36	14.26	2	1	33	13	1 081	399
5-14	4	0.89	4	0.89	10	1	4	1	182	41
15-44	123	13.12	168	17.92	34	1	83	9	3 434	364
45-59	12	3.98	17	5.64	56	1	11	4	119	56
60+	5	3.44	7	4.82	72	1	5	3	19	13
All Ages	*179*	*9.54*	*232*	*12.36*	*29.3*	*0.9*	*136*	*7*	*4 835*	*239*
	World									
0-4	36	11.20	37	11.52	1.5	0.5	33	10	1 104	357
5-14	4	0.73	4	0.73	10.0	1.0	4	1	187	36
15-44	174	13.92	250	20.00	33.9	1.6	108	9	3 593	300
45-59	22	7.04	33	10.56	56.2	1.7	20	6	135	43
60+	7	3.20	10	4.57	71.9	1.4	7	3	22	8
All Ages	*243*	*9.16*	*334*	*12.59*	*31.9*	*1.4*	*172*	*6*	*5 041*	*193*

Table 13 Epidemiological Estimates for HIV-AIDS, 1990, *females*

Age group (years)	*Incidence* Number ('000s)	*Incidence* Rate per 100 000	*Prevalence* Number ('000s)	*Prevalence* Rate per 100 000	*Avg. age at onset* (years)	*Avg. duration* (years)	*Deaths* Number ('000s)	*Deaths* Rate per 100 000	*DALYs* Number ('000s)	*DALYs* Rate per 100 000
	Established Market Economies									
0-4	1	3.20	1	4.89	2.5	2.0	0.0	1.4	17	64
5-14	0	0.20	0	0.30	10.0	2.0	0.0	0.1	3	6
15-44	8	4.60	18	10.00	35.0	2.0	4.0	2.2	899	488
45-59	1	1.60	2	3.40	57.0	2.0	1.0	1.3	144	218
60+	0	0.50	1	1.00	73.0	2.0	0.0	0.4	12	21
All Ages	*10*	*2.6*	*23*	*5.5*	*36.0*	*2.0*	*6.0*	*1.4*	*1 077*	*276*
	Formerly Socialist Economies of Europe									
0-4	0	2.70	0	2.90	1.5	0.5	0.0	2.3	10	73
5-14	0	0.20	0	0.20	10.0	1.0	0.0	0.2	2	7
15-44	0	0.10	0	0.20	33.5	1.0	0.0	0.1	13	17
45-59	0	0.10	0	0.10	55.5	1.0	0.0	0.0	1	4
60+	0	0.00	0	0.00	71.5	1.0	0.0	0.0	0	0
All Ages	*1*	*0.3*	*1*	*0.3*	*11.8*	*0.7*	*0.0*	*0.2*	*25*	*15*
	India									
0-4	0	0.30	0	0.30	1.5	0.5	0.0	0.3	5	8
5-14	0	0.00	0	0.00	10.0	1.0	0.0	0.0	1	1
15-44	0	0.00	0	0.10	33.5	1.0	0.0	0.0	140	70
45-59	0	0.00	0	0.00	55.5	1.0	0.0	0.0	5	11
60+	0	0.00	0	0.00			0.0	0.0	1	3
All Ages	*1*	*0*	*1*	*0*	*6.5*	*0.6*	*0.0*	*0.0*	*152*	*35*
	China									
0-4	0	0.00	0	0.00			0.0	0.0	0	0
5-14	0	0.00	0	0.00			0.0	0.0	0	0
15-44	0	0.00	0	0.00	33.5	1.0	0.0	0.0	3	1
45-59	0	0.00	0	0.00			0.0	0.0	0	0
60+	0	0.00	0	0.00			0.0	0.0	0	0
All Ages	*0*	*0*	*0*	*0*	*33.5*	*1.0*	*0.0*	*0.0*	*3*	*1*
	Other Asia and Islands									
0-4	0	0.20	0	0.20	1.5	0.5	0.0	0.2	3	7
5-14	0	0.00	0	0.00	10.0	1.0	0.0	0.0	0	0
15-44	0	0.00	0	0.00	33.5	1.0	0.0	0.0	69	43
45-59	0	0.00	0	0.00	55.5	1.0	0.0	0.0	3	9
60+	0	0.00	0	0.00			0.0	0.0	1	5
All Ages	*0*	*0*	*0*	*0*	*14.4*	*0.7*	*0.0*	*0.0*	*76*	*22*
	Sub-Saharan Africa									
0-4	34	72.30	35	75.10	1.5	0.5	30.0	64.1	1 090	2 296
5-14	4	5.40	4	5.60	10.0	1.0	4.0	6.4	167	238
15-44	101	95.00	139	131.20	33.5	1.0	84.0	78.5	2 474	2 384
45-59	7	29.80	9	41.10	55.5	1.0	6.0	27.3	146	719
60+	2	17.20	3	23.80	71.5	1.0	2.0	16.2	27	257
All Ages	*147*	*57.2*	*191*	*74.8*	*27.6*	*0.9*	*126.0*	*48.9*	*3 904*	*1 547*

Table 13 (continued)

Age group (years)	*Incidence* Number ('000s)	*Incidence* Rate per100 000	*Prevalence* Number ('000s)	*Prevalence* Rate per100 000	*Avg. age at onset* (years)	*Avg. duration* (years)	*Deaths* Number ('000s)	*Deaths* Rate per100 000	*DALYs* Number ('000s)	*DALYs* Rate per100 000
	Latin America and the Caribbean									
0-4	1	3.90	1	4.00	1.5	0.5	1.0	3.6	36	125
5-14	0	0.20	0	0.20	10.0	1.0	0.0	0.2	4	8
15-44	6	5.30	8	7.70	33.5	1.0	4.0	4.0	761	730
45-59	1	2.20	1	3.10	55.5	1.0	0.0	1.4	47	211
60+	0	1.50	0	2.20	71.5	1.0	0.0	1.1	9	63
All Ages	*8*	*3.4*	*10*	*4.7*	*31.3*	*0.9*	*6.0*	*2.6*	*857*	*387*
	Middle Eastern Crescent									
0-4	0	0.10	0	0.10	1.5	0.5	0.0	0.1	2	5
5-14	0	0.00	0	0.00	10.0	1.0	0.0	0.0	0	0
15-44	0	0.60	0	0.70	33.5	1.0	0.0	0.3	34	30
45-59	0	0.60	0	0.70	55.5	1.0	0.0	0.4	3	13
60+	0	0.20	0	0.20	71.5	1.0	0.0	0.1	0	0
All Ages	*1*	*0.4*	*1*	*0.4*	*36.2*	*1.0*	*0.0*	*0.2*	*39*	*15*
	Developed Regions									
0-4	1	2.62	1	2.62	2.5	0.5	0	0.0	27	67
5-14	0	0.00	0	0.00		0.0	0	0.0	5	6
15-44	8	3.15	18	7.08	35.0	2.0	4	1.6	912	350
45-59	1	1.02	2	2.04	57.0	1.8	1	1.0	145	156
60+	0	0.00	1	0.83			0	0.0	13	16
All Ages	*10*	*1.54*	*22*	*3.38*	*34.0*	*1.8*	*5*	*0.8*	*1 102*	*198*
	Developing Regions									
0-4	35	12.91	36	13.28	2	1	31	11.4	1 136	450
5-14	4	0.89	4	0.89	10	1	4	0.9	172	38
15-44	107	11.33	147	15.56	34	1	88	9.3	3 481	371
45-59	8	3.75	10	4.69	56	1	6	2.8	203	68
60+	2	1.35	3	2.02	72	1	2	1.3	38	26
All Ages	*156*	*7.70*	*200*	*9.87*	*27.3*	*0.9*	*131*	*6.5*	*5 031*	*268*
	World									
0-4	36	11.64	37	11.96	1.5	0.5	31	10.0	168	362
5-14	4	0.76	4	0.76	10.0	1.0	4	0.8	177	32
15-44	115	9.59	165	13.77	33.6	1.2	92	7.7	393	351
45-59	9	2.89	12	3.86	55.7	1.2	7	2.3	349	112
60+	2	0.74	4	1.49	71.5	1.0	2	0.7	51	23
All Ages	*166*	*6.35*	*222*	*8.49*	*27.7*	*1.0*	*136*	*5.2*	*1 133*	*231*

The cumulative build up of disease burden

For many disease conditions there may be a constant relation between incidence and the cumulative build up of infections as prevalence:

$$P=ID$$

where P = *prevalence*, I = *incidence* and D = *duration* of the illness. For HIV the ratio of prevalence to incidence varies considerably, from 3:1 to over 25:1 in different regions. An HIV epidemic results in a rapid cumulative increase of prevalence, which at any one time is strictly the source of future disability and mortality. For example if HIV incidence and therefore DALYs were reduced to zero at C, HIV prevalence would still provide a source of mortality, disability and disease burden up to 20 years into the future. In Figure 11 HIV incidence at A and C and therefore DALYs are similar. However the total burden of disease which has built up is almost ten times greater at C than A. The burden of disease is therefore not comparable between A and C, and an important consideration is to understand how the burden measure relates to HIV prevalence. This may not affect present prevention options but the reduction of mortality from prevalent cases presents a huge potential for reducing the disease burden, hypothetically to prevent mortality for most of 15-16 million HIV cases in 1995.

Therefore the table also shows "the present value of the future stream of disability free life lost" as a result of all HIV disease (HIV prevalence) in a year (World Bank 1993). For the illustrative purposes of the table, the calculations have been simplified, averaging HIV cases by age, sex and region, and prevalent cases are assumed to be evenly distributed throughout the incubation period. If HIV incidence were suddenly to stop in a year, Figure 11 shows the DALYs which would still be lost from future disability and mortality. This also captures the total disease burden which could be potentially prevented if all cases were cured in that year. Clearly an epidemic stopped at C rather than A, although with comparable HIV incidence and DALYs, would leave a much greater future burden of disease in terms of mortality and disability. The DALYs for HIV used in the GBD study well represent the disease burden from year to year, but a further consideration for many HIV epidemics is the disease prevalence which can be at very different levels for the same DALY value.

Secondary impacts and infections

DALYs are calculated from individual disability and mortality data, but further considerations stem from the relation of an individual HIV case to secondary social and economic impacts and infections. Previous sections in this chapter have highlighted that AIDS has a large impact beyond the morbidity and mortality of the individual. The burden of HIV can be seen as occurring at three levels:

1. The direct impact on the individual with HIV of disability and mortality, represented by the DALY measure.

Figure 11 Comparing DALYs for epidemic and stable disease incidence

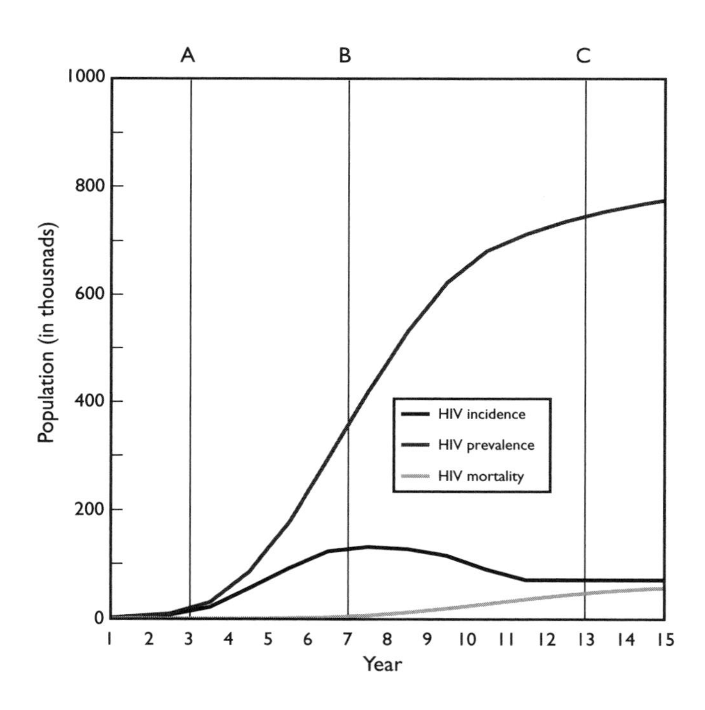

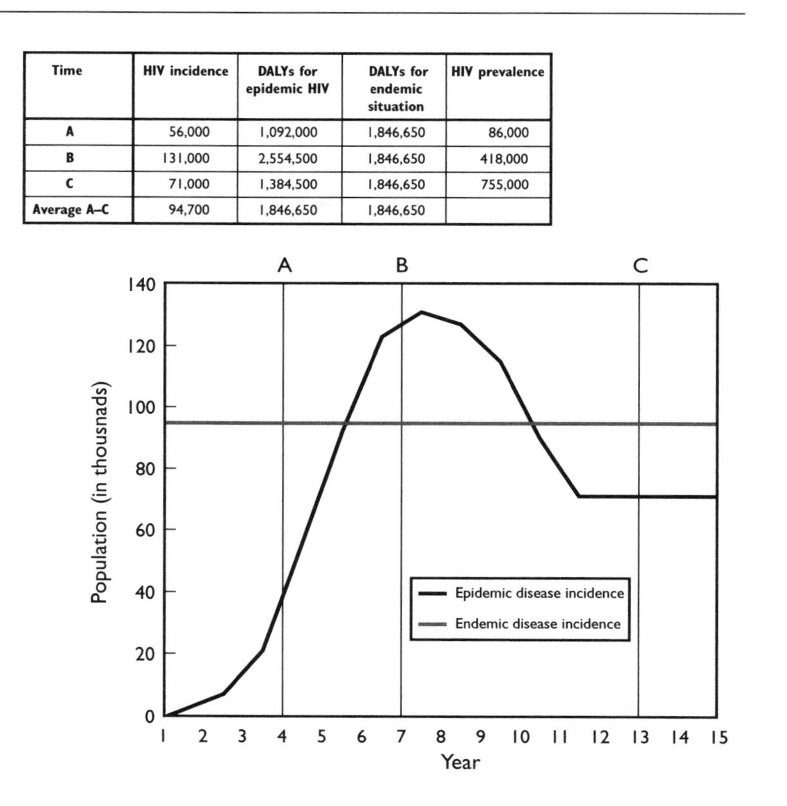

Time	HIV incidence	DALYs for epidemic HIV	DALYs for endemic situation	HIV prevalence
A	56,000	1,092,000	1,846,650	86,000
B	131,000	2,554,500	1,846,650	418,000
C	71,000	1,384,500	1,846,650	755,000
Average A–C	94,700	1,846,650	1,846,650	

Figure 12 Secondary impacts of HIV infection

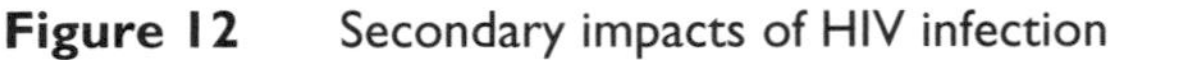

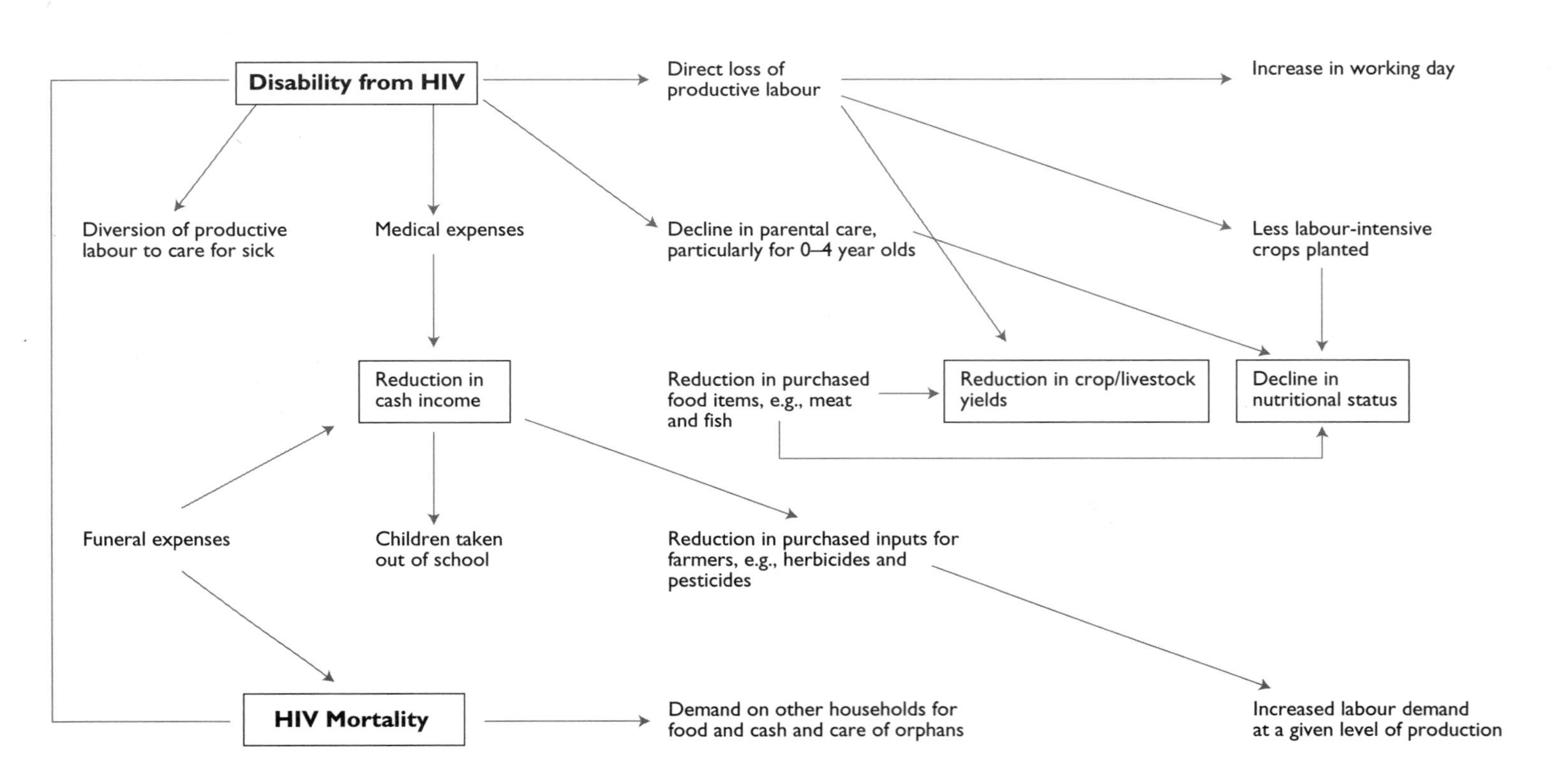

2. The secondary burden on health services, families and the community, of treatment and care of that individual.
3. The indirect impact in terms of lost labour, social and economic disruption.

Figure 12 shows the chains of secondary impacts which can stem from disability and mortality in an individual for a rural African epidemic, including medical expenses, diversion of productive labour and food reserves, withdrawal of children from school, and altered patterns of consumption and agricultural production. Although some studies have not shown for example a secondary impact of adult AIDS mortality on childrens' schooling (Over et al. 1993), or that AIDS dominated other adaptations required by households in severely affected areas (Barnett, Blaikie 1992), they also suggested that "in certain localized areas, AIDS is beginning to be the major determinant of socioeconomic change". An important consideration for HIV is to appreciate that the stream of disease burdens flows beyond mortality, morbidity and the DALY measure, to include extensive secondary social and economic impacts.

The final consideration for methods based on individual morbidity and mortality, is that for an infectious disease like HIV an index infection forms part of a chain of secondary infections. The importance of mixing patterns in generating HIV infection has been studied extensively (Gupta et al. 1989; Anderson et al. 1991; Seitz and Mueller 1994), and R_0 has been used to represent the average number of secondary infections produced from one index case in a susceptible population. The value of R_0 varies widely between groups and at different stages of the epidemic, Rowley et al. (1990) for example suggest R_0 varied in populations in Kenya from 2.9 to 6.5 from 1981 to 1986. In order to combat HIV effectively, it is important to prevent not just direct morbidity and mortality but the chains of secondary infection which sustain an epidemic. This generally emphasizes intervention early in an epidemic when DALYs may be small (Figure 11), as cases in 1990 not only produce a future stream of mortality and morbidity but the future infections producing further morbidity and mortality. Secondly it is important to intervene in groups most susceptible to infection due to their behaviour and central position in sustaining the epidemic. Similar to STDs, Over and Piot (1994) suggested that preventing an index HIV infection in a risk group can have dynamic benefits preventing a further five secondary infections over ten years. Furthermore these secondary disease chains extend to contribute to the burden of other important disease conditions, for example increasing trends in tuberculosis in North American cities and Africa, and will be analysed in the next section.

Public health priorities for HIV

Effective public health approaches to HIV

The first stage in evaluating interventions in terms of disease outcome is to understand the epidemiological rationale and evidence for their effects in reducing HIV incidence. At this level it is clear that effective intervention strategies exist to prevent HIV infection (Aggleton et al. 1994) and for care and limited intervention in the progression of HIV disease after infection (Weber, Merigan 1994). Interventions can be focused on four stages: modifying exposure in the environment, for example the screening of blood products and treatment of co-factors; behaviours which put humans at risk of infection; barrier methods which protect the risk situation, for example condoms; and care and limited prolongation of life after infection. In practice interventions combine these aspects, for example behavioural interventions are relevant to the proper use of condoms and improvements in well-being after infection.

The primary epidemiological basis for intervention priorities is to understand the associated behaviours and methods of HIV transmission, which were identified rapidly after the discovery of AIDS in 1981. Prevention activities are interventions before or during HIV exposure, whose major modes are through sexual activity, contact with infected blood or blood products, and from mother to child perinatally or during the postpartum period through breast feeding. Although the many economic and cultural aspects of HIV prevention have been described, in principle major practical public health methods of prevention related to the modes of transmission are simple and clear. Major activities involve: the provision of condoms, the promotion of safer sexual behaviours, the provision of a safe blood supply for transfusion, the provision of injection equipment and bleach for drug users, and the reduction of possible epidemiological and social co-factors of HIV infection, including STDs and poverty.

Economically, realistic options of care and prevention will vary widely between countries; for example AZT treatment costs US$3000 per year (World Bank 1993), and its priority for African countries, where expenditure on drugs is rarely more than US$5 per capita per year, is low (Foster 1994). Despite severe economic constraints (and limited DALY benefits) developing countries show a strong commitment to care, spending an estimated US$340 million in 1992, or twice that spent on prevention (World Bank 1993). The systematic evaluation of the costs and benefits of interventions is discussed at the end of this section.

Prevention of sexual transmission

At present the only major technology for the prevention of sexual transmission of HIV, which accounts for 80 per cent of new infections worldwide, is the condom. In principle condoms provide an effective physical barrier against nearly all STDs tested (Liskin et al. 1990),[10] and HIV (Cates et al., 1992), though breakage may be a problem in up to 10 per cent of cases particularly for anal sex.[11, 12] If used consistently and correctly condoms provide an effective protection method of the full sexual act, including the effect of cofactors for example STDs, and therefore condoms are at present regarded for both women and men as "the first line of defence" (Cates et al., 1992).

Public health programmes have focused on two priorities, firstly improving availability of condoms, and secondly improving their acceptability and use. There has been marked success in condom provision, with innovative methods like social marketing, for example in Zaire, using outlets from pharmacies, traditional healers, nightclubs to street vendors, increasing condom sales from 20,000 in 1987 to 18.3 million in 1991 (Mann et al. 1992). Similar approaches have been extended to ten more African countries, increasing condom provision from 5 to 40 million in two years. Increased condom provision has been paralleled by increased condom use in many situations, for example from a reported 10 per cent to 50 per cent in those aged 15-25 in the Netherlands (DeVries et al. 1989) and 11 per cent to 40 per cent in Tanzania (Mann et al. 1992), but there remains a substantial gap between knowledge, provision of condoms and their sustained use.

Prevention of blood-borne transmission

While small quantities of sera may play a role in sexual transmission, the major direct risk of blood-borne transmission is from blood transfusions and blood products, and injection practices associated with drug misuse and unsafe injections. Worldwide these may account for 5-10 per cent of infections (WHO 1993). In many EME countries the percentage is much higher due to IDU.

Infection from blood transfusions, blood products and unsafe injections are in principle largely preventable. Interventions to secure safe blood supplies involve three elements: the recruitment and retainment of low-risk donors,[23] the screening of donated blood products, and the reduction in unnecessary blood transfusions[24] (WHO 1993). In the EME, infections via this route have virtually ceased after an HIV antibody test was licensed in early 1985, despite AIDS becoming the leading cause of death in people with haemophilia in the USA (Mann et al. 1992). In developing countries securing safe blood supplies has shown to be feasible even where blood donor true HIV positives were as high as 15.6 per cent (Ryder 1992; EEC AIDS Task Force 1992; Watson-Williams and Kataaha 1990), though a WHO survey in 1991 showed some progress, with blood screening ranging from 50-99 per cent. The value of protecting blood has many other advantages in addition to HIV, including the risks of bacterial contamination, and transmission of other infectious agents including Hepatitis B, malaria, syphilis, Hepatitis C and cytomegalovirus, and these needs have been integrated into the Global Blood Safety Initiative.

Interventions among IDU have involved the provision of clean injection equipment, bleach and other cleaning materials, and behavioural campaigns to reduce equipment sharing, injection and sexual transmission between partners. These have shown considerable success: interventions reaching an estimated 90 per cent of IDUs in Sweden and Australia, 50 per cent in Thailand and 40 per cent in India (Mann et al. 1992) and impressive reductions in risk behaviour in Edinburgh (Robertson et al. 1988) and San Francisco (Guydish et al. 1990). The very rapid rises in HIV prevalence in IDUs requires quick and pre-emptive intervention responses if the bulk of HIV infections are to be prevented.

Prevention of transmission from mother to child

Wherever there is HIV infection from any transmission mode among women of child bearing age, HIV transmission from mother to child becomes an important issue. Most of the estimated one million child infections have occurred from maternal transmission before or during birth or in the postpartum period through breast feeding.[25] Children are also prone to infection through blood or blood products, most tragically for example in Romania. The current estimated risk of maternal transmission is 14 to 39 per cent (Gibb and Wara 1994), and an additional risk[26] of transmission via breastfeeding of 14 per cent (Dunn et al. 1992). Increased knowledge of risk factors including stage of infection of the mother, viral load, methods of delivery, and the effect of treatments for example zidovudine, are providing increasing scope for interventions.[27] Bottle-feeding is not recommended except in individual cases where safe and affordable, and in the context of the other health concerns of new-born children. Particularly in Africa the most effective method for preventing perinatal transmission is to prevent HIV-1 infection in women of child-bearing age[28] (Ryder and Temmerman 1991), and their partners.

Options for Care

Despite the lack of a cure there is a strong rationale for intervention after infection, among them the responsibility for care of the sick being one of the basic mandates of the medical profession, as well as the reduction of morbidity, the possible prolongation of life, and the prevention of further transmission of HIV. The medical management of HIV should aim to identify disease conditions,[29] provide treatment and retroviral therapy,[30] and administer primary/secondary prophylaxis[31] when indicated (Katabira and Wabitsch 1991), and clinical management guidelines and diagnostic criteria for different health care settings are well formulated (WHO 1993). However intervention possibilities for care relevant to DALY calculations showing an impact on mortality or morbidity are limited.

Perhaps this explains some of the scepticism in public health concerning evaluation based on economic methods. Even in poorer countries a strong commitment to care exists (the developing world spends twice as much on HIV care as HIV prevention), despite little DALY benefit. The public health perspective of an overall health package is required, which allows contact with populations at risk, provides them with benefits and care, and introduces public health activities for the prevention of further spread.

FUTURE INTERVENTION POSSIBILITIES

Future intervention possibilities will centre around the more intensive application of effective approaches developed over the last ten years, and possible future developments in the prevention, treatment or cure of HIV and AIDS. Possible important developments include: improvements in translating knowledge of HIV protection into sexual behaviour change; improved care and therapy to prolong life and reduce morbidity; rapid response and prevention to the early growth of epidemics not yet established; and the development, testing and provision of a prophylactic, therapeutic or perinatal vaccine. There are clinical trials in phase 1 or 2 of almost 30 candidate vaccines ongoing or ready to begin (Walker, Fast 1994).

The value of a curative vaccine is closely related to the number of prevalent HIV infections not included in the DALY method. Its priority for research is clear in terms of crude disease burden, as there are few potential interventions for any disease which could prevent 15-16 million deaths of those already infected by 1995 of future mortality. However by the time a vaccine is developed, the intensification of present interventions and the changing course of the epidemic could significantly alter the future burden of disease.

Some economic information on the costs and effectiveness of various prevention options are already available to public health decision makers; for example Moses et al. (1991) estimated condom programmes in high risk groups in Nairobi cost US$6 per HIV infection averted, and Bertozzi (1991) has estimated that blood screening in an African situation cost US$119 per infection averted. This compared to the estimated direct cost of health care per symptomatic HIV case, in Zaire ranging from US$132–US$1585, and in Tanzania from US$104 to $631 (Over et al. 1988). For example the inappropriateness of AZT as a public health strategy in Uganda, which would cost over 100 times the annual per capita health-care budget was shown by Rowley et al. (1990), and Haq (1988) estimated that treatment comparable to that provided in the United States for one AIDS patient would cost more than the annual budget of a rural health centre in Uganda.

OUTCOME MEASURES OF INTERVENTIONS

How effective are the interventions identified by public health in reducing life lost in relation to expenditure? Answering such a question involves several elements:

1. The identification of effective intervention strategies.
2. Measures of their impact in terms of incidence, mortality or morbidity.

3. Their quantification into a single DALY measure which allows comparison between interventions and costs.

The only comprehensive study of AIDS spending on prevention and care is described in Mann et al. (1992). Spending on prevention for 38 countries was extrapolated to regional populations to provide weighted per capita spending by region, and the cost and number of person years of care estimated. The cost of care included AIDS and not HIV infection, paediatric cases were not included, and prevention spending was extrapolated from National AIDS Control Programme spending estimates. The uneven geographical distribution of spending in relation to population and the number of HIV infections is apparent, with North America spending 67.5 per cent of the global total on care, and 40 times the per capita spending on prevention compared to Africa.

At the other end of the calculation, is the public health evaluation of effective interventions and their implementation after 15 years of experience, presented previously. Soderland et al. (1993) in a cost analysis of six prevention strategies, highlighted two important conceptual issues in their measurement:

1. HIV programmes were relatively new and cost estimates were therefore often unstable, for example condom social marketing costs declined over time, levelling out after three to five years.
2. Secondly, studies provide important information for operating interventions, but *the crucial problem of comparing "output measures" remains, for example units of blood with number of condoms.*

Evaluation studies therefore require a common currency to quantify outputs of public health priorities for comparison in terms of their reduction of loss of life.

Quantitative evaluation of burden

Quantitative measures of the disease outcomes of intervention strategies have generally had to rely on modelling of their impact on the HIV transmission process.[34] In addition to the problems of estimating HIV infections and deaths, these models require a quantitative structure for the HIV transmission process. Important parameters, for example the cofactor value of the presence of an STD or the impact of variable infectiousness, have a wide range of quantitative values.

Modelling studies have estimated that present interventions may already have prevented HIV prevalence in 1994 from being 30 to 40 per cent higher (FHI 1993) in severe African epidemics, and that the intensification of present intervention possibilities could avert an additional 57 per cent of HIV incidence between 1993 and 2000 (FH1 1993). This would have a comparable impact on reducing the DALY burden as DALYS are roughly proportional to HIV incidence standardized by age.

An association between interventions and a decline in HIV incidence can be shown in restricted studies where such a change is measurable, though declining HIV incidence can also occur without interventions. More importantly, interventions should occur at an early stage of an epidemic and may be associated with a rising incidence of disease and DALY burden. Deriving quantitative DALY estimates requires assumptions of the impact on HIV incidence of interruption in aspects of disease transmission, from awareness of HIV to the prevention of STD cofactors. Direct empirical data of such disease outcomes are likely to be incomplete, and, particlularly for sexual transmission, wide confidence intervals are required for research into effective interventions in public health and costing in health economics to be combined in the DALY evaluation of interventions.

Conclusions

In this chapter, we have presented each stage required in estimating the burden of HIV, from estimates of disease incidence, to the resulting stream of morbidity and mortality, and its quantification in terms of disability adjusted life years lost. The methods and results of the estimation process for HIV have been presented. Applying the DALY approach to measuring HIV in 1990 produced the following results:

1. HIV resulted in a total burden of 11 172 083 Disability-Adjusted Life Years lost (DALYs).
2. HIV ranked 28 worldwide among disease conditions, accounting for 0.81 per cent of the total burden of disease.
3. The HIV burden was heavily concentrated in SSA (75 per cent of global HIV DALYs), EME (11 per cent) and LAC (10 per cent), and to a lesser extent in India (2 per cent) and OAI (1 per cent), though the last two regional DALYs hide a rapidly increasing disease burden.
4. The large majority of the HIV DALYs were lost in ages 15-44 (70 per cent); males accounted for 51 per cent of total DALYs. Worldwide HIV ranked 27th among men and 31st among women as a cause of disease burden.
5. HIV was the 6th largest cause of burden in SSA in 1990.

HIV has emerged within 15 years as one of the major causes of disease worldwide. The burden may increase with new infections in Asia, and as people in other parts of the world with HIV increasingly develop AIDS. The burden of HIV continues to evolve from urban to rural areas, to South Asia, India, Cambodia, Vietnam, and Southern and West Africa, and to a lesser extent with proportional shifts to heterosexual infections in LAC and EME. By the year 2000 Asia will increase its share of the burden of HIV, but is unlikely to reach the highest rates in East and Central Africa.

There are a number of important considerations to be kept in mind when interpreting DALYs for HIV. The first is the problem of interpreting HIV DALYs for any point, in this study 1990, when HIV incidence is changing rapidly. This is particularly important for evaluating interventions which have an impact over an extended period, and could be improved with further studies for 1985, 1995, 2000. Control policies for HIV must consider where the epidemic is going, where it has come from, and how a point relates to the period disease measure. The second consideration relates to the build up of infections as HIV prevalence, which bears no simple relation to HIV incidence, and is strictly the source of future morbidity and mortality. Epidemics with similar HIV incidence may have very different HIV prevalence, resulting in different levels of mortality and disease burden not captured by the DALY method. When prevalence is used as the basis for the calculation of DALYs, HIV may become the major disease priority world-wide in any one year, as there are few conditions where a disease in 1995 provides the potential opportunity to prevent 15-16 million cases of future mortality.

Notes

1. The last naturally occurring case of smallpox occurred in Somalia in October 1977 and after a 2-year period in which no other cases (apart from laboratory accidents) were recorded. WHO formally announced in December 1979 the global eradication of smallpox.
2. HIV is used in this chapter to represent both HIV-1 accounting for 90 per cent of total infections, and HIV-2 which predominates in West Africa (De Cock, 1990), with signs of sporadic infection in parts of Europe, Latin America (Cortes et al. 1989; Veronesi et al. 1988), and North America (Ho et al. 1990)
3. Discounting is based on the economic concept of time preference, in relation to disease that "neither the individual nor the community are indifferent as to when the effects (i.e. they have a time preference) of disease occur" (Barnum 1987). A positive discounting rate used in this study assumes at the simplest level that "individuals prefer benefits now rather than in the future" (Murray 1994), and temporally near events are given greater weight than distant events. Future mortality and morbidity are therefore converted into present-value terms by reducing their value at a compound rate of 3 per cent per year. There has been considerable debate over the correct discount rate for health impacts, ranging from zero or negative to over 15 per cent (Barnum 1987), and the choice of 3 per cent is discussed in Murray (1994).
4. It reproduces often with rapid budding causing T-cell death, and over many years resulting in a continuous decline from approximately 900 CD4+ T cells/ml of blood (Kaslow, Francis, 1989) to less than 200/ml at end-stage disease.[2] Direct T4 lymphocyte death (between 1/100 and 1/10000 are directly infected) may be insufficient to explain the extreme cell depletion characteristic of AIDS, and other methods of pathogenesis including viral strain diversity (Nowak 1991), apoptosis, and autoimmune dysfunction have been suggested in vitro, resulting in the inability to respond to a host of viral, bacterial, fungal and parasitic infections, some of which are latent infections reactivated by immunosuppression (Redfield and Burke, 1988)
5. Following a WHO meeting of representatives of nine Central African nations in Bangui, Central African Republic in 1985.

6. Prior to 1983 conditions diagnosed as AIDS were assigned to ICD-9 No, 279.1 ("deficiency of cell- mediated immunity") as well as the ICD-9 codes of the diseases in the U.S. national case definition for AIDS ("Pnemocystis carinii" pneumonia, other AIDS defining infections, Kaposi sarcoma, non-Hodgkin's lymphoma, encephalopathy, and wasting syndrome).
7. The standard life expectancy is obtained from a Coale and Demeney "West" family model life table, with mortality level 26 and life expectancy of 82.5 for females, and life expectancy of 80 for males. Thus a man at 30 who dies loses of stream of lost life of 80-30 = 50 years (2.5 years less than a woman who dies at the same age).
8. The relative value of a life year lost has been modelled to emphasize young or middle-aged adult years, according to the exponential function:

   $$value\ of\ life\ year = ka\ exp(-Ba)$$

   where a is age and $B = 0.04$. The constant k is chosen so that the total number of DALYs is equivalent to uniform age weights. The function increases quickly from 0 to a peak at age 25 and then declines asymptotically toward 0. However an infant who dies loses all the years he or she is expected to live, and thus after cumulating loses the most crude life years, after discounting of future years the maximum DALY loss increases to age 10.
9. "We know how many condoms were shipped, we cannot document how many were actually used" (Hanenberg et al., 1994)
10. At least nine studies have shown the protective effect of condoms for both women and men against many bacterial STDs (Feldblum 1988; Stone et al. 1986), and viral STDs (Barlow, 1977; Cates et al. 1992)
11. Simulation of coitus have shown superficial irregularities but no pores in latex condoms and protection against HIV (Conant et al. 1986), although lower quality brands may show leakage of particles the same size as HIV in a minority of condoms (Carey et al., 1992)
12. Special stronger condoms have been developed particularly for anal sex, and further product development are possible in materials, the ratio of strength to sensitivity, and reusability.
13. Mass media campaigns appear to create awareness and set an agenda, while campaigns integrated into local activities, for example schools and using key community members, and interpersonal channels seem more likely to influence behaviour (Mann et al. 1992, p.337).
14. While substantial behaviour change to reduce HIV risk is achievable, some studies have reported problems in its maintenance, and a relapse into unsafe sexual behaviour for some men over a longer period of time (Adib et al., 1991; De Wit et al. 1993; Van den Hoek et al. 1990)
15. In particular risk indicators among men aged 30 and younger who entered the Amsterdam Cohort Study in 1984 and the Amsterdam Young Men's study in 1992, showed an increase in those practising anal receptive intercourse with one partner or less in the last six months from 39 per cent to 79 per cent, and a decrease in those with 10 partners or more from 13 per cent to 5 per cent (van Griensven et al., 1994), with similar trends reported in the San Francisco cohorts.

16. Despite its value as a technology, behavioural studies have highlighted the gap between the "method effectiveness" and the "user effectiveness" of condoms (Rosenberg et al. 1992; Trussell et al. 1990; Elias and Heise 1993). This includes problems of breakage and intermittent or improper use, but also of acceptability and the ability of women to negotiate use among their partners. The need for a protection method which women can control directly has therefore been emphasized.
17. A meta-analysis of ten studies (Rosenberg et al., 1992) suggested that the "user effectiveness" of condoms may be as low as 50 per cent.[3] There were problems in these studies, including weak definitions of exposure and overlap with the interval of barrier use, overlap of protection methods used, and differing outcome measures (Cates et al. 1992), and clinical trials of condoms and of their "user effectiveness" in vivo are lacking (Rosenberg 1992). A particular gap in condom coverage, is the necessity of women to negotiate condom use by their partners to protect themselves. While women from many backgrounds are successful in this (Elias, Heise 1993; Kline et al. 1992; Orubuloye et al. 1992; Plummer 1988), in important situations they lack the empowerment to protect the sexual act, presenting a risk to both women and men. In sex workers for example, Liskin et al. (1989) reported of six studies where the main reason condoms were not used was refusal among clients. Condoms also involve birth control which is not always wished, and have involved religious controversy which is particularly significant in extensive areas where the church may be a major provider of primary health care.
18. Although having a lower in vitro effect, it has been suggested that microbicide user effectiveness may be comparable to condoms in certain situations (Rosenberg et al. 1992). In vitro microbicides have been shown to be active against HIV (Wainberg 1990), and protected against HIV leaked through intentionally ruptured condoms (Reitmejer 1988). However in vivo studies have shown varied and inconsistent protection against HIV (Zekeng 1991, Niruthisard 1992), and particularly worrying are observations of lesions due to microbicide toxicity, which may increase the probability of HIV transmission (Kreiss 1992; Goeman, Perriens 1991).
19. This does not deter from the need for further product development for the value of chemical barriers to be realised, as condom lubricants or in situations where condoms are not acceptable.
20. Polyurethane and latex female condoms have been and shown to be impermeable to HIV in vitro (Drew et al. 1990)
21. There are at least two biologically plausible explanations of why STDs may facilitate HIV transmission (Laga et al., 1994). STD-related inflammatory responses and exudates from lesions increase the shedding of HIV in genital fluids, increasing the infectivity of HIV+ persons. Secondly, STD related lesions of the epithelial barriers of the genital tract may facilitate HIV infection, increasing the susceptibility of those not already HIV+.
22. In the early stages of an HIV epidemic, STDs may play an important role in driving epidemic growth, though it is not clear how they account for end HIV prevalence levels in the general adult population of 20-30 per cent, unless STD co-factors are broadly defined and STD prevalence is very high, or mixing patterns are extreme.

23. A focus on voluntary rather than paid donors has been suggested as central to international efforts to improve the safety of blood products. Donor deferral programs in the United States also resulted in a decrease in HIV prevalence in blood from first time donors by four times, and the recruitment of relatives to give blood on an emergency basis in developing countries has also been implemented.
24. Unnecessary blood transfusions have been reduced and when strict indications for use were followed in Africa, a 60 per cent decline in blood transfusion occurred (Mann et al. 1992)
25. Evidence of in utero infection includes the presence of virus in some babies' blood within hours or days after birth (Burgade 1992), and intrapartum transmission by the absence of virus detected by PCR in 50 per cent of infants in the first days after birth, and that firstborn discordant twins are more frequently infected than second born (Goedert et al. 1991).
26. Over and above transmission in utero or during delivery
27. Identification of HIV infection in women before or during pregnancy may provide advantages for both mother and baby. Recent research suggested that antiretroviral therapy using zidovudine during pregnancy, at delivery and during the new-born period reduced vertical transmission from 25 per cent in the placebo group compared to 8 per cent in the treated group (ACTG, 076 trial). Though such treatment is costly it may not need to be administered for an extended period as in use for HIV therapy. The risk of vertical transmission appears greatest shortly after initial HIV infection in the mother and during the latest stages of disease, probably due to increased viral load reflected by the presence of p24 antigen, and may increase transmission threefold (Newell, Peckham 1993). The timing of pregnancy and limited use of retroviral therapy may therefore reduce transmission in situations where risk is established.
28. Early HIV diagnosis in the child and interpretation is not straightforward, in part due to the presence of passively acquired maternal antibodies detected up to 18 months after birth, and delayed infection, virus or antigen expression, but upon diagnosis PCP prophylaxis may have benefits (Gibb,Wara 1994). HIV infected children should receive immunizations, except BCG in regions where TB prevalence is low, and satisfactory antibody reponses to measles vaccination occur although they may not continue with HIV progression (Lepage et al., 1992 . Care of HIV positive children involves PCP prophylaxis, treatment for encapsulated bacteria which causes significant morbidity, early immunizations against Haemophilus influenzae and streptococcus pneumoniae, and support for the affected families.
29. Diagnosis and treatment of opportunistic diseases and cancers has improved considerably in the developed world, and may result in a limited prolongation of life with HIV and particularly with AIDS.
30. Acute bacterial infections contribute significantly to morbidity and mortality in the developing world (Gilks et al. 1990, Taelman et al., 1990) and may also provide opportunities for an impact on the DALY burden via prophylaxis and treatment. The results of the Anglo-French Concorde study have provided a setback for antiretroviral treatment, with zidovudine delaying the onset of AIDS and increasing CD4 counts in the arm of the study with immediate

treatment, but not providing clear survival benefits. Furthermore, so far antiretroviral treatment has had implications only for a few patients in Africa.

31. Briefly the most important prophylactic approaches to reduce morbidity, has been primary and secondary PCP prophylaxis in the developed world (Public Health Service Task Force 1990), and primary prophylaxis of tuberculosis in Africa (Perriens et al. 1991)

32. The cost of providing condoms through social marketing for example was calculated at 0.07 US$ (1990) per condom sold in Ghana, 0.02 in Mexico, 0.15 in Cote d'Ivoire and 0.18 in Zimbabwe, of providing STD treatment in Mozambique and Kenya at 10 US$ per episode managed, of providing a needle exchange to drug users in the United States at 2.25 US$ per client contact, and of ensuring HIV safety per unit of blood produced in Uganda at 13.3 US$ and Zimbabwe at 3.9 US$ (WHO, GPA, 1993.2).

33. The prevention of mortality in a child for example saves 35 DALYs compared to approximately 30 DALYs at age 30 and 25 DALYs at age 40, and the burden is therefore greater in a younger population with a high fertility rate.

34. Moses et al. (1991) used a simple modelling framework to estimate that provision of STD care and condom prevention to a group of sex workers with 80 per cent HIV prevalence in Nairobi, Kenya, may have prevented 6000 to 10000 new cases of HIV taking into account mainly condom protection, at a cost of between US$8 and US$12 per HIV infection prevented.

References

Abel N et al. (1988) The impact of AIDS on food production systems in East and Central Africa over the next ten years: a programmatic paper, in Fleming A et al. *The Global Impact of AIDS*, London, John Wiley.

Adib S et al. (1991) Relapse in sexual behaviour among homosexual men: a 2-year follow-up from the Chicago MACS/CCS, *AIDS*, 5, 757–60.

Adjorlolo G (1992) Natural History of HIV-2, *VIII International Conference on AIDS*, Amsterdam, session 50.

Aggleton P et al. (1994) Risking Everything? Risk behaviour, behaviour change and AIDS, *Science*, 265, 341–345.

Ahmed S, Kheir E (1990) Sudanese sexual behaviour in the context of socio-cultural norms and transmission of HIV, *Anthropological studies relevant to the sexual transmission of HIV*, Denmark (U.S. Bureau of the Census, HIV database).

Alameda-Lozada J, Gonzalez-Martinez A (1989) Economic analysis of AIDS in Puerto Rico, *V International Conference on AIDS*, Montreal, abstract W.H.P5.

Anderson RM et al. (1991) The spread of HIV-1 in Africa: sexual contact patterns and the predicted demographic impact of AIDS *Nature*, 352, 581–587.

Anderson RM (1991) Mathematical models of the potential demographic impact of AIDS in Africa, *AIDS* 5 (suppl 1), S37–S44

Anderson RM, May RM, (1991) *Infectious diseases of humans: Dynamics and control*, Oxford, Oxford University Press.

Anzala O et al. (1995) Rapid progression to disease in African sex workers with HIV-1 infection, *Journal of Infectious Diseases*, 171, 686–9.

Anzala A, Wambugu P, Plummer FA (1991) Incubation time to symptomatic disease and AIDS in women with known duration of infection. *VII International Conference on AIDS*. Florence, abstract TUC103.

Asagba A, Andy J, Ayele T (1992) HIV sentinel surveillence in Nigeria, *Nigerian Bulletin of Epidemiology*, 2 (2), 10–13.

Asiimwe-Okiror G, Tembo G, Naamala W (1992) *AIDS surveillance report: June 1992*, Ministry of Health, AIDS Control Programme, Entebbe, Uganda.

Asiimwe-Okiror G et al. (1995) Declining HIV prevalence in women attending ANC sentinel surveillance sites, Uganda, 1989–1995, *IX International Conference on AIDS and STDs in Africa*, Kampala, Uganda.

Assefa A et al. (1994) Seroprevalence of HIV-1 syphilis antibodies in blood donors in Gonder, Ethiopia, 1989–1993 *Journal of AIDS*, 7, 1282–1285

Auerbach D et al. (1984) Cluster of cases of AIDS: patients linked by sexual contact. *American Journal of Medicine*, 76, 487–492.

Auvert B, Moore M, Bertrand W (1990) Dynamics of HIV infection and AIDS in central African cities, *International Journal of Epidemiology*, 19, 417–428

Avolio J, Rimoldi I, Arreseigor T (1993) Seroprevalence of HIV-1 in young men recruited for military service in Buenos Aires, Argentina, *IX International Conference on AIDS/STD*, Berlin, Abstract POCO6 2729.

Aylward RB et al. (1994) Validation of the proposed WHO staging system for HIV disease and infection in a cohort of intravenous drug users. *AIDS* 8:1129–1133.

Bagenda D et al. (1995) HIV-1 seroprevalence rates in women attending prenatal clinics in Kampala, Uganda, *IX International Conference on AIDS and STD in Africa,* Kampala, Abstract MoC016.

Bailey NJ (1957) *The mathematical theory of epidemics*, Charles Griffin, London.

Baltimore D, Feinberg MB (1989) HIV revealed: Towards a natural history of the infection *N Engl J Med* 321:1673–5.

Barnett T, Blaikie P (1992) *AIDS in Africa*, London, Belhaven Press.

Barnum H (1987) Evaluating healthy days of life gained from health projects, *Soc. Sci. Med.*, 24(10), 833–841.

Barongo L et al. (1992) The epidemiology of HIV-1 infection in urban areas, roadside settlements and rural villages in Mwanza region, Tanzania, *AIDS*, 6, 1521–1528.

Baroyan O, Rvachev L, Ivannikov Y (1977) *Modelling and prediction of Influenza epidemics in the USSR.*, Moscow: Gamaleia Institute of epidemiology and microbiology.

Batter V et al. (1994) High HIV incidence in young women masked by stable overall seroprevalence among childbearing women in Kinshasa, Zaire: estimating incidence for serial seroprevalence data, *AIDS* 8, 811–818.

Ben Salem N, Ben Rachid M, Hankins C (1993) Seroprevalence among women attending an antenatal clinic in Tunis, *VIII International Conference on AIDS in Africa*, abstract THPC077.

Bensilamene A, Rivjad M, Sekkat S (1987) Incidence of HIV in Morocco, *II International Symposium on AIDS and associated cancers in Africa*, Italy, Abstract TH84.

Berkley S, Okware S, Naamara W (1989) Surveillance for AIDS in Uganda, *AIDS*, 3, 79–85.

Berkley S et al. (1990) AIDS and HIV infection in Uganda — are more women infected than men? *AIDS*, 4, 1237–1242.

Berkley S (1991) Public Health significance of STDs for HIV infection in Africa, in Chen LC, Sepulveda J, Segal SJ *AIDS and Women's Reproductive Health*, Plenum Press, NY 1991.

Bernard Y, Camara B, Ferrus A (1994) Results of a serosurveillance study: prevalence of HIV, hepatitis B and syphilis among pregnant women in five sentinel sites in Haiti, *Haiti-Epidemiol*, 2, 30–40.

Bertozzi S, Harris J (1991) When is HIV screening of blood for transfusion cost-effective? Two models for use in Africa *VII International Conference on AIDS*, Italy.

Bertozzi S (1991) Combating HIV in Africa: a role for economic research, AIDS *5* (suppl 1), S45–S54.

Bertozzi S (1994) The impact of HIV/AIDS, Plenary Speech, *Xth International Conference on AIDS*, Yokohama, Japan.

Bhave G, Wagle U, Desai S (1992) HIV surveillance and prevention, *2nd International Conference on AIDS in Asia*, India, Abstract C401.

Bloom DE, Mahal AS (1997) Does the AIDS epidemic threaten economic growth? *Journal of Econometrics* 77: in press.

Bounds W et al (1988) A female condom (Fernshield): a study of its user acceptability, *British Journal of Family Planning*, 14, 83–87.

Brookmeyer R, Damiano A (1989) Statistical methods for short-term projections of AIDS incidence, *Statistics in Medicine*, 8, 23–24.

Brookmeyer R, Gail MH (1994) *AIDS Epidemiology: A Quantitative Approach*, Oxford University Press. Oxford.

Brookmeyer R, Gail MH (1986) Minimum size of the AIDS epidemic in the United States *Lancet*, Dec 6, 1320–1322

Brown T et al. (1994) The recent epidemiology of HIV and AIDS in Thailand, *AIDS*, 8 (suppl 2), S131–S141

Buchbinder SP et al. (1994) Long-term HIV-1 infection without immunologic progression. *AIDS*; 8:1123–1128.

Burgarde M, Mayaus M, Blanche S (1992) The use of viral culture and p24 antigen testing to diagnose HIV infection in neonates *New England Journal of Medicine*, 327, 1192–1197.

Bushaur N et al. (1995) Rising trend in the prevalence of HIV infection among blood donors, *Indian Journal of Medical Research*, in press.

Cameron D, Da Costa L, Gregory M (1989) Female to male transmission of HIV-1: risk factors for seroconversion in men, *Lancet*, 403–407.

Carael M et al. (1991) Overview and selected findings of sexual behaviour surveys, *AIDS*, *5* (suppl1), S65–74.

Carre N et al. (1994) Effect of age and exposure group on the onset of AIDS in heterosexual and homosexual HIV-infected patients. *AIDS*, 8:797–802.

Cates W, Stewart F, Trussel J (1992) Commentary: The quest for women's prophylactic methods — Hopes vs Science, *Am. J. Public Health*, 82, 1479–1482.

Centers for Disease Control (1982) Update on acquires immune deficiency syndrome (AIDS) — United States *MMWR*, 31(37):507–8, 513–14.

Centers for Disease Control (1986) Classification system for human T-lymphotropic virus type III/lymphadenopathy-associated virus infections *MMWR*, 35:334–339.

Centers for Disease Control (1987) HIV infectioncodes, official authorized addendum, ICD-9-CM (Revision No. 1), *MMWR*, 36 (S7), 1–20.

Centers for Disease Control (1991) HIV/AIDS Surveillance Report, Atlanta.

Centers for Disease Control (1991) Patterns of sexual behaviour change among homosexual/bisexual men — selected U.S. sites. 1987–90, *MMWR*, 40, 792–4.

Centers for Disease Control (1993a) Update: Mortality attributable to HIV infection/AIDS among persons aged 25–44 years — United States, 1990 and 1991, *MMWR*, 42, 25, 481–6.

Centers for Disease Control (1993b) Revised classification system for HIV infection and expanded surveillance case definitions for AIDS among adolescents and adults *MMWR*, 41:1–19.

Centers for Disease Control (1993c) Mortality attributable to HIV infection, MMMR, 42 (45), 869

Chaika N (1993) Syphilis morbidity in St Petersburg 1989–1993, *X Meeting of the International Society for STD research*, Finland.

Chin J, Lwanga S (1991) Estimation and projection of adult AIDS cases: a simple epidemiological model *Bulletin of WHO*, 69, 399–406.

Colebunders RL, Latif AS (1991) Natural history and clinical presentation of HIV-1 infection in adults. *AIDS*, 5(suppl 1):S103–12.

Curran J, Morgan W, Hardy A (1985) The epidemiology of AIDS: Current status and future prospects, *Science* 229, 1352–57.

Dean L, Meyer I (1995) HIV prevalence and sexual behaviour in a cohort of New York city gay men (Aged 18–24), *Journal of AIDS*, 8, 208–211.

De Cock K, Barrere B, Diaby L, Lafontaine M-F, Gnaore E, Porter A, Pantobe D, Lafontant G, Dago-Akribi A, Ette M, Odehouri K, Heyward W (1990) AIDS-the leading cause of adult death in the West African city of Abidjan, Cote d'Ivoire, *Science*, 249, 793–796.

Dempsey M (1947) Decline in tuberculosis. the death rate fails to tell the entire story, *American review of tuberculosis*, 56, 157–164.

Deschamps M (1988) AIDS in the Caribbean, *Archives of AIDS research*, 2, 51–56.

Diallo M, Traore V, Maran M (1992) STDs and HIV-1 and HIV-2 infection among pregnant women attending antenatal clinic in Abidjan, Cote d'Ivoire, *VII International conference on AIDS in Africa*, Cameroon, TP041.

Downs A, Salamina G, Ancell-Park R (1995) Incubation period of vertically acquired AIDS in Europe before widespread use of prophylactic therapies, *Journal of AIDS*, 9, 297–304.

Dunn D et al. (1992) Risk of human immunodeficiency virus type 1 transmission through breast-feeding, *Lancet*, 340, 585–588.

Edlin B, Irwin K, Faruque S (1994) Intersection epidemics: crack cocaine use and HVI-1 infection among inner-city young adults, *New England Journal of Medicine*, 331: 1422–1427.

El Alaqui A et al. (1993) Prevalence of anti-HIV antibodies in blood donors, *VIII International Conference on AIDS in Africa*, Marrakesh, abstract MPC079.

Elias C, Heise L (1994) Challenges for the development of female-controlled vaginal microbicides, *AIDS*, 8, 1–9.

European Centre for the Epidemiological monitoring of AIDS (1993) AIDS surveillance in Europe *Quarterly report* 40, St. Maurice.

European Collaborative Study (1994) Natural history of vertically acquired human immunodeficiency virus-1 infection *Pediatrics* 94:815–819.

Fayo Y, Viglianc R, Taboro M (1992) HIV prevalence among different communities in Argentina after 4 years of surveillance, *VII International Conference on AIDS*, Amsterdam, PoC 4064.

FHI Family Health International (1993) Simulation modeling of interventions to control the AIDS epidemic by Sokal D, Seitz S, Auvert B, Namara W, Stover j, Bernstein R. FHI Report, NC 27709 United States.

Fletcher RH, Fletcher SW, Wagner EH (1988) *Clinical Epidemiology: The Essentials* 2 ed., Baltimore, Williams and Wilkins.

Foster S (1994) Care and treatment of HIV disease in developing countries from a socioeconomic perspective, *AIDS*, 8 (suppl 1), S341–347.

Friedman S, Des Jarlais D, Wenston J (1994) New injectors remain at high risk of HIV infection, *X International Conference on AIDS/STDs*, Japan, abstract 073C.

Gail M, Rosenberg P (1992) Perspectives on using back-calculation to estimate HIV prevalence and project AIDS incidence, in Jewell N et al. *AIDS epidemiology: methodological issues*, Boston, Birkhauser.

Getchell J et al. (1987) HIV isolated from a serum sample collected in 1976 in Central Africa. *Journal of Infectious Diseases*, 156, 833–7.

Ghana Health Assessment Project Team (1981) A quantitative method of assessing the health impact of different diseases in less developed countries, *International Journal of Epidemiology* 10, 73–80.

Gibb D, Wara D (1994) Paediatric HIV infection, *AIDS*, 8 (suppl 1), S1–2.

Gillespie S (1989) The potential impact of AIDS on farming systems: a case-study from Rwanda, *Land Use Policy*, 6, 301–312.

Giraldo G, Serwadda D, Mugerwa R (1988) Seroepidemiology analyses on populations from Uganda and Tunisia — High and low risk African regions for HIV, *IV International Conference on AIDS*, Stockholm, Abstract 5038.

Godfried J et al. (1994) Risk behaviour and HIV infection among younger homosexual men, *AIDS*, 8 (suppl 1), S125–30.

Goedert J, Duliege A, Amos C (1991) High risk of HIV-1 infection for first-born twins *Lancet*, 338, 1471–1475.

Gottlieb M et al. (1981) Pneumocystis carinii pneumonia and mucosal candidiasis in previously healthy homosexual men: evidence of a new acquired cellular immunodeficiency. *New England Journal of Medicine*, 305: 1425–1431.

Gregson S, Garnett G, Anderson RM (1994) Is HIV-1 likely to become a leading cause of adult mortality in sub-Saharan Africa? *Journal of AIDS*, 7(8): 839–52

Graham NH et al. (1991) Effect of zidovudine and Pneumocytis carinii pneumonia prophylaxsis on progression of HIV-1 infection to AIDS. The Multicenter AIDS Cohort Study. *Lancet*; 338:265–9.

Grosskurth H et al. (1995) Impact of improved treatment of STDs on HIV infection in rural Tanyaniaö randomised controlled trial, *Lancet*, 346, 530–536.

Gupta S, Anderson RM, May RM (1989) Networks of sexual contacts: implications for the pattern of spread of HIV, *AIDS* 3: 807–817.

Guydish HR, Abramowitz A, Woods W (1990) Changes in needle-sharing behaviour among intravenous drug users: San Francisco, 1986–1988, *Am. J. Public Health* 80(8), 995–7.

Haq C (1988) Management of AIDS patients: case report from Uganda, in *AIDS in Africa — the social and policy impact* eds Miller, Rockwell, Lewiston, Edwin Mellen Press.

Hanenberg RS et al. (1994) Impact of Thailand's HIV-control programme as indicated by the decline of sexually transmitted diseases, *Lancet*, 344, 243–5.

Hardy A (1986) The economic impact of the first 10000 cases of AIDS in the United States, *JAMA* 255, 209–214

Harrera F, Gallardo M (1992) Nation-wide HIV-1 seroprevalence in Mexican blood donors, *VIII International Conference on AIDS*, Amsterdam, PoC4065.

Harry T, Bukbuk D, Idrisa A (1994) HIV among pregnant women: A worsening situation in Maiduguri, Nigeria, *IX International Conference on AIDS/STD*, Berlin, POC112861.

Hassene A, Paradis R, Moukaila A (1993) Rapid estimate of the prevalence of HVI/ AIDS in Niamey, Niger, *VIII International Conference on AIDS in Africa*, Marrakesh, abstract THPC087.

Hendriks J et al. (1993) The treatment-free incuation period of AIDS in a cohort of homosexual men, *AIDS*, 7, 231–239.

Hethcote HW, Yorke JA (1984) Gonorrhea: transmission dynamics and control, *Lect. Notes Biomath.*, 56, 1–105.

Hethcote H, Van Ark J (1992) *Lecture Notes in Biomathematics Modeling HIV transmission and AIDS in the United States*, Berlin, Springer-Verlag.

Hira S et al. (1989) Perinatal transmission of HVI-1 in Lusaka, Zambia, *V International Conference on AIDS*, Montreal, Abstract W.A.P.50.

Holmes K, Karon J, Kreiss J (1990) The increasing frequency of heterosexually acquired AIDS in the United States, 1983–1988, *Am J Public Health*, 80; 858–863.

Hyman J., Stanley E, (1988) Using mathematical models to understand the AIDS epidemic, *Mathematical Biosciences* 90, 415–473.

Ibotomba S, Brajachand (1992) Sentinel surveillance in Manipur, 2nd International Congress on Asia, India, Poster B352.

Indian Council of Medical research (1988) HIV infection — ongoing studies and future research plans, *Indian Council of Medical Research Bulletin*, 18, 109–119.

Jain M, John T, Keusch G (1994) A review of HIV infection in India, *Journal of AIDS*, 7, 1185–1194.

Jones DS et al. (1992) Epidemiology of transfusion associated acquired immunodeficiency syndrome in children in the United States, 1981–1989 *Pediatrics* 89:123–127.

John T et al. (1989) Prevalence of HIV-1 among voluntary blood donors, *Indian J Med Res*, 89, 1–3.

Johnson A, Gill O (1989) Evidence for recent changes in sexual behaviour in homosexual men in England and Wales, *Philos Trans R Soc Lond Biol*, 325, 153–161.

Joshi S, Chipkar S, Patil R (1992) HIV-1 and HIV-2 in Bombay, *2nd International Conference on AIDS*, India, Abstract B319.

Kapiga S., Shao J, Hunter P (1992) Contraceptive practice and HIV-1 infection among family planning clients in Dar es Salaam, Tanzania, *VIII International Conference on AIDS*, Amsterdam, PoC 4343.

Karon J, Dondero T, Curran J (1988) The projected incidence of AIDS and estimated prevalence of HIV infection in the United States, *J. of AIDS*, 1:542–550

Kaslow R, Francis D eds. (1989) *The epidemiology of AIDS: expression, occurrence and control of HIV-1 infection*, New York, Oxford University Press.

Katabira E, Wabitsch K (1991) Management issues for patients with HIV infection in Africa, *AIDS*, 5 (suppl 1), S149–156.

Kegeya-Kayondo J et al. (1994) HIV-1 incidence in adults and risk factors for seroconversion in a rural population in Uganda: 3 years of follow up, *X International Conference on AIDS/STD World Congress*, Japan, abstract 068C.

Khanboonruang C et al. (1994) HIV-1 incidence in adults in northern Thailand, *X International Conference on AIDS/STD*, Japan, abstract 038C.

Kigadye RM et al. (1993) Sentinel surveillance for HIV-1 among pregnant women in a developing country: 3 years experience and comparison with a population serosurvey. *AIDS* 7(6):849–55

Kingsley L, Zhou S, Bacellar H (1991) Temporal trends in HIV-1 seroconversion, 1984–89. A report from the MACS, *American Journal of Epidemiology*, 134, 331–9.

Kitayaporn D et al. (1993) HIV incidence determined retrospectively in drug-users in Bangkok, Thailand, IX International Conference on AIDS/IV STD World Congress. Berlin, (abstract WS-C09-2)

Kozlov A, Volkova G, Verevochkin S (1994) *New features of HIV/AIDS epidemic in Russia,* X International Conference on AIDS/STD, Japan, abstract 126C.

Ladner J, De Clercq A., Ukulikiyimfura C (1992) Seroprevalence de l'infection par le VIH-1 et counselling chez les femmes enceintes: Une etude de cohorte a Kigali, Rwanda, VII International Conference on ADIS in Africa, Yaounde, Cameroon, WP 179.

Laga M, Nzilambi N, Goeman J (1991) The interrelationship of sexually transmitted diseases and HIV infection: implications for the control of both epidemics in Africa, *AIDS 5* (suppl1), S55–S63.

Laga M et al. (1994) Condom promotion, sexually transmitted diseases treatment, and declining incidence of HIV-1 infection in female Zairian sex workers, *Lancet,* 344, 246–8.

Lang W et al. (1989) Patterns of T-lymphocyte change with human immunodeficiency virus infection from seroconversion to the development of AIDS. *Journal of AIDS*, 2:63–9.

Lemp G, Hirozawa A, Givertz D (1994) Seroprevalence of HIV and risk behaviours among young homosexual and bisexual men, *JAMA* 272, 440–454.

Lepage, Van de Perre P, Maellati P (1993) Mother to child transmission of HIV-1 and its determinants: a cohort study in Kigali, Rwanda. *American Journal of Epidemiology*, 137:589–599.

Lepage P, Hitimana DG (1991) Natural history and clinical presentation of HIV-1 infection in children. *AIDS*; 5:S117–S125.

Levy JA (1993) The transmission of HIV and factors influencing progression to AIDS. *American Journal of Medicine,* 95:86–100.

Lifson AR, Rutherford GW, Jaffe HW (1988) The natural history of human immunodeficiency virus infection. *J Infec Dis,* 158:1360–1367.

Lindan CP, Allen S, Serufilira A (1992) Predictors of mortality among HIV infected women in Kigali, Rwanda. *Annals of Internal Medicine*, 116:320–328.

Liskin L, Wharton C, Blackburn R (1990) Condoms-now more than ever, *Population Report*, 8, 1–36.

Lucas SB, Odida M, Wabinga H (1991) The pathology of severe morbidity and mortality caused by HVI infection in Africa, *AIDS*, 5(suppl 1), S143–S148.

Lucas SB et al. (1994) Contribution of tuberculosis to slim disease in Africa. *BMJ*, 308:1531–3.

Magazani K et al. (1993) Low and Stable HIV seroprevalence in pregnant women in Shaba Province, Zaire *Journal of AIDS*, 6, 419–423

Mann J, Tarantola D, Netter T eds. (1992) AIDS in the world: a global report, Cambridge, Massachusetts, Harvard University Press.

Martin J (1987) The impact of AIDS on gay male sexual behaviour patterns in New York city, *American Journal of Public Health*, 77, 578–581.

Mason C et al. (1885) Declining prevalence of HIV-1 infection in young Thai men, AIDS, 9, 1061–1065.

Mastro D, Limpakarnjanarat K (1995) Condom use in Thailand: how much is it slowing the HIV/AIDS epidemic? *AIDS*, 9, 523–525.

Mathiot C et al. (1990) HIV seroprevalence and male to female ration in central Afrcia. *Lancet*, 335, 672.

McKusick L et al. (1990) Longitudinal predictors of unprotected anal intercourse among gay men in San Francisco, *American Journal of Public Health*, 80, 978–83

McNeil (1983) *New York Review of Books*, July 21st 1983.

Medvedev ZA (1990) Evolution of AIDS policy in the Soviet Union. 1. Serological screening 1986–7. *British Medical Journal*, 300, 860–861.

Mertens T et al. (1994) Global estimates and epidemiology of HIV infections and AIDS, *AIDS*, 8 (suppl 1), S361–372.

Mertens T et al. (1994) Prevention indicators for evaluating the progress of national AIDS programmes, *AIDS* 8, 1359–1369.

Mertens T et al. (1995) Global estimates and epidemiology of HIV-1 infections and AIDS: further heterogeneity in spread and impact, *AIDS*, 9 (suppl A), S259–S272.

Miller E et al. (1995) Incidence of HIV infection in homosexual men in London, 1988–1994, *British Medical Journal*, 311, 545.

Mills A, Lee K (1993) *Health Economics research in developing countries,* Oxford, Oxford University Press.

Mohamed K, Kasule J, Makuyana D (1991) Seroprevalence of HIV amongst antenatal clinics in Greater Harare, Zimbabwe, *Central African Journal of Medicine*, 37, 10, 322–5

Morris M, Dean L (1994) Effect of sexual behaviour change on long-term HIV prevalence among homosexual men, *American Journal of Epidemiology*, 140, 3, 217–232.

Morris M et al. (1995) The relational determinants of condom use with commercial sex partners in Thailand, *AIDS*, 9, 507–515.

Morvan J et al. (1989) Enquete sero-epidemiologique sur les infections a HIV au Burundi entre 1980 et 1981, *Bulletin de la Societe de Pathologie exotique et de ses Filiales*, 82, 130–140.

Moses S et al. (1991) Controlling HIV in Africa: effectiveness and cost of an intervention in a high-frequency STD transmitter core group, *AIDS*, 5, 407–411

Moss AR, Bacchetti P (1989) Natural history of HIV infection. *AIDS*, 3:55–61.

Mulder DW et al. (1993) HIV-1 associated mortality in a rural Ugandan cohort: results at two year follow-up *IX International Conference on AIDS*. Berlin, [Abstract WS-C03-6].

Mulder DW et al. (1994) HIV-1 incidence and HIV-1 associated mortality in a rural Ugandan population cohort. *AIDS*; 8:87–92.

Mulder DW et al. (1995) Decreasing HIV-1 seroprevalence in young adults in a rural Ugandan cohort, *British Medical Journal*, 311, 833–6.

Murray CJ (1994) Quantifying the burden of disease: the technical basis for disability-adjusted life years, *Bulletin of the World Health Organization*, 72(3), 429–445.

Murray CJ, Lopez AD (1994) Global and regional cause-of-death patterns in 1990, *Bulletin of the World Health Organization*, 72(3), 447–480

Murray CJ, Lopez AD (1994) Quantifying disability: data, methods and results, *Bulletin of the World health Organization*, 72(3), 481–494

Murray CJ, Lopez AD, Jamison DT (1994) The global burden of disease in 1990: summary results, sensitivity analysis and future directions, *Bulletin of the World Health Organization*, 72(3), 495–509

Murray CJL, Lopez AD, eds. (1996) *The Global Burden of Disease*, Cambridge, Harvard University Press.

Nabarro D, McConnell C (1989) The impact of AIDS on socioeconomic development, AIDS 3 (suppl 1), S265–S272.

Nanu A, Sharma S, Bhasin I (1992) The AIIMS blood donor, *2nd International Congress on AIDS in Asia*, India, Poster A206

Nelson A et al. (1991) HIV-1 seropositivity and mortality at University Hospital, Kinshasa, Zaire, 1987 *AIDS*, 5, 583–586.

Nagelkerke NJ et al. (1990) Transition dynamics of HIV disease in a cohort of African prostitutes: a Markov model approach. *AIDS*; 4:743–747.

Namboze J (1993) *AIDS/HIV Update — Botswana*, WHO/Botswana, unpublished report.

N'Galy B, Ryder R (1988) Epidemiology of HIV infection in Africa, *Journal of AIDS*, 1, 551–558

Nkowane B (1988) The impact of HIV and AIDS on a primary industry: mining (A case study from Zambia) in *The Global Impact of AIDS* eds. Fleming AF et al., New York, Alan Liss.

Nzilambi N et al. (1988) The prevalence of infection with HIV over a 10-year period in rural Zaire. *New England Journal of Medicine*, 318, 276–79.

Opio A et al. (1995) Behaviour change? Results of a population survey in Uganda, *IX International Conference on AIDS and STDs in Africa,* Kampala, Uganda. Supplementary session on Declining HIV prevalence.

Osmond D (1993) HIV infection rate remians high in young homosexuals, *Am Fam Physician*, 48, 315.

Over M, Bertozzi S, Chin J (1989) Guidelines for rapid estimation of the direct and indirect costs of HIV infection in a developing country, *Health Policy*, 11, 169–186.

Over M et al. (1988) The direct and indirect cost of HIV infection in developing countries: the cases of Zaire and Tanzania in Fleming AF et al. eds *The Global Impact of AIDS*. New York. Alan R. Liss.

Over M, Mujinja P, Ainsworth M (1993) Economic impact of adult death from AIDS: overview of preliminary results from a random sample of households in Tanzania, *IX International Conference on AIDS/STD*, Berlin, abstract POD284200.

Over M, Piot P (1994) HIV infection and STDs, in Jamison D et al. *Disease control priorities in the developing world*, New York, Oxford University Press.

Over M (1984) Cost effective integration of immunization and basic health services in developing countries: the problem of joint costs, Discussion Paper No. 1, African-American issues Center, Boston University.

Pavri K (1990) HIV disease in India: an update, *Center AIDS Res Contro*l, 3, 30–34.

Perriens J, Mukadi Y, Nunn P (1991) Tuberculosis and HIV infection: implications for Africa, *AIDS*, 5 (suppl 1): S127–S133.

Peterson L, Gwinn M, Janssen R (1994) HIV-1 seroprevalence trends in the United States 1988–1992, *X International Conference on AIDS/STD World Congress*, Japan, abstract 123C.

Piot P et al. (1984) AIDS in a heterosexual population in Zaire, *Lancet* 2, 65–69.

Pizzo PA, Wilfert CM, and the Pediatric AIDS Siena Workshop II (1995) Markers and determinants of disease progression in children with HIV infection. *Journal of AIDS*; 8:30–44.

Plummer F, Simonson J, Cameron D (1991) Co-factors in femal to male transmission of HIV, *Journal of Infectious Diseases*, 163, 233–239.

Pradinaud R et al. (1989) L'infection par le HIV chez la mere et l'enfant en Guyane Francaise: etude epidemiologicque a propos de 44 femmes ayant eu 55 enfants., *Medecine Tropicale*, 49, 51–57.

Prevots D et al. (1994) The epidemiology of heterosexually acquired HIV infections and AIDS in western industrialized countries, *AIDS* , 8 (suppl 1), S109–S117.

Prost A, Prescott N (1984) Cost-effectiveness of blindness prevention by the onchocerciasis control programme in Upper Volta, *Bulletin of WHO*, 62, 795–802.

Public Health Service Task Force (1990) Anti-pneumocystic prophylaxis for patients infected with human immunodeficiency virus *AIDS Patient Care*, 4, 5–14.

Ravinathan R, Sukumar R, Ramalingam J (1992) Role of HIV screening in blood banks, *2nd International Congress on AIDS in Asia*, India, Abstract B333.

Rebagliato M et al. (1995) Trends in incidence and prevalence of HIV-1 infection in IDUs in Valencia, Spain, *Journal of AIDS*, 8, 297–301.

Rederick T, Mascola L, Eller A (1994) Progression of human immunodeficiency virus disease among infants and children infected perinatally with human immunodeficiency virus of through neonatal blood transfusion. *Pediatric Infectious Disease Journal*; 13:1091–1097.

Redfield RR, Wright DC, Tramont EC (1986) The Walter-Reed staging classification for HTLV-III/LAV infection. *New England Journal of Medicine*; 314, 131–132.

Redfield R, Burke D (1988) HIV infection: the clinical picture, *Scientific American*, 259, 70–78

Rhodes T, Holland J, Hartnoll R (1991) *Hard to reach or out of reach, an evaluation of an innovative model of the HIV outreach health education*, Tuffnell Press, London, 1991.

Rihad M, Mefalout L, Dehissy L (1992) STDs and HIV infections in four Morroccan centres, *VIII International Conference on AIDS/STDs*, Amsterdam, PoC4305

Robert C, Deglon B, Wintsch J (1990) Behavioural changes in IDU in Geneva: rise and fall of HIV infection 1980–1989, *AIDS*, 4, 657–660.

Robertson J, Skidmore C, Roberts J (1988) Infection in intravenous drug users: a follow-up study indicating changes in risk-taking behaviou, *British Journal of Addictions* 83, 387–91.

Rodrigues J et al. (1995) Risk factors for HIV infection in people attending clinics for STDs in India, *British Medical Journal*, 311, 283–6.

Rodrigues L et al. (1994) HIV sero surveillance in Brazil: a new epidemic emerges, *X International Conference on AIDS/STD World Congress*, Yokohama, abstract 072C.

Romeder J-M, McWhinnie JR (1977) Potential Years of Life Lost Between Ages 1 and 70: An indicator of premature mortality for health planning, *International Journal of Epidemiology*, 6, 143–151.

Rosenberg PS, Goedert JJ, Biggar RJ (1994) Effect of age at seroconversion on the natural AIDS incubation distribution. *AIDS*; 8:803–810.

Rosenberg M, Bollub E (1992) Commentary: methods women can use that may prevent STDs, including HIV, *American Journal of Public Health*, 82, 1473–8.

Rowley J, Anderson RM, NG T (1990) Reducing the spread of HIV infection in sub-Saharan Africa: some demographic and economic implications *AIDS* 4, 47–56.

Rudin C et al. (1990) HV-1, hepatitis and measles in Romanian children, *Lancet*, 336, 1592–93.

Rutherford GW et al. (1990) Course of HIV-1 infection in a cohort of homosexual and bisexual men: an 11 year follow-up study. *British Medical Journal*; 301:1183–8.

Ryder R., Nsa W, Hassig S. (1989) Perinatal transmission of HIV-1 to infants of seropositive women in Zaire, *New England Journal of Medicine* 320, 1637–1642.

Ryder R et al. (1990) Heterosexual transmission of HIV-1 among employees and their spouses at two large businesses in Zaire, *AIDS*, 4, 725–732

Ryder R, Temmerman (1991) The effect of HIV-1 infection during pregnancy and the prinatal period on maternal anc child health in Africa, *AIDS*, 5 (suppl 1) S75–86

Sakondhavat C (1990) The female condom, *Am J Public Health*, 80, 498.

Sawanpanyalert P et al. (1994) HIV-1 seroconversion rates among female commercial sex workers, Chang Mai, Thailand: a multi cross-sectional study, *AIDS*, 8, 825–829,

Schwartz JS, Dans PE, Kinosian BP (1988) HIV test evaluation, performance and use: Proposals to make good tests better. *Journal of the American Medical Association*. 259: 2574–79.

Scitovsky A (1988) Estimates of the direct and indirect costs of AIDS in the United States, in Fleming A et al. *The Global Impact of AIDS*, London, John Wiley.

Seitz S, Mueller G (1994) Viral load and sexual risk: epidemiological and policy implications for HIV/AIDS, in *Modelling the AIDS epidemic: Planning, policy and prediction* eds Kaplan E, Brandeau M, New York, Raven Press.

Selik R, Chu S, Buehler J (1993) HIV infection as leading cause of death among young adults in US cities and states, JAMA, June 16th, 269 (23), 2991–4.

Sewankambo N et al. (1994) Demographic impact of HIV infection in rural Rakai District, uganda: results of a population-based cohort study, *AIDS*, 8, 1707–1713.

Shepard D, Thompson M (1979) First principles of cost-effectiveness analysis in health, *Public Health Reports*, 94 (6), 535–543.

Simoes E, Babu P, John T (1987) Evidence for HTLV III infection in prostitutes in Tamil Nadu (India), *Indian Journal of Medical Research*, 1989; 89, 1–3.

Smallman-Raynor M, Cliff AD, Haggett P (1992) *The Atlas of AIDS*, Blackwell, Oxford.

Soderlund N et al. (1993) The costs of HIV prevention strategies in developing countries, *Bulletin of the World Health Organisation*, 71(5), 595–604

Sokal D, Buzingo T, Nitunga N, Kadende P, Standaert B (1993)Geographic and temporal stability of HIV seroprevalence among pregnant women in Bujumbura, Burundi, *AIDS* 7, 1481–4.

Stark K, Wirth D (1994) High HIV seroprevalence in injecting drug users in Warsaw, Poland, *Journal of AIDS*, 7, 877–878.

Stoneburner R et al. (1993) Insight into the infection dynamics of the AIDS epidemic: a birth cohort analysis of New York city AIDS mortality, *American Journal of Epidemiology*, 138, 12, 1093–1104.

Stoneburner R et al. (1995) HIV infection dynamics in Uganda deduced from surveillance data, unpublished (SEF/GPA/WHO).

Stoneburner R et al. (1995) HIV incidence dynamics underlying stable and declining HIV prevalence in Uganda, *IX International Conference on AIDS and STDs in Africa*, Kampala, Uganda. Supplementary session on Declining HIV prevalence.

Stover J, Wagman A (1992) *The costs of contraceptive social marketing programs implemented through the SOMARC project*, SOMARC special study, No.1, Washington DC, SOMARC, The Futures Group.

Taelman H., Bogart J, Batungwanayo J. (1990)Community acquired bacteraemia, fungaemia and parasitaemia in febrile adults infected with HIV in Central Africa *VI Internaational Conf AIDS in Africa*, Kinshasha,abstract FRTC2.

Taylor J et al. (1990) Estimating the distribution of times from HIV seroconversion to AIDS using multiple imputation, *Stat Med*, 9, 505–514.

Till M et al. (1993) HIV infection: Gender-related differences in presentation and progression. *IX International Conference on AIDS*. Berlin [Abstract PO-B01-0911].

Tindall B et al. (1988) Characterization of the acute clinical illness associated with human immunodeficiency virus infection. *Archives of Internal Medicine*; 148:945–9.

Tova PA et al. (1992) Prognostic factors and survival in children with perinatal HIV-1 infection. *Lancet*; 339:1249–1253.

Trussel J et al. (1990) Contraceptive failure in the United States: An Update, *Studies in Family Planning*, 21, 51–54.

Turner B et al. (1995) A population-based comparison of the clinical course of children and adults with AIDS, *AIDS*, 9, 65–72.

Un-eklabh T, Phutiprawan T (1988) Prevalence of HIV infection among Thai drug dependents *IV International Conference on AIDS*. Stockholm, (abstract 5524).

United States Bureau of the Census date, Centre for International Research: AIDS/HIV Surveillance Database. Washington D.C.

Valdespino J, Garcia M, Loo E (1992) HIV-1 in Mexico through national sentinel surveillanc system, An update, *VIII International Conference on AIDS*, PoC4063.

Van Griensven G, de Vroome E, Goudsmit J, Coutinho R (1989) Changes in sexual behaviour and the fall in incidence of HVI infection among homosexual men, *BMJ*, 298, 218–221.

Van Noren B, Boerna J, Sempebwa E (1989) Simplifying the evaluation of primary health care programmes, *Social Science and Medicine* 26, 1091–7.

Von Overbeck J et al. (1993) Progression and survival in HIV infection: does gender matter? *IX International Conference on AIDS*. Berlin [Abstract PO-B01-0909].

Von Overbeck J et al. (1993) Progression and survival in IDUs: different form hetero- or homosexually infected people with HIV? *IX International Conference on AIDS*. Berlin, Abstract PO-B01-0910.

Wagner H-U et al. (1993) General and HIV-1-associated morbidity in a rural Ugandan community, AIDS 7, 1461–1467

Walker M, Fast P (1994) Clinical trials of candidate AIDS vaccines, *AIDS* 8 (suppl 1), S213–236.

Watson-Williams E, Kataaha P (1990) Revival of the Ugandan blood transfusion system 1989: an example of international cooperation, *Transfus Sci*, 11, 179–184.

Wawer M, Sewankambo N, Gray R (1994) Trends in crude prevalence may not reflect incidence in communitites with mature epidemics, Waer M, Sewankambo N, Gray R, X International Conterence on AIDS/STD

Way P, Stanecki K (1991) The demographic impact of an AIDS epidemic on an African country: aplication of the iwgAIDS model, Center for International Research, U.S. Bureau of Census, Washington D.C., CIR staff paper 58.

Weber J, Merigan T (1994) Clinical treatment: Overview, *AIDS*, 8(suppl 1), S237–9.

Weinstock H et al. (1995) Trends in HIV prevalence among persons attending sTD clinics in the United States, 1988–1992, *Journal of AIDS*, 9, 514–522.

Wilkinson D (1994) Anonymous antenatal HIV seroprevalence surveys in rural Africa, *X International Conference on AIDS/STD*, Japan, Abstract 069C.

Wilson D, Mehryar A (1991) The role of AIDS knowledge, attitudes, beliefs and practices research in sub-Saharan Africa, *AIDS*, 5(suppl 1), 177–182.

Winkelstein W et al. (1987) The San Francisco men's health study: III. Reduction in HIV transmission among homosexual/bisexual men 1982–6 *American Journal of Public Health*, 77, 685–689.

Woody J, Buran J, Fox E (1988) HIV seroprevalence in Egypt and North East Africa, *IV International Conference on AIDS*, Stockholm, Abstract 5043.

World Bank (1992) *Tanzania AIDS Assessment and Planning Study*, Washington DC, The World Bank.

World Bank (1993) *World Development Report, 1993: Investing in Health,* Oxford University Press, New York.

WHO-EC Collaborating Centre (1994) *Surveillance of AIDS/HIV in Europe, 1984–1994*, European Center for the epidemiological monitoring of AIDS, Saint-Maurice, France.

World Health Organization (1985) Workshop on AIDS in central Africa, Bangui, 1–16.

World Health Organization (1990) AIDS: interim proposal for a WHO staging system for HIV infection and disease *Weekly Epidemiological Record* 65: 221–228.

World Health Organization (1991) *The AIDS epidemic and its demographic consequences; Proceedings of the UN/WHO workshop on modelling the demographic impact of the AIDS epidemic in pattern II countries*, New York, United Nations ST/ESA/SER.A/119.

World Health Organization (1993) Effective approaches to AIDS prevention, GPA, Geneva.

World Health Organization (1994) WHO case definition for AIDS surveillance in adults and adolescents, *Weekly Epidemiological Record*, 68, 37, 273–275

Zeng Y (1992) HIV infection and AIDS in China, *Archives of STD/HIV research,* 6, 4, 1–5.

Zhang L (1991) An epidemiological study on HIV inf Ruili County, Yunnan Province, Chung Hua Liu Hsing Hsueh Tsa Chih, 12, 1, 9–11 (U.S. Bureau of the Census).

Zhang L, Quing G, Lui G (1993) HIV/AIDS trends in Sichuan province, *IX International Conference on AIDS*, Berlin, Abstract PO-CO8-2781.

Chapter 10

Low Birth Weight

Kenji Shibuya
Christopher JL Murray

Introduction

Birth weight is considered as the single most important determinant of the chances of a newborn to survive and to experience healthy growth and development (World Health Organization 1980). Birth weight and gestational age can be considered as both morbidity indicators and mortality predictors since the incidence of both congenital anomalies and non-teratogenic perinatal conditions is significantly higher among low birth weight (LBW) newborns than in newborns with normal birth weights. The relationship between birth weight and mortality has been consistently shown. Although only a few studies on perinatal morbidity based on various classification and definition are available in developing countries, most of them suggest that LBW is a major contributor to infant morbidity. In a study in Kenya, for example, the major causes of morbidity were immaturity and respiratory distress syndrome (35.9 per cent), infections (33.4 per cent) and perinatal asphyxia, all of which were highly associated with LBW (Kasirye-Bainda and Musoke 1992). In India, 20 per cent of all newborns had perinatal conditions; LBW and infections were the most common cause of morbidity (Thirugnanasambandham et al. 1986).

Definition and Measurement

Definition of low birth weight

In general, low birth weight (LBW) is defined as a birth weight less than 2 500g consisting of both infants who are small for their gestational age (SGA or intrauterine growth retardation: IUGR) and preterm birth infants (premature). SGA infants are born at the expected time but are expected to be underdeveloped (term SGA), whereas preterm infants are born too early but are assumed to have developed appropriately for their gestational age (preterm AGA). Preterm birth and prematurity are often used interchangeably, although it seems more appropriate to use preterm to refer to age since prematurity describes function rather than chronological age. LBW can be further subclassified as very low birth weight (VLBW < 1500g) or extremely low birth weight (ELBW < 1000g). Both VLBW and ELBW have become major issues in studies of LBW in developed countries.

While preterm birth is usually defined as a gestational age of less than 37 weeks, SGA does not have any accepted standard definition. The following are commonly used definitions: birth weight lower than the 10th (or 5th) percentile for gestational age; birth weight less than 2500g and gestational age greater than or equal to 37 weeks; and birth weight less than 2 standard deviations below the mean value for gestational age (Kramer 1987). Among them, SGA is most commonly defined as an infant whose birth weight is clearly below average and below the 10th percentile for its gestational age.

The date of onset of the last normal menstrual period (LMP) is of clinical importance for determining fetal age. However, it is widely known that the estimation of the gestational age from LMP is fraught with error (Ahmed and Klopper 1986, Hertz et al. 1978, Treloar et al. 1969), although it proved to have greater validity than gestation based on physicians' estimates in the pre-ultrasonography era (Hammes and Treloar 1970). Using early second-trimester ultrasound determinations of the fetal biparietal diameter as the gold standard, Kramer and colleagues examined the validity of LMP-based gestational age. The positive predictive values of LMP gestational age estimates decreased from term (0.949) to preterm (0.775) to post-term (0.119) (Kramer et al. 1988).

In most developed countries there are other methods to estimate fetal age based on fetal size such as fundal height measurement, and ultrasonography measurement. Several simplified methods appropriate for community health workers in the developing countries have been proposed (Capurro et al. 1978, Narayanan et al. 1982). Chauham et al. (1992) suggested an interesting alternative for intrapartum assessment of fetal size. The maternal estimates of fetal size were equivalent in accuracy to clinical estimation by a physician or ultrasound estimates based on fetal measurement (Chauham et al. 1992). It should be noted, however, that these methods measure size, not fetal age (Hall 1990). In short, the variability of the methods available and difficulty in accurate estimation in developing countries make the estimation of gestational age difficult.

In regions where the majority of births occur outside health facilities, estimation of birth weight itself would be quite difficult. Several alternative measurements which are practical and relatively accurate have been proposed, such as mid-arm, chest and head circumferences (De Vaquera et al. 1983; Bhargava et al. 1985; Singh et al. 1988; World Health Organization 1993). Others have shown that neonatal body measurements can be used to screen preterm and SGA births with relatively high sensitivity and specificity (Raymond et al. 1994).

It is generally recognized that birth weight distribution is essentially normal (Gaussian), but slightly negatively skewed because of additional births in the lower tail (VLBW) (Wilcox and Russell 1983a,b). Although the cut-off point for LBW is arbitrarily defined as 2 500g, some researchers suggest a more practical definition of LBW for babies in developing countries such as a birth weight less than 2 000g (Ghosh and Berry 1962, Pethybridge et al. 1974). Since average birth weight in developing countries is low, a large proportion of LBW is actually mature neonates weighing between 2 000g and 2 500g (World Health Organization 1980). In these regions, the normal birth weight is lower than in developed countries and the birth weight-specific neonatal mortality might be lower. Most of the studies on LBW prevalence do not take into account ethnic or genetic factors, which are often confounded by socioeconomic and cultural factors (World Health Organization 1980). For example, Terry et al. compared the incidence of VLBW and neonatal mortality among various racial groups in the United States. Although VLBW was more common in West Indians than in the European and Pakistani groups, neonatal survival in West Indians was better than in any other groups (Terry et al. 1987).

Others have proposed an alternative criterion of LBW based on the assumption that the distribution of birth weight is actually a mixture of two components: the predominant (including about 95 per cent of the newborns and assumed to be normally distributed), and the residual (assumed to be mainly composed of newborns with a greater risk of mortality and forming the elevated left tail of the total distribution) (Chen et al 1991, Wilcox and Russell 1983c). They suggested that their criterion reduced the sex and ethnic differences in perinatal mortality among LBW categories. It is therefore important to evaluate LBW data in accordance with mortality level and other sociocultural factors.

International Classification of Diseases (ICD) codes for LBW

The ICD codes assigned to LBW in three consecutive revisions are summarized in Table 1.

ICD-8 did not make clear a distinction between preterm and SGA. LBW is classified as "Immaturity, unspecified (777)". LBW infants were further classified into slow fetal growth (IUGR) and short gestation (preterm) in the 9th Revision. In the 10th Revision, low birth weight is further differentiated according to extremely low birth weight (999 g or less) and other low birth weight (1000–2499 g).

SGA and preterm birth

The importance of the distinction between SGA and prematurity has been emphasized because of the difference in their causes and outcome (Kramer 1987, Mavalankar et al. 1982, Michilutte et al. 1992). However, because of the difficulty of accurately measuring gestational age, especially in developing countries, many studies have focused on LBW as if it were a single pathological entity. Although both types of LBW newborns have increased

Table 1 ICD codes for low birth weight

ICD-8	*ICD-9*	*ICD-10*
777 Immaturity, unqualified	**764 Slow fetal growth and fetal malnutrition**	**P05 Slow fetal growth and fetal malnutrition**
Immaturity NOS	764.0 "Light-for-dates" without mention of fetal malnutrition	P05.0 Light for gestational age P05.1 Small for gestational age
Prematurity NOS	764.1 "Light-for-dates" with sighns of fetal malnutrition	P05.1 Small for gestational age
Dysmaturity	764.2 Fetal malnutrition without mention of "light-for-dates"	P05.2 Fetal malnutrition without mention of light or small for gestational age
Low-birthweight infant	764.9 Fetal growth retardation, unspecified	P05.9 Slow fetal growth, unspecified
	765 Disorders relating to short gestation and unspecified low birthweight	**P07 Disorders related to short gestation and low birth weight, not elsewhere classified**
	765.0 Extreme immaturity	P07.0 Extremely low birth weight (Birth weight 999 g or less)
	765.1 Other preterm infants	P07.1 Other low birth weight (Birth weight 1000-2499 g)
		P07.2 Extreme immaturity (Less than 28 completed weeks of gestation)
		P07.3 Other preterm infants (28 completed weeks or more but less than 37 completed weeks of gestation)

risk of morbidity and mortality, preterm babies tend to have a greater risk of perinatal mortality than term SGA infants if congenital anomalies are excluded (Rush et al. 1976, 1978). The risk of developing other perinatal conditions such as respiratory distress syndrome, intracranial haemorrhage and infection is much higher in preterm infants (Table 2) (Dunn 1986). Preterm infants with immature organs tend to have a greater risk of mortality than SGA infants (Alberman 1990). Nevertheless, SGA itself is also a strong risk factor for perinatal mortality (Kramer et al. 1990). It should be noted that the two conditions sometimes coexist and thus SGA infants born preterm (preterm SGA) have a particularly high risk of mortality and morbidity.

The proportion of both conditions is different by region. In regions where the proportion of LBW is higher than 10 per cent, most of the LBW infants are SGA-LBW infants, while preterm birth remains unchanged (5–7 per cent). In contrast, when the LBW proportion is less than 10 per cent, preterm birth accounts for the majority of LBW (Villar and Belizan 1982).

Table 2 Hazards of low birth weight

	Preterm AGA	*SGA at term*
Congenital malformations	+	++
Transplacental infection	+	++
Intra-uterine infection	+	++
Respiratory difficulties		
Hyaline membrane disease	++	0
Meconium aspiration	+	++
Pulmonary haemmorhage	+	++
Apnoeeic attacks	++	+
Metabolic difficulties		
Hypoglycemia	+	++
Metabolic acidosis	+	++
Hypocalcemia	+	++
Jaundice, kernicterus	++	+
Alimentary difficulties		
Inability to suck or swallow	++	0
Functional intestinal obstruction, enterocolitis	++	+
Other hazrads		
Polycythemia	0	++
Anemia	++	0
Cerebral haemorrahge	++	0
Cerebral oedema, neuronal necroses	+	++
Retinopathy of prematurity	++	+
Sensorineural deafness	++	+
Liability to infection	++	+
Difficulty in maintaining body temperature	++	+
Withdrawal syndrome (maternal drug abuse)	+	++
Renal function	Urine concentration reduced	Normal

Source: Dunn 1986

Note: 0 = no hazard; + = low hazard; ++ = high hazard

A similar result was shown in a study of the secular trend of the LBW proportion in the United States which suggested that the reduction of LBW proportion was principally due to the reduction of SGA-LBW (Kessel et al. 1984). Although many studies in developing countries have not separated preterm birth from SGA (Mavalankar et al. 1992), limited data in the 1980s suggest considerable regional variations in the proportion of term SGA infants among all LBW infants (Table 3) (World Health Organization 1992).

The proportion of term SGA infants among all LBW infants varied from 40 to 60 per cent in LAC, 30 to 70 per cent in SSA, and about 30–50 per cent in EME. Higher proportions have been consistently reported from OAI and India with figures of about 75–85 per cent. In spite of the considerable difference in nutritional status of both mothers and infants between states or countries in IND and OAI, the consistently higher proportion of term SGA suggests the possible role of genetic or ethnic factor in these regions (World Health Organization 1980).

Table 3 Proportion of SGA among LBW, selected countries

Country	*Year*	*Study type*	*Sample size*	*Mean birth weight*	*Proportion of LBW*	*Proportion of term SGA among LBW infants*
Mexico	1984	Hospital	29001	3077g	8.2%	46%
Brazil	1984-86	Hospital	11171		7.6%	50%
India	1980-82	Hospital	2360	2772g	34.7%	81%
Philippines	1983-84	Community & Hospital	2139	3008g	10.7%	79%
Singapore	1984	Registration	41024	3168g	6.1%	62%
Thailand	1980	Hospital	1297	2995g	11.9%	75%
USA	1985	Registration			6.8%	41%
Canada	1986	Registration	364180	3378g	5.7%	42%
Ethiopia	1985	Hospital	3999		12.3%	62%
Nigeria	1983	Hospital	1191		16.4%	34%

Source: WHO database

Data sources for LBW proportions

The study of LBW is particularly important in developing countries because a higher proportion of infants are of low birth weight as compared with developed countries and the wide range of social and environmental conditions that affect birth weight which could potentially be improved through public health measures. The data collection methods currently used in the World Health Organization database are: (1) vital registration data, (2) community-based studies, (3) hospital-based studies, (4) WHO monitoring data (Health for All 2000 questionnaires), and (5) field office estimates (UNICEF). Most of the LBW data from developing regions are based on community or hospital-based estimates.

In addition to the definition bias mentioned before, selection bias might occur in the hospital-based prospective studies in regions where a considerable number of newborns are delivered at home and may not be included in the survey. Babies delivered in hospitals might have a lower likelihood of LBW. Only about one-third of births in the developing world take place in institutions (World Health Organization 1980). Even in a community-based retrospective survey which includes women whose babies were born outside hospitals, it is difficult to collect accurate information on birth weight from each woman because many infants are not weighed at birth, or because women have not been told their infants' weights and are subject to recall bias (Moreno and Goldman 1990). There are various confounding factors such as social class, residence (urban or rural), ethnicity, and other socioeconomic variables which could lead to an over or underestimate of the true magnitude of the LBW proportion. Comparisons are possible from these data, but great care is clearly required in making comparisons between countries or across regions (World Health Organization 1992).

REVIEW OF PAST STUDIES MEASURING DISEASE BURDEN

MORTALITY FROM LOW BIRTH WEIGHT

LBW is a significant contributor to neonatal deaths in both developed and developing countries. In the United States, LBW infants account for two-thirds of neonatal deaths and VLBW infants account for half of neonatal deaths (McCormick 1985). In developed regions where post-neonatal mortality has declined, neonatal mortality is the most significant component of infant mortality and the proportion of VLBW infants is a principle predicator of neonatal mortality (Lee et al. 1980). Although available data are limited in developing countries, LBW is one of the major causes of both infant and neonatal deaths, accounting for about 15–50 per cent of all neonatal deaths. For example, in a community-based study in Nigeria, 42 per cent of the infant deaths were associated with low birth weight. Infant mortality in LBW infants was 6 times as high as in normal birth weight babies (Ayeni and Oduntan 1978).

The relationship between birth weight and mortality has been studied repeatedly in developed countries. Mortality is very high in the VLBW babies, falls to a minimum within the range of the most frequent birth weights (i.e. 3 000–3 500g in developed countries), but rises again for the heaviest birth weights (Wilcox and Russell 1983c).

As mentioned before, preterm babies have a greater risk of death within the same birth weight group (Koops et al., 1982, McCormick 1985, Shapiro et al. 1980). The risk of neonatal death in LBW infants is 40 times higher than normal birth-weight infants and that of VLBW infants is almost 200 times higher (McCormick 1985, Shapiro et al. 1980). In the post-neonatal period, LBW infants continue to have an increased risk of death (Table 4) (Asworth and Feachem 1985, Koops et al., 1982).

Although the same relationship between birth weight and mortality is seen in both developing and developed countries, the chance of survival is quite different by region. For example, the risk of death among VLBW is about 90 per cent in some developing countries, suggesting that many VLBW infants die in such regions, whereas a significant proportion of VLBW infants survive in EME (Bergman and Juriso 1994, Marlow et al. 1987).

However, in a region where the proportion of LBW infants is high, the risk of neonatal or post-neonatal death, especially in those babies weighing 1 500–2 500g, might be lower than in the regions with a higher mean birth weight. Although there are insufficient birth-weight-specific mortality data to examine the risk of death from LBW in developing countries (Asworth and Feachem 1985), data from different regions on the relation-

Table 4 Neonatal and post-neonatal mortality rates by birth weight and gestational age

		Mortality rate			
Birth weight (g)	**Gestational age**	**Santa Maria Cauque**	**Delhi**	**North Arcot**	**New York City**
		Neonatal mortality rate per 1,000			
< 2500	Preterm	323	87	73	93
	Term (IUGR)	28	27	41	44
> 2500	Preterm	—	10	30	—
	Term (IUGR)	8	4	21	—
		Post-neonatal mortality per 1,000			
< 2500	Preterm	286	46	66	16
	Term (IUGR)	58	35	66	13
> 2500	Preterm	—	18	50	—
	Term (IUGR)	42	13	42	—

Source: Ashworth and Feachem 1985

ship between birth weight and perinatal mortality suggest that a high LBW proportion does not necessarily imply a high mortality rate in the 1 500–2 500g group (Table 5) (World Bank, unpublished data).

Contribution of LBW to morbidity and disability

LBW itself is regarded as a major risk factor for other perinatal conditions although the attributable risk of LBW to morbidity is not well established primarily because of definition bias and lack of population-based morbidity data (McCormick 1985). Recent studies have focused on the outcomes of VLBW infants in particular hospitals and there are few outcome studies for all LBW infants (Dunn 1986). Many survivors of LBW would suffer both immediate and long-term morbidity (Table 6) (Kliegman et al. 1990). Among the sequelae of LBW infants, most of the follow-up studies have focused on the relationship between LBW and long-term disability such as mental retardation, cerebral palsy, hearing impairment, visual impairment, and epilepsy because LBW infants have been shown to have a higher incidence of such major childhood disabilities. The Vancouver study of the sequelae of LBW infants gives a good estimate of the prevalence of disability among LBW infants (Dunn 1986). It was reported that 140 (41.8 per cent) of the 335 LBW babies developed some neurodevelopmental disability at 6.5 years. In contrast, only 15 (10.8 per cent) of 139 normal birth weight babies were found to have such a disability. It was shown that the frequency of neurological abnormality was inversely related to birth weight: the frequency at 1 year rose from 24 per cent in babies of birth weight 1 801–2 041g to 45 per cent in those below 1 360g. Although mental retardation was slightly more common among SGA children, cerebral palsy was more common among preterm children, the differences were not statistically significant.

Table 5 Birth weight specific perinatal mortality rates, selected countries

Country	Perinatal mortality rate					Proportion of LBW
	Total	1000-1500g	1500-2500g	2000-2500g	> 2500g	
Brazil, 1982	34	690	220	97	13	9%
India, 1988	79	567	291	55	23	44%
Tanzania, 1976-79	54	692	235	81	7	4%
Libya, 1982	27.5	705	282	81	7	4%

Source: Bobadilla, unpublished

Table 6 Sequelae of low birth weight

Immediate	*Late*
Birth asphyxia (Hypoxia-ischaemia)	Mental retardation Cerebral palsy Microcephaly Seizures Poor school performance
Intraventricular haemorrhage	Mental retardation Cerebral palsy Seizures Hydrocephalus
Sensorineural injury	Hearing-visual impairment Retinopathy of prematurity
Respiratory infection	Bronchopulmonary dysplasia Cor pulmonale Bronchospasm Malnutrition Respiratory infection
Necrotizing enterocolitis	Short bowel syndrome Malabsorption Malnutrition Infectious diarrhoea
Cholestatic liver disease	Cirrhosis Hepatic failure Carcinoma Malnutrition
Other	Sudden infant death syndrome Infections

Source: Kliegman et al. 1990

Table 7 Outcome of LBW infants, EME

Birth weight	*% survival*	*% disabled*
< 1500 g	65–85%	10–35%
1500–2500 g	> 90%	< 10%

Studies on birth prevalence of cerebral palsy (CP) and birth weight in three countries in EME consistently showed that CP prevalence rises as birth weight falls (Stanley and Blair 1991). In Western Australia, although there was no significant time trend for CP prevalence, there was a highly significant increase of CP rates among VLBW infants weighing less than 1 500g. The result coincides with the increasing number of low and very low birth weight infants surviving since the introduction of neonatal intensive care (Bhushan et al. 1993, Ehrnhaft et al. 1989, Powell et al. 1986). Among LBW newborns, those that were premature are reported to have a higher incidence of neurodevelopmental disability (Alberman et al. 1985, Veen et al. 1991).

Because of the relative size of the groups, however, the majority of disabled children were of heavier birth weight (Ehrnhaft et al. 1989). This fact, together with the probability that relatively more disability is seen in the lower birth weight groups, suggests that as mortality in the LBW and VLBW falls, the number of children who survive with a disability will rise. In developed countries, one may assume that more LBW children who develop a disability can survive due to the improvements in perinatal care. At the same time, we may assume that the same process is also likely to reduce the incidence of disability in larger or more mature babies who were previously disabled. For example, as the survival prospects for VLBW infants have improved significantly during the past 30 years, leading to a 70 per cent chance of survival of VLBW infants, the proportion of severely disabled babies has increased from 6.7 to 10.1 per 1 000 as neonatal care improved (Alberman et al. 1982). The results of some recent studies suggest that increased survival has not been associated with increased neurological disability in the last few years (McCormick 1985). Similar results have been reported in the EME region (Aylward et al. 1989, Kitchen et al. 1992, Robertson et al. 1992). This is still a controversial issue in developed countries, especially with regard to the effectiveness of neonatal intensive care.

In follow-up studies, there are possible biases in selection of the cohort and in measurement of exposure and outcome. Because of the variety of outcome criteria, it is sometimes difficult to analyse and compare results among studies (Aylward et al. 1989). Furthermore, it should be noted that many of the disabilities among SGA and preterm infants might exist prenatally and be confounded by factors such as chromosomal and congenital anomalies, cerebral lesions, and infections. It seems difficult to distinguish between babies affected in the prenatal period and those affected in the perinatal or neonatal period in the case of neurologic disability (Escobar et al. 1991).

Prevalence of reported impairments in relation to birth weight was 16.1 per cent in babies of 1 500g or less, 10.5 per cent in the group weighing 1 501g to 1 750g, and 7.1 per cent for those weighing 1 751g to 2 000g, if disabilities originating in the prenatal period were excluded (Alberman et al. 1985). Similar results are obtained from other studies. After correcting for the effect of congenital anomalies, Marlow et al. found that 20 per cent of the survivors of VLBW became disabled. In contrast, the chance of survival was 90 per cent in babies of more than 1 500g and 4.7 per cent were disabled among survivors (Marlow et al. 1987). Escobar et al. (1991) reviewed the published outcome studies in VLBW infants and found that the median incidence of cerebral palsy was 7.7 per cent and that of disability was 25 per cent among survivors. The reported figures for mortality and morbidity in the EME region are summarized in Table 7.

Unfortunately, there are no comparable follow-up studies on the relationship between LBW and disability in other regions. One study in Guatemala which followed SGA infants suggests that chronically malnourished SGA infants (symmetrical IUGR) scored the lowest in growth and mental development at three years of age (Villar et al. 1984). However, the probability of developing disability was not examined. It remains unclear whether it is possible to generalize these results from EME to developing countries. In addition, the difference in the proportion of SGA and prematurity might affect the risk of mortality and morbidity in different regions.

ESTIMATION OF BURDEN

ESTIMATION OF THE PROPORTION OF LBW BY REGION

Table 8 shows the WHO estimates of the number of live births and low birth weight infants by country based on an analysis from a variety of sources. In 1990, the WHO estimated that almost 25 million (17 per cent) of all infants born in 1990 weighed less than 2 500g and that more than 90 per cent of all LBW infants were born in developing countries (World Health Organization 1992).

Established Market Economies

Most of the WHO data are derived from vital registration. National proportions of LBW infants in Western Europe vary from 4 per cent to 7 per cent, with the lowest proportions in Scandinavian countries. A relatively higher figure is seen in the United Kingdom, especially among ethnic minorities, which is comparable to that of North America. Approximately 6 to 7 per cent of infants born in North America are LBW, while in Japan the figure is about 5.5 per cent. However, there are considerable socioeconomic and racial differences in North America. For example, in the United States, vital registration data in the mid-1980s suggested that the proportion of LBW in whites was about 5.6 per cent whereas in blacks it was more than twice that (12.4 per cent). The weighted average of Western Europe, North America and Japan leads to a proportion of LBW infants of 6 per cent.

Table 8 Estimated number of births of live infants and of LBW infants, by country, 1990 and estimated proportion of LBW infants, 1979, 1982 and 1990

Region and country or Territory	*Live births*	*Low birth weight infants*			
	(in '000s) 1990	(in '000s) 1990	Percentage 1979	1982	1990
Established Market Economies					
Australia	246	14	5.8	5.3	5.7
Austria	88	5	5.8	5.6	5.7
Belgium	118	7		5.6	5.9
Canada	356	20	6.4	6.0	5.6
Denmark	57	3	6.4	6.0	5.3
Finland	60	2	3.9	4.1	3.3
France	761	40	6.5	5.2	5.3
Germany, Fedral Republic of	863	52	6.7	5.5	6.0
Greece	117	6		5.9	5.1
Ireland	67	4		4.7	6.0
Italy	587	31	11.0	6.7	5.3
Japan	1390	79	5.1	5.2	5.7
Netherlands	192	8	4.0	4.0	4.2
New Zealand	55	3	4.9	5.3	5.5
Norway	53	2	4.2	3.8	3.8
Portugal	137	7		8.0	5.1
Spain	486	19			3.9
Sweden	109	5	3.6	4.0	4.6
Switzerland	78	4		5.2	5.1
United Kingdom	786	55	7.0	7.0	7.0
USA	3634	251	7.4	6.9	6.9
Formerly Socialist Economies of Europe					
Albania	74	7			9.5
Bulgaria	112	7			6.3
Former Czechoslovakia	217	13	6.1	6.2	6.0
German Democratic Republic	226	14	6.3	6.2	6.2
Hungary	123	11	11.7	11.8	8.9
Poland	588	46	8.0	7.6	7.8
Romania	358	25			7.0
USSR	5065	355	8.0	8.0	7.0
Yugoslavia	339	37	7.4	7.0	10.9
India					
	26985	8905	30.0	30.0	33.0
China					
	24288	2186	6.0	6.0	9.0

Table 8 *(continued)*

Region and country or Territory	*Live births*	*Low birth weight infants*			
	(In '000s) 1990	(in '000s) 1990	Percentage 1979	1982	1990
Other Asia and Islands					
Bangladesh	4796	2398	50.0	50.0	50.0
Bhutan	58				
Brunei Darussalam	7	1			14.3
Cambodia	322				
Democratic People's Republic of Korea	530				
Republic of Korea	670	60	8.0	9.2	9.0
Fiji	20	2			10.0
French Polynesia	5	<1			7.0
Guam	3	<1			8.0
Hong Kong	72	6	8.0	8.0	8.3
Indonesia	5091	713	18.0	14.0	14.0
Kiribati	2	<1			7.0
Lao People's Democratic Republic	187	34	18.0	18.0	18.2
Macao	8	<1			5.0
Malaysia	538	54	9.0	10.6	10.0
Mauritius	19	2		10.6	10.5
Mongolia	77	8		10.0	10.4
Myanmar	1252	200	20.0	20.0	16.0
Nepal	725				0.0
Papua New Guinea	131	30			22.9
Philippines	1988	298	19.5	19.5	15.0
Samoa	2	<1			6.0
Seychelles	2	<1			10.0
Singapore	47	3	11.2	7.0	6.4
Solomon Islands	12	2			20.0
Sri Lanka	369	92	21.0	27.0	24.9
Thailand	1158	151	13.0	38.0	13.0
Tonga	3	<1			3.0
Viet Num	2076	353		10.0	17.0
Vanuatu	6	<1			7.0
Sub-Saharan Africa					
Angola	472	90	18.7	18.7	19.1
Benin	229	34			14.8
Botswana	61	5		12.0	8.2
Burkina Faso	426	89			20.9
Burundi	261		13.5	13.5	
Cameroon	566	74	11.0	12.5	13.1
Cape Verde	15				
Central African Republic	138	21	23.0	23.0	15.2
Chad	249		10.5	10.5	
Comoros	26	2			7.7
Congo	105	17	15.0	15.0	16.2
Cote d'Ivore	603	84			13.9
Djibouti	19	2			10.5
Ethiopia	2424	388	13.1	13.1	16.0
Equatorial Guinea	16				

Table 8 *(continued)*

Region and country or Territory	*Live births*	*Low birth weight infants*			
	(in '000s) 1990	(in '000s) 1990	Percentage 1979	1982	1990
Sub-Saharan Africa ***(continued)***					
Gabon	49	6	13.0	13.0	12.2
Gambia	40	8			20.0
Ghana	665	93			14.0
Guinea	294	62			21.1
Guinea-Bissau	41	8			19.5
Kenya	1132	181	17.5	12.8	16.0
Lesotho	72	8	14.5	7.6	11.1
Madagascar	547	55	10.0	10.0	10.1
Malawi	494	99		12.0	20.0
Mali	472	80	12.7	12.7	16.9
Mauritania	94	10			10.6
Mozambique	699	140		15.7	20.0
Namibia	76	9			11.8
Niger	401			15.0	
Nigeria	5183	829	18.0	18.0	16.0
Reunion	13	1			7.7
Rwanda	368	63	17.0	19.9	17.1
Sao Tome and Principe	4	<1			
Senegal	328	36	9.9	9.9	11.0
Sierra Leone	201	34		17.0	16.9
Somalia	360	58			16.1
South Africa	1108	133	14.8	12.0	12.0
Sudan	1111	167	16.7	16.7	15.0
Swaziland	37	4			10.8
Togo	158	32		16.9	20.3
Uganda	985		10.0	10.0	
United Republic of Tanzania	1387	194	13.0	14.4	14.0
Zaire	1626	244	15.9	15.9	15.0
Zambia	433	56	14.2	14.2	12.9
Zimbabwe	399	56	15.0	15.0	14.0
Latin America and the Carribbean					
Antigua and Barbuda	1	<1			8.0
Argentina	670	54	6.0	6.0	8.1
Bahamas	5	<1			7.0
Barbados	4	<1	9.6	9.6	10.0
Bolivia	309	37		10.0	12.0
Brazil	4115	453	8.7	9.0	11.0
Chile	306	21	13.0	9.0	6.9
Colombia	878	88	10.0	10.0	10.0
Costa Rica	81	6	8.5	8.5	7.4
Cuba	188	15	10.1	9.2	8.0
Dominica	2	<1			10.0
Dominican Republic	214	32	15.4	15.4	15.0
Ecuador	338	44			13.0
El Salvador	191	21	12.8	12.8	11.0
Guadeloupe	7				
Guatemala	367	51	17.9	17.9	13.9

Table 8 *(continued)*

Region and country or Territory	*Live births*	*Low birth weight infants*			
	(in '000s) 1990	(in '000s) 1990	Percentage 1979	1982	1990
Latin America and the Carribbean ***(continued)***					
Guyana	20	3			15.0
Haiti	233	35	10.2	12.0	15.0
Honduras	198	18			9.1
Jamaica	56	6	9.6	8.0	10.7
Martinique	7	1			
Mexico	2466	296	11.7	11.7	12.0
Nicaragua	156	20			12.8
Panama	63	6	11.0	10.3	9.5
Paraguay	146	12			8.2
Perto Rico	64	6			9.4
Peru	647	71	9.0	9.0	11.0
Suriname	11	1	11.6	11.6	9.1
St Lucia	3	<1			8.0
St Vincent	3	<1			8.0
St Kitts and Nevis	1	<1			10.0
Trinidad and Tobago	32	3			9.4
Uruguay	54	4	10.0	8.3	7.4
Venezuela	582	52	11.0	9.3	8.9
Middle Eastern Crescent					
Afghanistan	888	178		20.0	20.0
Algeria	877	79	10.4	12.0	9.0
Bahrain	14	1			7.1
Cyprus	12	1			8.3
Egypt	1727	180	13.5	7.0	10.4
Iran (Islamic Republic of)	1830	165	14.0	14.0	9.0
Iraq	789	118	6.1	6.1	15.0
Israel	99	7	6.3	7.2	7.1
Jordan	157	4	7.3	7.3	2.5
Kuwait	55	4			7.3
Lebanon	83	9	12.0	12.0	10.8
Libyan Arab Jamahiriya	199				
Malta	5	<1	4.2	4.2	
Morocco	858	77		8.6	9.0
Oman	67	10		16.0	14.9
Pakistan	5451	1363	21.0	27.0	25.0
Qatar	11	1			9.1
Saudi Arabia	594	43			7.2
Syrian Arab Republic	550	60			10.9
Tunisia	239	19	7.3	7.3	7.9
Turkey	1579	126		7.5	8.0
United Arab Emirates	34	2		6.7	5.9
Yemen	602	117			19.4

Source: World Health Organization

Formerly Socialist Economies of Europe

National proportions in FSE are around 6 to 8 per cent, with relatively higher proportions in Poland and Hungary. Since more than two-thirds of live births occur in the Former Soviet Union (FSU), the representative figure for the region is based on data predominantly from the FSU (7 per cent). This figure is consistent with other countries in FSE except for two countries mentioned above.

India

Community-based studies in the 1980s, which mainly covered rural or low socioeconomic populations have consistently suggested high LBW proportions in India, with figures of 20 per cent to 56 per cent. After excluding the small sample size studies, the remaining data yield an overall estimate of about 35 per cent. Recently UNICEF estimated a LBW proportion of 39.3 per cent derived from multiple studies covering both poor urban and rural areas. There are other hospital-based studies whose results vary between 14 per cent and 53 per cent. This compilation of data suggests a figure of about 30 per cent. Since a considerable proportion of births occurs outside the hospitals in the region, a reasonable estimate is around 35 per cent.

China

Both community- and hospital-based studies in the 1980s suggested a fairly low proportion of LBW infants at 3 per cent to 5 per cent for China as a whole. A more recent community-based study in 1987 and the WHO monitoring data showed higher values of 9 per cent and 9.8 per cent respectively. In spite of the validity of the monitoring data, a weighted estimate would be around 6 per cent for the region.

Other Asia and Islands

This heterogeneous region has considerable variations in national proportions of LBW. The lowest proportion is seen in Eastern Asia at about 5 per cent, which is comparable to EME. In South-Eastern and Southern Asian countries, higher LBW proportions have been consistently reported with figures of more than 20 per cent. An extremely high figure of 50 per cent was reported for Bangladesh. Vital registration data and community and hospital-based studies from the countries included in Table 9 were used to estimate the overall LBW proportion of the region.

The regional estimate was around 22 per cent. This figure is higher than the previous estimate used by the World Bank (1993) because of the inclusion of data from Bangladesh where a considerable proportion of births in OAI occurs.

Sub-Saharan Africa

Estimated national LBW proportions in SSA are generally lower than in India and range between 10 and 20 per cent. Higher proportions have been

Table 9 Estimated proportion of LBW infants in OAI, 1990

Country	*Livebirths* (in millions)	*Proportion of LBW* *(per cent)*
Bangladesh	4.8	41
Indonesia	5.1	15.9
Malaysia	0.5	9.2
Myanmar	1.3	17.5
South Korea	0.7	9.2
Thailand	1.2	12.7
Vietnam	2.1	18.7

Table 10 Estimated proportion of LBW infants in SSA, 1990.

Country	*Livebirths* (in millions)	*Proportion of LBW* *(per cent)*
Angola	0.5	18.5
Burkina Faso	0.4	16.8
Cameroon	0.6	12.5
Ethiopia	2.4	12.4
Kenya	1.1	16
Mali	0.5	15.4
Mozambique	0.7	15.6
Nigeria	5.2	16.5
Rwanda	0.4	17.5
South Africa	1.1	12 (blacks: 14.2 whites: 10.6)
Tanzania	1.4	13.7
Zaire	1.6	14.7
Zambia	0.4	11.3

reported in West and East Africa, where about 16 per cent of livebirths are LBW. Southern Africa has a lower proportion of 12 per cent. The proportion of LBW infants in SSA appears to be fairly constant throughout the region. The overall LBW estimates are derived mainly from the reliable hospital-based studies in the countries shown in Table 10.

The aggregate estimate of the proportion of LBW infants in SSA was 14.9 per cent. However, once again this value needed to be adjusted upward since the majority of births occur outside hospitals in SSA. Thus, the figure of 16 per cent has been used as an appropriate estimate of LBW proportion in the region.

Latin America and the Caribbean

Vital registration and hospital-based surveys mandate most of the national proportions of LBW between 9 per cent and 12 per cent. Higher values are reported in some Caribbean countries, Guatemala and Guyana, around 14 to 17 per cent. The totality of these data suggest an estimated proportion of 11 per cent. However, this figure may well underestimate the LBW proportion among the rural poor population in the region. For example, vital registration data from Brazil, where about one-third of live births in LAC occur, suggest that the LBW proportion in the rural area is 14.8 per cent, while that in the urban area is 10.5 per cent. The proportion was 13.9 per cent in a community-based retrospective study in Peru which covered the rural poor population. If we take into account the possible selection bias of the hospital-based study, a figure of 13 per cent seems reasonable as the best estimate.

Middle Eastern Crescent

Although there is some variation in the proportion of LBW infants across countries in this region it is not as much as OAI. The reported national proportions of LBW infants are lower than those in OAI and vary from 6 to 15 per cent. Pakistan has the highest value at about 25 per cent. There are no community-based studies available from the WHO database. Many of the regional estimates are derived from UNICEF field estimates or WHO monitoring data. For the estimation of the regional LBW proportion, the prospective hospital-based studies from the countries shown in Table 11 were used.

The available data suggest an overall figure of 16.5 per cent LBW for MEC; however, no hospital-based data are available for countries such as Algeria and Morocco which have a relatively large number of livebirths and a lower proportion of LBW infants. Thus, the figure was adjusted downward to 16 per cent.

Worldwide, more than 24 million infants (17 per cent of all livebirths) born in 1990 weighed less than 2 500 g and more than 90 per cent of them were born in developing regions. Despite the slight improvement in the proportion of LBW infants since the late 1970s, the number of LBW babies has increased along with the rise in the number of births. The total number of LBW infants is highest in India (38 per cent of the world total), followed by SSA (17 per cent), OAI (15 per cent), MEC (13 per cent), LAC (7 per cent), China (6 per cent), and EME and FSE (4 per cent).

Estimation of mortality and disability

Mortality estimates by region

The category defined in the ICD as "conditions originating in the perinatal period" includes a variety of conditions. For the purpose of the Global Burden of Disease Study, overall mortality from all perinatal conditions

Table 11 Estimated proportion of LBW infants in MEC, 1990

Country	*Livebirths* (in millions)	*Proportion of LBW (per cent)*
Egypt	1.7	12.7
Tunisia	0.2	7.6
Iran	1.8	4.8
Iraq	0.8	8
Saudi Arabia	0.6	7
Turkey	1.6	7
Yemen	0.6	26.5
Pakistan	5.4	26

(760–799 of ICD) was assumed to be the residual of all neonatal deaths after subtracting other common causes of neonatal death such as neonatal infections and congenital anomalies. The underlying assumption is that most deaths from perinatal conditions occur in the neonatal period (within the first month of life). The previous version of the estimates was made in this way. Since LBW, birth asphyxia and infection are considered to be leading causes of neonatal deaths in developing countries (Costello 1993), we have tried to estimate the burden for each of them individually. Because of the significant overlap with estimates of burden from infectious diseases, estimation of burden from perinatal infection was not separately done. Among all perinatal causes of death, deaths due to LBW and birth asphyxia only are estimated in this and in Chapter 11 in this volume.

To estimate the number of deaths due to LBW, one approach is to apply the set of cause-specific death rates to all liveborns or case-fatality rates to LBW cases using DISMOD. For EME, FSE and some LAC, reported vital registration data for the category of "certain conditions originating in the perinatal period" are available from the WHO database and classified as follows (Basic Tabulation List codes):

- 45 Certain conditions originating in the perinatal period (760–779)
- 450 Maternal conditions affecting fetus or newborn (760)
- 451 Obstetric complications affecting fetus or newborn (761–763)
- 452 Slow fetal growth, fetal malnutrition and immaturity (764, 765)
- 453 Birth trauma
- 454 Hypoxia, birth asphyxia and other respiratory conditions (768–770)
- 455 Haemolytic disease of fetus or newborn (773).

From the total number of deaths and corresponding cause-specific death rates from LBW for almost all EME and FSE, and some LAC countries can be estimated. For China, both vital registration data for selected areas and data from Disease Points Surveillance are useful sources of mortality estimates. It should be noted that the calculations using proportion of LBW as incidence and cause-specific death rates derived from the vital registration data are based on live births rather than deliveries. Thus, a small bias can occur with regard to the case of stillbirths.

For other regions (IND, MEC, OAI and SSA) where the LBW proportion is considerably high (16 per cent), data on birth-weight specific mortality are very scarce and almost all of them come from hospital-based studies with various sample sizes. However, the overall mortality is considered to be higher than in the other four regions (EME, FSE, CHN and LAC). In SSA, one study at a tertiary hospital suggests that mortality of LBW infants was 11.8 per cent (53.5 per cent for VLBW) compared to 5.3 per cent in normal birth weight infants (Okoji and Oruamabo 1992). In rural areas, mortality was quite high and, before the introduction of simple neonatal care, was 90 per cent for VLBW and 70 per cent for those weighing 1 500–1 999g (Bergman and Jurisoo 1994). In India, one study at a tertiary hospital also shows higher mortality among LBW infants (55 per cent for LBW 1 500g and 74 per cent for VLBW) although the sample was small and more than half of LBW was VLBW because of the nature of the hospital (Njokanma and Fabule 1994). Another study comparing the mortality and morbidity of LBW among tertiary hospitals, district hospitals and villages consistently showed no significant difference between the three levels of the health care system. Neonatal mortality was 21, 18, and 18 per cent, respectively (Das et al. 1993). It may be possible to estimate the mortality level in such cases based on a few hospital-based studies and extrapolation from the historical data in EME. However, this process may lead to overestimation. As pointed out earlier, the higher proportion of LBW does not necessarily mean a higher risk of death among neonates with a birth weight of 2 000–2 500 which represent the largest share of LBW. It should be noted that application of mortality data from EME to other regions with a higher proportion of SGA infants may lead to overestimation of mortality from LBW. However, the studies have suggested the predominant effect of birth weight over gestational age on mortality (McCormick 1985, Das et al 1993). Thus, the effect of gestational age on the overall LBW mortality estimate may not be as significant.

Another possible source of overestimation is comorbidity. Since LBW is not a disease, there are multiple factors and diseases which contribute to LBW incidence. For example, there is an inverse relationship between birth prevalence and mortality from congenital anomalies and the infants' birth weights. The higher risk of congenital anomalies among LBW infants contributes to their excess mortality and morbidity. Other diseases such as diarrhoeal diseases and respiratory infections are also more common in LBW infants.

Finally, the most fundamental source of overestimation is the comparatively high incidence of LBW in these four regions. The simple application of reported mortality rates, for example, to IND, results in an estimated number of deaths from LBW which exceeds the total neonatal deaths estimate. Thus, to estimate the number of deaths from LBW in MEC, OAI, IND and SSA, instead of applying the mortality rates derived from limited studies to incidence, an alternative approach was applied. That is, the proportion of LBW mortality (BTL code 452) among total mortality from perinatal conditions (45) except infection was estimated from the available vital registration data in EME, FSE, LAC, CHN, MEC and OAI. After excluding countries with small death numbers and obvious outliers, the relative proportion of LBW deaths (BTL code 452) and birth trauma, asphyxia and other respiratory conditions (codes 453 and 454) was estimated as follows:

$$\text{Log}\ (\%D_{453\ \&\ 454}) = 4.9738 - 0.40377\ \text{Log}\ (\%\text{LBW})$$

where $\%D_{453\ \&\ 454}$ is the proportion of deaths classified coded to 453 and 454 among the number of deaths in 453, 453 and 454, and $\%LBW$ is the proportion of LBW in a given region. It is reasonable to assume that the relative proportion of deaths from LBW increases as the proportion of LBEW in a region increases. For OAI, MEC, IND and SSA, the relative proportion of LBW deaths was derived from this formula assuming that the proportion of other perinatal causes of death (BTL codes 451 and 455) was constant across the regions: based on the vital registration data, 15 per cent of all deaths due to perinatal conditions was attributable to maternal and obstetrical conditions or haemolytic disease. It should be noted that since this estimate was derived from high income countries, the result may be somewhat biased in the low-income regions.

Applying the formula to the estimated proportion of LBW by region, the relative proportions of LBW mortality (452) and birth trauma, asphyxia and other respiratory conditions (453 and 454) by region were calculated and are shown in Table 12.

The estimated proportion of LBW mortality was then applied to the estimated number of deaths from perinatal conditions to get the total number of death from LBW.

Estimates of the number of deaths from conditions arising during the perinatal period were based on vital registration data for EME, FSE and LAC, and were adjusted as described in Chapter 3, Volume I of this Series (Murray and Lopez 1996). For China the number of low-birth weight deaths was derived from the Disease Surveillance Point system; the strengths and weaknesses of this sample registration system are described in Murray and Lopez (1996). For OAI, SSA and MEC mortality estimates were based on the epidemiological estimates for low birth weight and birth asphyxia presented in this chapter and Chapter 11 of this volume. Mortality estimates for all six developing regions were then subjected to the neonatal adjustment algorithm which is described in detail in Chapter 3 (pages 163–169) in The Global Burden of Disease (Murray and Lopez 1996).

Table 12 Estimated mortality from LBW by region, 1990.

Region	*Proportion LBW* (per cent)	*Proportion of LBW death (452)* (per cent)	*Proportion of death from other causes (453* and 454*)* (per cent)
EME	6	33.6	66.4
FSE	7	37.9	62.1
CHN	6	33.6	66.4
IND	35	69.1	20.9
SSA	16	56.6	43.4
OAI	22	62.2	37.8
MEC	16	56.6	43.4
LAC	13	52.5	47.5

**BTL codes in ICD-9*

Estimation of disability from LBW by region

For the purpose of estimating disability from LBW, several assumptions were made. First, based on past studies in EME, the probability of developing a disability in LBW survivors is considered to be quite different for LBW and VLBW. We then estimate the relative proportion of total LBW cases for each of these two groups and apply the probability to annual LBW numbers for each group to get the total number of disabled children. Second, it is assumed that the distribution of birth weight is constant within a region. In a region with high LBW prevalence, the proportion of VLBW is likely to be lower because of the higher risk of death and the predominance of SGA-LBW. In fact, limited data from the WHO database suggest a lower proportion of VLBW among all LBW infants in developing countries than in EME.

If we can assume that the distribution of birth weight is exactly normal and if the mean birth weight and variance are available, we can apply the following formula to get the proportion of VLBW among all LBW:

$$\%VLBW = \frac{\int_0^{500} f(x)dx}{\int_0^{2500} f(x)dx} \times 100$$

where x is a given birth weight, $f(x)$ is the normal distribution function defined as

$$f(x) = \frac{1}{\sqrt{2\pi\sigma}} exp[^{-(x-\mu)^2}/_{2\sigma^2}]$$

with mean birth weight μ and variance σ. However, this assumption underestimates the VLBW proportion because of the "residual" component in the lower tail (Chen et al., 1991; Wilcox and Russell, 1983c). In fact, if we apply this formula to data from the USA, VLBW would be less than 1 per cent. This estimate is quite implausible. Instead, direct estimation from the actual data was undertaken. For this purpose, studies on birth weight distribution were selected from the WHO database on the basis of study design, sample size, and consistency with the overall LBW proportion (Table 13).

For EME and IND, sufficient data are available although almost all studies in India are hospital-based. The proportion of VLBW was relatively consistent within each region, being 10–17 per cent in EME and 3–10 per cent in IND. For FSE, MEC, OAI and SSA, not enough data are available although in LAC the data suggest that the proportion of VLBW was between the level of IND and EME. Recent data in CHN suggest the proportion of VLBW is very low at around 5 per cent (Ji 1992). For the purpose of these estimates, the proportion of LBW and VLBW was assumed to be: 15 per cent for EME and FSE; 10 per cent for LAC, OAI, MEC. 7.5 per cent for IND and SSA; and 6 per cent for CHN.

Finally, the probabilities of developing a disability among survivors were assumed to be similar to those suggested from past studies in EME. No comparable studies are available in other regions. In all regions, these were assumed to be 5–7 per cent for LBW and 25 per cent for VLBW. Thus, assuming that the probability of developing a disability among VLBW survivors is 5 times higher than that of LBW (McComick 1985), the overall probabilities of developing a disability among surviving LBW infants were calculated as shown in Table 14.

Because of the assumption of a lower proportion of VLBW and of higher mortality in developing countries, the overall risk of developing a disability is slightly higher in developed countries. However, the data from EME where the majority of LBW babies are preterm would tend to overestimate the disability burden in other regions since SGA is the predominant cause of LBW in the developing regions.

Congenital anomalies also contribute to disabilities among surviving LBW infants. Generally, the contribution of congenital anomalies as a cause of childhood disabilities increases as the mortality due to perinatal conditions falls. We have assumed that the proportion of congenital anomalies among disabled LBW infants depends primarily on the mortality level in a region. The assumed proportions of congenital anomalies among disabled LBW infants used in these estimates were as follows: 80 per cent for EME, FSE and CHN; 55 per cent for LAC, MEC and OAI; 40 per cent for IND and SSA. This assumption was based on the fact that the contribution of congenital anomalies to childhood disability increases as the mortality level of a region decreases.

As mentioned above, LBW infants suffer both immediate and long-term morbidity. In the calculation of disabilities among LBW survivors, the ma-

Table 13 Cumulative distribution of birthweight, by region, 1990

Region *Country/region*	*Year*	*Type of survey*	*Sample size*	*Mean birth weight*	*<1500g*	*<2000g*	*<2500g*	*<3000g*	*%VLBW*
EME									
Canada	1986	R	364 180	3 378	0.9	1.9	5.7	21.3	15.8
USA	1988	R	3 909 510		1.2		6.9		17.4
Denmark	1987	R	56 221	3 400	0.7	1.9	5.7	21.0	12.3
Finland	1985	R	62 796	3 550	0.6	1.6	4.0	13.8	15.0
Iceland	1983	T	4 342	3 532	0.5	1.5	3.3	11.9	15.2
Norway	1983	R	49 830	3 513	0.5	1.5	4.2	15.1	11.9
Sweden	1983	R	91 319	3 490	0.7	1.7	4.5	16.0	15.6
England and Wales	1985	R	642 089	3 320	0.7	1.8	5.9	23.9	11.9
Greece	1985	R	116 481	3 290	0.9	2.1	6.0	24.5	15.0
Italy	1981	R	623 103	3 330	0.7	1.5	5.2	21.9	13.5
Portugal	1985	R	130 492	3 330	0.6	1.4	5.4	22.8	11.1
Austria	1985	R	87 440	3 320	0.8	2.0	5.8	22.3	13.8
Belgium	1981-82	R	242 658	3 300	0.6		5.7		10.5
Germany	1985	R	586 155	3 360	0.8	2.0	5.7	21.6	14.0
Switzerland	1979-85	R	518 770	3 300	0.7	1.8	5.4	23.4	13.0
Japan	1987	R	1 346 437	3 150	0.5	1.3	5.7	34.1	8.8
Australia	1980-86	R	142 571	3 380	0.7	1.6	4.6	19.7	15.2
New Zealand	1985	R	51 798		0.8	1.9	5.5	20.4	14.5
FSE									
former Czechoslovakia	1984	R	227 784	3 320	0.7	1.8	5.8	23.5	12.1
Hungary	1989	R	123 304	3 184	1.3	3.2	9.2	31.6	14.1
Poland	1985	R	677 576		0.9	2.7	7.8	28.9	11.5
IND									
Bihar, Bokaro	1976-77	H	5 340		1.7	9.6	45.4	86.6	3.7
Bihar, Ghatsila	1978-83	H	5 138		2.9	9.8	24.5		11.8
Delhi, New Delhi	1983	H	26 418	2 730	1.9	5.9	29.1	70.3	6.5
Delhi, New Delhi	1986	H	6 718	2 620	4.5	12.5	38.7	77.0	11.6
Harayana	1982-85	C	3 515	2 774	1.8	8.8	27.6	82.2	6.5
Maharashtra, Pune	1984-85	H	8 931	2 490	4.1	14.0	52.8	87.9	7.8
Maharashtra, Pune	1984	H	3 095	2 830	0.7	3.3	20.3	68.9	3.4
Orissa, Rourkela	1983	H	3 550	2 724	1.4	5.1	26.1	69.5	5.4
Orissa, Rourkela	1986	H	3 368	2 726	1.3	4.9	25.1	69.4	5.2
Uttar Pradesh, Vranasi	1979-80	H	4 415		4.3	12.3	36.5		11.8
Uttar Pradesh, Vranasi	1979-80	H	4 183		2.8	10.4	34.7		8.1
CHN									
Beijing	1977	H	4 000		0.3	0.9	6.6	34.5	4.5
Shanghai	1968-79	R			0.2	0.8	4.4		4.5
OAI									
Indonesia	1978-80	H	13 080		1.3	2.7	9.4	41.4	13.8
Malaysia	1984	R	221 916	3 120	0.5	1.9	9.2	38.5	5.4
Philippines	1981	H	3 066		5.2	10.3	36.4	60.0	14.3
Singapore	1985	R	42 484	3 160	0.6	1.7	7.0	34.6	8.6
Thailand	1983	R	164 338	2 980	0.7	2.6	12.7	50.8	5.5
SSA									
Ethiopia	1977-83	H	6 813	3 039	0.7		11.1	45.4	6.3
Tanzania	1980-83	H	4 201	2 946	1.3	3.5	13.2	49.7	9.8

Table 13 *(continued)*

Region *Country/region*	*Year*	*Type of survey*	*Sample size*	*Mean birth weight*	*<1500g*	*<2000g*	*<2500g*	*<3000g*	*%VLBW*
SSA *(continued)*									
Zimbabwe	1982-84	H	4 850	2 990	3.0	7.2	18.5	45.2	16.2
Lesotho	1983	H	10 794	3 070	1.2	2.7	10.5	44.0	11.4
South Africa	1982	R	35 993		1.4	3.6	12.0		11.7
LAC									
Costa Rica	1977-80	H	21 062		0.8	2.3	7.2		11.1
Panama	1980	H	6 527		0.8	2.6	9.8		8.2
Cuba	1981	R	136 211	3 160	0.9	2.5	9.8	35.6	9.2
Puerto Rico	1984	R	63 257		1.0	2.6	9.1	33.0	11.0
Brazil	1980-82	H	8 867	3 042	1.8	4.2	12.9	42.0	14.0
Chile	1985	R	248 879	3 170	0.9	2.0	6.4	26.0	14.1
Uruguay	1983	H	53 405	3 270	1.0	2.4	7.3	26.6	13.7
MEC									
Israel	1985	R	99 376	3 240	1.1	2.5	7.5	28.1	14.7
Saudi Arabia	1983	H	27 396		0.7	2.6	5.5		12.7
Tunisia	1989	H	5 419		1.5	3.3	7.6		19.7

* H=hospital-based, C=community-based, R=registration

Source: World Heath Organization, 1992

Table 14 Estimated probabilities of developing a disability among LBW survivors, by region

Region	*Proportion of LBW ≥1500g (%)*	*Probability of disability among LBW ≥1500g (%)*	*Proportion of VLBW survivors (%)*	*Probability of disability in VLBW survivors (%)*	*Probability of disability among all LBW (%)*
EME and FSE	85	5	15	25	8%
LAC, OAI and MEC	90	5	10	25	6%
IND and SSA	92.5	5	7.5	25	6%
CHN	94	5	6	25	6%

Table 15 Prevalence of neurodevelopmental disability among LBW survivors

Type of disability	*Prevalence (per cent)*
Mental retardation (IQ < 70)	9.0
Cerebral Palsy	8.1
Minimal cerebral dysfunction	18.2
Epilepsy	4.2
Hearing loss	3.6
Visual defects	4.8

Source: Dunn 1986

Table 16 Disability weights for low birth weight — treated and untreated forms

	Age (years)				
Disability Weights	*0-4*	*5-14*	*15–44*	*45–59*	*60+*
Treated	0.256	0.256	0.256	0.256	0.256
Untreated	0.291	0.291	0.291	0.291	0.291

see Murray and Lopez 1996

Table 17 Per cent distribution of cases across the seven disability classes

Dis Class	*I*	*II*	*III*	*IV*	*V*	*VI*	*VII*
Untreated							
0-4	38	12	0	6	20	13	12
Treated							
0-4	38	12	5	9	17	9	10

see Murray and Lopez 1996

Table 18 Per cent of cases in each region that are treated

	Male	*Female*
EME	80	80
FSE	60	60
IND	15	15
CHN	20	20
OAI	15	15
SSA	5	5
LAC	35	35
MEC	30	30

see Murray and Lopez 1996

jor sequela was defined as neurodevelopmental disability such as mental retardation and cerebral palsy. The result of the Vancouver study (Dunn 1986) was used to estimate the type of disability among LBW survivors. After excluding congenital anomalies and congenital disorders, the prevalence of each neurodevelopmental disability was estimated as shown in Table 15. After adjusting for the overlap, about 35 per cent of disabled children had severe neurodevelopmental sequela including cerebral palsy (CP) and mental retardation (MR). There was no significant difference in the prevalence of these disabilities between SGA and preterm infants.

In the calculation of disability-adjusted life years (DALYs), different disability weights were used for treated and untreated cases (Table 16). These weights are the weighted average of the disability weights for LBW in each of the seven severity classes of disability; the estimated proportion of LBW infants in each disability class is shown in Table 17. These disability weights were derived from person-trade off health state preference measurements conducted at the World Health Organization in August 1995. (For a more detailed description of the person-trade off exercise and the methods used to derive the disability weights see Murray (1996).)

Next, the adjustment factors (the ratio of treated cases among all cases) were applied to the estimated number of cases in each region (Table 18). These adjustment factors were estimated based on information about the available health infrastructure and access to perinatal care by region. The overall disability weight for a region is the weighted average of treated and untreated cases.

Under these assumptions, the estimates for deaths, Years of Life Lost (YLLs) and DALYs due to LBW are shown in Tables 19 and 20.

BURDEN AND INTERVENTION

A reduction in the incidence of LBW would have a significant effect on reducing infant mortality and morbidity. Many studies have focused on risk factors associated with low birth weight (Da Vanzo et al. 1984, Ferraz et al. 1990, Kamaladoss et al. 1992, Mavalankar et al. 1992). Table 21 summarizes risk factors for low birth weight, grouped by time periods (Sinclair 1991). It should be noted that the LBW proportion is confounded by a complex interaction between socioeconomic, genetic and cultural factors, especially in the case of SGA-LBW (Kliegman et al. 1990). The majority of preterm births in both developing and developed countries remain unexplained. Some reproductive complications such as amniotic fluid infection and premature rupture of membranes may be related although the initiating events of preterm labour cannot be identified in the majority of cases (Amon et al. 1987; Thomsen et al. 1987).

Kramer (1987) extensively reviewed past studies on the determinants of LBW. In developing countries, major determinants of SGA were specific racial origin, poor gestational nutrition, low pre-pregnancy weight, short maternal stature, and malaria. In developed countries, cigarette smoking was the most important factor, followed by poor nutrition and low pre-pregnancy weight. Based on these findings, Kramer recommended a number of public health interventions (Table 22).

In developing regions where SGA-LBW is predominant, a substantial proportion of LBW births may be averted by improving maternal nutrition status, anaemia and antenatal care including health education (Mavalankar et al. 1992, Oruamabo and John 1989) whereas an effective anti-smoking strategy is one of the primary interventions to reduce preterm infants in developed countries. It is well recognized that improvements in

Table 19 Epidemiological estimates for low birth weight, 1990, males

Age group (years)	*Incidence* Number ('000s)	*Incidence* Rate per100 000	*Prevalence* Number ('000s)	*Prevalence* Rate per100 000	*Avg. age at onset* (years)	*Avg. duration* (years)	*Deaths* Number ('000s)	*Deaths* Rate per100 000	*YLLs* Number ('000s)	*YLLs* Rate per100 000	*DALYs* Number ('000s)	*DALYs* Rate per100 000
	Established Market Economies											
0-4	2	7	9	35	0.0	68.1	6	21	197	746	197	746
5-14	0	0	19	35	–	–	0	0	0	0	0	0
15-44	0	0	64	35	–	–	0	0	0	0	0	0
45-59	0	0	23	35	–	–	0	0	0	0	0	0
60+	0	0	21	35	–	–	0	0	0	0	0	0
All Ages	*2*	*1*	*136*	*35*	*0.0*	*68.1*	*6*	*1*	*197*	*50*	*197*	*50*
	Formerly Socialist Economies of Europe											
0-4	2	11	8	56	0.0	62.8	3	24	103	752	103	752
5-14	0	0	15	56	–	–	0	0	0	0	0	0
15-44	0	0	43	56	–	–	0	0	0	0	0	0
45-59	0	0	15	56	–	–	0	0	0	0	0	0
60+	0	0	12	56	–	–	0	0	0	0	0	0
All Ages	*2*	*1*	*93*	*56*	*0.0*	*62.8*	*3*	*2*	*103*	*63*	*103*	*63*
	India											
0-4	77	128	382	639	0.0	58.8	164	289	5 475	9 157	5 475	9 157
5-14	0	0	650	639	–	–	0	0	0	0	0	0
15-44	0	0	1,281	639	–	–	0	0	0	0	0	0
45-59	0	0	304	639	–	–	0	0	0	0	0	0
60+	0	0	190	639	–	–	0	0	0	0	0	0
All Ages	*77*	*17*	*2,807*	*639*	*0.0*	*58.8*	*164*	*32*	*5 475*	*1 246*	*5 475*	*1 246*
	China											
0-4	5	8	25	42	0.0	64.1	24	42	818	1 357	818	1 357
5-14	0	0	41	42	–	–	0	0	0	0	0	0
15-44	0	0	128	42	–	–	0	0	0	0	0	0
45-59	0	0	30	42	–	–	0	0	0	0	0	0
60+	0	0	20	42	–	–	0	0	0	0	0	0
All Ages	*5*	*1*	*244*	*42*	*0.0*	*64.1*	*24*	*4*	*818*	*140*	*818*	*140*
	Other Asia and Islands											
0-4	12	28	60	137	0.0	60.6	91	206	3 067	7 009	3 067	7 009
5-14	0	0	115	137	–	–	0	0	0	0	0	0
15-44	0	0	220	137	–	–	0	0	0	0	0	0
45-59	0	0	47	137	–	–	0	0	0	0	0	0
60+	0	0	28	137	–	–	0	0	0	0	0	0
All Ages	*12*	*4*	*469*	*137*	*0.0*	*60.6*	*91*	*22*	*3 067*	*894*	*3 067*	*894*
	Sub-Saharan Africa											
0-4	28	59	139	293	0.0	51.1	127	193	4 327	9 113	4 327	9 113
5-14	0	0	206	293	–	–	0	0	0	0	0	0
15-44	0	0	304	293	–	–	0	0	0	0	0	0
45-59	0	0	60	293	–	–	0	0	0	0	0	0
60+	0	0	31	293	–	–	0	0	0	0	0	0
All Ages	*28*	*11*	*740*	*293*	*0.0*	*51.1*	*127*	*37*	*4 327*	*1 715*	*4 327*	*1 715*

Table 19 *(continued)*

Age group (years)	Incidence Number ('000s)	Incidence Rate per100 000	Prevalence Number ('000s)	Prevalence Rate per100 000	Avg. age at onset (years)	Avg. duration (years)	Deaths Number ('000s)	Deaths Rate per100 000	YLLs Number ('000s)	YLLs Rate per100 000	DALYs Number ('000s)	DALYs Rate per100 000
	Latin America and the Caribbean											
0-4	10	36	51	178	0.0	63.4	16	56	550	1 916	550	1 916
5-14	0	0	93	178	–	–	0	0	0	0	0	0
15-44	0	0	186	178	–	–	0	0	0	0	0	0
45-59	0	0	40	178	–	–	0	0	0	0	0	0
60+	0	0	25	178	–	–	0	0	0	0	0	0
All Ages	*10*	*5*	*394*	*178*	*0.0*	*63.4*	*16*	*6*	*550*	*248*	*550*	*248*
	Middle Eastern Crescent											
0-4	18	44	90	220	0.0	61.5	101	204	3 428	8 328	3 428	8 328
5-14	0	0	144	220	–	–	0	0	0	0	0	0
15-44	0	0	250	220	–	–	0	0	0	0	0	0
45-59	0	0	49	220	–	–	0	0	0	0	0	0
60+	0	0	30	220	–	–	0	0	0	0	0	0
All Ages	*18*	*7*	*563*	*220*	*0.0*	*61.5*	*101*	*30*	*3 428*	*1 337*	*3 428*	*1 337*
	Developed Regions											
0-4	4	10	17	42	0.0	66.1	9	22	300	748	300	748
5-14	0	0	34	42	–	–	0	0	0	0	0	0
15-44	0	0	107	41	–	–	0	0	0	0	0	0
45-59	0	0	38	41	–	–	0	0	0	0	0	0
60+	0	0	33	40	–	–	0	0	0	0	0	0
All Ages	*4*	*1*	*229*	*41*	*0.0*	*66.1*	*9*	*2*	*300*	*54*	*300*	*54*
	Developing Regions											
0-4	150	59	747	296	0	58.3	523	207	17 665	6 998	17 665	6 998
5-14	0	0	1 249	279	–	–	0	0	0	0	0	0
15-44	0	0	2 369	253	–	–	0	0	0	0	0	0
45-59	0	0	530	176	–	–	0	0	0	0	0	0
60+	0	0	324	223	–	–	0	0	0	0	0	0
All Ages	*150*	*8*	*5 219*	*278*	*0.0*	*58.3*	*523*	*28*	*17 665*	*941*	*17 665*	*941*
	World											
0-4	154	48	764	238	0.0	60.6	532	166	17 965	5 591	17 965	5 591
5-14	0	0	1 283	233	–	–	0	0	0	0	0	0
15-44	0	0	2 476	198	–	–	0	0	0	0	0	0
45-59	0	0	568	182	–	–	0	0	0	0	0	0
60+	0	0	357	163	–	–	0	0	0	0	0	0
All Ages	*154*	*6*	*5 448*	*205*	*0.0*	*60.6*	*532*	*20*	*17 965*	*677*	*17 965*	*677*

Table 20 Epidemiological estimates for low birth weight, 1990, females

Age group (years)	*Incidence* Number ('000s)	Rate per100 000	*Prevalence* Number ('000s)	Rate per100 000	*Avg. age at onset* (years)	*Avg. duration* (years)	*Deaths* Number ('000s)	Rate per100 000	*YLLs* Number ('000s)	Rate per100 000	*DALYs* Number ('000s)	Rate per100 000
	Established Market Economies											
0-4	2	7	9	35	0.0	73.8	5	17	152	608	152	608
5-14	0	0	18	35	–	–	0	0	0	0	0	0
15-44	0	0	62	35	–	–	0	0	0	0	0	0
45-59	0	0	24	35	–	–	0	0	0	0	0	0
60+	0	0	29	35	–	–	0	0	0	0	0	0
All Ages	*8*	*0*	*142*	*35*	*0.0*	*73.8*	*5*	*1*	*152*	*37*	*152*	*37*
	Formerly Socialist Economies of Europe											
0-4	1	11	7	56	0.0	70.7	2	19	77	589	77	589
5-14	0	0	15	56	–	–	0	0	0	0	0	0
15-44	0	0	42	56	–	–	0	0	0	0	0	0
45-59	0	0	17	56	–	–	0	0	0	0	0	0
60+	0	0	20	56	–	–	0	0	0	0	0	0
All Ages	*1*	*1*	*102*	*56*	*0.0*	*70.7*	*2*	*1*	*77*	*32*	*77*	*32*
	India											
0-4	73	128	362	639	0.0	59.7	169	313	5 750	10 145	5 750	10 145
5-14	0	0	609	639	–	–	0	0	0	0	0	0
15-44	0	0	1 171	639	–	–	0	0	0	0	0	0
45-59	0	0	294	639	–	–	0	0	0	0	0	0
60+	0	0	185	639	–	–	0	0	0	0	0	0
All Ages	*73*	*18*	*2 620*	*639*	*0.0*	*59.7*	*169*	*35.00*	*5 750*	*1 402*	*5 750*	*1 402*
	China											
0-4	5	8	24	42	0.0	66.9	22	39	738	1 274	738	1 274
5-14	0	0	38	42	–	–	0	0	0	0	0	0
15-44	0	0	119	42	–	–	0	0	0	0	0	0
45-59	0	0	27	42	–	–	0	0	0	0	0	0
60+	0	0	22	42	–	–	0	0	0	0	0	0
All Ages	*0*	*0*	*22*	*42*	–	–	*0*	*0*	*738*	*135*	*738*	*135*
	Other Asia and Islands											
0-4	12	28	57	137	0.0	64.5	73	173	2 494	5 941	2 494	5 941
5-14	0	0	11	0	–	–	0	0	0	0	0	0
15-44	0	0	218	137	–	–	0	0	0	0	0	0
45-59	0	0	48	137	–	–	0	0	0	0	0	0
60+	0	0	31	137	–	–	0	0	0	0	0	0
All Ages	*12*	*3*	*464*	*137*	*0.0*	*64.5*	*73*	*18*	*2 494*	*735*	*2 494*	*735*
	Sub-Saharan Africa											
0-4	28	59	138	3	0.0	54.1	122	191	4 168	8 863	4 168	8 863
5-14	0	0	205	3	–	–	0	0	0	0	0	0
15-44	0	0	312	3	–	–	0	0	0	0	0	0
45-59	0	0	65	293	–	–	0	0	0	0	0	0
60+	0	0	37	293	–	–	0	0	0	0	0	0
All Ages	*389*	*11*	*5 833*	*293*	*0.0*	*54.1*	*122*	*0*	*4 168*	*1 616*	*4 168*	*1 616*

Table 20 *(continued)*

Age group (years)	*Incidence* Number ('000s)	Rate per100 000	*Prevalence* Number ('000s)	Rate per100 000	*Avg. age at onset* (years)	*Avg. duration* (years)	*Deaths* Number ('000s)	Rate per100 000	*YLLs* Number ('000s)	Rate per100 000	*DALYs* Number ('000s)	Rate per100 000
	Latin America and the Caribbean											
0-4	10	36	49	178	0.0	67.3	12	44	421	1 522	421	1 522
5-14	0	0	90	178	–	–	0	0	0	0	0	0
15-44	0	0	2 059	178	–	–	0	0	0	0	0	0
45-59	0	0	42	178	–	–	0	0	0	0	0	0
60+	0	0	30	178	–	–	0	0	0	0	0	0
All Ages	*10*	*4*	*396*	*178*	*0.0*	*67.3*	*12*	*5*	*421*	*189*	*421*	*189*
	Middle Eastern Crescent											
0-4	18	44	87	220	0.0	64.1	98	206	3 324	8 367	3 324	8 367
5-14	0	0	136	220	–	–	0	0	0	0	0	0
15-44	0	0	236	220	–	–	0	0	0		0	0
45-59	0	0	49	220	–	–	0	0	0	0	0	0
60+	0	0	34	220	–	–	0	0	0	0	0	0
All Ages	*18*	*7*	*542*	*220*	*0.0*	*64.1*	*98*	*30*	*3 324*	*1 348*	*3 324*	*1 348*
	Developed Regions											
0-4	3	8	16	42	0.0	16.4	7	18	230	601	230	601
5-14	0	0	33	43	–	–	0	0	0	0	0	0
15-44	0	0	104	41	–	–	0	0	0	0	0	0
45-59	0	0	41	42	–	–	0	0	0	0	0	0
60+	0	0	49	41	–	–	0	0	0	0	0	0
All Ages	*3*	*0*	*243*	*37*	*0.0*	*16.4*	*7*	*1*	*230*	*35*	*230*	*35*
	Developing Regions											
0-4	146	54	717	265	0	60	496	183	16 897	6 234	16 897	6 234
5-14	0	0	1 089	243	–	–	0	0	0	0	0	0
15-44	0	0	4 115	436	–	–	0	0	0	0	0	0
45-59	0	0	525	246	–	–	0	0	0	0	0	0
60+	0	0	339	229	–	–	0	0	0	0	0	0
All Ages	*146*	*7*	*6 785*	*335*	*0.0*	*60.3*	*496*	*24*	*16 897*	*834*	*16 897*	*834*
	World											
0-4	149	48	733	237	0.0	59.4	503	163	17 126	5 538	17 126	5 538
5-14	0	0	1 122	213	–	–	0	0	0	0	0	0
15-44	0	0	4 219	352	–	–	0	0	0	0	0	0
45-59	0	0	566	182	–	–	0	0	0	0	0	0
60+	0	0	388	144	–	–	0	0	0	0	0	0
All Ages	*149*	*6*	*7 028*	*269*	*0.0*	*59.4*	*503*	*19*	*17 126*	*655*	*17 126*	*655*

Table 21 Risk factors for low birth weight

I. Demographic risks
1. Age (<17; >34)
2. Race / Ethnicity
3. Low socieconomic status
4. Unmarried
5. Low level of education

II. Medical risks predating pregnancy
1. Parity (0 or >4)
2. Low weight for height
3. Genitourinary anomalies / surgery
4. Selected diseases such as diabetes, chronic hypertension
5. Nonimmune status for selected infections, such as rubella
6. Poor obstetric history, including previous low birth weight infant, multiple spontaneous abortions
7. Maternal genetic factors (such as low maternal weight at own birth)

III. Medical risks in current pregnancy
1. Multiple pregnancy
2. Poor weight gain
3. Short interpregnancy interval
4. Hypotension
5. Hypertension / pre-eclampsia / toxemia
6. Selected infections such as symptomatic bacteriuria, rubella, and cytomegalovirus
7. First or second trimester bleeding
8. Placental problems such as placenta previa, abruptio placenta
9. Hyperemesis
10. Oligohydroamniosis / polyhydroamniosis
11. Anaemia / abnormal haemoglobin
12. Isoimmunization
13. Fetal anomalies
14. Incompetent cervix
15. Spontaneous premature rupture of membranes

IV. Behavioural and environmental risks
1. Smoking
2. Poor nutritional status
3. Alcohol and other substance abuse
4. DES exposure and other toxic exposures, including occupational hazards
5. High altitude

V. Health care risks
1. Absent or inadequate prenatal care
2. Iatrogenic prematurity

VI. Evolving concepts of risks
1. Stress (physical and psychosocial)
2. Uterine irritability
3. Events triggering uterine contraction
4. Cervical changes detected before onset of labour
5. Selected infections such as mycoplasma and chlamydia trachomatis
6. Inadequate plasma volume expansion
7. Progesterone deficiency

Source: Sinclair 1991

Table 22 Public health interventions for the prevention of LBW

	Developed countries	*Developing countries*
Intrauterine growth	Anti-smoking efforts, Selective caloric supplementation before and during pregnancy, Delayed child-bearing in young adolescents, Improved maternal education, Selective improvements in nutrition, Selective improvements in socioeconomic conditions, New vaccines to prevent communicable diseases.	Caloric supplementation before and during pregnancy, Malaria prophylaxis or treatment Anti-smoking efforts, Efforts to reduce tobacco chewing Delayed child-bearing in young adolescents, Improved maternal education, General Improvements in nutrition, General improvements in socioeconomic conditions, Improved sanitation and water supplies.
Gestational duration	Anti-smoking efforts, Selective caloric supplementation before and during pregnancy, Delayed child-bearing in young adolescents, Improved maternal education, Selective improvements in nutrition,	Caloric supplementation before pregnancy, Delayed child-bearing in young adolescents, Improved maternal education, General improvements in socioeconomic conditions.

Source: Kramer 1987

socioeconomic status and maternal education are highly correlated with the reduction of infant mortality as a whole. For the specific interventions for reducing LBW, clinical trials to examine their efficacy have been conducted in several regions including developing countries. However, the beneficial effects of a nutritional and anti-smoking program on fetal or infant survival and development have not yet been determined with confidence (Garner et al. 1992). For example, a meta-analysis of clinical trials of protein-energy supplementation suggests that these programs result in a small increase in fetal growth (29.5g increase in mean birth weight) but do not necessarily lead to a reduction of LBW incidence and other long-term benefits (Garner et al. 1992, Kramer 1993). Another meta-analysis suggests that there are no significant effects of anti-smoking programmes on the reduction of both SGA and preterm incidence (Lumley 1993). Since most of these clinical trials are from EME and differ in terms of the study population, design, allocation methods and control for confounding factors, it is unknown whether generalization of these results to high LBW proportion regions is appropriate.

Another important strategy to reduce LBW is through early identification of pregnant women at high risk of giving birth to LBW infants (Narayanan 1986). In developed regions, where the majority of LBW is due to preterm births, early identification and prompt treatment of preterm delivery are important elements of a prevention strategy. The relationship between availability of perinatal care and infant mortality has been repeatedly proposed (Gortmaker 1979, Narayanan 1986). A recent review of the published literature in the United States, however, suggested that prenatal care has not been demonstrated to improve birth outcomes significantly (Fiscella 1995). More detailed efficacy studies should be undertaken to determine the cost-effectiveness of such specific primary and secondary interventions, especially in developing regions.

Several interventions have been shown to improve the likelihood of surviving for LBW infants. For example, breast-feeding has been shown to reduce the risk of infections among LBW infants in prospective controlled studies (Narayanan et al. 1980, 1983). Others have shown that it was possible to care for VLBW babies at home through appropriate interventions within the context of primary health care (Whitelaw and Sleath 1985). After the introduction of the "kangaroo method" (constant contact of the baby's skin with the skin on the mother's chest), the chance of survival improved from 10 per cent to 50 per cent among VLBW babies (Bergman and Jurisoo 1994). In the developed regions, the efficacy of community-based educational programs has been demonstrated (Resnick et al. 1987, Ross 1984). For example, a randomized study to evaluate the effects of a simple educational curriculum focussing on child development as well as family support and paediatric follow-up showed that the intervention group had significantly higher mean IQ scores than the control group (The Infant Health and Development Program 1990). These studies suggest that relatively simple interventions could improve the health outcomes of LBW infants.

Conclusions

Low birth weight is a major cause of infant mortality and morbidity in both developing and developed countries. It imposes significant burden on the affected children, in the form of immediate perinatal sequelae or life-long disability. LBW is, however, not a single pathological entity but the consequence of multiple factors. It is also important to take into account relevant factors such as mortality level and genetic/ethnic composition in order to evaluate the true magnitude of the LBW burden. Both LBW prevalence and the likelihood of an adverse outcome from LBW could potentially be reduced through public health interventions. For this purpose, the efficacy and cost-effectiveness of each intervention in reducing LBW should be carefully examined in future research.

ACKNOWLEDGEMENT

We would like to posthumously acknowledge Dr. Jose-Louis Bobadilla for his contribution on the burden of LBW to the *World Development Report 1993*, on which this paper is based.

REFERENCES

Ahmed AG, Klopper A (1986) Estimation of gestational age by last menstrual period, by ultrasound scan and SP1 concentration: Comparisons with date of delivery. *British Journal of Obstetrics and Gynaecology*, 93:122–127.

Alberman E, Benson J, Kani W (1985) Disabilities in survivors of low birthweight. *Archives of Disease in Childhood*, 60:913–919.

Alberman E, Benson J, McDonald A (1982) Cerebral palsy and severe educational subnormality in low birthweight children: A comparison of births in 1951–53 and 1970–73. *Lancet*, 1:606–608.

Alberman E (1990) Low birth weight and prematurity. In: Pless IB (ed.) *Epidemiology of childhood disorders*. New York, Oxford University Press.

Amon E, Anderson GD, Sibal BM, et al. (1987) Factors responsible for preterm delivery of the immature newborn infant (< 1000g). *American Journal of Obstetrics and Gynecology*, 157:738–742.

Asworth A, Feachem RG (1985) Interventions for the control of diarrhoeal diseases among young children: prevention of low birth weight. *Bulletin of the World Health Organization*, 63:165–184.

Ayeni O, Oduntan SO (1978) The effects of sex, birthweight, birth order and maternal age on infant mortality in a Nigerian community. *Annals of Human Biology*, 5:353–358.

Aylward GP, Pfeiffer SI, Wright A, et al. (1989) Outcome studies of low birth weight infants published in the last decade: a meta-analysis. *Journal of Pediatrics*, 115:515–520.

Bergman NJ, Jurisoo LA (1994) The 'kangaroo-method' for treating low birth weight babies in a developing country. *Tropical Doctor*, 24:57–60.

Bhargava SK, Ramji S, Kumar A, et al. (1985) Mid-arm and chest circumference at birth as predictors of low birth weight and neonatal mortality in the community. *British Medical Journal*, 291:1617–1619.

Bhargava SK, Sachdev HPS, Iyer PUS (1985) Current status of infant growth measurements in the perinatal period in India. *Acta Paediatrica Scandinavica*, 319 (suppl.):103–110.

Bhushan V, Paneth N, Kiely JL (1993) Impact of improved survival of very low birth weight infants on recent secular trends in the prevalence of cerebral palsy. *Pediatrics*, 91:1094–1100.

Capurro H, Konichezky S, Fonsea D, et al. (1978) A simplified method of diagnosis of gestational age in the newborn infant. *Journal of Pediatrics*, 93:120–122.

Chauham SP, Lutton PM, Bailey KJ, et al. (1992) Intrapartum clinical, sonographic, and parous patients estimate of newborn birth weight. *Obstetrics and Gynecology*, 79:956–958.

Chen R, Wax Y, Lusky A, et al. (1991) A criterion for a standardized definition of low birthweight. *International Journal of Epidemiology*, 20:180–186.

Costello AM (1993) Perinatal health in developing countries. *Transaction of Royal Society in Tropical Medicine and Hygiene*, 87:1–2.

Da Vanzo J, Habicht JP, Butz WP (1984) Assessing socioeconomic correlates of birthweight in peninsular Malaysia: ethnic differences and changes over time. *Social Science and Medicine*, 118:387–404.

Das BK, Mishra RN, Mishra OP, et al. (1993) Comparative outcome of low birth weight babies. *Indian Pediatrics*, 30:15–21.

De Vaquera MVD, Townsend JW, Arroyo JJ, et al. (1983) The relationship between arm circumference at birth and early mortality. *Journal of Tropical Pediatrics*, 29: 167–174.

Dunn HG, ed. (1986) *Sequelae of low birthweight; The Vancouver study*. Spastics Mc Jeith Press, *Clinics in Developmental Medicine*, No.95/96. Oxford: Blackwells Scientific Publications.

Ehrenhaft PM, Wagner JL, Herdman RC (1989) Changing prognosis for very low birth weight infants. *Obstetrics and Gynecology*, 74:528–535.

Escobar GJ, Littenberg B, Petitti DB (1991) Outcome among surviving very low birthweight infants: a meta-analysis. *Archives of Disease in Childhood*, 66:204–211.

Fedrick J (1986) Antenatal identification of women at high risk of spontaneous preterm birth. *British Journal of Obstetrics and Gynaecology*, 83:351–354.

Ferraz EM, Gray RH, Cunha TM (1990) Determinants of preterm delivery and intrauterine growth retardation in North-East Brazil. *International Journal of Epidemiology*, 19:101–108.

Fiscella (1995). Does prenatal care improve birth outcomes? a critical review. *Obstetrics and Gynecology*, 85:468–479.

Garner P, Kramer MS, Chalmers I (1992) Might efforts to increase birthweight in undernourished women do more harm than good? *Lancet*, 340:1021–1023.

Ghosh S, Berry S (1962) Standards of prematurity for North Indian babies. *Indian Journal of Child Health*, 11:210–212.

Gortmaker SL (1979) The effects of prenatal care upon the health of the newborn. *American Journal of Public Health*, 69:653–660.

Hall MH (1990) Definitions used in relation to gestational age. *Paediatric and Perinatal Epidemiology*, 4:123–128.

Hammes LR, Treloar AE (1970) Gestational interval from vital records. *American Journal of Public Health*, 60:1496–1505.

Hertz RH, Sokol RJ, Knoke JD, et al. (1978) Clinical estimation of gestational age: Rules for avoiding preterm delivery. *American Journal of Obstetrics and Gynecology*, 131:395–402.

Ji X (1992) Perinatal care in China. *Early Human Development*, 29:203–206.

Kamaladoss T, Abel R, Sampathkumar V (1992) Epidemiological correlates of low birth weight in rural Tamil Nadu. *Indian Journal of Pediatrics*, 59:299–304.

Kasirye-Bainda E, Musoke FN (1992) Neonatal morbidity and mortality at Kenyatta National Hospital newborn unit. *East African Medical Journal*, 69:360–365.

Kessel SS, Villar J, Berendes HW, et al. (1984) The changing pattern of low birth weight in the United States: 1970–80. *JAMA*, 251:1978–1982.

Kitchen WH, Rickards Al, Doyle LW, et al. (1992) Improvement in outcome for very low birthweight children: apparent or real? *Medical Journal of Australia*, 157:154–158.

Kliegman RM, Rottman CJ, Behrman RE (1990) Strategies for the prevention of low birth weight. *American Journal of Obstetrics and Gynecology*, 162:1073–1083.

Koops BL, Morgan LJ, Battaglia FC (1982) Neonatal mortality risk in relation to birth weight and gestational age: update. *Journal of Pediatrics*, 101:969–977.

Kramer MS, McLean FH, Boyd ME, et al. (1988) The validity of gestational age estimation by menstrual dating in term, preterm, and postterm gestations. *JAMA*, 260:3306–3308.

Kramer MS, Olivier M, Mclean FH, et al. (1990) Impact of intrauterine growth retardation and body proportionality on fetal and neonatal outcome. *Pediatrics*, 86:707–713

Kramer MS (1993) Balanced protein/energy supplementation in pregnancy. In: Enkin MW, Keirse MJNC, Renfrew MJ, Neilson JP (eds.) *Pregnancy and Childbirth Module. 'Cochrane Database of Systematic Reviews': Review No.07141.* Oxford, Updata Software.

Kramer MS (1987) Determinants of low birth weight: methodological assessment and meta-analysis. *Bulletin of the World Health Organization*, 65:663–737.

Lee K, Paneth M, Gartner LM, et al. (1980) The very low-birth-weight rate: principal predictor of neonatal mortality in industrialized populations. *Journal of Pediatrics*, 97:759–764.

Lumley J (1993) Strategies for reducing smoking in pregnancy. In: Enkin MW, Keirse MJNC, Renfrew MJ, Neilson JP (eds.) *Pregnancy and Childbirth Module 'Cochrane Database of Sytematic Reviews': Review No. 03312.* Oxford, Updata Software.

Marlow N, D'Souza SW, Chiswick ML (1987) Neurodevelopmental outcome in babies weighing less than 2001 g at birth. *British Medical Journal*, 294:1582–1586.

Mavalankar DV, Gray RH, Trivedi CR (1992) Risk factors for preterm and term low birthweight in Ahmedabad, India. *International Journal of Epidemiology*, 21:362–272.

McCormick MC (1985) The contribution of low birth weight to infant mortality and childhood morbidity. *New England Journal of Medicine*, 312:82–90.

Michilutte R, Ernst JM, Moore ML, et al. (1992) A comparison of risk assessment models for term and preterm low birthweight. *Preventive Medicia*, 21:98–109.

Moreno L, Goldman N (1990) An assessment of survey data on birthweight. *Social Science and Medicine*, 31:491–500.

Murray CJL (1996) Rethinkg DALYs. In: Murray CJL and Lopez AD, eds. *The global burden of disease: a comprehensive assessment of mortality and disability from diseases, injuries, and risk factors in 1990 and projected to 2020.* Cambridge, Harvard University Press.

Murray CJL and Lopez AD (1996) *The global burden of disease: a comprehensive assessment of mortality and disability from diseases, injuries, and risk factors in 1990 and projected to 2020.* Cambridge, Harvard University Press.

Narayanan I, Dua K, Prabhakar AK, et al. (1982) A simple method of assessment of gestational age at birth. *Pediatrics*, 69:27–32.

Narayanan I, Prakash K, Bala S, et al. (1980) Partial supplementation with expressed breast-milk for prevention of infection in low-birth-weight infants. *Lancet*, 2:561–563.

Narayanan I, Prakash K, Verma RK, et al. (1983) Administration of colostrium for the prevention of infection in the low birth weight infant in a developing country. *Journal of Tropical Pediatrics*, 29: 197–200.

Narayanan I (1986) Care of the low birthweight infant in developing countries. *Annals of Tropical Paediatrics*, 6:11–15.

Njokanma F, Fabule D (1994) Outcome of referred neonates weighing less than 2500g. *Tropical and Geographic Medicine*, 46:172–174.

Okoji GO, Oruamabo RS (1992) Survival in very low birth infants at the University of Port-Harcourt Teaching Hospital, Nigeria. *West African Journal of Medicine*, 11:1–6.

Oruamabo RS, John CT (1989) Antenatal care and fetal outcome, especially low birthweight, in Port Harcourt, Nigeria. *Annals of Tropical Paediatrics*, 3:173–177.

Pethybridge RJ, et al. (1974) Some features of the distribution of birth weight of human infants. *British Journal of Preventive and Social Medicine*, 28:10–18.

Powell TG, Pharoah PO, Cooke RW (1986) Survival and morbidity in geographically defined populations of low birth weight infants. *Lancet*, 1:539–543.

Raymond EG, Tafari N, Troendle F, et al. (1994) Development of a practical screening tool to identify preterm, low-birthweight neonates in Ethiopia. *Lancet*, 344:524–527.

Resnick MB, Eyler FD, Nelson RM, et al. (1987) Developmental intervention for low birth weight infants: improved early development outcome. *Pediatrics*, 80:68–74.

Robertson CM, Hrynchyshyn GJ, Ethes PC, et al. (1992) Population-based study of the incidence, complexity, and severity of neurologic disability among survivors weighing 500 through 1250 grams at birth: a comparison of two birth cohorts. *Pediatrics*, 90:750–755.

Ross GS (1984) Home intervention for premature infants of low-income families. *American Journal of Orthopsychiatry*, 54:263–270.

Rush RW, Davey DA, Segall ML (1978) The effect of preterm delivery on perinatal mortality. *British Journal of Obstetrics and Gynecology*, 85:806–811.

Rush RW, Keirse MJNC, Howat P, et al (1976) Contribution of preterm delivery to perinatal mortality. *British Medical Journal*, 2: 965–968.

Shapiro S, McCormick MC, Starfield BH, et al. (1980) Relevance of correlates of infant deaths for significant morbidity at 1 year of age. *American Journal of Obstetrics and Gynecology*, 136:363–373.

Sinclair JC (1991) Epidemiology of prematurity. *International Journal of Technology Assessment in Health Care*, 7(suppl.):2–8.

Singh M, Paul VK, Deorari AD, et al. (1988) Simple tricolored measuring tapes for identification of low birthweight babies by community health workers. *Annals of Tropical Paediatrics*, 8:87–91.

Stanley FJ, Blair E (1991) Why have we failed to reduce the frequency of cerebral palsy? *Medical Journal of Australia*, 154:623–626.

Stewart AL, Reynolds EOR, Lipscomb AP (1981) Outcome for infants of very low birth weight: survey of world literature. *Lancet*, 1:1038–1040.

Tambyraja RL (1991) The prematurity paradox of the small Indian baby. *Indian Journal of Pediatrics*, 58:415–419.

Terry PB, Condie RG, Bissenden JG, et al. (1987) Ethnic differences in incidence of very low birthweight and neonatal deaths among normally formed infants. *Archives of Disease in Childhood*, 62:709–711.

The Infant Health and Development Program. (1990) Enhancing the outcomes of low-birth-weight, premature infants. *JAMA*, 263:3035–3042.

Thirugnanasambandham C, Gopaul S, Sivakumar T (1986) Pattern of early neonatal morbidity: observations in a referral maternity hospital. *Journal of Tropical Pediatrics*, 32:203–205.

Thomsen AC, Morup L and Brogaard Hansen K (1987) Antibiotic elimination of group-B streptococci in uterine in prevention of preterm labour. *Lancet*, 1:591–593.

Treloar AE, Behn BG, Cowan DW (1969) Analysis of gestational interval. *American Journal of Obstetrics and Gynecology*, 99:34–45.

Veen S, Ens-Dokkum MH, Schreuder A, et al. (1991) Impairments, disabilities, and handicaps of very preterm and very-low-birthweight infants at five years of age. *Lancet*, 338:33–36.

Verloove-Vanhorick SP, Veen S, Ens-Dokkum MH, et al. (1994) Sex differentials in disability and handicap at five years of age in children of very short gestation. *Pediatrics*, 93:576–579.

Victoria CG, Barros FC, Vaughan JP, et al. (1987) Birthweight and infant mortality: A longitudinal study of 5914 Brazilian chldren. *International Journal of Epidemiology*, 16:239–245.

Villar J, Belizan JM (1982) The relative contribution of prematurity and fetal growth retardation to low birth weight in developing and developed societies. *American Journal of Obstetrics and Gynecology*, 143:793–798.

Villar J, Smeriglio V, Martorell R, et al. (1984) Heterogeneous growth and mental development of intrauterine growth-retarded infants during the first 3 years of life. *Pediatrics*, 74:783–791.

Whitelaw A, Sleath K (1985) Myth of the marsupial mother: home care of very low birth weight babies in Bogota, Colombia. *Lancet*, 1:1206–1208.

Wilcox AJ, Russell IT (1983a) Birthweight and perinatal mortality: I. On the frequency distribution of birthweight. *International Journal of Epidemiology*, 12:314–318.

Wilcox AJ, Russell IT (1983b) Birthweight and perinatal mortality: III. Towards a new method of analysis. *International Journal of Epidemiology*, 15:188–196.

Wilcox JW, Russell IT (1983c) Birthweight and perinatal mortality: II. On weight-specific mortality. *International Journal of Epidemiology*, 12:319–325.

Williams RL, Creasy RK, Cunningham GC, et al. (1982) Fetal growth and perinatal viability in California. *Obstetrics and Gynecology*, 59:624–632.

World Bank. (1993) *World Development Report 1993: Investing in health*. Oxford, Oxford University Press.

World Health Organization Collaborative Study of Birth Weight Surrogates. (1993) Use of simple anthropometric measurements to predict birth weight. *Bulletin of the World Health Organization*, 71:157–163.

World Health Organization. (1980) The incidence of low birth weight: a critical review of available information. *World Health Statistics Quarterly*, 33:197–224.

World Health Organization. (1984) The incidence of low birthweigt: an update. *Weekly Epidemiological Record*, 59:205–221.

World Health Organization (1992) *Low birth weight. A tabulation of available information*. WHO/MCH/92.2.

Chapter 11

Birth Asphyxia

Kenji Shibuya
Christopher JL Murray

Introduction

Among perinatal insults, asphyxia at birth is the major cause of mortality and morbidity in neonates. Signs of asphyxia of the fetus are not uncommon and can be detected during labour, delivery or the early neonatal period. In developed countries, the incidence of birth asphyxia has declined with the improvement of fetal monitoring and obstetrical management. Past studies suggest that incidence varies from 0.4 to 5 per cent, and more recently from 0.29 to 0.9 per cent in full term infants (Airede 1991, Tafari 1985). However, birth asphyxia continues to be one of the major causes of mortality among babies, together with other perinatal conditions such as respiratory distress syndrome and immaturity. In developing countries, birth asphyxia accounts for 20–50 per cent of neonatal deaths and is one of the leading causes of perinatal and early neonatal mortality in many regions. For example, a study in eight African countries showed that the incidence of birth asphyxia diagnosed by low Apgar score at a tertiary hospital was 22.9 per cent of liveborns (Kinoti 1993). The perinatal risk factors for birth asphyxia which are potentially preventable through proper monitoring, diagnosis and management are still predominant in developing countries (Table 1) (Donn and Nagile 1986). It should be noted that a high incidence of maternal risk factors such as malnutrition and preeclampsia also contribute to the high incidence of birth asphyxia.

Definition and Measurement

Definition of birth asphyxia

Birth asphyxia has been defined in a variety of ways in past studies, but is actually difficult to define and measure (Hall 1989). There is no gold standard about how best to identify fetuses at risk for asphyxia or how to diagnose asphyxia in utero or at birth (Jacobs and Phibbs 1989, Marrin

Table 1 Conditions associated with birth asphyxia

Maternal	*Placental*	*Fetal*	*Neonatal*
Analgesics/Anesthetics	Abruption	Abnormal presentation	Anesthetics
Diabetes	Infarct	Arrhythmia	Anomalies
Hypertension/ Pre-eclampsia	Insufficiency	Infection	CNS injury
Severe illness	Postmaturity Previa	Multiple pregnancy Prolonged labour	Prematurity/LBW* Infection

Source: Donn and Nagile 1986
*Low Birth Weight

and Paes 1989, Sykes et al. 1982). As no direct measure of asphyxia is available, definitions used in developed countries for asphyxia are summarized as follows:

Late deceleration (fetal heart rate)
Moderate/severe meconium
Apgar score 0–3 at 1 minute
Apgar score 0–3 at 5 minutes
Neonatal encephalopathy (seizures and recurrent apnea)
Umbilical cord blood acid-base status: pH < 7.20
(metabolic acidosis)

Recent studies have highlighted the limitations of most of these markers. The Apgar score has been commonly used as the indicator of birth asphyxia. The 1-minute score is thought to have the greater predictive value for neonatal mortality and the 5-minute score the greater predictive value for later neurological abnormalities. Although the relationship between the Apgar score and later disability such as cerebral palsy (CP) has been demonstrated, it has been shown to have limited predictive value (Freeman and Nelson 1988, Low et al. 1975, Marrin and Paes 1989, Ruth and Raivio 1976, Sykes et al. 1982). In a large prospective study, Nelson and Ellenberg (1981) found that 12 per cent of children among those who had Apgar scores of 0 to 3 at 10, 15 or 20 minutes subsequently had a disability whereas 80 per cent of those who had Apgar scores of 0 to 3 at 10 minutes or later were free of major disability (Table 2).

Low (1990) compared the adequacy of markers of birth asphyxia with umbilical cord acidosis which is thought be an indicator of severity of hypoxia. The predictive value of each marker is relatively low (Table 3). Neither traditional clinical signs nor electronic monitoring are reliable indicators of asphyxia (Hall 1989, Freeman and Nelson 1988, Ruth and Raivio 1976). The predictive value of neonatal seizures for the severity of hypoxia is low although neonatal seizures are strongly associated with later disability. It may be that many markers which describe poor condition at

Table 2 Death rate and proportion developing cerebral palsy in infants weiging more that 2 500 grams who have an Apgar score below 4 at 1 minute to 20 minutes after birth

Age (min)	*Death in first year (%)*	*Cerebral palsy (%)*
1	3	0.7
5	8	0.9
10	18	5
15	48	9
20	59	57

Source: Nelson and Ellenberg 1981

Table 3 Adequacy of markers of birth asphyxia*

Markers of Birth Asphyxia	*Sensitivity (%)*	*False positive (%)*
Late deceleration fetal heart rate	50	> 50
Moderate/severe meconium	32	95
Apgar score 0–3 at 1 minute	46	84
Apgar score 0–3 at 5 minutes	8	73
Neonatal encephalopathy (seizures and recurrent apnea)	23	79

Source: Low 1990

*These markers are compared to the umbilical artery buffer base

birth may reflect factors other than birth asphyxia (Low et al. 1975, Paneth and Stark 1983). For example, low Apgar scores may be due to other perinatal factors such as: asphyxia, drugs, trauma, hypovolemia, infection and congenital anomalies (Paneth and Kiely 1984).

Birth asphyxia is perhaps best defined as hypoxia of sufficient severity and duration to produce metabolic acidosis. However, most of the markers cannot capture both components of asphyxia and are poor predictors of later disability (Freeman and Nelson 1988, Ruth and Raivio 1976). It is well recognized that considered in isolation, most of the independent markers of biologic risks are not predictive of later outcomes such as cerebral palsy and mental retardation because these current measures do not provide insight into the duration, severity, or the adaptive ability of the fetus to respond to hypoxic insults (Freeman and Nelson 1988, Paneth and Stark 1983, Torfs et al. 1990).

Among the various indicators of birth asphyxia, the most reliable indicator of later neurological abnormality for the full term newborn free from congenital or genetic abnormality is hypoxic-ischaemic encephalopathy (HIE), a condition indicative of that fact that the infant has suffered sufficient asphyxia to cause brain injury (Ellenberg and Nelson 1988,

Levene et al. 1986, Sarnat and Sarnat 1976, Tafari 1985). The severity of HIE is a more reliable indicator of adverse outcome than a low Apgar score or acidosis (Levene et al. 1986). HIE is usually classified as mild, moderate and severe as follows (Sarnat and Sarnat 1976):

Mild (Grade I) neonatal encephalopathy;
Neonates with hyperalertness, staring (decreased frequency of blinking without enhanced visual tracking responses), normal or decreased spontaneous motor activity, and a lower threshold for all stimuli including easily elicited Moro reflex.

Moderate (Grade II) neonatal encephalopathy;
Neonates with lethargy, slight increased stimuli threshold, decreased spontaneous movement accompanied by hypotonia, suppressed primitive reflexes, and predominantly parasympathetic responses.

Severe (Grade III) neonatal encephalopathy;
Flaccid newborns with stupor, absent primitive reflexes, and few seizures.

In spite of these findings, traditional markers remain important in clinical measurement, because they help direct attention to early neonatal status (Rosen 1985). Since there is large variation in the definition of birth asphyxia, it is difficult to obtain the incidence of birth asphyxia based on the strict criteria for each region.

In developing countries where a considerable proportion of deliveries occur outside hospitals with the assistance of traditional birth attendants (TBAs) or unskilled relatives, the diagnosis of birth asphyxia can only be made by clinical signs (Raina and Kumar 1989, Shah 1990). Despite progress in the training of TBAs, the attention given to birth asphyxia remains inadequate (World Health Organization 1978). It is difficult for TBAs without training or equipment to accurately assess the physical condition of babies during delivery and after birth. For example, the recording of time which is one of the important elements of measuring an Apgar score is impossible in communities where watches are often not available and, if available, wall clocks often lack a second-hand (Palme 1985). Scoring systems (Apgar, Chamerlain or DeSouza) are difficult to evaluate and interpret for illiterate TBAs. Therefore, the true magnitude of mortality and morbidity from birth asphyxia in developing countries is very difficult to estimate. However, severe asphyxia is considered to be more common and more often fatal in these regions than in developed regions (Tafari 1985).

ICD codes for birth asphyxia

In the ICD-8, birth asphyxia is classified in the broader category of "Anoxic and hypoxic conditions not elsewhere classified (776)" which includes: hyaline membrane disease (776.1); respiratory distress syndrome

Table 4 ICD-codes for birth asphyxia

ICD-8
776 Anoxic and hypoxic conditions not elsewhere classified
776.3 Foetal distress
776.4 Intra-uterine asphyxia
776.9 Asphyxia of newborn unspecified
ICD-9
768 Intrauterine hypoxia and birth asphyxia
768.0 Fetal death from asphyxia or anoxia before labour or at unspecified time
768.1 Fetal death from asphyxia or anoxia during labour
768.2 Fetal distress before onset of labour, in liveborn infant
768.3 Fetal distress first noted during labour, in liveborn infant
768.4 Fetal distress, unspecified as to time of onset, in liveborn infant
768.5 Severe birth asphyxia
768.6 Mild or moderate birth asphyxia
768.9 Unspecified birth asphyxia in liveborn infant
ICD-10
P20 Intrauterine hypoxia
P20.0 Intrauterine hypoxia first noted before onset of labour
P20.1 Intrauterine hypoxia first noted during labour and delivery
P20.9 Intrauterine hypoxia, unspecified
P21 Birth asphyxia
P21.0 Severe birth asphyxia
P21.1 Mild or moderate birth asphyxia
P21.9 Birth asphyxia, unspecified

776.2); fetal distress (776.3); intra-uterine anoxia (776.4); and asphyxia of newborn unspecified (776.5). There is no clear distinction among the last three categories. The Ninth revision of the ICD defines birth asphyxia more clearly based on clinical signs such as fetal heart rate, acidosis, and neurologic involvement. A single category was assigned to asphyxic conditions: "Intrauterine hypoxia and birth asphyxia" (768). In the 10th revision, intrauterine and birth asphyxia are further divided into "Intrauterine hypoxia (P20)" and "Birth asphyxia (P21)". Birth asphyxia is classified as severe, mild, moderate, and unspecified asphyxia, which are primarily based on traditional clinical signs such as heart rate, respiration, skin colour, muscle tone and one-minute Apgar score (Table 4). Although ICD-10 makes a clear distinction between asphyxia in utero and at birth, the term "birth asphyxia" in this paper includes both groups of asphyxia.

Methods for the measurement of mortality and morbidity from birth asphyxia

In regions where reliable vital registration data are available, they can be used for the assessment of mortality to obtain cause-specific death rates for the general population. For developing regions where vital registration is incomplete or absent, the assessment of mortality is based on community- and hospital-based surveys. The limited studies in developing countries have consistently shown that birth asphyxia is one of the leading causes of neonatal deaths. For example, in China, a hospital-based study showed that birth asphyxia is the single most important cause of neonatal deaths and accounts for more than 50 per cent of all neonatal deaths (Min-yi et al. 1989). A community-based study in Bangladesh suggests that the major cause of early neonatal deaths was very small size at birth (54 per cent), birth asphyxia/trauma (26 per cent), and neonatal tetanus (8 per cent) (Fauveau et al. 1990). However, these studies should be interpreted with caution because of the indirect or less reliable measures of birth asphyxia, differences in classification of causes of death, and selection bias.

Longitudinal studies provide reliable data for mortality and morbidity among asphyxiated infants. There have been a number of longitudinal studies in countries in the Established Market Economies, most of which have focused on the relationship between birth asphyxia and consequent disability. The typical sequelae in severely asphyxiated neonates include mental retardation (MR), cerebral palsy (CP), seizures, hearing impairment, and visual defects. It is usually impossible, however, to identify a single perinatal causative factor and its effect on later sequelae (Task Force on Joint Assessment of Prenatal and Perinatal Factors Associated with Brain Disorders 1985). Furthermore, one has to take into account the role of potential confounding factors in longitudinal studies, such as outcome variables, age at the time of measurement and study population (full-term versus term or mixed population) (Aylward 1993). Although many of these studies have defined the outcomes as MR and CP, these indicators often have a lower prevalence than others and thus may preclude the accurate assessment of relationships. The duration of follow-up period also affects the study results. For example, many types of disability may not be apparent until later in life whereas more severe disability such as CP can be detected at younger ages. Stanley and Blair pointed out the difficulty of conducting epidemiological studies on birth asphyxia due to the confounding factors, low incidence of outcome and selection bias (Stanley and Blair 1992).

Nevertheless, estimates based on longitudinal studies reflect the best available data on mortality and morbidity of asphyxiated children. Unfortunately, no comparable studies on the sequelae of birth asphyxia are available in developing countries. It is unknown whether a higher incidence of birth asphyxia in developing countries results in a higher prevalence of disability since there are more new cases and a higher possibility of disability, or a lower prevalence because of a higher mortality of neonates with birth asphyxia.

Review of past studies measuring disease burden and empirical data

Incidence of birth asphyxia

In EME, incidence defined by hypoxic-ischaemic encephalopathy (HIE) varies between 2 and 9 per 1 000 births and exhibits a declining trend. Hull and Dodd examined the trend of HIE incidence over a 13-year period and found that overall the incidence of HIE decreased from 7.7 per 1 000 in the period 1976–80 to 4.6 per 1 000 in 1984–88. This fall of HIE incidence was consistent with the reduction of perinatal mortality (Hull and Dodd 1991). During the period, the proportion of mild to severe HIE cases increased from 34 per cent to 40 per cent, suggesting an increase in survival probability among severely asphyxiated infants.

In developing countries, there are very few available data on the incidence of birth asphyxia, although data suggest much higher frequency. Table 5 shows the incidence of birth asphyxia in selected countries. Unfortunately, the definition and the measurement of birth asphyxia varies among studies. Recent hospital-based studies in developing countries suggest that the incidence of birth asphyxia is between 1 and 30 per cent of live births. Since many deliveries occur outside of hospitals, the true magnitude of birth asphyxia is still unknown and may be even higher. Extrapolation of historical data in EME during the 1950s and 1960s suggests that the current incidence of moderate to severe asphyxia in some developing countries could be at least 30 per 1 000 live births (Tafari 1985). This figure is comparable to the results of a recent study in Nigeria, although stricter criteria (HIE) were used as the definition of birth asphyxia. (Airede 1991).

Mortality and morbidity from birth asphyxia

Birth asphyxia is considered to be the major cause of neuro-developmental disability such as cerebral palsy (CP). However, there is increasing evidence to suggest that the association between birth asphyxia and cerebral palsy has been overestimated (Freeman and Nelson 1988). Although obstetrical interventions which aim to reduce birth asphyxia such as fetal monitoring and caesarean section have been increasingly used and have consequently led to a reduction in the incidence of neonatal seizures, the prevalence of CP has not changed significantly (Freeman and Nelson 1988, Paneth and Kiely 1984, Pharaoh et al. 1987). In a study in Western Australia, only about 8 per cent of cases with cerebral palsy were found to be associated with birth asphyxia (Blair and Stanley 1988). Another cohort study of 50000 births in 1959–1966 shows that majority of asphyxiated infants did not develop CP, and that the majority of children with CP had not experienced asphyxia (Nelson and Ellenberg 1986). Furthermore, the majority of children with cerebral palsy did not have any of these signs in

Table 5 Incidence of birth asphyxia: overview of studies by region

Region	*Period*	*Type of study*	*Incidence per 1,000*	*Definition of birth asphyxia*	*Reference*
EME					
Canada	1960–62	Hospital-based	15.4	Hypoxic-ischemic encephalopathy	Cry et al. 1984
Canada	1978–80	Hospital-based	10.4	Hypoxic-ischemic encephalopathy	Cry et al. 1984
Sweden	1973–79	Hospital-based	2.6 1.7 for full term, 16 for premature	low Apgar score (5min<3)	Ergander et al. 1983
United States	1978–86	Hospital-based	61 for (<2 000g), 22 for (>2 000g)	FHR, Umbilical blood, low Apgar, etc.	Low et al. 1990a
United States	1987–89	Hospital-based	27	Umbilical blood	Low et al. 1990b
IND					
Chandigrah	1987–89	Hospital-based	97.5	low Apgar score (1min<6)	Bhakoo et al. 1989
New Delhi	1981–88	Hospital-based	76	low Apgar score (1min<6)	Kumari et al. 1993
SSA					
Nigeria	1987–89	Hospital-based	26.5	Hypoxic-ischemic encephalopathy	Airede 1991
8 African countries*	1991	Hospital-based	229	low Apagr score	Kinoti 1993
CHN					
China	1989	Hospital-based	18.7	low Apgar score	Xu 1990
OAI					
Malaysia	1989	Hospital-based	18.7	FHR, Meconium, low Apgar, apnea, etc.	Boo and Lye 1992
Hong-Kong	1985–87	Hospital-based	2.9 (severe asphyxia)	low Apgar score (1min<3)	Lam and Yeung 1992
MEC					
Kuwait	1989	Hospital-based	9.4	Hypoxic-ischemic encephalopathy	Al-Alfy et al. 1990

*Kenya, Lesotho, Mauritius, Seychelles, Swaziland, Tanzania, Uganda and Zambia

the neonatal period (Pharaoh et al., 1990). Therefore, it appears that the contribution of asphyxia to overall cerebral palsy is less than was previously thought. Some researchers suggest that birth asphyxia might be the early manifestation of cerebral palsy among babies who are already affected by other antenatal conditions (Blair and Stanley 1988, Pharaoh et al. 1990).

Although a relatively small proportion of childhood disability is attributable to birth asphyxia, infants with birth asphyxia have a greater risk of mortality or morbidity than those without the condition. A review of data from 14 different studies in EME between 1966 and 1983 revealed rates of term asphyxiated babies varying from 4 per cent to 61 per cent for mortality and from 3.6 per cent to 57.1 per cent for disability (Table 6) (Brann 1985).

As mentioned above, hypoxic-ischaemic encephalopathy (HIE) is a more reliable indicator of adverse neurological outcome than a low Apgar score or acidosis and its sensitivity is 96 per cent (Levene et al. 1986). For example, if asphyxia is defined as an Apgar score 0-3 at 5 minutes, only 0.7 per cent of full-term infants will develop CP (Nelson and Ellenberg 1981). The relationship between birth asphyxia defined by HIE and neurodevelopmental outcome among full-term infants has repeatedly been studied in EME. Robertson and colleagues followed 174 asphyxiated children for 8 years (Table 7) (Robertson et al. 1989, Levene 1991). Among neonates with HIE, moderate to severe cases were shown to have more adverse outcomes than those with mild asphyxia. The incidence of severe disability or death in the moderate HIE group was between 15 and 27 per cent. In the severe HIE group, the majority of cases had very poor prognosis.

Recent studies on the sequelae of HIE are summarized in Table 8. Most of the studies are consistent with the findings of Robertson and colleagues. The variation seems to be due to differences in the duration of follow-up, study population and sample size. A meta-analysis of these studies also showed that 25 per cent of moderate and 90 to 100 per cent of severe HIE cases will have neurologic disability (Costello and Manandhar 1990, Levene et al. 1988). No comparable data are available from other regions. Difficulties in ascertaining the severity and duration of asphyxia and lack of follow-up studies preclude assessment of the extent and distribution of the HIE sequelae (Tafari 1985, Shah 1990).

Estimation of mortality and disability due to birth asphyxia

Estimation of mortality

For EME, FSE and some LAC countries, reported vital registration data for the category of ìcertain conditions originating in the perinatal periodî are available from the WHO database and classified as follows according to the Basic Tabulation List (BTL) of ICD-9 (BTL numbers preceed the description of each condition):

Table 6 Incidence of moderate or severe long-term neurologic sequelae (LTNS) (cerebral palsy and/or mental retardation) in surviving term-asphyxiated infants

Reference	*Definition of asphyxia*	*LTNS in survivors (%)*	*Mortality (%)*
Drage 1966	0-3 Apgar at 1 min. 0-3 Apgar at 5 min.	3.6 7.4	23 50
Dweck 1974	0-3 Apgar at 1 min.	33.0	61
Brown 1974	0-2 Apgar at 1 min. or 0-4 at 5 min. or IPPV*	26.0	22
Steiner 1975	0-1 Apgar at 15 min.	28.0	44
Sarnat 1976	0-4 Apgar at 1 or 5 min.	31.0	10
Scott 1976	0 Apgar at 1min. or 1-2 at 20 min. IPPV*	25.0	52
Thomson 1977	0 Apgar at 1 min. or 0-3 at 5 min.	10.3	50
De Souza 1978	0 Apgar at 1 min. or onset of breathing after 5 min.	8.0	4
Nelson 1977 1979 1981	0-3 Apgar at 5 min. 0-3 at 10 min. 0-3 at 15 min. 0-3 at 20 min.	4.7 16.7 36.0 57.1	15.5 34.4 52.5 59.0
Mulligan 1980	IPPV* more than 1 min.	27.0	19.0
Fitzharinge 1981	0-5 Apgar at 5 min. or IPPV* more than 2 min.	47.0	–
Finer 1981	0-3 Apgar at 5 min.	28.0	7.0
Storz 1982	0-5 Apgar at 5 min. or IPPV*	22.0	–
Finer 1983	0-5 Apgar at 5 min. or IPPV*	16.3	0
Ergander 1983	0-3 Apgar at 5 min.	22.0	21.0
Robertson (unpublished)	0-5 Apgar at 1 or 5 min. IPPV*	14.7	3.5

* IPPV = intermittent positive pressure ventilation

Source: Brann 1985

Table 7 Outcome of 100 full-term infants with hypoxic-ischaemic encephalopathy (HIE)

Severity of HIE	*% dead*	*% disabled*
Mild	0	0
Moderate	5	15
Severe	82	18

Source: Robertson et al. 1989

Table 8 Hypoxic-ischaemic encephalopathy (HIE) and outcome

		Proportion disabled or dead, by severity of HIE			
Reference	**n**	**Mild**	**Moderate**	**Severe**	**Duration of follow-up**
Sarnat and Sarnat 1976	21	–	25	100	1 year
Finer et al. 1981	89	0	15	92	3.5 years
Robertson and Finer 1985	200	0	27	100	3.5 years
Low et al. 1985	42	–	27	50	1 year
Levene et al. 1986	122	1	25	75	Median 2.5 years
Robertson et al. 1989	174	0	20	100	8 years

Source: Levene 1991; Robertson et al. 1989

Table 9 Estimated proportion of all perinatal deaths attributed to birth asphyxia

Region	*Per cent*
EME	66.4
FSE	62.1
IND	20.9
CHN	66.4
OAI	37.8
SSA	43.4
LAC	47.5
MEC	43.4

45 Certain conditions originating in the perinatal period (760–779)
- 450 Maternal conditions affecting fetus or newborn (760)
- 451 Obstetric complications affecting fetus or newborn (761–763)
- 452 Slow fetal growth, fetal malnutrition and immaturity (764, 765)
- 453 Birth trauma
- 454 Hypoxia, birth asphyxia and other respiratory conditions (768–770)
- 455 Haemolytic disease of fetus or newborn (773).

The number of deaths assigned to BTL code 454 (hypoxia, birth asphyxia and other respiratory conditions) was estimated as follows. To begin with, it is important to note that among the causes of death included within BTL code 454 are respiratory distress syndrome and other respiratory conditions which are likely to be more prevalent in developed countries. Indeed, in EME, a considerable proportion of deaths classified under 454 are actually due to these two conditions. The relative proportion of deaths from birth asphyxia may be much higher in developing regions.

However, since this proportion is unavailable for other regions, the estimated number of deaths actually refers to the broader category of hypoxia and asphyxia rather than to birth asphyxia itself.

From the vital registration data, the total number of deaths and corresponding cause-specific death rates from deaths classified under 454 for almost all of EME and FSE, and some LAC countries can be estimated. For China, both vital registration data of selected areas and data from the Disease Surveillance Points were useful in the estimation of mortality rates. In other regions (IND, MEC, OAI and SSA) data on mortality from birth asphyxia are very scarce and thus, cause-specific death rates and case-fatality rates from birth asphyxia needed to be estimated. Application of the reported mortality rates in EME to other regions would lead to an underestimation of mortality from birth asphyxia in developing countries. Therefore, for the estimation of the number of deaths from birth asphyxia in MEC, OAI, IND and SSA, instead of applying EME mortality rates to incidence, an alternative approach described in the chapter on low birth weight was applied. (Please see Chapter 10 in this volume for a complete description of the model used to estimate the proportion of deaths from perinatal conditions attributable to 453 and 454 in each region.) Applying the model described in Chapter 10 to the estimated proportion of LBW by region, the relative proportions of birth trauma, asphyxia and other respiratory conditions (453 and 454) by region were shown in Table 9.

Estimation of disability due to birth asphyxia

Disability from birth asphyxia defined as neurodevelopmental disability including cerebral palsy and mental retardation, was estimated by the models for all regions. For this purpose, the incidence of birth asphyxia, the probability of developing disability among asphyxiated neonates, and the severity of disability from asphyxia needs to be estimated.

The incidence of birth asphyxia defined by hypoxic-ischaemic encephalopathy (HIE) was assumed to lie somewhere between the incidence in EME (0.5–1 per cent of live births) as the lower bound and that in SSA (around 3 per cent of live births) as the upper bound. Specifically, HIE incidence was estimated to be 1 per cent for EME and FSE and 3 per cent for all other developing regions. The assumption of constant incidence for developing regions may overestimate the incidence of birth asphyxia in the lower mortality regions such as China and LAC since the incidence of birth asphyxia is thought to be correlated with the level of perinatal mortality (Hull and Dodd 1991). However, the estimate of 3 per cent was applied to all developing regions since actual incidence data on HIE for all regions were not available and the hospital-based studies no doubt underestimate the regional incidence. It should be noted that the incidence rate was based on live births and that this will lead to an underestimation of the incidence of birth asphyxia which will also occur in the case of stillbirths. However, stillbirths do not contribute to HIE and subsequent disability and have no effect on the estimation of disability.

Table 10 Severity distribution of hypoxic-ischemic encephalopathy (HIE)

	Distribution of severity of HIE (%)		
Investigator	**Mild**	**Moderate**	**Severe**
Developed regions			
Finer et al., 1981	35%	50%	15%
Robertson & Finer, 1985	60%	25%	15%
Levene et al., 1986	63%	20%	17%
Robertson et al., 1989	32%	52%	16%
Average	*48%*	*37%*	*16%*
Developing regions			
Airede, 1991	55%	20%	25%
Al-Alfy et al., 1990	49%	23%	28%
Average	*52%*	*22%*	*27%*

The proportion of disabled children among survivors was assumed to be constant across regions: 0 per cent for mild HIE; 25 per cent for moderate HIE; and 100 per cent for severe HIE. For EME and FSE, the severity distribution of HIE was estimated from longitudinal studies in EME: 48 per cent for mild HIE; 37 per cent for moderate HIE; and 16 per cent for severe HIE. For other regions, evidence from two studies in developing countries was used: 52 per cent for mild; 22 per cent for moderate; and 27 per cent for severe HIE (see Table 10). That is, severe cases are assumed to be more prevalent in the developing regions.

The type of disability among disabled infants was derived from an eight-year follow-up study (Robertson et al. 1989, Levene 1991). Among the cohort of 174 asphyxiated children, 23 were disabled and 16 of these (70 per cent) had either cerebral palsy (CP) or mental retardation (MR). Other disabilities such as deafness and seizures were observed in 7 children. Considering the higher proportion of moderate HIE cases in this study, the proportion of CP and MR to 60 per cent and this proportion was applied to the estimated number of disabled cases to get the incidence of CP and MR among survivors of birth asphyxia. Under these assumptions, the estimation of disability among asphyxiated neonates was derived from DISMOD. The model may overestimate the disability burden if the actual mortality rate of asphyxiated babies of the same HIE severity is much higher in developing countries than that in EME (Bhushan 1994).

DISABILITY WEIGHT

There are only a few follow-up studies which describe the severity of each neurological disability. Finer et al. (1981) followed 89 infants with hypoxic-ischaemic encephalopathy. The distribution of disability severity was: 40 per cent babies of mild handicap, 35 per cent in the group of mod-

Table 11 Per cent distribution of cases across the seven disability classes, all ages

Disability class	*I*	*II*	*III*	*IV*	*V*	*VI*	*VII*
Untreated	26	8	0	8	22	20	16
Treated	26	9	6	12	22	13	12

Source: Murray and Lopez (1996)

erate handicap, and 25 per cent for those of severe handicap (Finer et al. 1981). Even though the contribution of birth asphyxia to total childhood disability, considerable proportion of moderate and severe HIE cases will have serious sequelae.

Different disability weights were used for each region taking into account the difference in access to medical treatment, rehabilitative technology and special training services. Actual disability weights used were based on the person trade-off method as described in *The Global Burden of Disease* (Murray and Lopez 1996). The assumed disability weights were 0.4213 for the treated and 0.4793 for the untreated cases. The distribution of treated and untreated cases across the seven disability classes are shown in Table 11. The adjustment factor (the ratio of treated cases among all cases) was then applied as follows: 0.8 for EME; 0.6 for FSE; 0.35 for LAC; 0.3 for MEC; 0.2 for CHI; 0.15 for OAI, and IND; and 0.05 for SSA. The overall disability weight for a region is the weighted average of disability weights for treated and untreated cases. The final disability weights by region were as follows: 0.433 for EME; 0.445 for FSE; 0.459 for LAC; 0.462 for MEC; 0.468 for CHI; 0.471 for OAI and IND; and 0.476 for SSA. Under these assumptions, the estimated number of deaths, Years of Life Lost (YLLs), Years Lived with Disability (YLDs), and Disability-Adjusted Life Years (DALYs) due to birth asphyxia are shown in Table 12.

Burden and Intervention

A primary intervention for preventing birth asphyxia is to identify and treat high risk pregnancies. There are many risk factors which are considered to be associated with birth asphyxia (Table 1). Many of the potentially preventable risk factors such as low birth weight, maternal conditions and infection are still predominant in developing countries. In India, a case-control study on the risk of birth asphyxia showed that major risk factors are primigravidity, history of perinatal death, pre-eclampsia, and antepartum haemorrhage (Daga et al. 1990).

In many cases, asphyxia at birth is a continuation of the process of intrapartum asphyxia. Thus, identification of fetuses at risk is an important element of prevention. In developed countries, many methods are available to monitor and evaluate the fetal well-being and growth in utero such as ultrasonography, electronic fetal heart monitoring, and fetal blood gas sampling. In developing countries, however, these technologies are often unavailable, especially in rural areas. Even at a referral hospital, abnormal fetal heart rate and signs of meconium passage may be the only possible way to detect intrapartum asphyxia (Daga et al. 1990).

Although various scoring systems have been proposed to determine the risk of asphyxia, identification of a fetus at risk is difficult and risk factors are often unpredictable. Moreover, several randomized trials have shown that the efficacy of each monitoring method to prevent birth asphyxia is not very high. Therefore, primary prevention programs should be supported by skilled obstetrical care and a strong referral system. It is often argued that limited access to appropriate perinatal care contributes to the excess mortality and morbidity in developing countries. In such circumstances the role of traditional birth attendants or community midwives is of great importance (Tafari 1985; Costello and Manandhar 1990). However, in training programs of TBAs, less attention has been paid to the management of birth asphyxia (Mangay-Maglacas and Simmons 1986). An evaluation study of the practice of TBAs in rural India suggested that TBAs should be trained to manage birth asphyxia and be provided with equipment for rescucitation (Raina and Kumar 1989). More intensive efforts to resuscitate the asphyxiated babies such as assisted ventilation and brain protection are widely implemented in developed countries (Costello and Manandhar 1990, Svenningsen et al. 1982). However, the efficacy and cost-effectiveness of such interventions in developing countries is still to be determined.

CONCLUSIONS

Although the relationship between birth asphyxia and long-term disability is still unclear, birth asphyxia is a major cause of perinatal deaths in developed countries. It is also likely to contribute greatly to excess mortality and morbidity in developing countries. However, there are reliable epidemiological studies of birth asphyxia and its sequelae in such regions. Understanding the nature of birth asphyxia and examining the efficacy and cost-effectiveness of available interventions is a priority in preventing the global burden of birth asphyxia.

Table 12a Epidemiological estimates for birth asphyxia, 1990, males.

Age group (years)	*Incidence* Number ('000s)	Rate per100 000	*Prevalence* Number ('000s)	Rate per100 000	*Avg. age at onset* (years)	*Avgerage duration* (years)	*Deaths* Number ('000s)	Rate per100 000	*YLLs* Number ('000s)	Rate per100 000	*YLDs* Number ('000s)	Rate per100 000	*DALYs* Number ('000s)	Rate per100 000
Established Market Economies														
0–4	9	36	47	177	0.0	68.1	12	41	396	1 500	5	20	401	1 520
5–14	0	0	94	177	–	–	0	0	0	1	26	48	26	49
15–44	0	0	326	177	–	–	0	0	0	0	59	32	59	32
45–59	0	0	117	177	–	–	0	0	0	0	11	16	11	16
60+	0	0	107	177	–	–	0	0	0	0	3	5	3	5
All Ages	*9*	*2*	*691*	*177*	*0.0*	*68.1*	*12*	*3*	*396*	*102*	*104*	*27*	*500*	*128*
Formerly Socialist Economies of Europe														
0–4	5	36	24	177	0.0	62.8	5	41	176	1 279	3	21	179	1 299
5–14	0	0	48	177	–	–	0	0	0	0	14	50	14	50
15–44	0	0	135	177	–	–	0	0	0	0	32	41	32	41
45–59	0	0	48	177	–	–	0	0	0	0	6	22	6	22
60+	0	0	37	177	–	–	0	0	0	0	1	3	1	3
All Ages	*5*	*3*	*292*	*177*	*0.0*	*62.8*	*5*	*3*	*176*	*106*	*55*	*33*	*231*	*139*
India														
0–4	78	131	390	651	0.0	58.8	87	153	2 889	4 833	48	81	2 938	4 913
5–14	0	0	663	651	–	–	0	0	0	0	232	228	232	228
15–44	0	0	1 306	651	–	–	0	0	0	0	535	267	535	267
45–59	0	0	310	651	–	–	0	0	0	0	93	196	93	196
60+	0	0	194	651	–	–	0	0	0	0	0	0	0	0
All Ages	*78*	*18*	*2 863*	*651*	*0.0*	*58.8*	*87*	*17*	*2 889*	*658*	*908*	*207*	*3 797*	*864*
China														
0–4	38	64	189	313	0.0	64.1	67	114	2 245	3 726	23	39	2 268	3 765
5–14	0	0	304	313	–	–	0	0	0	0	113	116	113	116
15–44	0	0	959	313	–	–	0	0	0	0	260	85	260	85
45–59	0	0	227	313	–	–	0	0	0	0	48	66	48	66
60+	0	0	153	313	–	–	0	0	0	0	8	16	8	16
All Ages	*38*	*7*	*1 832*	*313*	*0.0*	*64.1*	*67*	*10*	*2 245*	*384*	*452*	*77*	*2 697*	*461*

Table 12a (continued)

Age group (years)	*Incidence* Number ('000s)	Rate per100 000	*Prevalence* Number ('000s)	Rate per100 000	*Avg. age at onset* (years)	*Avgerage duration* (years)	*Deaths* Number ('000s)	Rate per100 000	*YLLs* Number ('000s)	Rate per100 000	*YLDs* Number ('000s)	Rate per100 000	*DALYs* Number ('000s)	Rate per100 000
Other Asia and Islands														
0–4	37	84	183	417	0.0	60.6	43	97	1 445	3 302	23	52	1 467	3 353
5–14	0	0	351	417	–	–	0	0	0	0	109	129	109	129
15–44	0	0	671	417	–	–	0	0	0	0	251	156	251	156
45–59	0	0	142	417	–	–	0	0	0	0	46	136	46	136
60+	0	0	84	417	–	–	0	0	0	0	1	6	1	6
All Ages	*37*	*11*	*1 431*	*417*	*0.0*	*60.6*	*43*	*11*	*1 445*	*421*	*430*	*125*	*1 874*	*547*
Sub–Saharan Africa														
0–4	75	158	372	784	0.0	51.1	82	124	2 782	5 859	47	98	2 829	5 957
5–14	0	0	551	784	–	–	0	0	0	0	224	319	224	319
15–44	0	0	813	784	–	–	0	0	0	0	517	499	517	499
45–59	0	0	159	784	–	–	0	0	0	0	48	236	48	236
60+	0	0	82	784	–	–	0	0	0	0	0	0	0	0
All Ages	*75*	*30*	*1 977*	*784*	*0.0*	*51.1*	*82*	*24*	*2 782*	*1 103*	*837*	*332*	*3 618*	*1 434*
Latin America and the Caribbean														
0–4	21	73	105	365	0.0	63.4	54	184	1 817	6 325	13	44	1 829	6 369
5–14	0	0	190	365	–	–	0	0	0	0	61	117	61	117
15–44	0	0	381	365	–	–	0	0	0	0	140	135	140	135
45–59	0	0	81	365	–	–	0	0	0	0	26	117	26	117
60+	0	0	52	365	–	–	0	0	0	0	4	25	4	25
All Ages	*21*	*10*	*809*	*365*	*0.0*	*63.4*	*54*	*20*	*1 817*	*820*	*243*	*110*	*2 060*	*930*
Middle Eastern Crescent														
0–4	43	105	215	521	0.0	61.5	48	96	1 615	3 923	26	63	1 641	3 987
5–14	0	0	341	521	–	–	0	0	0	0	125	192	125	192
15–44	0	0	594	521	–	–	0	0	0	0	289	254	289	254
45–59	0	0	116	521	–	–	0	0	0	0	53	239	53	239
60+	0	0	71	521	–	–	0	0	0	0	3	25	3	25
All Ages	*43*	*17*	*1 337*	*521*	*0.0*	*61.5*	*48*	*14*	*1 615*	*630*	*497*	*194*	*2 112*	*824*

Table 12a (continued)

Age group (years)	*Incidence*		*Prevalence*		*Avg. age at onset* (years)	*Avgerage duration* (years)	*Deaths*		*YLLs*		*YLDs*		*DALYs*	
	Number ('000s)	Rate per100 000	Number ('000s)	Rate per100 000			Number ('000s)	Rate per100 000	Number ('000s)	Rate per100 000	Number ('000s)	Rate per100 000	Number ('000s)	Rate per100 000
Developed Regions														
0–4	14	35	71	177	0.0	66.6	17	42	572	1 424	8	20	580	1 444
5–14	0	0	142	176	–	–	0	0	0	1	39	49	40	49
15–44	0	0	461	177	–	–	0	0	0	0	90	35	91	35
45–59	0	0	165	177	–	–	0	0	0	0	17	18	17	18
60+	0	0	144	177	–	–	0	0	0	0	4	5	4	5
All Ages	*14*	*3*	*983*	*177*	*0.0*	*66.6*	*17*	*3*	*572*	*103*	*158*	*28*	*731*	*131*
Developing Regions														
0–4	292	116	1 454	576	0.0	60.6	381	151	12 792	5 067	180	71	12 972	5 139
5–14	0	0	2 400	537	–	–	0	0	0	0	864	193	864	193
15–44	0	0	4 724	504	–	–	0	0	0	0	1 992	213	1 992	213
45–59	0	0	1 035	344	–	–	0	0	0	0	315	105	315	105
60+	0	0	636	438	–	–	0	0	0	0	16	11	16	11
All Ages	*292*	*16*	*10 249*	*546*	*0.0*	*60.6*	*381*	*20*	*12 792*	*682*	*3 367*	*179*	*16 160*	*861*
World														
0–4	306	95	1 525	475	0.0	60.9	398	124	13 364	4 159	188	58	13 552	4 218
5–14	0	0	2 542	461	–	–	0	0	0	0	903	164	904	164
15–44	0	0	5 185	415	–	–	0	0	0	0	2 082	167	2 083	167
45–59	0	0	1 200	384	–	–	0	0	0	0	332	106	332	106
60+	0	0	780	356	–	–	0	0	0	0	20	9	20	9
All Ages	*306*	*12*	*11 232*	*423*	*0.0*	*60.9*	*398*	*15*	*13 365*	*504*	*3 525*	*133*	*16 890*	*636*

Table 12b Epidemiological estimates for birth asphyxia, 1990, females

Age group (years)	*Incidence* Number ('000s)	Rate per100 000	*Prevalence* Number ('000s)	Rate per100 000	*Avg. age at onset* (years)	*Avgerage duration* (years)	*Deaths* Number ('000s)	Rate per100 000	*YLLs* Number ('000s)	Rate per100 000	*YLDs* Number ('000s)	Rate per100 000	*DALYs* Number ('000s)	Rate per100 000
Established Market Economies														
0–4	9	66	44	177	0.0	73.8	8	29	269	1 074	5	20	274	1 094
5–14	0	0	90	177	–	–	0	0	0	1	24	48	25	49
15–44	0	0	317	177	–	–	0	0	0	0	56	31	56	31
45–59	0	0	120	177	–	–	0	0	0	0	10	15	10	15
60+	0	0	150	177	–	–	0	0	0	0	4	5	4	5
All Ages	*9*	*2*	*721*	*177*	*0.0*	*73.8*	*8*	*2*	*270*	*66*	*100*	*25*	*370*	*91*
Formerly Socialist Economies of Europe														
0–4	5	36	23	177	0.0	70.7	3	28	115	878	3	21	118	899
5–14	0	0	47	177	–	–	0	0	0	0	13	49	13	49
15–44	0	0	133	177	–	–	0	0	0	0	30	40	30	40
45–59	0	0	53	177	–	–	0	0	0	0	6	19	6	19
60+	0	0	64	177	–	–	0	0	0	0	2	5	2	5
All Ages	*5*	*3*	*320*	*177*	*0.0*	*70.7*	*3*	*2*	*115*	*48*	*53*	*22*	*169*	*70*
India														
0–4	74	131	369	652	0.0	59.7	82	153	2 801	4 942	46	81	2 847	5 022
5–14	0	0	621	652	–	–	0	0	0	0	220	231	220	231
15–44	0	0	1 194	652	–	–	0	0	0	0	507	277	507	277
45–59	0	0	300	652	–	–	0	0	0	0	92	201	92	201
60+	0	0	188	652	–	–	0	0	0	0	0	0	0	0
All Ages	*74*	*18*	*2 672*	*651*	*0.0*	*58.8*	*87*	*17*	*2 801*	*683*	*865*	*211*	*3 666*	*894*
China														
0–4	36	63	181	313	0.0	66.9	80	143	2 701	4 662	22	39	2 724	4 700
5–14	0	0	283	313	–	–	0	0	0	0	107	119	107	119
15–44	0	0	889	313	–	–	0	0	0	0	247	87	247	87
45–59	0	0	202	313	–	–	0	0	0	0	46	71	46	71
60+	0	0	162	313	–	–	0	0	0	0	12	23	12	23
All Ages	*36*	*7*	*1 717*	*313*	*0.0*	*66.9*	*80*	*13*	*2 701*	*492*	*434*	*79*	*3 136*	*572*

Table 12b (continued)

Age group (years)	*Incidence* Number ('000s)	Rate per100 000	*Prevalence* Number ('000s)	Rate per100 000	*Avg. age at onset* (years)	*Avgerage duration* (years)	*Deaths* Number ('000s)	Rate per100 000	*YLLs* Number ('000s)	Rate per100 000	*YLDs* Number ('000s)	Rate per100 000	*DALYs* Number ('000s)	Rate per100 000
Other Asia and Islands														
0–4	35	84	175	417	0.0	64.5	34	81	1 176	2 800	22	52	1 197	2 851
5–14	0	0	335	417	–	–	0	0	0	0	104	130	104	130
15–44	0	0	666	417	–	–	0	0	0	0	240	151	240	151
45–59	0	0	146	417	–	–	0	0	0	0	44	127	44	127
60+	0	0	95	417	–	–	0	0	0	0	8	34	8	34
All Ages	*35*	*11*	*1 417*	*417*	*0.0*	*64.5*	*34*	*9*	*1 176*	*346*	*419*	*123*	*1 594*	*469*
Sub–Saharan Africa														
0–4	74	158	368	783	0.0	54.1	82	129	2 804	5 961	46	98	2 850	6 060
5–14	0	0	547	783	–	–	0	0	0	0	222	318	222	318
15–44	0	0	832	783	–	–	0	0	0	0	512	482	512	482
45–59	0	0	173	783	–	–	0	0	0	0	66	298	66	298
60+	0	0	100	783	–	–	0	0	0	0	0	0	0	0
All Ages	*74*	*29*	*2 020*	*783*	*0.0*	*54.1*	*82*	*23*	*2 804*	*1 087*	*847*	*328*	*3 650*	*1 415*
Latin America and the Caribbean														
0–4	20	73	101	365	0.0	67.3	37	132	1 251	4 521	12	44	1 263	4 565
5–14	0	0	185	365	–	–	0	0	0	0	59	116	59	116
15–44	0	0	380	365	–	–	0	0	0	0	135	130	135	130
45–59	0	0	85	365	–	–	0	0	0	0	25	107	25	107
60+	0	0	61	365	–	–	0	0	0	0	7	40	7	40
All Ages	*20*	*9*	*812*	*365*	*0.0*	*67.3*	*37*	*14*	*1 251*	*562*	*238*	*107*	*1 489*	*669*
Middle Eastern Crescent														
0–4	42	105	207	521	0.0	64.1	46	97	1 567	3 943	25	63	1 592	4 006
5–14	0	0	323	521	–	–	0	0	0	0	121	195	121	195
15–44	0	0	559	521	–	–	0	0	0	0	279	260	279	260
45–59	0	0	116	521	–	–	0	0	0	0	52	232	52	232
60+	0	0	81	521	–	–	0	0	0	0	8	54	8	54
All Ages	*42*	*17*	*1 286*	*521*	*0.0*	*64.1*	*46*	*14*	*1 567*	*635*	*485*	*197*	*2 052*	*832*

Table 12b (continued)

Age group (years)	*Incidence*		*Prevalence*		*Avg. age at onset* (years)	*Avgerage duration* (years)	*Deaths*		*YLLs*		*YLDs*		*DALYs*	
	Number ('000s)	Rate per100 000	Number ('000s)	Rate per100 000			Number ('000s)	Rate per100 000	Number ('000s)	Rate per100 000	Number ('000s)	Rate per100 000	Number ('000s)	Rate per100 000
Developed Regions														
0–4	101	265	67	175	0.0	72.1	11	29	385	1 007	8	20	392	1 027
5–14	0	0	137	178	–	–	0	0	0	0	37	48	38	49
15–44	0	0	450	177	–	–	0	0	0	0	86	34	86	34
45–59	0	0	173	177	–	–	0	0	0	0	16	16	16	16
60+	0	0	214	177	–	–	0	0	0	0	6	5	6	5
All Ages	*101*	*16*	*1 041*	*160*	*0.0*	*72.1*	*11*	*2*	*385*	*59*	*153*	*24*	*538*	*83*
Developing Regions														
0–4	614	227	1 401	517	0.0	60.1	361	133	12 299	4 538	173	64	12 473	4 602
5–14	0	0	2 294	512	–	–	0	0	0	0	833	186	833	186
15–44	0	0	4 520	479	–	–	0	0	0	0	1 921	203	1 921	203
45–59	0	0	1 022	479	–	–	0	0	0	0	325	153	325	153
60+	0	0	687	463	–	–	0	0	0	0	35	23	35	23
All Ages	*614*	*30*	*9 924*	*490*	*0.0*	*60.1*	*361*	*18*	*12 299*	*607*	*3 287*	*162*	*15 587*	*770*
World														
0–4	716	231	1 468	475	0.0	61.8	372	120	12 684	4 101	181	59	12 865	4 160
5–14	0	0	2 431	463	–	–	0	0	0	0	870	166	871	166
15–44	0	0	4 970	415	–	–	0	0	0	0	2 007	167	2 007	167
45–59	0	0	1 195	384	–	–	0	0	0	0	341	110	341	110
60+	0	0	901	335	–	–	0	0	0	0	41	15	41	15
All Ages	*716*	*27*	*10 965*	*420*	*0.0*	*61.8*	*372*	*14*	*12 684*	*485*	*3 441*	*132*	*16 125*	*617*

References

Airede AI (1991) Birth asphyxia and hypoxic-ischaemic encephalopathy: incidence and severity. *Annals of Tropical Paediatrics,* 11:331–335.

Al-Alfy AJ et al. (1990) Term Infant Asphyxia in Kuwait. *Annals of Tropical Paediatrics,* 10(4): 355–61.

Aylward GP (1993) Perinatal asphyxia: effects of biologic and environmental risks. *Clinincs in Perinatology,* 2:433–449.

Bhakoo ON et al. (1989) Lessons from Improved Neonatal Survival at Chandigarh. *Indian Pediatrics* 26(3): 234–40.

Bhushan V (1994) Cerebral palsy and birth asphyxia: myth and reality. *Indian Journal of Pediatrics,* 61:49–56.

Blair E, Stanley FJ (1988) Intrapartum asphyxia: a rare cause of cerebral palsy. *Journal of Pediatrics,* 112:515–519.

Boo NY and Lye MS (1992) Factors Associated with Clinically Significant Perinatal Asphyxia in the Malaysian Neonates; A Case-Control Study. *Journal of Tropical Pediatrics* 38(6): 284–289.

Brann AW (1985) Factors during neonatal life that influence brain disorders. In: Freeman JM (ed.) *Prenatal and perinatal factors associated with brain disorders.* NIH Publication No. 85–1149, pp 263–358.

Brown JK et al. (1974) Neurological Aspects of Perinatal Asphyxia. *Developmental Medicine and Child Neurology* 16(5): 567–80.

Costello AM, Manandhar DS (1990) Perinatal asphyxia in less developed countries. *Archives of Disease in Childhood Fetal & Neonatal Edition,* 7:F1–3.

Cyr RM et al. (1984) Changing Patters of Birth Asphyxia and Trauma over 20 Years. *American Journal of Obstetrics and Gynecology* 148(5): 490–8.

Daga AS, Daga SR, and Patole K (1990) Risk assessment in birth asphyxia. *Journal of Tropical Pediatrics,* 36:34–39.

De Souza SW and Richards B (1978) Neurological Sequelae in Newborn Babies after Perinatal Asphyxia. *Archives of Disease in Childhood* 53(7): 564–9.

Donn SM, Nagile RA (1986) Prevention of post-asphyxial hypoxic-ischaemic encephalopathy. *Indian Journal of Pediatrics,* 53:573–586.

Drage JS et al. (1966) The Apgar Scores as An Index of Infant Morbidity. *Developmental Medicine Child Neurology* 8(2): 141–8.

Dweck HS et al. (1974) Development Sequelae in Infants Having Suffered Severe Perinatal Asphyxia. *American Journal of Obstetrics and Gynecology* 119(6): 811–5.

Ellenberg JH,Nelson KB (1988) Clusters of perinatal events identifying infants at high risk for death or disability. *Journal of Pediatrics,* 113:546–552.

Ergander U et al. (1983) Severe Neonatal Asphyxia. Incidence and Prediction of Outcome in the Stockholm Area. *Acta Paediatrica Scandinavica* 72(3): 321–5.

Fauveau V, Wojtyniak B, Mostafa G, et al. (1990) Perinatal mortality in Matlab, Bangladesh: a community-based study. *International Journal of Epidemiology,* 19:606–612.

Finer NN et al. (1981) Hypoxic-ischemic encephalopathy in term infants: perinatal factors and outcome. *Journal of Pediatrics* 98(1): 112–7.

Finer NN et al. (1983) Factors Affecting Outcome in Hypoxic-ischemic Encephalopathy in Term Infants. *American Journal of Disease of Children* 137(1): 21–5.

Fitzhardinge PM et al. (1981) The Prognostic Value of Computerized Tomography as and Adjunct to the Assessment of the Term Infant with Post-Asphyxial Encephalopathy. *Journal of Pediatrics* 99(5): 777–81.

Freeman JM, Nelson KB (1988) Intrapartum asphyxia and cerebral palsy. *Pediatrics,* 82:240–249.

Hall DMB (1989) Birth asphyxia and cerebral palsy. *British Medical Journal,* 299:279–282.

Hull J, Dodd KL (1991) Falling incidence of hypoxic-ischaemic encephalopathy in term infants. *British Journal of Obstetrics and Gyneacology,* 99:386–391.

Jacobs MM, Phibbs RH (1989) Prevention, recognition, and treatment of perinatal asphyxia. *Clinics in Perinatology,* 16:785–807.

Kinoti SN (1993) Asphyxia of the Newborn in East, Central, and Southern Africa. East African Medical Journal 70(7): 422–33.

Kumari S et al. (1993) Trends in neonatal outcome with low Apgar scores. *Indian Journal of Pediatrics* 60(3): 415–22.

Lam BC and Yeung CY (1992) Perinatal Features of Birth Asphyxia and Neurologic Outcome. *Acta Paediatrica Japonica* 34(1): 17–22.

Levene MI (1991, suppl.) Outcome after asphyxia and ciculatory disturbances in the brain. *International Journal of Technology Assessment in Health Care,* 1:113–117.

Levene MI, Bennet MJ and Punt J (1988) *Fetal and neonatal neurology and neurosurgery.* Edinburgh: Churchill Livingstone.

Levene MI, Sands C, Grindulis H, et al. (1986) Comparison of two methods of predicting outcome in perinatal asphyxia. *Lancet,* 1:67–69.

Low J (1990) The significance of fetal asphyxia in regard to motor and cognitive deficits in infancy and childhood. In: Tejani N, (ed.) *Obstetrical Events and Development in Sequelae.* Boca Raton, CRC Press.

Low J et al. (1975) Clinical characteristics of pregnancies complicated by intrapartum fetal asphyxia. *American Journal of Obstetrics and Gynecology,* 121:452–459.

Low J et al. (1985) The Relationship Between Perinatal Asphyxia and Newborn Encephalopathy. *American Journal of Obstetrics and Gynecology* 152(3): 256–60.

Low J et al. (1990a) Intrapartum Asphyxia in the Preterm Fetus less than 2000 gm. *American Journal of Obstetrics and Gynecology* 162(2): 378–82.

Low J et al. (1990b) The Association of Intrapartum Asphyxia in the Mature Fetus with Newborn Behavior. *American Journal of Obstetrics and Gynecology* 163(4): 1131–5.

Mangay-Maglacas A, Simmons J (1986) *The potential role of the traditional birth attendant.* WHO Offset Publication No.95, Geneva.

Marrin M, Paes BA (1989) Birth asphyxia: Does the Apgar score have diagnostic value? *Obstetrics and Gynecology,* 72:120–123.

Min-yi T, Yan-ning Z, Hang X, et al. (1989) Clincopathological analysis of causes of perinatal death. *Chinese Medical Journal,* 102:672–678.

Mulligan JC et al. (1980) Neonatal Asphyxia. II. Neonatal Mortality and Long-Term Sequelae. *Journal of Pediatrics* 96(5): 903–7.

Murray CJL and Lopez AD, eds. (1996) *The global burden of disease: a comprehensive assessment of mortality and disability from diseases, injuries, and risk factors in 1990 and projected to 2020.* Cambridge, Harvard University Press.

Nelson KB, Broman SH (1977) Perinatal Risk Factors in Children with Serious Motor and Mental Handicaps. *Annals of Neurology* 2(5): 371–7.

Nelson KB, Ellenberg JH (1979) Neonatal Signs as Predictors of Cerebral Palsy. *Pediatrics* 64(2): 225–32.

Nelson KB, Ellenberg JH (1981) Apgar score as predictor of chronic neurologic disability. *Pediatrics,* 68(1):36–44.

Nelson KB, Ellenberg JH (1986) Antecedents of cerebral palsy. *New England Journal of Medicine,* 315:81–86.

Palme C. "State of the art" in workshop participating countries: A report of a survey. In: Sterky HG, Tafari N, Tunnel R (eds.) *Breathing and warmth at birth, judging the appropriateness of technology.* Swedish Agency for Research Cooperation with Developing Countries, Stockholm, pp 29–32.

Paneth N, Kiely J (1984) The frequency of cerebral palsy: A review of population studies in industrial nations since 1950. In: Stanley F, Alberman E (eds.) *The Epidemiology of the Cerebral Palsies.* Philadelphia, JB Lippincott, pp 46–56.

Paneth N, Stark RI (1983) Cerebral palsy and mental retardation in relation to indicators of perinatal asphyxia. *American Journal of Obstetrics and Gynecology,* 147:960–966.

Pharaoh PO et al. (1990) Birthweight specific trends in cerebral palsy. *Archives of Disease in Childhood,* 65:602–606.

Pharaoh POD et al. (1987) Trends in birth prevalence of cerebral palsy. *Archives of Disease in Childhood,* 62:379–384.

Raina N, Kumar V (1989) Management of birth asphyxia by traditional birth attendants. *World Health Forum,* 10:243–246.

Robertson C, Finer N (1985) Term Infants with Hypoxic-Ischemic Encephalopathy: Outcome at 3.5 years. *Developmental Medicine and Child Neurology* 27(4): 473–84.

Robertson CMT, Finer N, Grace MGA (1989) School performance of survivors of neonatal encephalopathy associated with birth asphyxia at term. *Journal of Pediatrics,* 114(5):753–760.

Rosen MG (1985) Factors during labour and delivery that influence brain disorders. In: Freeman JM (ed.) *Prenatal and perinatal factors associated with brain disorders.* NIH Publication No. 85–1149, pp 237–261.

Ruth VJ, Raivio KO (1976) Perinatal brain damage: predictive value of metabolic acidosis and the Apgar score. *British Medical Journal,* 297:24–27.

Sarnat HB, Sarnat MS (1976) Neonatal encephalopathy following fetal distress. A clinical and lectroencephalographic study. *Archives of Neurology,* 33:696–705.

Scott H (1976) Outcome of Very Severe Birth Asphyxia. *Archives of Disease in Childhood* 51(9): 712–6.

Shah PM (1990) Birth asphyxia: a crucial issues in the prevention of developmental disabilities. *Midwifery,* 6:99–107.

Stanley FJ, Blair E (1982) Cerebral palsy. In: Pless IB, (ed.) *Epidemiology of childhood disorders.* New York, Oxford University Press, pp473–497.

Steiner H and Neligan G (1975) Perinatal Cardiac Arrest: Quality of Survivors. *Archives of Disease in Childhood* 50(9): 696–702.

Storcz J and Mestyan J (1982) Long-term Prognosis of Asphyxic Neonates from an Intensive care Unit. Intrauterine Related Infants at High Risk of Cerebral Palsy. *Acta Paediatrica Academiae Scientiarum Hungaricae* 23(3): 361–74.

Svenningsen NW, Blennow G, Lindroth M, et al. (1982) Brain-oriented intensive care treatment in severe neonatal asphyxia. Effects of phenobarbital protection. *Archives of Disease in Childhood,* 57:176–183.

Sykes GS, Molloy PM, Jhonson P, et al. (1982) *Lancet,* 1:494–496.

Tafari N (1985) Epidemiology of birth asphyxia. In: Sterkey HG, Tafari N, Tunnell R (eds.) *Breathing and warmth at birth, judging the appropriateness of technology.* Swedish Agency for Research Cooperation with Developing Countries, Stockholm, pp45–49.

Task Force on Joint Assessment of Prenatal and Perinatal Factors Associated with Brain Disorders (1985) National Institute of Health Report on causes of mental retardation and cerbral palsy. *Pediatrics,* 76:457–458.

Thomson AJet al. (1977) Quality of Survival After Severe Birth Asphyxia. *Archives of Disease in Childhood* 52(8): 620–6.

Torfs CP, van den Berg BJ, Oechsli FW, et al. (1990) Prenatal and perinatal factors in the etiology of cerebral palsy. *Journal of Pediatrics,* 116:615–619.

World Health Organization (1978) *Traditional birth attendants. A field guide to their training, evaluation and articulation with health services.* WHO Offset Publication No.44, Geneva.

Xu J (1990) 126 Small Gestational Age Infants. Clinical Characteristics and Long-Term Observation (Chinese). *Chinese Medical Journal* 72(8): 459–61.

Chapter 12

Congenital Anomalies

Kenji Shibuya
Christopher JL Murray

Introduction

During the 20th century, infant mortality has declined significantly in both developing and developed countries. Demographers have distinguished between endogenous infant mortality which refers mainly to mortality from congenital anomalies and other conditions originating in the perinatal period and exogenous infant mortality which refers to infections and postnatal accidents that are largely preventable and treatable (Shyrock and Siegel 1976). As mortality from exogenous causes has declined over the last few decades, endogenous causes, such as congenital anomalies, account for a greater proportion of total perinatal mortality.

In developed countries where perinatal mortality rates have reached about 10 per 1 000 births, congenital malformations, birth asphyxia and very low birth weight account for the majority of perinatal deaths. Therefore, the contribution of congenital anomalies to premature deaths and to morbidity is quite substantial both because they occur early in life (resulting in large numbers of potential years of life lost) and because the disability that results from them is relatively severe (Powell-Griner and Woolbright 1990). For example, in the United States, congenital anomalies were the fifth leading cause of potential years of life lost before age 65 in 1984, contributing six per cent of the total years lost in that year (Centers for Disease Control 1986). Even in developing countries, where perinatal deaths are primarily due to conditions arising during the perinatal period, such as low birth weight, complicated delivery, birth asphyxia and infections, congenital anomalies account for a large proportion of the disability and mortality associated with perinatal conditions.

Despite the great advances in diagnostic technology, epidemiological studies and research, the etiology of the vast majority of congenital anomalies is not yet well understood. Table 1 lists the twenty factors which are assumed to cause congenital anomalies in humans (Leck 1994). There are well-known risk factors for several congenital anomalies. For example,

Table 1 Teratogens and their effects on the frequency of malformations

Teratogen	*Main defects caused*	*Estimated risk difference*
	Infections	
Cytomegarovirus infection	Deafness; brain damage; eye disorder	8% of maternal seroconversion in pregnnancy
Herpes simplex	Brain damage; eye disorder; cutaneous scara	Not known
Rubella	Eye and heart defects; deafness; brain damage	90% after serologically confirmed infection of mother in first 10 weeks of pregnancy
Toxoplasmosis	Brain damage; eye disorder; deafness	30-40% after maternal seroconversion in pregnancy without treatment
Varicella-zoster	Brain damage; eye disorder; cutaneous scara	2% after clinical varicella infection of mother
Venezuelan equine encephalitis	Brain damage	Not known
	Other Maternal Diseases	
Phenyketonuria	Brain damage; cardiac defects	Microcephaly in 8.5% of infants of phenyketonurics with blood phenylalanine >1.2 nmol/L
Insulin-dependent diabetes mellitus	Cardiovascular and central nervous defects; caudal regression	Major defects in 8% of infants of affected women who did not receive special care during early pregnency
	Medications	
Androgens and progestins	Anomalies of external genitalia	Mild clitoridal hypertrophy in 20% and more marked virilization in 9% of female infants after norethindrone in first trimester; risks with other drugs not known but seem to be lower. Hypospadiasis in 0.6% of male infants after progestines in early pregnancy
Anticonvulsants	Spina bifida after valproate; oral clefts; cardiovascular defects	4% overall, but varies with number and nature of anticonvulsants used
Coumarin derivatives	Nasal hypoplasia; epiphyseal stripping; brain damage	Nasal hypoplasia/epiphyseal stippling in 8% after use in first trimester; brain damage in 5% after use in second trimester
Diethylstilbestrol	Genital anomalies	Testicular anomalies, epididymal cysts, or penile hypoplasia in 20% of males, and ridges in cervix and/or vagina in 40% of females after dose increasing from 5 to 150 mg between 7 and 34 weeks gestation

Table 1 *(continued)*

Teratogen	*Main defects caused*	*Estimated risk difference*
	Medications	
Folic acid antagonists (aminopterin, methotrexate)	Carniofacial defects	40% after amnipterin in first 10 weeks of pregnancy; not known for methotrexate
Lithium	Cardiac defects, especially Ebstein's anomaly	3%
Retinoids	Microtia/anotia; central nervous, cardio-aortic, and thymic defects	20% after isotretinoin in first trimester
Thalidomide	Reduction deformities of limbs and ears	50% after use in first 8 weeks of pregnancy
	Other Chemical Agents	
Cocaine	Urinary tract defects	Major defects in 5% of users of cocaine with/without other drugs
Ethyl alcohol	Brain damage; cardiac and joint defects	30% of infants of women with manifest chronic alcoholism
Methylmercury	Brain damage	6% of infants in fishing village where seafood was contaminated
	Miscellaneous Influences	
Hypoxia	Persitant ductus arteriosus; perhaps atrial septal defect	1-5% of school children born and living > 4km above sea level
Iodine deficincy	Brain damage; deafness	40% of surviving infants in iodine-deficint area whose mothers' blood total throxine was < 25 ng/mL
Ionizing radiation	Brain damage	Microcephaly in 70% after estimated dose > 1.5 gray from atomic bombs in first 18 weeks of pregnancy

(*Source:* Leck 1994)

older maternal age and family histories are highly associated with Down syndrome. Kalter and Warkany estimated that single genes and major chromosomal abnormalities account for 13.5 per cent of the total anomalies and that major environmental factors (including medications as well as diabetes mellitus and infections) account for 5 per cent of the total. Thus, only 18 per cent of the total congenital anomalies are attributable to specific factors (Kalter and Warkany 1983).

Table 2 Classification of major congenital anomalies according to successive revisions of the International Classification of Diseases

Type of congenital anomaly	*ICD-7 categories*	*ICD-8 categories*	*ICD-9 categories*	*ICD-10 categories*
Central nervous system	750-53	740-43	740-42	Q00-07
Anencephalus	750	740	740	Q00
Spina bifida	751	741	741	Q05
Other CNS anomalies	752, 753	742, 743	742	
Cardiovascular system	754	746, 747	745-47	Q20-28
Respiratory system		748	748	Q30-34
Digestive system	755, 756	749-51	749-51	Q35-45
Cleft lip and palate	755	749	749	Q35-37
Atresia				
Oesophageal	756	750	750	Q39
Anorectal	756	751	751	Q42
Urinary system	757	753	753	Q60-64
Musculoskelatal system	759	754-56	754-56	Q65-79
Abdominal wall defects		756	756	Q79
Down syndrome		759	758	Q90
All other	Other codes (758)	Other codes (744-5, 752, 757-8)	Other codes (743-4, 752, 757, 759)	Other codes (Q10-18, Q50-56, Q80-89, Q91-99)

Definition and Measurement

According to the International Classification of Diseases (ICD), congenital anomalies are defined primarily according to the localization-oriented anatomical classification, rather than the etiology or pathogenesis-oriented classification. Some congenital diseases are excluded. For example, some congenital endocrine and metabolic disorders, such as congenital cretinism and phenylketonuria, or congenital infections, such as congenital rubella and toxoplasmosis, are included in other categories. ICD codes for congenital anomalies are summarized in Table 2.

Congenital anomalies are usually classified by cause, although most of the etiology of congenital anomalies is not yet well understood. Causes are divided into the following broad categories: monogenic (caused by single major mutant genes), chromosomal, environmental, and multifactorial (Czeizel 1988). They are often further classified as either major or minor, based on their impact on mortality and morbidity.

Birth prevalence of congenital anomalies

Incidence and prevalence

It should be noted that the term incidence often used in the study of congenital anomalies is not truly identical to the incidence used in epidemiology. It is virtually impossible to calculate the incidence rate of congenital anomalies because either the numerator (number of new events in a certain period time) or the denominator (number of population at risk) cannot be accurately calculated with currently available methods (Borman and Cryer 1990, Sever 1983).

Ideally, the following information should be available to obtain an exact birth prevalence of congenital anomalies in a region: it is necessary to record all the births (as a denominator) in a region or community, not just those occurring in particular hospitals; all congenital anomalies (as a numerator) should be recorded; finally, data should be recorded not only at birth but also later in a follow-up study. Obviously, it is difficult for many countries to meet these data requirements, especially for developing countries, where most of the data are hospital-based, and a considerable proportion of births occur outside the hospitals.

Data sources for birth prevalence

The birth prevalence of congenital anomalies can be estimated from either registration and birth certificates or hospital and community based studies. These are further classified as: prospective recording of information about all pregnancies; recording of malformations observed at birth; registration of children found to be malformed at birth or at any time after birth; and retrospective studies of hospital records (Weatherall et al. 1984).

Most of the developed countries have had registration systems of congenital anomalies since the late 1960s and early 1970s. The vital registration systems in these countries are fairly complete and provide a relatively accurate estimate of birth prevalence. Since 1974, international co-operation has been promoted to monitor birth defects. The International Clearinghouse for Birth Defects Monitoring Systems (ICBDMS) has collected data on the birth prevalence of 22 types of major congenital anomalies in Established Market Economies (15 countries and 19 regions), Formerly Socialist Economies of Europe (Former Czechoslovakia and Hungary), China (Sichuan), Latin America and the Caribbean (Mexico and 28 other Latin American countries) and the Middle Eastern Crescent (Israel) (ICBDMS 1991).

Since most of the developing countries do not have accurate vital registration systems, hospital or community-based studies are important sources of information. Unfortunately, while community-based studies provide the highest quality of estimates, there are few such studies conducted in developing countries. Thus, hospital-based studies are often used to estimate birth prevalence. However, these hospital-based studies should be interpreted with caution, as there may have been selection bias in the

Table 3 Birth prevalence of congenital anomalies, selected countries

Region	*Country/ Region*	*Year*	*Prevalence per 1 000*	*Study design*	*Source*
EME	France	1979-83	20.1	Registration system	Roth et al. 1987
	Italy	1978-84	23.0	Population based registry system	Calzolari et al. 1987
	Japan	1970-90	12.8	Hospital-based, retrospective	Imaizumi et al. 1991
	New Zealand	1990-91	43.0	Hospital-based, surveillance system	Tuohy et al. 1993
	Spain	1876-86	20.2	Hospital-based, surveillance system	Martinez-Frias et al. 1989
	USA	1980-82	35.0	Population-based surveilance	Brewster and Heim 1985
MEC	Liberia		22.4	Hospital-based, prospective	Njoh et al. 1991
	Pakistan		21.0	Hospital-based, prospective	Jalil et al. 1993
	Tunisia	1983-84	39.6	Hospital-based, prospective	Khrouf et al. 1986
IND	Lucknow	1981-84	20.0	Hospital-based, prospective	Agarwel et al. 1991
	Maharashata	1985-86	27.2	Hospital-based, prospective	Chaturvedi and Banerjee 1989
	Punjab	1983-89	36.0	Hospital-based, retrospective	Verma et al. 1991
	Varanasi	1978-79	20.8	Hospital-based, prospective	Chinara and Singh 1982
OAI	Indonesia	1985-90	9.0	Hospital-based, retrospective	Masloman et al. 1991
	Singapore	1982-89	24.7	Hospital-based, retrospective	Ho 1991
	Singapore	1986-88	15.1	Hospital-based, case-control study	Thein et al. 1992
SSA	Zaire	1985	14.0	Hospital-based, prospective	Ekanem and Chong 1985

Note: EME=Established Market Economies; MEC=Middle Eastern Crescent; IND=India; OAI=Other Asia and Islands; SSA=Sub-Saharan Africa.

estimation process. Table 3 summarizes the results of hospital-based studies of congenital anomalies in selected countries.

The overall birth prevalence of congenital disorders, including those classified as minor anomalies or not classified as congenital anomalies according to ICD codes , is generally estimated to be in the range of 20–60 per 1000 live births. Across the eight regions of the world, the average birth prevalence of congenital disorders is approximately 30 per 1 000 live births. The incidence of severe congenital disorders, disorders that can cause early death or life-long chronic disease, ranges from about 14 to 43 per 1 000 live births (Modell and Bulyzhenkov 1988). Birth prevalence of severe congenital anomalies ranges between 8 and 15 per 1 000 births (Table 4). The most common anomalies are usually those of the central nervous system and of the cardiovascular system.

Unfortunately, the calculation of birth prevalence of congenital anomalies depends on a number of factors that are by no means uniform. First of all, the classification or definition system used can differ greatly among countries. For example, even though according to the ICD classification

Table 4 Estimated birth prevalence of congenital anomalies

Type of disorder	*All disorders per 1 000 births*	*Severe disorders per 1 000 births*
Congenital malformations	17-30	8-15
Chromosomal aberrations	4-9	2-5
Menderian disorders	4-7	4-7
Hemoglobinopathies	0-16	0-18
Total	25-62	14-43

Source: Modell and Bulyzhenkov 1988

hereditary disorders should not be counted as congenital anomalies, some countries might include certain hereditary disorders in their estimates of prevalence of congenital anomalies. As a result, the birth prevalences calculated using these different classification systems are likely to be somewhat different (Leck 1994, Oakley 1986). In addition, the diagnostic capabilities and ascertainment techniques available will also influence the calculation of birth prevalence. While certain anomalies, such as neural tube defects and cleft lip, are easily identifiable, others are more difficult to detect. Therefore, especially in developing countries which lack more advanced detection technology and techniques, a large number of anomalies are not reported, and birth prevalence figures are often underestimated (Leck 1994, Oakley 1986).

Mortality from congenital anomalies

Congenital anomalies are now among the leading causes of perinatal and infant deaths in most of the developed, and in some of the developing countries. In LAC, congenital anomalies account for between 2 per cent and 27 per cent of all infant deaths, and rank among the five leading causes of infant deaths (PAHO 1986).

The proportion of perinatal and infant deaths due to congenital anomalies increases if the reduction of perinatal and infant mortality rates through socioeconomic development is faster than the reduction of mortality due to congenital anomalies. Most of the developed countries have followed this pattern. Kalter analysed the long-term temporal trends in stillbirth and neonatal deaths rates and congenital anomalies using data from hospital-based reports from 1950 in EME (Kalter 1991). In the last 50 years, perinatal mortality has declined steadily, decreasing by 65–80 per cent, whereas the proportion of congenital anomalies among perinatal deaths has increased by up to 30 per cent. Similar trends have been observed in other regions. However, the timing and pace of the increase in the proportion of congenital anomalies as a cause of perinatal mortality differs across the regions. In India, published hospital-based studies in the 1980s suggest that the proportion of congenital anomalies varies from 5.5

per cent to 20.7 per cent; however, one study suggests that the prevalence of congenital anomalies increased from 1977 to 1986 (Singh et al. 1990). In OAI, the prevalence of congenital anomalies varies significantly by country. For example, congenital anomalies account for 30.7 per cent of early neonatal deaths in Thailand (Pengsaa and Taksaphan 1987) but only 2 per cent in rural Bangladesh, as estimated in a community-based study (Fauveau et al. 1990). In SSA, 4.3 per cent of early neonatal deaths were due to congenital anomalies (Abudu et al. 1988).

In developed countries, among all congenital anomalies, those of the cardiovascular system and the central nervous system are the major causes of death in the early period of life. However, the proportion of infant deaths due to anomalies other than those of the cardiovascular system varies within the same region. For example, analysis of the trend of mortality due to different types of congenital anomalies for the period 1976–1985 in four populations in EME, United States, England and Wales, Scotland, and Sweden— suggests that anomalies of the cardiovascular system have been the leading cause of infant deaths, and that the proportion of infant deaths due to anomalies of the cardiovascular system remain relatively constant in all countries. On the other hand, the proportion of infant deaths due to anomalies of the central nervous system declined dramatically in all countries except the United States (primarily due to the acceptance of selective abortion after the diagnosis of the anomaly) (Powell-Griner and Woolbright 1990).

The majority of deaths from congenital anomalies occur in the first year of life, particularly within the first month of life. Figure 1 shows the proportion of the number of deaths due to congenital anomalies in each age group. Leck (1994) has estimated the cumulative mortality of a cohort of malformed infants based on the mortality schedule from England and Wales, assuming that 2.5 per cent of all infants have severe anomalies. The cumulative proportion of death is 2 per cent at birth, and rises to 7 per cent after 1 week, and to 10 per cent after 1 month. About 13 per cent of affected infants die within one year. Of course, the risk of death depends on the type of anomaly. For example, the proportion dead within one year varies from 100 per cent for anencephaly to 16 per cent for Down syndrome. Although infants with severe congenital anomalies have a greater risk of death, a considerable proportion of children with anomalies in EME will live, albeit with chronic disability. Unfortunately, comparable studies are not available for other regions. It is likely that the chance of survival for those infants is lower in developing countries.

Review of Empirical Data

In this chapter, ten relatively severe congenital anomalies for which data are available from ICBDMS were used to estimate the disease burden from congenital anomalies by region. The anomalies included in the estimation process were: anencephaly, spina bifida, congenital heart disease, Down

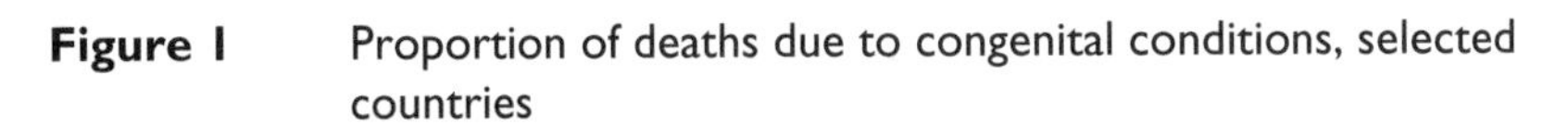

Figure 1 Proportion of deaths due to congenital conditions, selected countries

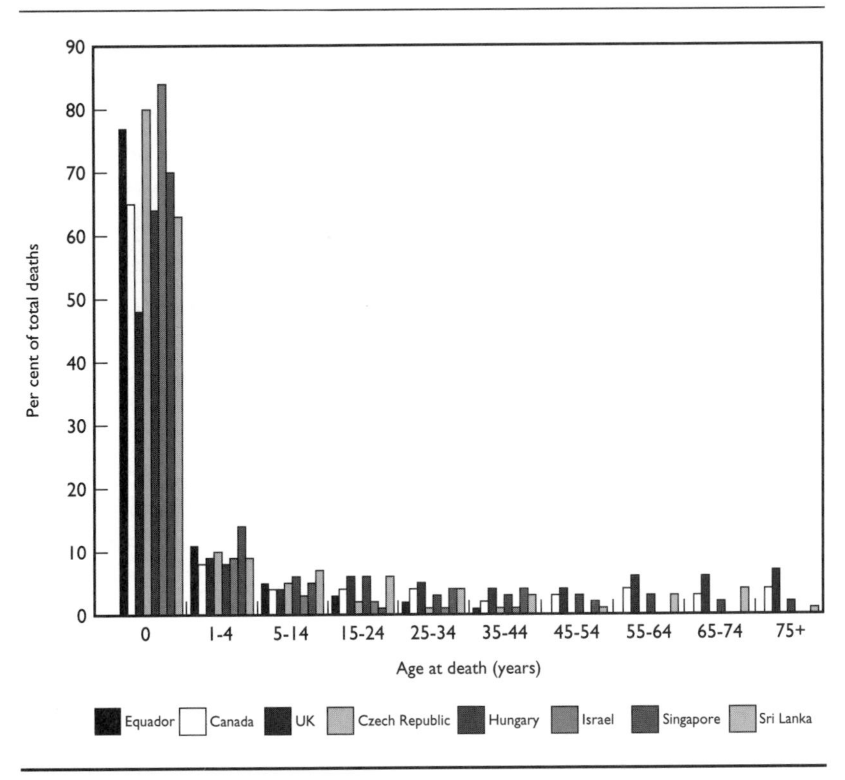

syndrome, cleft lip, cleft palate, abdominal wall defects, oesophageal atresia, anorectal atresia, and renal agenesis or dysgenesis.

BIRTH PREVALENCE AND MORTALITY OF MAJOR CONGENITAL ANOMALIES

1. Neural tube defects (anencephaly and spina bifida)

Birth prevalence of neural tube defects varies markedly, especially for anencephaly. This variation between regions can be explained by genetic and environmental factors as well as the difference in the availability of prenatal screening followed by selective abortion. Neural tube defects in EME have shown a considerable decrease in prevalence at birth, especially since the early 1970s. Although introduction of perinatal screening is the most important factor, some studies suggest that the improvement of environmental factors, such as nutrition, may also contribute to the reduction in neural tube defects (Cuckle et al. 1989, Cuckle and Wald 1987, Leck 1983).

Reported birth prevalence data are available for EME, FSE, CHN and LAC from the ICBDMS database. Since neural tube defects (NTDs) are easily recognizable at birth (and prevalence has been frequently reported from developing countries), published studies which are mainly hospital-based were used to estimate the prevalence for other regions.

In the case of China, only data from Sichuan were available from the ICBDMS database. These limited data suggested high NTD birth prevalence, ranging from 0 in Tibet, to 105.54 per 1000 in Hibei, and that prevalence tends to decline from North to South and from East to West (Chinese Birth Defects Monitoring Program 1990). To estimate the prevalence of NTDs in China, data from this study was used.

Reported rates in India are generally higher than those in EME, and vary from 0.9 per 1 000 in Calcutta, to 8.7 per 1 000 in Chandigarh. On average, in past studies, prevalence is 5.5 per 1 000 (Chaturvedi and Banerjee 1989, Choudhury et al. 1989, Chouhan et al. 1985, Sharma and Gulati 1992, Sood et al. 1991, Verma et al. 1991). A recent study in Karnakata indicated a very high prevalence of 11 per 1 000 (Kulkarni et al. 1987, 1989). Although selection bias might explain the higher prevalence (since there is no reporting system and all studies are hospital-based), the average figure seems to be plausible for a regional estimate.

Earlier studies showed lower rates of NTDs in blacks than in whites (Cornell et al. 1983, Milunsky and Alpert 1978). For example, in Cape Town, birth prevalence of NTDs in whites was 7 times higher than in blacks (Cornell et al. 1983). However, a recent study suggested that the prevalence of NTDs in blacks was similar to that in whites in the Transkei district (Ncayiyana 1986); reported prevalence is in the range of 0.76 to 7.0 per 1000 (Airede 1992, Anyebuno et al. 1993, Ekanem and Chong 1985, Sayed et al. 1989).

Of the countries in MEC, only Israel has continuously reported the birth prevalence of neural tube defects, as well as other major congenital anomalies. Recent reported rates are comparable to those in EME. There are also several recent hospital-based studies available from Turkey, Kuwait, Libya and Egypt, with rates varying from 1 per 1 000 to 4.5 per 1 000 (Al-Awadi et al. 1984, Guvenc et al. 1993, Khrouf et al. 1986, Kishan et al. 1985, Posaci et al. 1992). Even though the region is heterogeneous, the rates are relatively low. The median prevalence from the available data was used for the calculation. Published data from OAI (a heterogeneous region with some low mortality countries such as Singapore) showed relatively lower birth prevalence of neural tube defects than MEC (Tan et al. 1984). We have extrapolated the rate suggested from the MEC data to the OAI region. The reported birth prevalence for specific countries and cities is summarized in Tables 5 and 6.

Many studies have consistently shown that there is female predominance of neural tube defects with a male/female ratio of 0.6–0.8. However, if NTDs are subdivided, the sex ratios according to the site of the lesion vary, with the highest ratio in anencephalus, suggesting the impor-

Table 5 Birth prevalence of neural tube defects anomalies in developed regions, 1988

Region	Birth prevalence per 10 000		
	Anencephaly	Spina bifida (including encephalocele)	Hydrocephaly
EME			
Atlanta	3.3	0	3.5
Australia	3.6	0	3.8
Canada	3.5	0	5.1
Central-East France	0.5	0	3.1
Denmark	2.g	0	2.4
Italy (Emilia-Romagna)	0.4	0	2.2
England & Wales	0.6	0	2
Finland	0.7	0	1.8
Italy (IPIMC)	0.9	0	4.2
Japan	6.5	0	5.6
New Zealand	1.6	0	3.6
Norway	2.6	0	4.8
Paris	0.7	0	2.9
Spain	2.5	0	4
Strasbourg	3.7	0	6
Sweden	0.7	0	2.1
Tokyo	9.2	0	2.5
United States	2.1	0	5.8
FSE			
Czechoslovakia	1.1	0	2.3
Hungary	1.8	0	3.6

tance of the effect of the mode of formation of the neural tube. Overall, studies have reported a male /female sex ratio of 0.73 (0.66 for anencephaly and 0.86 for spina bifida) (Seller 1987, James 1986).

An anencephalic infant is usually stillborn or expires soon after birth. The case-fatality rate at birth for these infants is 1. Spina bifida was considered a lethal condition in the past. The few survivors were often mentally retarded, as a result of hydrocephalus and meningitis. However, the introduction of a new surgical approach at birth and effective methods of controlling progressive hydrocephalus has improved prospects for survival. Now, provided this new surgical approach is implemented at birth, many infants with spina bifida survive,, although they are often significantly handicapped (Gross et al. 1983; Hunt 1990; Laurence 1974; McLaughlin et al. 1985). Laurence (1974) compared the survival of an unoperated series and an operated series. Of 100 liveborn cases only 17 can expect to survive into their teenage years without an operation; whereas with aggressive operative treatment, 50 out of 100 can expect to survive although they were more severely disabled. No data are available for other regions.

Table 6 Birth prevalence of neural tube defects in developing regions

Region	*Study type*	*Year*	*Number of births*	*Birth prevalence per 10 000*		
				Anencephaly	**Spina bifida (including encephalocele)**	**Hydrocephaly**
CHN						
CBDMP*	H	1986-1987	1243284	15.2	12.2	9.17
Sichuan	H	1988	65100	6.3	5.5	6.3
IND						
Karnakata	H	1984	2000	65	45	—
Karnakata	H	1985-87	3500	51	54.6	—
East Delhi	H	1988-90	9220	39	27.1	—
Rohtak	H	1984-88	16554	26	48	—
Calcutta	H	1988	115851	4.9	5.6	—
Jaipur	H	1985	28511	56	53	—
Punjab	H	1983-89	10000	36	11	—
Lucknow	H	1981-84	9633	22.8	21.8	—
Rural Maharashata	H	1985-86	3000	13.2	13.2	—
				19.6	19.4	—
SSA						
Ghana	H	1993	19094	8.4	3.1	—
Nigeria	H	1987-90	5977	3.3	65.7	—
Transkei	H	1980-84	9142	17.5	43.8	—
Cape Town whites & blacks	H	1980	21042	2.8	4.8	—
Zaire	H		23512	5.9	7.7	11.48
PNMS**	H	1984	17487	1.8	5.8	2.1
				5.9	12.8	—
LAC						
Mexico	H	1988	40903	16.6	20.1	3.9
South America (ECLAMC***)	H	1988	188363	5.7	9.2	6.2
				7.6	11.1	5.8
MEC						
Izmir, Turkey	H	1980-90	82720	15	7.4	—
Eastern Turkey	H	1985-90	5240	38	—	—
Libya	H	1982-84	48974	6.5	3.6	—
Kuwait	H	1983	36138	13.3	—	—
Israel	H	1988	17479	1.7	2.9	2.9
Tunisia	H	1983-84	10000	6	16	9

*Chinese Births Defects Monitoring Program (Xiao et al. 1990)
**Peninsula Maternity and Neonatal Service
***Latin American Collaborative Study of Congenital Malformations

2. *Congenital heart disease*

Unlike anomalies such as neural tube defects and clefts, congenital heart disease (CHD) is often not recognizable at birth. Birth prevalence of CHD is affected by the differences in ascertainment methods, case definitions, length of follow-up, diagnostic exclusions and degree of paediatric cardiology expertise (Roth et al. 1987; Ferencz 1990). Early estimates of the birth prevalence of CHD of 3 to 5 per 1 000 live births would seem to be an underestimate mainly because of inadequate ascertainment (MacMahon et al. 1953; Pleydell 1960; Mustacchi et al. 1963). Even in countries with good health care systems, only 40 to 50 per cent of CHD is diagnosed within one week after birth, and only 50 to 60 per cent of CHD is diagnosed within the first month of life (Hoffman and Christianson 1978; Laursen 1980; Hoffman 1990). New diagnostic techniques, such as two-dimensional and Doppler echocardiography, have increased the reported rates of CHD. More recent studies in developed regions suggest higher birth prevalence and are relatively consistent, ranging from 4 to 10 per 1 000 (Table 7). Even though very little data are available from developing countries, it may well be that there is no significant effect of genetic or environmental factors on the birth prevalence of CHD, and that the difference in prevalence is primarily due to differences in diagnostic practices.

Although a significant sex differential has been documented for several congenital heart defects (Czeizel et al. 1972, Samanek 1994, Shinebourne et al. 1976, Vesterby et al. 1987), a recent population-based study suggests that there is no significant difference between the sex ratio in the total population of live born children and that in children born with a heart defect (Samanek 1994).

Advances in surgery have significantly decreased the mortality of CHD in developed countries since the introduction of cardiopulmonary bypass for paediatric cardiac surgery in the 1950s. In the 1940–50s, studies of the natural history of CHD showed that nearly half of babies with CHD died by their first birthday (Hoffman 1968). A recent population-based cohort study suggests that both age at surgery and operative mortality have decreased significantly over the last 30 years (Morris and Menashe 1991).

3. *Down syndrome*

There is some variation in the reported birth prevalence of Down syndrome, although not as great as that of neural tube defects (Table 8) (ICBDMS 1991). As mentioned before, the difference in the proportion of mothers of older age (>35 years of age) and lower fertility rates among older mothers may explain the variation, as well as the difference in the extent of the perinatal screening program. The birth prevalence of Down syndrome in EME has decreased from about 1.5 per 1 000 in the 1950s, to about 1.3 per 1 000 in the 1980s (Holmes 1978, Lowry et al. 1976)

An excess of males among Down syndrome cases has been reported in many studies. Recent studies based on complete ascertainment suggest that Down syndrome was more common in males than females, with a male-to-female ratio of 1.2 –1.4 (Iselius and Lindsten 1986, Staples et al. 1991, Stoll et al. 1990).

The life expectancy of babies born with Down syndrome has improved dramatically over the past few decades (Table 9) (Mastroiacovo et al.

Table 7 Birth prevalence of congenital heart defects in EME

Region	*Year of birth*	*Total live birth*	*Birth prevalence per 1 000*
Birmingham, United Kingdom	1940-49	194 216	3.2
Gothenburg, Sweden	1941-50	58 105	6.3
Olmstead County, Sweden	1944-50	8 716	5.9
Northamptonshire, United Kingdom	1944-57	60 890	3.2
Finland	1945-63	—	8.0
New York, USA	1946-53	5 638	5.5
Toronto, Canada	1948-49	134 367	5.7
Japan	1948-54	16 144	7.0
San Francisco, USA	1949-51	47 137	5.9
Birmingham, United Kingdom	1950-52	55 539	4.2
Olmstead County, Sweden	1950-69	32 393	5.7
Gothenburg, Sweden	1951-60	58 314	7.7
Leiden, Netherlands	1951-62	1 817	8.3
Uppsala, Sweden	1952-61	48 500	6.0
Hawaii, USA	1953-54	1 922	4.7
British Colombia, Canada	1955-60	228 787	4.2
Balckpool, United Kingdom	1957-71	57 979	6.0
Minnesota, USA	1957	8 546	5.4
San Francisco, USA	1959-66	19 044	8.8
Liverpool, United Kingdom	1960-64	80 641	4.7
Liverpool, United Kingdom	1960-69	163 692	6.6
Liverpool, United Kingdom	1960-69	160 480	5.5
Denmark	1963-73	5 249	6.1
Budapest, Hungary	1963-65	52 569	7.1
Szolnok County, Hungary	1963	2 259	10.2
Szolnok County, Hungary	1963-65	5 644	11.9
Bas-Rhin, France	1979-83	66 068	3.4
Bohemia, Czech Republic	1980	91 823	6.4
Baltimore-Washington, USA	1981-82	368 889	4.1
Sweden	1981	94 778	7.6

(*Source:* Samanek 1989; Hoffman 1990)

1992). In the 1940–50s, the proportion surviving to age five was 40 per cent. Recent studies however have consistently shown the improvement in life expectancy of cases: now about 80–90 per cent will survive to five years of age (Baird and Sadovnick 1987, Bell et al. 1989, Malone 1988). The major causes of death in Down syndrome infants are respiratory infection and complications of congenital heart disease (Balarajan et al. 1982, Bell et al. 1989, Deaton 1973, Mulcahy 1979, Thase 1982) and the

Table 8 Birth prevalence of Down syndrome, 1988

Country/Region	*Birth prevalence per 10 000*
Australia	12.4
Canada	13.8
Denmark	7.8
Finland	8.0
France, Central-East	10.4
France, Paris	13.5
Italy (Emilia-Romagna)	16.2
Italy	12.5
Japan	5.7
Japan, Tokyo	11.0
Mexico	13.7
New Zealand	9.8
Norway	10.9
Sweden	11.2
United Kingdom, England & Wales	6.1
United States (1,200 hospitals)	9.7
USA, Atlanta	9.8

(*Source:* ICBDMS 1991)

Table 9 Reported survival of children with Down syndrome

Location	*Years*	*Sample size*	*Cumulative 5-year survival (%)*	*Congenital heart disease + (%)*
Birmingham, UK	1942-52	252	40.3	
London, UK	1944-56	725	39.7	
Victoria, Australia	1948-57	729	49.4	
Massachusetts, USA	1950-66	2421	65.4 (female) 71.9 (male)	29.9 27.2
Western Australia	1966-76	231	74.8 (survival at 4 years)	34.2
Salford, UK	1961-77	50	76.8	
Japan hospitals	1966-75	1052	87.1	41.4
British Columbia	1952-81	1341	81.5	28.9
Western Australia	1976-84	149	89	36.2
Queensland, Australia	1976-85	366	81	
Italy	1976-84	917	76.4	18.5
Denmark	1980-85	278	73.7	

(*Source:* Mastroiacovo et al. 1992)

dramatic improvement in survival is attributable to the effective interventions for these conditions as well as active case management (Fryers 1986, Malone 1988).

4. Cleft lip and palate

Facial clefts are one of the most common congenital anomalies, and are easily recognized at birth. Birth prevalence of clefts usually ranges from 1 to 5 per 1 000 live births (ICBDMS 1991, Vanderas 1987). The birth prevalence of cleft lip with or without cleft palate is about 1 per 1 000 and the birth prevalence of cleft palate alone is about 0.5 per 1 000 (Table 10). Although these rates are reasonably constant during the observation period, there are some variations, especially in cleft lip. Both genetic factors and environmental factors are considered to affect the incidence of clefts (Emanuel et al. 1973, ICBDMS 1991, Leck 1969, Tyan 1982, Vanderas 1987). Genetic factors seems to be of more importance in total cleft lip than in cleft palate. In terms of the sex ratio of birth prevalence of facial clefts, many studies suggest that males outnumber females, especially in cleft lip, for which the average male to female ratio is in the range of 1.1–1.6 (Vanderas 1987).

Unfortunately, there are few studies published in OAI, MEC and IND. Two hospital-based studies in MEC (Saudi Arabia and Iran) showed much higher values than those of other countries (Borkar et al. 1993; Taher 1992). It is unclear whether these results were due to selection bias or to genetic and environmental factors. More systematic reporting in Israel suggests that birth prevalence of clefts is not very high. A hospital-based study in India (Chaturvdi and Banerjee 1989) also showed a very high prevalence of total cleft lip. However, it may be reasonable to assume that birth prevalence of facial clefts in these genetically heterogeneous regions falls within the range of the observed prevalence mentioned above.

Prognosis of facial clefts is considered to be excellent if no serious malformations are associated with it. It is well known that many syndromes involve facial clefts (Jones 1988). Cleft palate is more often associated with other malformations than cleft lip. For example, in the EUROCAT data for 1986 to 1988, the proportion of associated anomalies was 20.5 per cent for cleft palate cases and 14.5 per cent for cleft lip cases (EUROCAT 1991). In the developed regions, most of the deaths among children with facial cleft are attributable to associated congenital anomalies, and the majority of deaths occur early in the life. A large cohort study suggests that 95 per cent of deaths occur in the first year of life (Mackeprang and Hay 1972). In regions where surgical repair is not easily available and a considerable number of cleft cases are untreated, malnutrition and infection might contribute to the excess mortality. However, no data are available for developing regions to substantiate this.

Table 10 Birth prevalence of selected congenital anomalies

Region	*Birth prevalence per 10 000*						
	Oesophageal atresia	**Anorectal atresia**	**Cleft plalate**	**Total cleft lip**	**Hypospadias**	**Abdominal wall defects**	**Limb reduction defects**
EME	**2.2**	**2.9**	**6.3**	**9.9**	**17.6**	**3.4**	**4.4**
Australia	2.8	2.8	5.4	8.5	19.7	3.8	4.9
Canada		5.8	5.3	12.7	21.9	6.4	4.8
Denmark	2.2	1.9	6.9	15.9	14.9	2.7	
Finland	1.0	1.7	12.2	8.2	7.3	1.5	4.0
France, Central-East	3.1	3.5	6.4	6.8	10.4	3.3	4.3
France, Paris	0.7	1.0	3.4	6.0	9.9	4.4	4.4
France, Strasbourg	2.2	2.2	11.2	6.0	30.0	3.7	6.0
Italy (Emilia-Romagna)	3.1	2.6	6.6	5.3	22.8	1.8	6.6
Italy (IPIMC)	3.2	3.2	5.0	6.7	26.3	1.7	5.1
Japan	2.0	4	5.9	15.3	2.1	4.2	2.5
Japan, Tokyo	3.7	6.1	7.4	23.3	3.7	1.8	4.3
New Zealand	2.4	2.2	7.3	7.6	10.7	2.7	2.9
Norway	2.6	1.4	5.2	14.9	20.7	4.5	5.5
Spain	0.4	2.5	3.6	4.7	18.4	1.3	7
Sweden	2.8	3.6	6.9	11.6	17.2	1.0	5.6
United Kingdom, England & Wales	1.0	2.0	3.9	7.6	15.7	6.4	4.3
USA	2.4	3.5	5.3	8.6	33.7	4.2	3.5
USA, Atlanta	1.6	2.2	4.6	9.0	31.7	6.0	3.8
FSE	**1.6**	**2.1**	**4.6**	**9.9**	**22.4**	**1.9**	**4.2**
Czech Republic	1.6	2.7	6.1	11.1	21.9	1.9	4.1
Hungary	1.5	1.4	3.1	8.6	22.8	1.8	4.2

Table 10 *(continued)*

Region	*Birth prevalence per 10 000*						
	Oesophageal atresia	**Anorectal atresia**	**Cleft plalate**	**Total cleft lip**	**Hypospadias**	**Abdominal wall defects**	**Limb reduction defects**
CHN							
Sichun	**0.6**	**2.3**	**1.1**	**15.1**	**2.3**	**2.9**	**4.8**
LAC	**2.7**	**4**	**4.75**	**12.85**	**5.8**	**3.6**	**6.7**
Mexico	2.2	3.9	2.2	14.7	3.7	4.2	7.8
South America	3.2	4.1	7.3	11	7.9	3	5.6
Median Prevalence per 10 000	**2-3**	**3**	**5**			**2-4**	**4-6**

Source: ICBDMS 1988

5. *Abdominal wall defects*

Abdominal wall defects consist of several groups of malformations. The two main groups are omphalocele and gastroschisis, which are reported in the ICBDMS database. Birth prevalence of abdominal wall defects is relatively constant— approximately 2–4 cases per 10 000 births according to the ICBDMS database (Table 10). Minor variations are probably due to differences in ascertainment and definition, and to the inclusion of umbilical hernia. Secular trends in several countries in EME suggest that prenatal diagnosis and selective abortion seem to have contributed to the decrease in birth prevalence of abdominal wall defects. Very little data are available for other regions. However, it is reasonable to assume that there may not be significant difference in birth prevalence among regions since there is no exogenous cause established for the majority of abdominal wall defects (ICBDMS 1991).

Omphalocele and gastroschisis are acute emergencies of the neonatal period (Grosfeld et al. 1981, Mabogunje and Mahour 1984, Mahour et al. 1973). Most deaths from abdominal wall defects occur in the first year of life (Mabogunje and Mahor 1984). Surgical advances have reduced mortality from abdominal wall defects significantly since the 1960s. While survival rates in the 1950s and 1960s ranged from 41 per cent to 62 per cent (Eckstein 1963, Jones 1969, Smith and Leix 1966), data from recent studies in North America suggest that, on average, about 87 per cent of infants with gastroschisis and 63 per cent of infants with omphalocele survive (Grosfeld and Weber 1982). A more recent study shows an overall survival rate of 75 per cent (Kohn and Shi 1990).

Although mortality from both omphalocele and gastroschisis has been declining over the past decades, mortality from omphalocele is still considerably higher than that from gastroschisis, primarily because major chromosomal and associated anomalies adversely affect the survival of omphalocele cases (Grosfeld et al. 1981, Mabogunje and Mahour 1984, Mayer et al. 1980). No comparable data exist for other regions. However, historical data in developed regions suggest that abdominal wall defects are highly lethal with a mortality rate of more than 90 per cent.

6. *Oesophageal atresia and anorectal atresia*

Birth prevalence of both oesophageal and anorectal atresia reported in the ICBDMS database is relatively constant, at around 3 per 10 000 in most regions (Table 10). Few data are available for other regions. Three studies from India indicated that birth prevalence of oesophageal atresia was 2 to 5.2 per 10,000 births, and that of anorectal atresia was 4 to 6.6 per 10 000 (Agarwel et al. 1991, Chaturvedi and Banerjee 1989, Verma et al 1991). However, these are all hospital-based studies at referral hospitals and therefore may not be representative. The available data suggest that there is no significant difference in birth prevalence among regions.

Oesophageal atresia is an emergency condition, and a life-saving operation has to be performed. In EME, mortality from oesophageal atresia has been declining over the past decades, to the point where more than 80 per cent of cases will survive (Manning et al. 1986, Sillen et al. 1988, Strodel et al. 1979). A considerable proportion of the deaths that do occur are attributable to associated severe anomalies. If the infants without other severe anomalies survive surgery, the prognosis is considered to be good, at least in developed regions. However, extrapolation of the historical data in EME suggests that mortality in developing countries is considerably higher. In fact, the survival rate of oesophageal atresia at a tertiary hospital in India was 4.6 per cent in the 1970s and 45.7 per cent in the late 1980s (Sharma et al. 1993). Since access to tertiary hospitals is quite limited for infants with severe anomalies in these regions, mortality levels may well be higher than that observed in EME in the 1950s.

Mortality from anorectal atresia in developed countries is also primarily due to associated severe anomalies, and the prognosis for those without such associated severe anomalies is good. However, in developing regions, there are several problems associated with the management of neonatal intestinal obstruction, including delay of diagnosis and treatment and lack of health personnel and equipment (Adeyemi 1989). In addition, other perinatal conditions, such as low birth weight and malnutrition, contribute to excess mortality among infants with interstitial atresia in developing countries. Even after treatment, the mortality rate of anorectal atresia was more than 30 per cent in Nigeria (Morgan 1979).

7. Renal agenesis or dysgenesis

Birth prevalence of this lethal anomaly varies considerably. This variation may be due to differences in ascertainment, inclusion criteria, or frequency of autopsy (Table 10). Higher rates are constantly reported from the Unites States, Canada, and France, whereas a very low rate is reported from China (Sichuan). In EME the recent upward trend of birth prevalence is due to better reporting of cases of renal dysgenesis. Thus, regional variation could well be primarily due to difference in ascertainment of the anomaly rather than difference in actual birth prevalence.

Considerations in calculating DALYs and Estimation of DALYs

Estimation of birth prevalence

Birth prevalence data for major congenital anomalies were available for EME, FSE, LAC and CHN from the ICBDMS database, and these data were used to estimate the number of cases. For other regions, published data for each anomaly are quite limited and usually come from hospital-based studies. The use of such data may be subject to bias. Thus, for most conditions, if the birth prevalence did not vary significantly across regions or if genetic and/or environmental factors did not greatly affect birth prevalence of congenital anomalies (i.e. congenital heart disease, abdominal wall defects, oesophageal atresia and anorectal atresia), data from the developed countries were extrapolated to estimate the prevalence in developing regions.

In the case of neural tube defects and facial clefts, the regional variation was incorporated in the estimation process of birth prevalence. If the variation in birth prevalence of an anomaly was partly explained by a clinical intervention such as selective abortion, historical data from the developed countries before the introduction of such interventions were used. Down syndrome is a case in point. However, application of historical data from developed countries may underestimate the risk of Down syndrome in developing countries with high fertility rates, since one of the main reasons for declining birth prevalence of Down syndrome in developed countries is low fertility of older mothers. Although considerable variation of birth prevalence of renal agenesis/dysgenesis has been observed, it was assumed that the primary cause of the large variation was of differences in diagnostic techniques detection. Thus, in lieu of a more reliable alternative, the average birth prevalence of congenital anomalies in EME has been applied to SSA, IND, MEC and OAI.

Under these assumptions, the number of cases for each congenital anomaly was calculated using DISMOD. Only age-specific incidence rates for age 0 were used in the model, since congenital anomalies occur only at birth. (As noted above, the term "incidence of congenital anomalies" actually means the birth prevalence.) In addition, we assume that the remission rate is 0: if a baby is born with a certain congenital anomaly, then he/she will live with certain degree of disability for the rest of his/her life until death, or the time of surgical repair.

ESTIMATION OF MORTALITY

Mortality estimates for congenital anomalies for the Global Burden of Disease Study were made using the neonatal adjustment algorithm described in more detail by Murray and Lopez (1996). In most regions, 85 per cent of neonatal deaths are due to a limited number of causes namely congenital syphilis, neonatal tetanus, conditions arising during the perinatal period, and congenital anomalies. To obtain estimates of deaths from these causes, we first estimated the number of neonatal deaths in each region and then required that the sum of deaths from congenital syphilis, neonatal tetanus, conditions arising during the perinatal period and congenital anomalies during the neonatal period must equal 85 per cent of estimated neonatal deaths.

The demographic analyses undertaken by the World Bank for the 1993 World Development Report provided estimates of deaths at ages 0–4 years and the probability of death between birth and age 5, for each of the eight WDR regions; estimates of mortality at ages 0–4 years for more detailed age-groups, such as neonatal death, infant death and childhood death were not undertaken. In all regions, neonatal deaths are an important fraction of all infant deaths and can easily be under-estimated unless reliable bounds on the neonatal mortality rate are derived. We therefore estimated neonatal deaths by taking advantage of the recent survey data collected through the Demographic and Health Surveys Programme (Sullivan et al. 1994). For 28 of these national surveys in developing countries, estimates of the probability of death between birth and one month, birth and 1 year and birth and 5 years have been calculated for males and females separately.

Not all deaths from conditions arising during the perinatal period or from congenital anomalies occur within the first month of life. Based on data from EME and FSE countries with detailed vital registration information on the timing of deaths from these two causes, it was estimated that 65 per cent of congenital deaths in children under age 5 occur within one month of birth. We then summed deaths from conditions arising during the perinatal period, congenital anomalies expected in the first month, neonatal tetanus deaths and congenital syphilis deaths. The estimates of deaths from each of these conditions were then proportionately adjusted so that their total was equal to 85 per cent of the estimated neonatal deaths in a given region.

For EME, FSE, and LAC, vital registration data provide the cause-specific mortality rates for congenital anomalies of the central nervous system and of the heart and large vessels. Since there are no comparable data for other regions, we used the historical mortality data in developed countries to estimate mortality from all congenital anomalies in developing regions. It may be reasonable to use these data since the survival rate for major congenital anomalies, except inevitably lethal ones, has increased due to the advances in surgery. In addition, congenital anomalies are endogenous causes of infant deaths, and are less responsive to improvements in environmental factors than exogenous causes of mortality, such as infections. For anomalies other than neural tube defects and congenital heart defects, model estimates were used for all regions (see Murray and Lopez 1996 for more detail).

The availability of treatment, especially surgery, affects mortality from major congenital anomalies. For spina bifida, congenital heart disease and Down syndrome, natural history or mortality data before the introduction of common surgical procedures are available (almost no interventions). For oesophageal and anorectal atresia, abdominal wall defects, and cleft lip and palate, the change of mortality through the improvement of surgical interventions in EME during the past decades was also examined. These data were then extrapolated to estimate case-fatality rates of anomalies in SSA and IND as the upper bound and the cause-specific death rates were then calculated using DisMod. The cause-specific death rates for four other regions (CHN, LAC, MEC and OAI) were assumed to fall in between those of the developed regions (EME and FSE) and those of the regions with the highest mortality (IND and SSA) and then proportionally distributed among the four diseases. The estimated birth prevalence in selected countries for some congenital anomalies is shown in Table 11.

Disability

In most of the developing regions, data on disability among children with congenital anomalies are quite limited. The distribution of disability may vary by region because of differences in access to, and the utilization of, clinical and rehabilitative services, as well as differences in the actual prevalence of anomalies. If we take into consideration the fact that more infants with severe congenital anomalies die and less infants have access to medical interventions (especially surgery) in developing regions than in developed regions, we may assume that the degree of disability associated with congenital anomalies in developing regions is less severe than in developed regions. Conversely, if birth prevalence of a non-fatal but severe congenital anomaly is much higher, the prevalence of disability may be higher. Because of the limited data, it is unknown which assumption is more appropriate.

Clinical intervention affects the duration of disability imposed by surgically correctable anomalies such as facial clefts and congenital heart disease. We have taken into account the effects of surgery for the calculation of the burden of disability. In addition, measures of the availability of and access to medical interventions for each region were also incorporated into the final calculation of disease burden. For anomalies for which surgery will save the life of the child but will lead to a disability (spina bifida), different disability weights were used for developed and developing regions (a higher disability weight was used for developed regions). Table 11 shows for congenital anomalies the distribution of cases across the seven classes of disability, separately for treated and untreated cases; Table 12 depicts the estimated proportion of cases for each anomaly that receive treatment.

Surgically correctable anomalies

Infants with anomalies for which emergency surgery is needed during the neonatal period (oesophageal atresia, anorectal atresia and abdominal wall defects) have relatively good prognoses if they survive surgery. It is reasonable to conclude that they will die if they do not undergo surgery. In developed regions, many of them will survive without significant disability. For survivors, the duration of disability is assumed to be 0 since surgery is conducted during the neonatal period. In developing regions, many infants will die because of lack of access to surgery, or from complications arising from surgery. For these anomalies, most of the DALYs lost may be due to premature deaths.

Congenital heart disease, with the exception of fatal cases, is slightly different from the anomalies mentioned above, since infants with CHD may not die during the neonatal period and will not manifest symptoms until their heart failure becomes severe. It is assumed that, in EME, the duration of disability is the average age at surgery if operated, or life-long if unoperated. The same assumption was made for clefts: infants with clefts

Table 11 Proportion of congenital anomalies in each disability class, treated and untreated forms.

Disability class	*I*	*II*	*III*	*IV*	*V*	*VI*	*VII*
Untreated cases							
Abdominal wall defects	0	0	0	0	0	0	100
Anencephaly	0	0	0	0	0	0	100
Anorectal atresia	0	0	0	0	0	0	100
Oesophageal atresia	0	0	0	0	0	0	100
Renal agenesis	0	0	0	0	0	0	100
Cleft lip	0	81	13	6	0	0	0
Cleft palate	0	0	58	42	0	0	0
Treated cases							
Abdominal wall defects	0	0	0	0	0	0	0
Anencephaly	0	0	0	0	0	0	0
Anorectal atresia	0	0	0	0	0	0	0
Oesophageal atresia	0	0	0	0	0	0	0
Renal agenesis	0	0	0	0	0	0	0
Cleft lip	90	10	0	0	0	0	0
Cleft palate	92	8	0	0	0	0	0

who are not operated on will live with disability for the rest of their life. Estimates of severity distribution of disability associated with chronic heart failure and otitis media/hearing impairment (see Murray and Lopez 1994) were used for CHD and clefts, respectively.

Other anomalies

Infants with spina bifida or Down syndrome will have severe life-long disability even if surgical interventions allow them to survive. As mentioned above, different disability weights were applied for spina bifida

Table 12 Estimated per cent of congenital anomalies cases that are treated, by region.

	EME	*FSE*	*IND*	*CHN*	*OAI*	*SSA*	*LAC*	*MEC*
Abdominal wall defects	0	0	0	0	0	0	0	0
Anencephaly	0	0	0	0	0	0	0	0
Anorectal atresia	0	0	0	0	0	0	0	0
Oesophageal atresia	0	0	0	0	0	0	0	0
Renal agenesis	0	0	0	0	0	0	0	0
Cleft lip	90	85	50	70	40	20	70	60
Cleft palate	90	85	50	70	40	20	70	60

based on follow-up data which compared disability between operated and un-operated cases (Laurence 1974).

It is well known that infants with Down syndrome will have mental retardation, which will progress as age increases. Thus, the degree of disability would change in accordance with chronological age. However, we have applied identical disability weights for all age groups because of the lack of data. The distribution of disability level is primarily determined by standard intelligence tests. For example, using the Stanford-Binet Intelligence Scale, the distribution of severity of mental retardation among 217 Down syndrome children was almost normally distributed (Morgan 1979). If we apply the results of the study, the overall weight will be 0.374.

Again, there are few studies on the prevalence and severity distribution of mental retardation in developing countries. One study in India showed the distribution of the degree of mental retardation was slightly skewed towards the severe retardation group (Parikh and Goyel 1990). The estimated disability weight was 0.528, which is intuitively high for the associated disability of Down syndrome. It should be noted that these kinds of studies are subject to selection bias and are not necessarily representative of all cases. Thus, the disability weight derived from EME data was applied to all regions. For Down syndrome survivors, the duration of disability is assumed to be life-long.

Tables 13–22 summarize the epidemiological estimates for congenital anomalies and include incidence and prevalence rates, average age at onset and average duration of the anomaly, as well as the number of deaths, Years of Life Lost (YLLs), Years Lived with Disability (YLDs) and Disability-Adjusted Life Years (DALYs) due to each condition separately.

As expected, DALYs lost from surgically correctable anomalies, such as congenital heart disease and clefts, are primarily due to premature deaths, both in developed and developing regions. In contrast, almost half of the DALYs lost from spina bifida which are not completely correctable are due to disability in developed regions, but to premature deaths in developing regions. In spite of the high mortality of Down syndrome in developing regions, the disability component in total DALYs lost is still considerably high. Admittedly, the estimation probably underestimates the true burden imposed by congenital anomalies because we only include the major and severe anomalies for which data on morbidity and mortality are available. Some anomalies, such as limb reduction defects, will increase the burden of disability rather than that of premature deaths, both in developing and developed regions.

BURDEN AND INTERVENTION

As noted in this chapter, there is considerable uncertainty about the causes of the majority of birth defects. If the cause of an anomaly is known, identifiable, and preventable, primary prevention programs can be effective. In developed countries, genetic counselling and prenatal diagnosis are available in routine clinical practice, especially for the cases with advanced maternal age and abnormal serum alpha-fetoprotein (AFP) screening test. Studies have shown that such interventions contribute to the decrease of birth prevalence of defects of the central nervous system, and of babies born with Down syndrome to elderly mothers (Wetherall 1982).

In all countries, primary prevention programs that are inexpensive and culturally feasible within the primary health care sector should be implemented. For example, PAHO (1984) recommends the following actions as part of primary prevention strategies:

- Discourage pregnancies in women over 40 in linkage with plans for health education;
- Reduce levels of exposures to mutagens and teratogens by immunization, control of radiation and teratogenic medication, and public education on the risk of drinking alcohol during pregnancy;
- Promote proper nutrition in women of childbearing age and in pregnant mothers.

Although it is still controversial, some researchers have shown that a deficiency of folic acid and other vitamins is a possible etiologic factor in neural tube defects (Bower and Stanley 1989, Laurence et al. 1980). There are also several recent studies which have shown the effectiveness of vitamin supplementation for the prevention of NTDs (Czeizel 1993, Milunsky et al. 1989, MRC Vitamin Study Research Group 1991, Mulinare et al. 1988). For example, Czeizel showed that periconceptual multivitamin supplementation can reduce not only the incidence of neural tube defects, but also that of other congenital anomalies in a randomized controlled trial (Czeizel 1993, Czeizel and Dudas 1992). Promotion of proper nutrition is also important to prevent cretinism, which is caused by iodine-deficiency.

Counselling and assessment of risk factors associated with congenital anomalies such as diabetes mellitus, alcoholism and smoking are also an essential component of primary prevention strategies (Eskes et al. 1992). Kitzmiller et al. showed that one major congenital anomaly occurred in 1.2 per cent of infants of diabetic women treated before conception compared with 10.9 per cent in the postconception treatment group. They conclude that education and intensive management of diabetic women before and during pregnancy will prevent excess rates of congenital anomalies (Kitzmiller et al. 1991). Elixhauser et al. (1993) showed that the preconception care of diabetic women is more cost-effective than prenatal care only. It should be noted, however, that primary prevention programs may not affect the majority of congenital anomalies, especially those for which no risk indicators or large-scale prenatal detection methods are available (PAHO 1984).

Consequently, early identification and accurate diagnosis followed by prompt treatment are essential for effective secondary prevention programs. Training health personnel, in genetics, congenital anomalies, and

Table 13 Epidemiological estimates for anencephaly, age group 0-4 years, 1990.

Region	Incidence		Prevalence		Deaths		YLLs		YLDs		DALYs	
	Number ('000s)	Rate per100 000	Number ('000s)	Rate per100 000	Number (years)	Rate (years)	Number ('000s)	Rate per100 000	Number ('000s)	Rate per100 000	Number ('000s)	Rate per100 000
Males												
EME	1	3.99	0	0.04	1	3.99	35	134	0	0.00	35	134
FSE	0	2.20	0	0.02	0	2.20	10	74	0	0.00	10	74
IND	18	30.68	0	0.31	18	30.68	612	1,024	0	0.00	612	1,024
CHN	15	25.00	0	0.33	15	25.02	506	840	0	0.00	506	840
OAI	8	17.40	0	0.23	8	17.37	257	587	0	0.00	257	587
SSA	5	9.60	0	0.13	5	9.57	154	325	0	0.00	154	325
LAC	3	11.67	0	0.12	3	11.67	113	393	0	0.00	113	393
MEC	8	18.50	0	0.25	8	18.53	258	627	0	0.00	258	627
Developed	1	3.38	0	0.03	1	3.38	45	113	0	0.00	45	113
Developing	58	27.01	1	0.27	57	22.40	1,900	753	0	0.00	1,900	753
World	58	21.64	1	0.22	58	18.02	1,945	605	0	0.00	1,945	605
Females												
EME	2	6.19	0	0.06	2	6.19	52	207	0	0.00	52	207
FSE	0	3.58	0	0.04	0	3.58	16	120	0	0.00	16	120
IND	28	48.66	0	0.49	28	48.66	940	1,658	0	0.00	940	1,658
CHN	24	41.30	0	0.34	24	41.33	808	1,395	0	0.00	808	1,395
OAI	12	28.00	0	0.23	12	27.97	401	956	0	0.00	401	956
SSA	7	15.9	0	0.13	7	15.85	255	543	0	0.00	255	543
LAC	5	18.77	0	0.19	5	18.77	175	634	0	0.00	175	634
MEC	12	29.70	0	0.25	12	29.69	401	1,009	0	0.00	401	1,009
Developed	2	5.29	0	0.05	2	5.29	68	177	0	0.00	68	177
Developing	88	28.76	1	0.29	88	32.36	2,981	1,100	0	0.00	2,981	1,100
World	90	29.00	1	0.26	90	29.02	3,048	986	0	0.00	3,048	986

disability management is the first step. Clinical and diagnostic resources are needed for accurate diagnosis of congenital anomalies. Mass screening and genetic counselling programs for specific congenital anomalies which are relatively simple and cheap would be feasible in most countries. For example, in Hungary, orthopaedic screening of new-borns has resulted in the almost total elimination of dislocation of the hip, which was the most common congenital anomaly in the country (Czeizel 1988). In a study of economic appraisal of screening for congenital dislocation of the hip (CDH), screening of CDH was compared with the treatment cost resulting from no screening. The result showed that such a screening program is highly cost-effective (Fulton and Barer 1984).

Certain serious congenital disorders, such as congenital hypothyroidism and phenylketonuria, can be diagnosed biochemically in the newborn and treated to prevent the development and manifestation of the disease, provided the treatment begins early. If mass screening with blood tests is applicable and cost-effective within the existing health system, programs such as newborn screening for congenital metabolic disorders and carrier screening for haemoglobinopathies should be implemented. In Mediterranean countries, large-scale carrier screening with simple blood tests and

Table 14a Epidemiological estimates for spina bifida, 1990 *males*.

Age group (years)	*Incidence* Number ('000s)	*Incidence* Rate per 100 000	*Prevalence* Number ('000s)	*Prevalence* Rate per 100 000	*Avg. age at onset* (years)	*Avgerage duration* (years)	*Deaths* Number ('000s)	*Deaths* Rate per 100 000	*YLLs* Number ('000s)	*YLLs* Rate per 100 000	*YLDs* Number ('000s)	*YLDs* Rate per 100 000	*DALYs* Number ('000s)	*DALYs* Rate per 100 000
Established Market Economies														
0-4	2	6.79	6	20.96	0.5	68.12	1	2.39	21	79.93	35	131.60	56	212
5-14	0	0.00	11	20.99	–	–	0	0.17	3	6.39	0	0.00	3	6
15-44	0	0.00	35	19.01	–	–	0	0.06	3	1.78	0	0.00	3	2
45-59	0	0.00	12	17.86	–	–	0	0.02	0	0.33	0	0.00	0	0
60+	0	0.00	11	17.53	–	–	0	0.02	0	0.13	0	0.00	0	0
All Ages	*2*	*0.46*	*74*	*18.99*	*0.5*	*68.12*	*1*	*0.22*	*28*	*7.19*	*35*	*8.59*	*63*	*16*
Formerly Socialist Economies of Europe														
0-4	1	5.61	2	17.01	0.5	62.80	1	6.88	32	231.22	23	163.83	54	395
5-14	0	0.00	2	8.78	–	–	0	0.33	3	12.33	0	0.00	3	12
15-44	0	0.00	6	7.66	–	–	0	0.06	1	1.77	0	0.00	1	2
45-59	0	0.00	2	7.52	–	–	0	0.02	0	0.27	0	0.00	0	0
60+	0	0.00	2	7.39	–	–	0	0.02	0	0.14	0	0.00	0	0
All Ages	*1*	*0.72*	*14*	*8.66*	*0.5*	*62.80*	*1*	*0.66*	*37*	*22.16*	*23*	*13.64*	*59*	*36*
India														
0-4	18	30.27	39	65.10	0.5	58.78	11	18.04	360	601.73	260	435.30	620	1,037
5-14	0	0.00	58	57.02	–	–	0	0.47	18	17.71	0	0.00	18	18
15-44	0	0.00	109	54.35	–	–	0	0.02	1	0.74	0	0.00	1	1
45-59	0	0.00	26	53.77	–	–	0	0.03	0	0.41	0	0.00	0	0
69+	0	0.00	16	53.37	–	–	0	0.05	0	0.31	0	0.00	0	0
All Ages	*18*	*4.12*	*247*	*56.30*	*0.5*	*58.78*	*11*	*2.56*	*380*	*86.38*	*260*	*59.23*	*640*	*146*
China														
0-4	12	20.19	28	47.07	0.5	64.10	6	9.74	197	327.02	179	297.05	376	624
5-14	0	0.00	38	39.50	–	–	1	0.93	34	34.73	0	0.00	34	35
15-44	0	0.00	109	35.58	–	–	0	0.02	2	0.64	0	0.00	2	1
45-59	0	0.00	26	35.37	–	–	0	0.00	0	0.04	0	0.00	0	0
60+	0	0.00	17	35.35	–	–	0	0.00	0	0.00	0	0.00	0	0
All Ages	*12*	*2.08*	*219*	*37.37*	*0.5*	*64.10*	*7*	*1.17*	*233*	*39.76*	*179*	*30.58*	*412*	*70*

Table 14a *(continued)*

Age group (years)	*Incidence* Number ('000s)	Rate per100 000	*Prevalence* Number ('000s)	Rate per100 000	*Avg. age at onset* (years)	*Avgerage duration* (years)	*Deaths* Number ('000s)	Rate per100 000	*YLLs* Number ('000s)	Rate per100 000	*YLDs* Number ('000s)	Rate per100 000	*DALYs* Number ('000s)	Rate per100 000
Other Asia and Islands														
0-4	4	9.39	8	18.99	0.5	60.64	3	6.06	90	204.62	60	136.15	149	341
5-14	0	0.00	10	12.35	–	–	0	0.51	16	19.13	0	0.00	16	19
15-44	0	0.00	16	9.75	–	–	0	0.01	1	0.43	0	0.00	1	0
45-59	0	0.00	3	9.48	–	–	0	0.02	0	0.26	0	0.00	0	0
60+	0	0.00	2	9.21	–	–	0	0.04	0	0.24	0	0.00	0	0
All Ages	*4*	*1.20*	*39*	*11.51*	*0.5*	*60.64*	*3*	*0.91*	*106*	*31.04*	*60*	*17.38*	*166*	*45*
Sub-Saharan Africa														
0-4	10	20.86	29	61.93	0.5	51.13	2	4.47	72	152.00	136	285.96	205	438
5-14	0	0.00	47	66.37	–	–	0	0.25	6	9.22	0	0.00	6	9
15-44	0	0.00	87	64.85	–	–	0	0.01	0	0.40	0	0.00	0	0
45-59	0	0.00	13	64.35	–	–	0	0.03	0	0.44	0	0.00	0	0
60+	0	0.00	7	63.22	–	–	0	0.08	0	0.47	0	0.00	0	0
All Ages	*10*	*3.93*	*163*	*64.63*	*0.5*	*51.13*	*2*	*0.92*	*79*	*31.39*	*136*	*53.61*	*215*	*85*
Latin America and the Carrihean														
0-4	5	17.20	12	40.73	0.5	63.40	3	9.40	91	316.74	72	252.35	163	569
5-14	0	0.00	16	30.59	–	–	0	0.59	12	22.07	0	0.00	12	22
15-44	0	0.00	27	26.32	–	–	0	0.09	3	2.75	0	0.00	3	3
45-59	0	0.00	6	25.17	–	–	0	0.00	0	0.07	0	0.00	0	0
60+	0	0.00	4	25.11	–	–	0	0.04	0	0.19	0	0.00	0	0
All Ages	*5*	*2.23*	*64*	*29.00*	*0.5*	*63.40*	*3*	*1.40*	*105*	*47.56*	*72*	*32.70*	*178*	*80*
Middle Eastern Crescent														
0-4	4	10.01	8	18.96	0.5	61.49	2	5.68	79	191.84	60	145.83	139	338
5-14	0	0.00	11	17.10	–	–	0	0.24	6	9.12	0	0.00	6	9
15-44	0	0.00	18	15.59	–	–	0	0.02	1	0.50	0	0.00	1	1
45-59	0	0.00	3	15.02	–	–	0	0.02	0	0.33	0	0.00	0	0
60+	0	0.00	2	14.59	–	–	0	0.06	0	0.35	0	0.00	0	0
All Ages	*4*	*1.61*	*42*	*16.41*	*0.5*	*61.49*	*3*	*0.99*	*86*	*33.39*	*60*	*23.41*	*146*	*57*

Table 14a *(continued)*

Age group (years)	*Incidence* Number ('000s)	Rate per 100 000	*Prevalence* Number ('000s)	Rate per 100 000	*Avg. age at onset* (years)	*Avgerage duration* (years)	*Deaths* Number ('000s)	Rate per 100 000	*YLLs* Number ('000s)	Rate per 100 000	*YLDs* Number ('000s)	Rate per 100 000	*DALYs* Number ('000s)	Rate per 100 000
Developed Regions														
0-4	3	7.41	8	19.60	0.5	18.9	2	3.93	53	131.78	57	142.65	110	274
5-14	0	0.00	14	16.85	–	–	0	0.22	7	8.40	0	0.00	7	8
15-44	0	0.00	41	15.74	–	–	0	0.06	5	1.78	0	0.00	5	2
45-59	0	0.00	14	14.87	–	–	0	0.02	0	0.31	0	0.00	0	0
60+	0	0.00	12	14.93	–	–	0	0.02	0	0.13	0	0.00	0	0
All Ages	*3*	*0.54*	*88*	*15.92*	*0.5*	*18.9*	*2*	*0.35*	*65*	*11.64*	*57*	*10.30*	*122*	*22*
Developing Regions														
0-4	53	21.13	125	49.32	1	59	26	10.48	888	351.94	767	303.87	1 656	656
5-14	0	0.00	180	40.36	–	–	2	0.55	92	20.51	0	0.00	92	21
15-44	0	0.00	346	36.93	–	–	0	0.03	8	0.85	0	0.00	8	1
45-59	0	0.00	77	25.40	–	–	0	0.01	0	0.16	0	0.00	0	0
60+	0	0.00	47	32.52	–	–	0	0.03	0	0.18	0	0.00	0	0
All Ages	*53*	*2.84*	*775*	*41.30*	*0.5*	*59.4*	*29*	*1.56*	*989*	*52.71*	*767*	*40.88*	*1 756*	*94*
World														
0-4	56	17.53	132	41.20	0.5	57.2	28	8.73	941	292.97	824	256.57	1 766	550
5-14	0	0.00	194	35.21	–	–	3	0.48	98	17.87	0	0.00	98	18
15-44	0	0.00	387	30.97	–	–	0	0.03	13	1.01	0	0.00	13	1
45-59	0	0.00	90	28.93	–	–	0	0.02	1	0.25	0	0.00	1	0
60+	0	0.00	59	27.16	–	–	0	0.03	0	0.17	0	0.00	0	0
All Ages	*56*	*2.12*	*863*	*32.54*	*0.5*	*57.2*	*31*	*1.18*	*1 054*	*39.70*	*824*	*31.06*	*1 878*	*71*

Table 14b Epidemiological estimates for spina bifida, 1990 *females*.

Age group (years)	*Incidence* Number ('000s)	Rate per100 000	*Prevalence* Number ('000s)	Rate per100 000	*Avg. age at onset* (years)	*Avgerage duration* (years)	*Deaths* Number ('000s)	Rate per100 000	*YLLs* Number ('000s)	Rate per100 000	*YLDs* Number ('000s)	Rate per100 000	*DALYs* Number ('000s)	Rate per100 000
Established Market Economies														
0-4	3	10.74	9	35.44	0.5	73.76	1	3.04	26	101.86	53	211.13	78	313
5-14	0	0.00	19	36.73	–	–	0	0.13	2	4.90	0	0.00	2	5
15-44	0	0.00	63	35.16	–	–	0	0.06	3	1.74	0	0.00	3	2
45-59	0	0.00	23	34.41	–	–	0	0.07	1	1.06	0	0.00	1	1
60+	0	0.00	29	33.74	–	–	0	0.05	0	0.29	0	0.00	0	0
All Ages	*3*	*0.66*	*142*	*34.95*	*0.5*	*73.76*	*1*	*0.25*	*32*	*7.88*	*53*	*12.99*	*85*	*21*
Formerly Socialist Economies of Europe														
0-4	2	13.51	4	34.17	0.5	70.70	1	7.96	35	267.43	35	263.80	70	531
5-14	0	0.00	7	26.78	–	–	0	0.32	3	12.10	0	0.00	3	12
15-44	0	0.00	18	23.86	–	–	0	0.06	1	1.72	0	0.00	1	2
45-59	0	0.00	7	22.50	–	–	0	0.02	0	0.31	0	0.00	0	0
60+	0	0.00	8	22.08	–	–	0	0.03	0	0.19	0	0.00	0	0
All Ages	*2*	*0.73*	*44*	*18.22*	*0.5*	*70.70*	*1*	*0.49*	*40*	*16.39*	*35*	*14.27*	*74*	*31*
India														
0-4	27	48.24	79	138.63	0.5	59.67	9	15.21	294	518.36	395	696.74	689	1,215
5-14	0	0.00	136	142.75	–	–	1	0.64	23	24.20	0	0.00	23	24
15-44	0	0.00	247	134.65	–	–	0	0.24	13	7.33	0	0.00	13	7
45-59	0	0.00	59	128.60	–	–	0	0.26	2	4.04	0	0.00	2	4
60+	0	0.00	36	124.99	–	–	0	0.29	1	1.98	0	0.00	1	2
All Ages	*27*	*6.67*	*557*	*135.72*	*0.5*	*59.67*	*10*	*2.41*	*333*	*81.13*	*395*	*96.29*	*728*	*177*
China														
0-4	19	33.11	58	99.43	0.5	66.93	4	7.37	144	248.92	285	491.80	429	741
5-14	0	0.00	93	103.21	–	–	1	1.16	39	43.53	0	0.00	39	44
15-44	0	0.00	275	96.85	–	–	0	0.03	3	0.97	0	0.00	3	1
45-59	0	0.00	62	96.29	–	–	0	0.00	0	0.05	0	0.00	0	0
60+	0	0.00	50	96.24	–	–	0	0.00	0	0.00	0	0.00	0	0
All Ages	*19*	*3.50*	*538*	*98.05*	*0.5*	*66.93*	*5*	*0.99*	*186*	*33.98*	*285*	*51.96*	*471*	*86*

Table 14b *(continued)*

Age group (years)	Incidence Number ('000s)	Incidence Rate per100 000	Prevalence Number ('000s)	Prevalence Rate per100 000	Avg. age at onset (years)	Avgerage duration (years)	Deaths Number ('000s)	Deaths Rate per100 000	YLLs Number ('000s)	YLLs Rate per100 000	YLDs Number ('000s)	YLDs Rate per100 000	DALYs Number ('000s)	DALYs Rate per100 000
Other Asia and Islands														
0-4	6	15.39	20	48.33	0.5	64.47	2	4.48	64	153.04	95	226.70	159	380
5-14	0	0.00	39	48.39	1–	–	1	0.74	22	27.81	0	0.00	22	28
15-44	0	0.00	70	43.60	–	–	0	0.10	5	2.92	0	0.00	5	3
45-59	0	0.00	14	40.81	–	–	0	0.13	1	2.01	0	0.00	1	2
60+	0	0.00	9	39.15	–	–	0	0.14	0	1.05	0	0.00	0	1
All Ages	*6*	*1.90*	*152*	*44.73*	*0.5*	*64.47*	*3*	*0.80*	*92*	*27.15*	*95*	*28.03*	*187*	*55*
Sub-Saharan Africa														
0-4	16	34.30	56	118.13	0.5	54.11	2	4.40	71	150.49	226	480.19	297	631
5-14	0	0.00	90	129.33	–	–	0	0.30	8	11.26	0	0.00	8	11
15-44	0	0.00	136	127.53	–	–	0	0.09	3	2.60	0	0.00	3	3
45-59	0	0.00	28	125.10	–	–	0	0.29	1	4.55	0	0.00	1	5
60+	0	0.00	15	121.61	–	–	0	0.38	0	2.74	0	0.00	0	3
All Ages	*16*	*6.25*	*325*	*125.80*	*0.5*	*54.11*	*2*	*0.96*	*83*	*32.08*	*226*	*87.55*	*309*	*120*
Latin America and the Caribbean														
0-4	8	27.34	22	77.94	0.5	67.34	3	9.72	91	328.28	113	406.64	203	735
5-14	0	0.00	39	76.68	–	–	0	0.63	12	23.87	0	0.00	12	24
15-44	0	0.00	73	69.98	–	–	0	0.14	4	4.22	0	0.00	4	4
45-59	0	0.00	16	66.64	–	–	0	0.05	0	0.79	0	0.00	0	1
60+	0	0.00	11	66.07	–	–	0	0.12	0	0.77	0	0.00	0	1
All Ages	*8*	*3.40*	*160*	*71.85*	*0.5*	*67.34*	*3*	*1.43*	*108*	*48.35*	*113*	*50.54*	*220*	*99*
Middle Eastern Crescent														
0-4	7	16.47	19	48.69	0.5	64.09	2	4.11	56	139.69	96	242.27	152	382
5-14	0	0.00	32	51.24	–	–	0	0.31	7	11.71	0	0.00	7	12
15-44	0	0.00	51	47.73	–	–	0	0.13	4	4.03	0	0.00	4	4
45-59	0	0.00	10	45.00	–	–	0	0.23	1	3.63	0	0.00	1	4
60+	0	0.00	7	43.69	–	–	0	0.15	0	0.99	0	0.00	0	1
All Ages	*7*	*2.65*	*119*	*48.26*	*0.5*	*64.09*	*2*	*0.83*	*68*	*27.58*	*96*	*39.02*	*164*	*67*

Table 14b *(continued)*

Age group (years)	Incidence Number ('000s)	Incidence Rate per100 000	Prevalence Number ('000s)	Prevalence Rate per100 000	Avg. age at onset (years)	Avgerage duration (years)	Deaths Number ('000s)	Deaths Rate per100 000	YLLs Number ('000s)	YLLs Rate per100 000	YLDs Number ('000s)	YLDs Rate per100 000	DALYs Number ('000s)	DALYs Rate per100 000
Developed Regions														
0-4	4	11.69	13	35.00	0.5	20.0	2	4.74	61	158.79	88	229.24	148	388
5-14	0	0.00	26	33.32	–	–	0	0.20	6	7.37	0	0.00	6	7
15-44	0	0.00	81	31.83	–	–	0	0.06	4	1.73	0	0.00	4	2
45-59	0	0.00	30	30.76	–	–	0	0.05	1	0.83	0	0.00	1	1
60+	0	0.00	37	30.23	–	–	0	0.04	0	0.26	0	0.00	0	0
All Ages	*4*	*0.69*	*187*	*28.71*	*0.5*	*20.0*	*2*	*0.34*	*72*	*11.06*	*88*	*13.47*	*159*	*25*
Developing Regions														
0-4	83	30.71	253	93.32	1	62	21	7.81	719	265.42	1,210	446.30	1,929	712
5-14	0	0.00	429	95.68	–	–	3	0.66	112	24.96	0	0.00	112	25
15-44	0	0.00	851	90.10	–	–	1	0.11	32	3.42	0	0.00	32	3
45-59	0	0.00	189	88.51	–	–	0	0.14	5	2.15	0	0.00	5	2
60+	0	0.00	128	86.40	–	–	0	0.14	1	0.97	0	0.00	1	1
All Ages	*83*	*4.11*	*1,850*	*91.33*	*0.5*	*61.7*	*26*	*1.27*	*870*	*42.94*	*1,210*	*59.72*	*2,079*	*103*
World														
0-4	88	28.36	266	86.12	0.5	59.6	23	7.43	780	252.25	1,297	419.49	2,077	672
5-14	0	0.00	455	86.53	–	–	3	0.60	118	22.38	0	0.00	118	22
15-44	0	0.00	932	77.74	–	–	1	0.10	37	3.06	0	0.00	37	3
45-59	0	0.00	219	70.35	–	–	0	0.11	5	1.74	0	0.00	5	2
60+	0	0.00	165	61.16	–	–	0	0.10	2	0.65	0	0.00	2	1
All Ages	*88*	*3.36*	*2,036*	*77.91*	*0.5*	*59.6*	*28*	*1.07*	*942*	*36.03*	*1,297*	*49.63*	*2,239*	*86*

Table 15a Epidemiological estimates for congenital heart anomalies, 1990 *males*.

Age group (years)	*Incidence* Number ('000s)	Rate per100 000	*Prevalence* Number ('000s)	Rate per100 000	*Avg. age at onset* (years)	*Avgerage duration* (years)	*Deaths* Number ('000s)	Rate per100 000	*YLLs* Number ('000s)	Rate per100 000	*YLDs* Number ('000s)	Rate per100 000	*DALYs* Number ('000s)	Rate per100 000
Established Market Economies														
0-4	32	119.90	114	434.00	0.0	68.1	6	21.40	188	714.31	328	1 245.00	517	1 959
5-14	0	0.00	246	462.00	–	–	0	0.80	15	28.87	0	0.00	15	29
15-44	0	0.00	824	448.00	–	–	1	0.70	38	20.79	0	0.00	38	21
45-59	0	0.00	284	430.00	–	–	0	0.70	6	9.70	0	0.00	6	10
60+	0	0.00	249	411.00	–	–	1	1.20	4	6.12	0	0.00	4	6
All Ages	*32*	*8.1*	*1 717*	*440*	*0.0*	*68.1*	*9*	*2.2*	*252*	*64.60*	*328*	*84.12*	*581*	*149*
Formerly Socialist Economies of Europe														
0-4	17	120.10	53	387.00	0.0	62.8	5	34.80	161	1 170.99	169	1 224.69	330	2 396
5-14	0	0.00	111	407.00	–	–	0	1.00	10	37.40	0	0.00	10	37
15-44	0	0.00	302	396.00	–	–	1	0.90	22	28.65	0	0.00	22	29
45-59	0	0.00	103	382.00	–	–	0	0.40	1	5.31	0	0.00	1	5
60+	0	0.00	78	371.00	–	–	0	0.40	0	2.36	0	0.00	0	2
All Ages	*17*	*10*	*647*	*392*	*0.0*	*62.8*	*6*	*3.6*	*195*	*118.03*	*169*	*101.93*	*364*	*220*
India														
0-4	74	125.00	171	286.00	0.0	58.8	24	39.80	793	1 326.44	745	1 246.80	1 539	2 573
5-14	0	0.00	282	277.00	–	–	3	2.50	97	94.85	0	0.00	97	95
15-44	0	0.00	524	261.00	–	–	2	0.90	57	28.46	0	0.00	57	28
45-59	0	0.00	114	239.00	–	–	1	2.40	17	35.10	0	0.00	17	35
60+	0	0.00	63	211.00	–	–	1	3.30	6	20.75	0	0.00	6	21
All Ages	*74*	*17*	*1 153*	*262*	*0.0*	*58.8*	*30*	*6.9*	*970*	*220.64*	*745*	*169.65*	*1 715*	*390*
China														
0-4	79	132.00	251	417.00	0.0	64.1	11	18.60	376	624.80	814	1 350.50	1 190	1 975
5-14	0	0.00	429	443.00	–	–	2	2.10	76	78.42	0	0.00	76	78
15-44	0	0.00	1 314	429.00	–	–	3	1.00	98	32.01	0	0.00	98	32
45-59	0	0.00	300	413.00	–	–	0	0.20	2	2.35	0	0.00	2	2
60+	0	0.00	196	400.00	–	–	0	0.00	0	0.00	0	0.00	0	0
All Ages	*79*	*14*	*2 490*	*426*	*0.0*	*64.1*	*16*	*2.8*	*552*	*94.37*	*814*	*139.03*	*1 366*	*233*

Table 15a *(continued)*

Age group (years)	*Incidence* Number ('000s)	Rate per100 000	*Prevalence* Number ('000s)	Rate per100 000	*Avg. age at onset* (years)	*Avgerage duration* (years)	*Deaths* Number ('000s)	Rate per100 000	*YLLs* Number ('000s)	Rate per100 000	*YLDs* Number ('000s)	Rate per100 000	*DALYs* Number ('000s)	Rate per100 000
Other Asia and Islands														
0-4	52	120.00	144	330.00	0.0	60.6	14	31.10	459	1 048.85	530	1 211.15	989	2 260
5-14	0	0.00	273	325.00	–	–	1	1.70	54	64.56	0	0.00	54	65
15-44	0	0.00	492	306.00	–	–	1	0.80	37	23.16	0	0.00	37	23
45-59	0	0.00	95	279.00	–	–	1	1.80	9	26.97	0	0.00	9	27
60+	0	0.00	52	258.00	–	–	1	2.60	3	15.80	0	0.00	3	16
All Ages	*52*	*15*	*1 056*	*308*	*0.0*	*60.6*	*17*	*5.1*	*563*	*164.13*	*530*	*154.54*	*1 093*	*319*
Sub-Saharan Africa														
0-4	62	131.00	127	268.00	0.0	51.1	7	15.00	242	508.68	591	1 243.83	832	1 753
5-14	0	0.00	177	253.00	–	–	1	1.90	49	70.42	0	0.00	49	70
15-44	0	0.00	236	228.00	–	–	1	0.80	26	25.02	0	0.00	26	25
45-59	0	0.00	37	183.00	–	–	1	2.80	8	41.60	0	0.00	8	42
60+	0	0.00	10	99.00	–	–	1	5.00	3	31.85	0	0.00	3	32
All Ages	*62*	*25*	*588*	*233*	*0.0*	*51.1*	*10*	*4.1*	*329*	*130.30*	*591*	*234.07*	*919*	*364*
Latin America and the Caribbean														
0-4	35	123.00	118	409.00	0.0	63.4	6	21.80	211	733.20	361	1 256.49	571	1 990
5-14	0	0.00	225	431.00	–	–	1	1.70	33	63.26	0	0.00	33	63
15-44	0	0.00	431	413.00	–	–	0	0.40	14	13.30	0	0.00	14	13
45-59	0	0.00	86	387.00	–	–	0	0.40	1	5.53	0	0.00	1	6
60+	0	0.00	53	369.00	–	–	0	2.10	2	11.39	0	0.00	2	11
All Ages	*35*	*16*	*912*	*411*	*0.0*	*63.4*	*8*	*3.6*	*260*	*117.45*	*361*	*162.84*	*621*	*280*
Middle Eastern Crescent														
0-4	53	128.00	138	334.00	0.0	61.5	13	31.60	440	1 069.52	534	1 297.15	974	2 367
5-14	0	0.00	221	338.00	–	–	1	2.10	51	77.63	0	0.00	51	78
15-44	0	0.00	363	319.00	–	–	1	0.90	32	28.04	0	0.00	32	28
45-59	0	0.00	65	292.00	–	–	1	3.50	8	36.77	0	0.00	8	37
60+	0	0.00	37	271.00	–	–	1	3.60	3	21.67	0	0.00	3	22
All Ages	*53*	*21*	*824*	*321*	*0.0*	*61.5*	*16*	*6.4*	*534*	*208.30*	*534*	*208.25*	*1 068*	*417*

Table 15a *(continued)*

Age group (years)	*Incidence* Number ('000s)	Rate per100 000	*Prevalence* Number ('000s)	Rate per100 000	*Avg. age at onset* (years)	*Avgerage duration* (years)	*Deaths* Number ('000s)	Rate per100 000	*YLLs* Number ('000s)	Rate per100 000	*YLDs* Number ('000s)	Rate per100 000	*DALYs* Number ('000s)	Rate per100 000
Developed Regions														
0-4	49	122.06	167	416.01	0.0	21.3	11	27.40	350	870.84	497	1 238.04	847	2 109
5-14	0	0.00	357	442.40	–	–	0	0.00	26	31.76	0	0.00	26	32
15-44	0	0.00	1 126	432.51	–	–	2	0.77	60	23.09	0	0.00	60	23
45-59	0	0.00	387	415.63	–	–	0	0.00	8	8.43	0	0.00	8	8
60+	0	0.00	327	401.17	–	–	1	1.23	4	5.15	0	0.00	4	5
All Ages	*49*	*8.82*	*2 364*	*425.33*	*0.0*	*21.3*	*14*	*2.52*	*447*	*80.49*	*497*	*89.42*	*944*	*170*
Developing Regions														
0-4	355	140.63	949	375.93	0	60	75	29.71	2 521	998.58	3 574	1 415.97	6 095	2 415
5-14	0	0.00	1 607	359.42	–	–	9	2.01	360	80.52	0	0.00	360	81
15-44	0	0.00	3 360	358.42	–	–	8	0.85	264	28.18	0	0.00	264	28
45-59	0	0.00	697	231.32	–	–	4	1.33	46	15.10	0	0.00	46	15
60+	0	0.00	411	282.74	–	–	4	2.75	17	11.90	0	0.00	17	12
All Ages	*355*	*18.92*	*7 024*	*374.36*	*0.0*	*59.8*	*100*	*5.33*	*3 208*	*170.96*	*3 574*	*190.51*	*6 782*	*361*
World														
0-4	404	125.74	1 116	347.33	0.0	55.1	86	26.77	2 870	893.36	4 071	1 267.17	6 942	2 161
5-14	0	0.00	1 964	356.31	–	–	9	1.63	386	69.96	0	0.00	386	70
15-44	0	0.00	4 486	358.90	–	–	10	0.80	324	25.94	0	0.00	324	26
45-59	0	0.00	1 084	347.01	–	–	4	1.28	53	17.08	0	0.00	53	17
60+	0	0.00	738	337.21	–	–	5	2.28	21	9.82	0	0.00	21	10
All Ages	*404*	*15.22*	*9 388*	*353.77*	*0.0*	*55.1*	*114*	*4.30*	*3 655*	*137.74*	*4 071*	*153.43*	*7 727*	*291*

Table 15b Epidemiological estimates for congenital heart anomalies, 1990 *females*.

Age group (years)	*Incidence* Number ('000s)	Rate per100 000	*Prevalence* Number ('000s)	Rate per100 000	*Avg. age at onset* (years)	*Avgerage duration* (years)	*Deaths* Number ('000s)	Rate per100 000	*YLLs* Number ('000s)	Rate per100 000	*YLDs* Number ('000s)	Rate per100 000	*DALYs* Number ('000s)	Rate per100 000
Established Market Economies														
0-4	30	119.90	113	452.00	0.0	73.8	4	17.90	150	597.92	317	1 263.04	466	1 861
5-14	0	0.00	245	484.00	–	–	0	0.70	13	26.13	0	0.00	13	26
15-44	0	0.00	851	475.00	–	–	1	0.50	25	14.00	0	0.00	25	14
45-59	0	0.00	315	464.00	–	–	0	0.60	6	8.64	0	0.00	6	9
60+	0	0.00	382	452.00	–	–	1	1.10	5	5.51	0	0.00	5	6
All Ages	*30*	*7.4*	*1 907*	*468*	*0.0*	*73.8*	*7*	*1.7*	*199*	*48.79*	*317*	*77.73*	*515*	*127*
Formerly Socialist Economies of Europe														
0-4	16	119.30	54	412.00	0.0	70.7	4	29.70	131	998.14	164	1 248.37	295	2 247
5-14	0	0.00	115	436.00	–	–	0	0.90	9	32.61	0	0.00	9	33
15-44	0	0.00	320	427.00	–	–	0	0.50	11	14.03	0	0.00	11	14
45-59	0	0.00	125	415.00	–	–	0	0.30	2	5.23	0	0.00	2	5
60+	0	0.00	149	409.00	–	–	0	0.40	1	2.44	0	0.00	1	2
All Ages	*16*	*8.7*	*763*	*422*	*0.0*	*70.7*	*5*	*2.6*	*153*	*62.91*	*164*	*67.55*	*317*	*130*
India														
0-4	71	125.00	160	282.00	0.0	59.7	19	34.40	664	1 171.44	712	1 256.54	1 376	2 428
5-14	0	0.00	258	271.00	–	–	3	3.30	116	122.26	0	0.00	116	122
15-44	0	0.00	464	253.00	–	–	2	1.10	60	32.47	0	0.00	60	32
45-59	0	0.00	108	235.00	–	–	1	3.10	22	48.12	0	0.00	22	48
60+	0	0.00	61	212.00	–	–	1	4.10	8	27.75	0	0.00	8	28
All Ages	*71*	*17*	*1 051*	*256*	*0.0*	*59.7*	*27*	*6.6*	*870*	*212.16*	*712*	*173.66*	*1 582*	*386*
China														
0-4	77	133.00	251	433.00	0.0	66.9	7	11.70	230	396.19	800	1 381.25	1 030	1 777
5-14	0	0.00	420	464.00	–	–	2	1.90	64	71.08	0	0.00	64	71
15-44	0	0.00	1 284	452.00	–	–	4	1.50	140	49.44	0	0.00	140	49
45-59	0	0.00	282	438.00	–	–	0	0.20	2	3.46	0	0.00	2	3
60+	0	0.00	222	429.00	–	–	0	0.00	0	0.00	0	0.00	0	0
All Ages	*77*	*14*	*2 459*	*448*	*0.0*	*66.9*	*3*	*2.4*	*437*	*79.58*	*800*	*145.92*	*1 237*	*226*

Table 15b *(continued)*

Age group (years)	*Incidence* Number ('000s)	Rate per100 000	*Prevalence* Number ('000s)	Rate per100 000	*Avg. age at onset* (years)	*Avgerage duration* (years)	*Deaths* Number ('000s)	Rate per100 000	*YLLs* Number ('000s)	Rate per100 000	*YLDs* Number ('000s)	Rate per100 000	*DALYs* Number ('000s)	Rate per100 000
Other Asia and Islands														
0-4	50	120.00	142	339.00	0.0	64.5	8	19.80	284	677.41	517	1 231.49	802	1 909
5-14	0	0.00	274	341.00	–	–	1	1.60	48	59.65	0	0.00	48	60
15-44	0	0.00	516	323.00	–	–	1	0.60	29	18.03	0	0.00	29	18
45-59	0	0.00	104	298.00	–	–	1	1.80	10	27.68	0	0.00	10	28
60+	0	0.00	63	277.00	–	–	1	2.30	4	16.11	0	0.00	4	16
All Ages	*50*	*15*	*1 099*	*324*	*0.0*	*64.5*	*12*	*3.4*	*374*	*110.26*	*517*	*152.28*	*891*	*263*
Sub-Saharan Africa														
0-4	61	130.00	131	278.00	0.0	54.1	7.0	14.70	237	503.56	597	1 270.21	834	1 774
5-14	0	0.00	186	267.00	–	–	2.0	2.30	60	86.28	0	0.00	60	86
15-44	0	0.00	259	244.00	–	–	1.0	0.60	18	17.22	0	0.00	18	17
45-59	0	0.00	45	204.00	–	–	1.0	3.40	12	53.84	0	0.00	12	54
60+	0	0.00	15	118.00	–	–	1.0	4.20	4	28.25	0	0.00	4	28
All Ages	*61*	*24*	*636*	*247*	*0.0*	*54.1*	*1.0*	*4*	*331*	*128.27*	*597*	*231.59*	*928*	*360*
Latin America and the Caribbean														
0-4	34	123.00	120	432.00	0.0	67.3	5	18.60	174	629.11	351	1 269.84	526	1 899
5-14	0	0.00	234	461.00	–	–	1	1.40	26	52.04	0	0.00	26	52
15-44	0	0.00	462	444.00	–	–	1	0.80	25	24.07	0	0.00	25	24
45-59	0	0.00	98	421.00	–	–	0	0.60	2	8.94	0	0.00	2	9
60+	0	0.00	69	408.00	–	–	0	1.70	2	10.35	0	0.00	2	10
All Ages	*34*	*15*	*982*	*441*	*0.0*	*67.3*	*7*	*3.2*	*229*	*103.02*	*351*	*157.82*	*581*	*261*
Middle Eastern Crescent														
0-4	51	128.00	133	335.00	0.0	64.1	9	22.90	309	778.56	523	1 315.88	832	2 094
5-14	0	0.00	210	339.00	–	–	1	2.40	55	88.46	0	0.00	55	88
15-44	0	0.00	344	321.00	–	–	1	0.80	27	24.83	0	0.00	27	25
45-59	0	0.00	66	297.00	–	–	1	3.20	11	50.42	0	0.00	11	50
60+	0	0.00	43	277.00	–	–	1	3.90	4	25.82	0	0.00	4	26
All Ages	*11*	*21*	*796*	*323*	*0.0*	*64.1*	*13*	*5.2*	*406*	*164.60*	*523*	*211.95*	*929*	*377*

Table 15b *(continued)*

Age group (years)	Incidence Number ('000s)	Incidence Rate per100 000	Prevalence Number ('000s)	Prevalence Rate per100 000	Avg. age at onset (years)	Avgerage duration (years)	Deaths Number ('000s)	Deaths Rate per100 000	YLLs Number ('000s)	YLLs Rate per100 000	YLDs Number ('000s)	YLDs Rate per100 000	DALYs Number ('000s)	DALYs Rate per100 000
Developed Regions														
0-4	46	120.42	167	437.17	0.0	22.4	8	20.94	281	735.54	481	1 258.00	762	1 994
5-14	0	0.00	360	466.92	–	–	0	0.00	22	28.35	0	0.00	22	28
15-44	0	0.00	1 171	460.74	–	–	1	0.39	36	14.01	0	0.00	36	14
45-59	0	0.00	440	449.87	–	–	0	0.00	7	7.60	0	0.00	7	8
60+	0	0.00	531	438.99	–	–	1	0.83	6	4.59	0	0.00	6	5
All Ages	*46*	*7.08*	*2 669*	*410.59*	*0.0*	*22.4*	*10*	*1.54*	*351*	*54.06*	*481*	*73.93*	*832*	*128*
Developing Regions														
0-4	344	126.91	937	345.69	0	62	55	20.29	1 898	700.33	3 501	1 291.75	5 400	1 992
5-14	0	0.00	1 582	352.78	–	–	10	2.23	370	82.52	0	0.00	370	83
15-44	0	0.00	3 329	352.47	–	–	10	1.06	299	31.63	0	0.00	299	32
45-59	0	0.00	703	329.64	–	–	4	1.88	59	27.81	0	0.00	59	28
60+	0	0.00	473	319.04	–	–	4	2.70	21	14.17	0	0.00	21	14
All Ages	*344*	*16.98*	*7 024*	*346.78*	*0.0*	*62.4*	*83*	*4.10*	*2 647*	*130.70*	*3 501*	*172.86*	*6 149*	*304*
World														
0-4	390	126.11	1 104	356.99	0.0	57.7	63	20.37	2 179	704.68	3 982	1 287.58	6 161	1 992
5-14	0	0.00	1 942	369.52	–	–	10	1.90	392	74.57	0	0.00	392	75
15-44	0	0.00	4 500	375.42	–	–	11	0.92	334	27.89	0	0.00	334	28
45-59	0	0.00	1 143	367.44	–	–	4	1.29	67	21.46	0	0.00	67	21
60+	0	0.00	1 004	372.94	–	–	5	1.86	27	9.86	0	0.00	27	10
All Ages	*390*	*14.92*	*9 693*	*370.85*	*0.0*	*57.7*	*93*	*3.56*	*2 999*	*114.73*	*3 982*	*152.35*	*6 981*	*267*

Table 16a Epidemiological estimates for Down syndrome, 1990 *males.*

Age group (years)	*Incidence* Number ('000s)	Rate per 100 000	*Prevalence* Number ('000s)	Rate per 100 000	*Avg. age at onset* (years)	*Avgerage duration* (years)	*Deaths* Number ('000s)	Rate per 100 000	*YLLs* Number ('000s)	Rate per 100 000	*YLDs* Number ('000s)	Rate per 100 000	*DALYs* Number ('000s)	Rate per 100 000
Established Market Economies														
0-4	6	7.00	25	35.00	0.5	68.12	1	20.50	26	98.55	121	460.40	147	559
5-14	0	0.00	52	35.00	10.0	59.16	0	0.00	3	4.85	0	0.00	3	5
15-44	0	0.00	178	35.00	35.0	38.97	0	0.00	3	1.44	0	0.00	3	1
45-59	0	0.00	61	35.00	55.0	18.73	0	0.00	5	7.65	0	0.00	5	8
60+	0	0.00	50	35.00	70.0	7.93	0	0.00	3	4.44	0	0.00	3	4
All Ages	*6*	*0.5*	*366*	*35.0*	*0.5*	*68.12*	*2*	*1.4*	*39*	*9.98*	*121*	*31.11*	*160*	*41*
Formerly Socialist Economies of Europe														
0-4	2	11.30	9	56.00	0.5	62.80	0	24.10	12	87.26	43	312.31	55	400
5-14	0	0.00	18	56.00	10.0	53.83	0	0.00	3	12.33	0	0.00	3	12
15-44	0	0.00	49	56.00	35.0	34.31	0	0.00	1	1.77	0	0.00	1	2
45-59	0	0.00	16	56.00	55.0	16.48	0	0.00	2	8.54	0	0.00	2	9
60+	0	0.00	11	56.00	70.0	7.25	0	0.00	0	1.23	0	0.00	0	1
All Ages	*2*	*0.9*	*104*	*56.0*	*0.5*	*62.80*	*1*	*1.8*	*19*	*11.67*	*43*	*25.99*	*62*	*38*
India														
0-4	23	128.00	77	639.00	0.5	58.78	5	289.00	166	276.93	330	551.40	495	828
5-14	0	0.00	133	639.00	10.0	53.30	2	0.00	57	56.04	0	0.00	57	56
15-44	0	0.00	211	639.00	35.0	33.98	3	0.00	76	38.09	0	0.00	76	38
45-59	0	0.00	42	639.00	55.0	15.76	0	0.00	0	0.63	0	0.00	0	1
60+	0	0.00	26	639.00	70.0	7.22	0	0.00	0	0.00	0	0.00	0	0
All Ages	*23*	*17.0*	*489*	*639.0*	*0.5*	*58.78*	*9*	*32*	*299*	*68.11*	*330*	*75.03*	*629*	*143*
China														
0-4	21	8.40	75	42.00	0.5	64.10	3	41.50	92	152.95	313	519.64	405	673
5-14	0	0.00	124	42.00	10.0	55.63	1	0.00	36	37.51	0	0.00	36	38
15-44	0	0.00	350	42.00	35.0	35.00	2	0.00	58	19.01	0	0.00	58	19
45-59	0	0.00	76	42.00	55.0	16.05	0	0.00	2	3.24	0	0.00	2	3
60+	0	0.00	50	42.00	70.0	6.96	0	0.00	0	0.00	0	0.00	0	0
All Ages	*21*	*0.9*	*675*	*42.0*	*0.5*	*64.10*	*6*	*3.7*	*189*	*32.31*	*313*	*53.49*	*502*	*86*

Table 16a *(continued)*

Age group (years)	Incidence Number ('000s)	Incidence Rate per100 000	Prevalence Number ('000s)	Prevalence Rate per100 000	Avg. age at onset (years)	Avgerage duration (years)	Deaths Number ('000s)	Deaths Rate per100 000	YLLs Number ('000s)	YLLs Rate per100 000	YLDs Number ('000s)	YLDs Rate per100 000	DALYs Number ('000s)	DALYs Rate per100 000
Other Asia and Islands														
0-4	14	27.50	53	137.00	0.5	60.64	3	206.00	86	196.05	204	466.23	290	662
5-14	0	0.00	104	137.00	10.0	54.65	1	0.00	21	24.97	0	0.00	21	25
15-44	0	0.00	180	137.00	35.0	35.33	1	0.00	26	16.08	0	0.00	26	16
45-59	0	0.00	35	137.00	55.0	16.68	0	0.00	0	0.00	0	0.00	0	0
60+	0	0.00	21	137.00	70.0	7.42	0	0.00	0	0.00	0	0.00	0	0
All Ages	*14*	*3.5*	*393*	*137.0*	*0.5*	*60.64*	*4*	*22*	*133*	*38.67*	*204*	*59.49*	*337*	*98*
Sub-Saharan Africa														
0-4	19	59.00	70	293.00	0.5	51.13	1	193.00	50	106.20	262	550.84	312	657
5-14	0	0.00	110	293.00	10.0	48.25	1	0.00	29	41.63	0	0.00	29	42
15-44	0	0.00	137	293.00	35.0	32.13	1	0.00	35	33.49	0	0.00	35	33
45-59	0	0.00	23	293.00	55.0	15.64	0	0.00	0	0.67	0	0.00	0	1
60+	0	0.00	12	293.00	70.0	7.02	0	0.00	0	0.00	0	0.00	0	0
All Ages	*19*	*11.0*	*352*	*293.0*	*0.5*	*51.13*	*3*	*37*	*115*	*45.40*	*262*	*103.66*	*376*	*149*
Latin America and the Caribbean														
0-4	9	35.80	35	178.00	0.5	63.40	1	56.00	48	167.99	139	483.49	187	651
5-14	0	0.00	66	178.00	10.0	56.04	0	0.00	14	26.24	0	0.00	14	26
15-44	0	0.00	124	178.00	35.0	36.87	0	0.00	7	7.07	0	0.00	7	7
45-59	0	0.00	25	178.00	55.0	18.12	0	0.00	2	8.19	0	0.00	2	8
60+	0	0.00	15	178.00	70.0	7.89	0	0.00	0	0.54	0	0.00	0	1
All Ages	*9*	*4.6*	*265*	*178.0*	*0.5*	*63.40*	*2*	*6*	*71*	*32.13*	*139*	*62.66*	*210*	*95*
Middle Eastern Crescent														
0-4	14	44.20	49	220.00	0.5	61.49	3	204.00	87	212.46	205	499.25	293	712
5-14	0	0.00	78	220.00	10.0	55.59	1	0.00	25	38.70	0	0.00	25	39
15-44	0	0.00	116	220.00	35.0	35.89	1	0.00	31	27.57	0	0.00	31	28
45-59	0	0.00	20	220.00	55.0	16.88	0	0.00	0	0.00	0	0.00	0	0
60+	0	0.00	12	220.00	70.0	7.40	0	0.00	0	0.00	0	0.00	0	0
All Ages	*14*	*7.1*	*276*	*220.0*	*0.5*	*61.49*	*4*	*30*	*144*	*56.22*	*205*	*80.15*	*350*	*136*

Table 16a *(continued)*

Age group (years)	*Incidence* Number ('000s)	Rate per100 000	*Prevalence* Number ('000s)	Rate per100 000	*Avg. age at onset* (years)	*Avgerage duration* (years)	*Deaths* Number ('000s)	Rate per100 000	*YLLs* Number ('000s)	Rate per100 000	*YLDs* Number ('000s)	Rate per100 000	*DALYs* Number ('000s)	Rate per100 000
Developed Regions														
0-4	9	21.23	34	84.18	0.5	32.4	1	2.83	38	94.68	164	409.64	202	504
5-14	0	0.00	71	87.60	–	–	0	0.20	6	7.38	0	0.00	6	7
15-44	0	0.00	227	87.30	–	–	0	0.05	4	1.54	0	0.00	4	2
45-59	0	0.00	77	83.01	–	–	1	0.54	7	7.91	0	0.00	7	8
60+	0	0.00	61	74.84	–	–	0	0.60	3	3.61	0	0.00	3	4
All Ages	*9*	*1.53*	*470*	*84.57*	*0.5*	*32.4*	*2*	*0.44*	*58*	*10.48*	*164*	*29.59*	*223*	*40*
Developing Regions														
0-4	101	39.98	360	142.60	1	60	16	6.24	530	209.81	1 453	575.46	1 982	785
5-14	0	0.00	616	137.69	–	–	5	1.09	183	40.84	0	0.00	183	41
15-44	0	0.00	1 118	119.27	–	–	8	0.81	234	24.96	0	0.00	234	25
45-59	0	0.00	221	73.26	–	–	0	0.10	5	1.53	0	0.00	5	2
60+	0	0.00	136	93.80	–	–	0	0.01	0	0.05	0	0.00	0	0
All Ages	*101*	*5.38*	*2 451*	*130.62*	*0.5*	*59.5*	*29*	*1.52*	*951*	*50.68*	*1 453*	*77.42*	*2 404*	*128*
World														
0-4	109	34.06	394	122.55	0.5	57.4	17	5.26	568	176.67	1 617	503.30	2 185	680
5-14	0	0.00	686	124.51	–	–	5	0.91	189	34.21	0	0.00	189	34
15-44	0	0.00	1 345	107.64	–	–	8	0.62	238	19.04	0	0.00	238	19
45-59	0	0.00	298	95.41	–	–	1	0.26	12	3.83	0	0.00	12	4
60+	0	0.00	197	90.18	–	–	1	0.23	3	1.38	0	0.00	3	1
All Ages	*109*	*4.12*	*2 921*	*110.07*	*0.5*	*57.4*	*31*	*1.17*	*1 009*	*38.03*	*1 617*	*60.94*	*2 626*	*99*

Table 16b Epidemiological estimates for Down syndrome, 1990 *females*.

Age group (years)	*Incidence* Number ('000s)	Rate per 100 000	*Prevalence* Number ('000s)	Rate per 100 000	*Avg. age at onset* (years)	*Avgerage duration* (years)	*Deaths* Number ('000s)	Rate per 100 000	*YLLs* Number ('000s)	Rate per 100 000	*YLDs* Number ('000s)	Rate per 100 000	*DALYs* Number ('000s)	Rate per 100 000
Established Market Economies														
0-4	5	7.00	19	35.00	0.5	73.76	1	16.60	20	78.09	92	368.84	112	447
5-14	0	0.00	39	35.00	10.0	64.30	0	0.00	2	3.79	0	0.00	2	4
15-44	0	0.00	137	35.00	35.0	43.00	0	0.00	2	1.16	0	0.00	2	1
45-59	0	0.00	49	35.00	55.0	21.54	0	0.00	5	7.65	0	0.00	5	8
60+	0	0.00	53	35.00	70.0	8.67	0	0.00	2	2.34	0	0.00	2	2
All Ages	*5*	*0.40*	*297*	*35.00*	*0.5*	*73.76*	*1*	*1.10*	*31*	*7.55*	*92*	*22.70*	*123*	*30*
Formerly Socialist Economies of Europe														
0-4	2	11.30	7	56.00	0.5	70.70	0	18.90	9	68.01	33	251.76	42	320
5-14	0	0.00	14	56.00	10.0	61.54	0	0.00	1	3.42	0	0.00	1	3
15-44	0	0.00	39	56.00	35.0	40.51	0	0.00	1	1.15	0	0.00	1	1
45-59	0	0.00	14	56.00	55.0	19.82	0	0.00	3	9.22	0	0.00	3	9
60+	0	0.00	15	56.00	70.0	8.11	0	0.00	0	1.04	0	0.00	0	1
All Ages	*2*	*0.80*	*89*	*56.00*	*0.5*	*70.70*	*1*	*1.20*	*14*	*5.70*	*33*	*13.62*	*47*	*19*
India														
0-4	17	128.00	60	639.00	0.5	59.67	3	313.00	110	194.35	250	441.58	360	636
5-14	0	0.00	102	639.00	10.0	54.83	1	0.00	55	57.36	0	0.00	55	57
15-44	0	0.00	152	639.00	35.0	35.90	2	0.00	63	34.51	0	0.00	63	35
45-59	0	0.00	31	639.00	55.0	16.85	0	0.00	0	0.78	0	0.00	0	1
60+	0	0.00	19	639.00	70.0	7.40	0	0.00	0	0.00	0	0.00	0	0
All Ages	*17*	*18.0*	*365*	*639.0*	*0.5*	*59.67*	*7*	*35.00*	*228*	*55.69*	*250*	*61.03*	*479*	*117*
China														
0-4	17	8.40	57	42.00	0.5	66.93	3	39.20	93	159.91	251	432.38	343	592
5-14	0	0.00	89	42.00	10.0	58.79	1	0.00	43	47.77	0	0.00	43	48
15-44	0	0.00	222	42.00	35.0	38.43	3	0.00	84	29.69	0	0.00	84	30
45-59	0	0.00	41	42.00	55.0	18.19	0	0.00	3	5.04	0	0.00	3	5
60+	0	0.00	32	42.00	70.0	7.69	0	0.00	0	0.00	0	0.00	0	0
All Ages	*17*	*0.00*	*441*	*42.00*	*0.5*	*66.93*	*7*	*0.00*	*223*	*40.73*	*251*	*45.68*	*474*	*86*

Table 16b *(continued)*

Age group (years)	Incidence Number ('000s)	Incidence Rate per100 000	Prevalence Number ('000s)	Prevalence Rate per100 000	Avg. age at onset (years)	Avgerage duration (years)	Deaths Number ('000s)	Deaths Rate per100 000	YLLs Number ('000s)	YLLs Rate per100 000	YLDs Number ('000s)	YLDs Rate per100 000	DALYs Number ('000s)	DALYs Rate per100 000
Other Asia and Islands														
0-4	11	27.50	42	137.00	0.5	64.47	1	173.00	45	106.83	159	379.72	204	487
5-14	0	0.00	82	0.00	10.0	57.93	0	0.00	16	20.41	0	0.00	16	20
15-44	0	0.00	149	137.00	35.0	38.12	1	0.00	15	9.70	0	0.00	15	10
45-59	0	0.00	31	137.00	55.0	18.47	0	0.00	0	0.00	0	0.00	0	0
60+	0	0.00	20	137.00	70.0	7.84	0	0.00	0	0.00	0	0.00	0	0
All Ages	*11*	*3.4*	*324*	*137.00*	*0.5*	*64.47*	*2*	*18.00*	*77*	*22.59*	*159*	*46.95*	*236*	*70*
Sub-Saharan Africa														
0-4	16	59.00	58	3.00	0.5	54.11	1	191.00	41	86.89	219	465.01	260	552
5-14	0	0.00	91	3.00	10.0	50.75	1	0.00	29	42.11	0	0.00	29	42
15-44	0	0.00	123	3.00	35.0	34.01	1	0.00	20	19.04	0	0.00	20	19
45-59	0	0.00	24	293.00	55.0	16.65	0	0.00	0	0.92	0	0.00	0	1
60+	0	0.00	14	293.00	70.0	7.30	0	0.00	0	0.00	0	0.00	0	0
All Ages	*16*	*11.0*	*309*	*293.00*	*0.5*	*54.11*	*3*	*0.00*	*91*	*35.16*	*219*	*84.78*	*309*	*120*
Latin America and the Caribbean														
0-4	7	35.80	27	178.00	0.5	67.34	1	44.00	39	139.56	108	391.44	147	531
5-14	0	0.00	51	178.00	10.0	59.55	0	0.00	12	22.69	0	0.00	12	23
15-44	0	0.00	97	178.00	35.0	39.59	0	0.00	10	9.33	0	0.00	10	9
45-59	0	0.00	19	178.00	55.0	19.78	0	0.00	3	11.39	0	0.00	3	11
60+	0	0.00	13	178.00	70.0	8.34	0	0.00	0	0.00	0	0.00	0	0
All Ages	*7*	*4.4*	*207*	*178.00*	*0.5*	*67.34*	*2*	*5.00*	*63*	*28.07*	*108*	*48.65*	*171*	*77*
Middle Eastern Crescent														
0-4	11	44.20	39	220.00	0.5	64.09	2	206.00	61	154.74	161	405.74	223	560
5-14	0	0.00	60	220.00	10.0	58.26	1	0.00	31	49.39	0	0.00	31	49
15-44	0	0.00	84	220.00	35.0	38.40	1	0.00	27	25.12	0	0.00	27	25
45-59	0	0.00	15	220.00	55.0	18.49	0	0.00	0	0.00	0	0.00	0	0
60+	0	0.00	10	220.00	70.0	7.82	0	0.00	0	0.00	0	0.00	0	0
All Ages	*11*	*7.1*	*208*	*220.00*	*0.5*	*64.09*	*4*	*30.00*	*119*	*48.25*	*161*	*65.35*	*280*	*114*

Table 16b *(continued)*

Age group (years)	*Incidence* Number ('000s)	Rate per 100 000	*Prevalence* Number ('000s)	Rate per 100 000	*Avg. age at onset* (years)	*Avgerage duration* (years)	*Deaths* Number ('000s)	Rate per 100 000	*YLLs* Number ('000s)	Rate per 100 000	*YLDs* Number ('000s)	Rate per 100 000	*DALYs* Number ('000s)	Rate per 100 000
Developed Regions														
0-4	6	16.75	25	66.54	0.5	29.2	1	2.23	29	74.63	126	328.58	154	403
5-14	0	0.00	53	69.35	–	–	0	0.10	3	3.66	0	0.00	3	4
15-44	0	0.00	176	69.34	–	–	0	0.04	3	1.16	0	0.00	3	1
45-59	0	0.00	63	64.43	–	–	1	0.53	8	8.13	0	0.00	8	8
60+	0	0.00	68	56.15	–	–	0	0.33	2	1.95	0	0.00	2	2
All Ages	*6*	*0.98*	*386*	*59.39*	*0.5*	*29.2*	*2*	*0.30*	*45*	*6.86*	*126*	*19.31*	*170*	*26*
Developing Regions														
0-4	79	29.10	283	104.59	1	62	11	4.22	389	143.38	1 149	423.72	1 537	567
5-14	0	0.00	474	105.77	–	–	5	1.10	186	41.42	0	0.00	186	41
15-44	0	0.00	827	87.55	–	–	7	0.75	220	23.29	0	0.00	220	23
45-59	0	0.00	161	75.54	–	–	0	0.20	6	3.03	0	0.00	6	3
60+	0	0.00	108	73.15	–	–	0	0.00	0	0.00	0	0.00	0	0
All Ages	*79*	*3.89*	*1 854*	*91.54*	*0.5*	*62.1*	*24*	*1.18*	*801*	*39.53*	*1 149*	*56.70*	*1 949*	*96*
World														
0-4	85	27.58	309	99.89	0.5	59.6	12	3.97	417	134.89	1 274	411.97	1 691	547
5-14	0	0.00	528	100.43	–	–	5	0.95	189	35.88	0	0.00	189	36
15-44	0	0.00	1 003	83.69	–	–	7	0.60	223	18.59	0	0.00	223	19
45-59	0	0.00	224	72.04	–	–	1	0.30	14	4.64	0	0.00	14	5
60+	0	0.00	176	65.51	–	–	0	0.15	2	0.88	0	0.00	2	1
All Ages	*85*	*3.26*	*2 240*	*85.71*	*0.5*	*59.6*	*26*	*0.99*	*845*	*32.34*	*1 274*	*48.74*	*2 119*	*81*

Table 17 Epidemiological estimates for cleft lip, age group 0–4 years, 1990.

Region	Incidence		Prevalence		Deaths		YLLs		YLDs		DALYs	
	Number ('000s)	Rate per100 000	Number ('000s)	Rate per100 000	Number ('000s)	Rate per100 000	Number ('000s)	Rate per100 000	Number ('000s)	Rate per100 000	Number ('000s)	Rate per100 000
Males												
EME	6	22.15	25	94.07	0	0.92	8	31	5	17.26	13	48
FSE	3	22.20	13	94.06	0	1.49	7	50	3	19.85	10	70
IND	14	23.43	56	93.76	1	1.16	23	39	25	41.45	48	80
CHN	22	37.29	85	141.73	0	0.73	15	25	29	48.11	44	73
OAI	10	22.56	41	94.69	1	1.14	17	39	20	46.08	37	85
SSA	12	24.56	44	93.32	0	0.44	7	15	28	59.21	35	74
LAC	8	29.47	35	121.02	0	1.25	12	42	11	37.92	23	80
MEC	10	24.07	39	94.03	0	0.93	13	32	15	36.93	28	69
Developed	*9*	*22.17*	*38*	*94.07*	*0*	*1.12*	*15*	*37*	*7*	*18.15*	*22*	*56*
Developing	*76*	*30.26*	*301*	*119.10*	*3*	*1.03*	*87*	*34*	*128*	*50.76*	*215*	*85*
World	**85**	**26.54**	**338**	**105.33**	**3**	**0.95**	**102**	**32**	**135**	**42.15**	**238**	**74**
Females												
EME	4	16.27	17	68.66	0	1.02	9	34	3	12.86	12	47
FSE	2	16.09	9	68.70	0	0.98	4	33	2	14.77	6	48
IND	10	17.06	39	68.03	0	0.75	15	26	17	30.32	32	56
CHN	22	37.77	82	141.52	0	0.48	9	16	29	49.20	38	65
OAI	7	16.59	29	69.54	0	0.58	8	20	14	34.42	23	54
SSA	9	18.67	33	71.03	0	0.33	5	11	22	46.02	27	57
LAC	6	21.83	25	89.96	0	0.95	9	32	8	28.48	17	61
MEC	7	17.96	28	69.87	0	0.68	9	23	11	27.85	20	51
Developed	*6*	*16.21*	*26*	*68.67*	*0*	*1.00*	*13*	*34*	*5*	*13.52*	*18*	*47*
Developing	*60*	*22.31*	*236*	*87.00*	*2*	*0.60*	*56*	*21*	*101*	*37.17*	*156*	*58*
World	**67**	**21.56**	**262**	**84.74**	**2**	**0.65**	**68**	**22**	**106**	**34.25**	**174**	**56**

genetic counselling programs have greatly reduced the incidence of thalassemia major (Modell and Bulyzhenkov 1988).

In developed countries, maternal serum AFP screening is conducted routinely. However, AFP screening has relatively low predictive value and is usually followed by ultrasound and amniocentesis to confirm diagnosis (Holtxman 1990). Chromosomal analysis or karyotyping for genetic disorders such as Down syndrome requires well-equipped clinical facilities as well as specialists. This is also the case with routine ultrasonography for screening of congenital anomalies. For example, in the study of developed countries, routine ultrasonography is shown to be not cost-effective, and should be carried out only in selected high risk patients (Kock 1989). There are several prerequisites for a screening program to be successful: capacity to alter clinical management; cost-effectiveness; reliable means of assessment; and capacity to handle problems (Simpson 1991). Thus, the implementation of these programs depends on the health impact of the congenital anomalies, the efficacy and cost-effectiveness of each intervention, and the existing health resources.

Table 18 Epidemiological estimates for cleft palate, age group 0–4 years, 1990.

Region	Incidence		Prevalence		Deaths		YLLs		YLDs		DALYs	
	Number ('000s)	Rate per100 000	Number ('000s)	Rate per100 000	Number ('000s)	Rate per100 000	Number ('000s)	Rate per100 000	Number ('000s)	Rate per100 000	Number ('000s)	Rate per100 000
						Males						
EME	3	11.22	14	51.23	0	0.62	5	21	3	13.21	9	34
FSE	1	8.21	5	37.37	0	0.99	5	33	2	12.28	6	46
IND	6	9.25	24	39.68	0	0.78	15	26	21	35.28	37	61
CHN	1	2.15	5	8.75	0	0.49	10	16	3	5.45	13	22
OAI	4	8.89	18	40.16	0	0.76	11	26	18	40.21	29	66
SSA	5	9.67	19	39.20	0	0.29	5	10	25	53.61	30	64
LAC	2	8.66	11	38.07	0	0.83	8	28	6	21.89	14	50
MEC	4	9.48	16	39.88	0	0.62	9	21	12	30.20	21	51
Developed	*4*	*10.19*	*19*	*46.48*	*0*	*0.75*	*10*	*25*	*5*	*12.89*	*15*	*38*
Developing	*22*	*8.60*	*93*	*36.66*	*2*	*0.68*	*58*	*23*	*86*	*34.13*	*144*	*57*
World	**26**	**8.03**	**111**	**34.61**	**2**	**0.63**	**68**	**21**	**91**	**28.42**	**159**	**50**
						Females						
EME	3	13.31	15	60.79	0	1.02	9	34	4	15.91	13	50
FSE	1	9.66	6	44.33	0	0.98	4	33	2	14.84	6	48
IND	6	11.03	27	47.14	0	0.75	15	26	24	42.25	38	68
CHN	2	2.65	6	10.61	0	0.48	9	16	4	6.77	13	23
OAI	4	10.69	20	48.27	0	0.58	8	20	21	49.16	29	69
SSA	6	11.94	23	48.70	0	0.33	5	11	32	67.66	37	79
LAC	3	10.37	13	45.72	0	0.95	9	32	7	26.56	16	59
MEC	5	11.53	19	48.29	0	0.68	9	23	15	37.10	24	60
Developed	*5*	*12.06*	*21*	*55.13*	*0*	*1.00*	*13*	*34*	*6*	*15.54*	*19*	*49*
Developing	*25*	*9.35*	*108*	*39.80*	*2*	*0.60*	*56*	*21*	*102*	*37.79*	*158*	*58*
World	**30**	**9.68**	**129**	**41.69**	**2**	**0.65**	**68**	**22**	**108**	**35.04**	**177**	**57**

Although considerable burden due to congenital anomalies could be reduced through primary and secondary prevention, a significant proportion of disability may be difficult to prevent, primarily because many congenital anomalies have unknown etiologies. Furthermore, as the infant mortality from congenital anomalies decreases with progress in diagnosis and treatment, the number of surviving infants with a disability due to severe congenital anomalies might increase. For example, a study of changes in infant morbidity during a period of substantial decreases in mortality showed that the change in morbidity was attributable to a reduction of minor congenital anomalies or developmental delay: the proportion of surviving children with severe or moderate congenital anomalies or developmental delay did not change during that period (Shapiro et al. 1983).

Thus, tertiary prevention including rehabilitation and special education is another recommended step to reduce the burden of congenital anomalies. For developmental disabilities such as mental retardation, deafness and blindness, the effectiveness of early intervention programs has been argued. However, these disabilities are actually difficult to assess, especially in developing countries, unless the magnitude of the problem is

Table 19 Epidemiological estimates for abdominal wall defects, age group 0–4 years, 1990.

Region	*Incidence*		*Prevalence*		*Deaths*		*YLLs*		*YLDs*		*DALYs*	
	Number ('000s)	Rate per 100 000	Number ('000s)	Rate per 100 000	Number ('000s)	Rate per 100 000	Number ('000s)	Rate per 100 000	Number ('000s)	Rate per 100 000	Number ('000s)	Rate per 100 000
						Males						
EME	1	3.79	0	0.00	0	0.00	5	20	0	0.00	5	20
FSE	0	0.00	0	0.00	0	0.00	3	20	0	0.00	3	20
IND	1	1.67	0	0.00	1	1.67	23	39	0	0.00	23	39
CHN	1	1.66	0	0.00	0	0.00	13	22	0	0.00	13	22
OAI	1	2.29	0	0.00	0	0.00	14	33	0	0.00	14	33
SSA	0	0.00	0	0.00	0	0.00	7	15	0	0.00	7	15
LAC	1	3.48	0	0.00	0	0.00	8	29	0	0.00	8	29
MEC	1	2.43	0	0.00	1	2.43	19	47	0	0.00	19	47
Developed	*1*	*2.49*	*0*	*0.00*	*0*	*0.00*	*8*	*20*	*0*	*0.00*	*8*	*20*
Developing	*5*	*1.98*	*0*	*0.00*	*2*	*0.79*	*86*	*34*	*0*	*0.00*	*86*	*34*
World	**5**	**1.56**	**0**	**0.00**	**3**	**0.93**	**94**	**29**	**0**	**0.00**	**94**	**29**
						Females						
EME	1	3.99	0	0.00	0	0.00	10	40	0	0.00	10	40
FSE	1	7.61	0	0.00	0	0.00	6	46	0	0.00	6	46
IND	1	1.76	0	0.00	1	1.76	19	34	0	0.00	19	34
CHN	1	1.73	0	0.00	0	0.00	10	17	0	0.00	10	17
OAI	0	0.00	0	0.00	0	0.00	9	21	0	0.00	9	21
SSA	0	0.00	0	0.00	0	0.00	7	15	0	0.00	7	15
LAC	1	3.61	0	0.00	0	0.00	8	29	0	0.00	8	29
MEC	0	0.00	0	0.00	0	0.00	10	25	0	0.00	10	25
Developed	*2*	*5.24*	*0*	*0.00*	*0*	*0.00*	*16*	*42*	*0*	*0.00*	*16*	*42*
Developing	*3*	*1.11*	*0*	*0.00*	*1*	*0.37*	*63*	*23*	*0*	*0.00*	*63*	*23*
World	**5**	**1.62**	**0**	**0.00**	**2**	**0.65**	**80**	**26**	**0**	**0.00**	**80**	**26**

understood through public awareness. Rehabilitation services are regarded as highly specialized and costly. Thus, it is difficult for developing countries to implement such services without strong government will and financial support. In LAC, as the magnitude of disability has increased, low cost projects have been implemented which provide early intervention combined with teaching, training and therapy carried out at home or at an institution (Thorburn 1986). Although the effectiveness of such programs has not yet been measured, integration of such programs into the existing primary health care system is an effective way to increase community awareness of disabled children, and to contribute to the sustainable activities for reducing the burden of those children (Simeonesson 1991).

Conclusions

Congenital anomalies are a significant public health issue in developed as well as developing countries, where socioeconomic development and improvements in health and sanitation have reduced the incidence of communicable diseases. The demands for health services dealing with

Table 20 Epidemiological estimates for oesophageal atresia, age group 0–4 years, 1990.

Region	Incidence		Prevalence		Deaths		YLLs		YLDs		DALYs	
	Number ('000s)	Rate per100 000	Number ('000s)	Rate per100 000	Number ('000s)	Rate per100 000	Number ('000s)	Rate per100 000	Number ('000s)	Rate per100 000	Number ('000s)	Rate per100 000
Males												
EME	1	4.39	0	0.00	0	0.38	3	13	0	0.00	3	13
FSE	0	3.20	0	0.00	0	0.50	2	17	0	0.00	2	17
IND	3	5.18	0	0.00	0	0.79	16	27	0	0.00	16	27
CHN	1	1.32	0	0.00	0	0.12	2	4	0	0.00	2	4
OAI	2	4.99	0	0.00	0	0.67	10	23	0	0.00	10	23
SSA	3	5.44	0	0.00	0	0.30	5	10	0	0.00	5	10
LAC	2	5.53	0	0.00	0	0.58	6	20	0	0.00	6	20
MEC	4	9.48	0	0.00	0	0.95	13	32	0	0.00	13	32
Developed	*2*	*3.98*	*0*	*0.00*	*0*	*0.42*	*6*	*14*	*0*	*0.00*	*6*	*14*
Developing	*14*	*5.61*	*0*	*0.00*	*2*	*0.61*	*52*	*21*	*0*	*0.00*	*52*	*21*
World	**16**	**4.90**	**0**	**0.00**	**2**	**0.53**	**57**	**18**	**0**	**0.00**	**57**	**18**
Females												
EME	1	4.39	0	0.00	0	0.53	4	18	0	0.00	4	18
FSE	0	3.18	0	0.00	0	0.43	2	15	0	0.00	2	15
IND	3	5.20	0	0.00	0	0.69	13	23	0	0.00	13	23
CHN	1	1.33	0	0.00	0	0.09	2	3	0	0.00	2	3
OAI	2	5.00	0	0.00	0	0.45	6	15	0	0.00	6	15
SSA	3	5.43	0	0.00	0	0.29	5	10	0	0.00	5	10
LAC	2	5.51	0	0.00	0	0.60	6	20	0	0.00	6	20
MEC	5	11.53	0	0.00	0	0.52	7	18	0	0.00	7	18
Developed	*2*	*3.98*	*0*	*0.00*	*0*	*0.50*	*6*	*17*	*0*	*0.00*	*6*	*17*
Developing	*14*	*5.34*	*0*	*0.00*	*1*	*0.42*	*39*	*14*	*0*	*0.00*	*39*	*14*
World	**16**	**5.17**	**0**	**0.00**	**1**	**0.43**	**45**	**15**	**0**	**0.00**	**45**	**15**

congenital anomalies and consequent disability will continue to rise. Despite the recent advances in etiology and diagnosis of congenital anomalies, the vast majority of them are not yet well understood. The continuous global monitoring system and comparable data collection to assess the true magnitude of the problem are essential to focussing interventions aimed at reducing the burden of congenital anomalies.

REFERENCES

Abudu OO, Uguru V, Lude O (1988) Contribution of congenital malformations to perinatal mortality in Lagos, Nigeria. *International Journal of Gynaecology and Obstetrics*, 27:63–67.

Adeyemi D (1989) Neonatal intestinal obstruction in a developing tropical country: patterns, problems, and prognosis. *Journal of Tropical Pediatrics*, 35:66–70.

Agarwel SS, Singh U, Singh PS et al. (1991) Prevalence and spectrum of congenital malformations in a prospective study at a teaching hospital. *Indian Journal of Medical Research Section A-Infectious Diseases*, 4:413–419.

Airede KI (1992) Neural tube defects in the middle belt of Nigeria. *Journal of Tropical Pediatrics*, 38:27–30.

Table 21 Epidemiological estimates for anorectal atresia, age group 0–4 years, 1990.

Region	Incidence		Prevalence		Deaths		YLLs		YLDs		DALYs	
	Number ('000s)	Rate per100 000	Number ('000s)	Rate per100 000	Number ('000s)	Rate per100 000	Number ('000s)	Rate per100 000	Number ('000s)	Rate per100 000	Number ('000s)	Rate per100 000
						Males						
EME	2	5.79	0	0.06	0	0.13	1	4	0	0.00	1	4
FSE	1	4.20	0	0.04	0	0.17	1	6	0	0.00	1	6
IND	4	6.22	0	0.06	0	0.59	12	20	0	0.00	12	20
CHN	3	5.05	0	0.05	0	0.14	3	5	0	0.00	3	5
OAI	3	5.99	0	0.06	0	0.32	5	11	0	0.00	5	11
SSA	3	6.52	0	0.07	0	0.22	4	8	0	0.00	4	8
LAC	2	8.19	0	0.08	0	0.26	3	9	0	0.00	3	9
MEC	3	6.39	0	0.06	0	0.44	6	15	0	0.00	6	15
Developed	*2*	*5.25*	*0*	*0.05*	*0*	*0.15*	*2*	*5*	*0*	*0.00*	*2*	*5*
Developing	*17*	*6.92*	*0*	*0.07*	*1*	*0.37*	*32*	*13*	*0*	*0.00*	*32*	*13*
World	**20**	**6.09**	**0**	**0.06**	**1**	**0.31**	**34**	**10**	**0**	**0.00**	**34**	**10**
						Females						
EME	1	5.79	0	0.06	0	0.18	2	6	0	0.00	2	6
FSE	1	4.17	0	0.04	0	0.14	1	5	0	0.00	1	5
IND	4	6.24	0	0.06	0	0.51	10	17	0	0.00	10	17
CHN	3	5.11	0	0.05	0	0.11	2	4	0	0.00	2	4
OAI	3	6.00	0	0.06	0	0.22	3	7	0	0.00	3	7
SSA	3	6.51	0	0.07	0	0.22	4	7	0	0.00	4	7
LAC	2	8.17	0	0.08	0	0.27	3	9	0	0.00	3	9
MEC	3	6.42	0	0.06	0	0.25	3	9	0	0.00	3	9
Developed	*2*	*5.23*	*0*	*0.05*	*0*	*0.17*	*2*	*6*	*0*	*0.00*	*2*	*6*
Developing	*17*	*6.23*	*0*	*0.06*	*1*	*0.27*	*25*	*9*	*0*	*0.00*	*25*	*9*
World	**19**	**6.11**	**0**	**0.06**	**1**	**0.26**	**27**	**9**	**0**	**0.00**	**27**	**9**

Al-Awadi S, Farag TI, Teebi AS, et al. (1984) Anencephaly: disappearing in Kuwait? *Lancet*, 2:701–702.

Anyebuno M, Amofa G, Peprah S, et al. (1993) Neural tube defects at Korle Bu Teaching Hospital, Accra, Ghana. *East African Medical Journal*, 70:572–574.

Baird PA, Sadovnick AD (1987) Life expectancy in Down syndrome. *Journal of Pediatrics*, 110:849–854.

Balarajan R, Donnan SPB, Adelstein AM (1982) Mortality and cause of death in Down syndrome. *Journal of Epidemiology and Community Health*, 36:127–129.

Bell JA, Pearn JH, Firman D (1989) Childhood deaths in Down syndrome. Survival curves and causes of death from a total population study in Queensland, Australia, 1976 to 1985. *Journal of Medical Genetics*, 26:764–768.

Borkar AS, Mathur AK, Mahaluxmivala S (1993) Epidemiology of facial clefts in the central province of Saudi Arabia. *British Journal of Plastic Surgery*, 46:673–675.

Borman B, Cryer C (1990) Fallacies of international and national comparison of disease occurrence in the epidemiology of neural tube defects. *Teratology*, 42:405–412.

Table 22 Epidemiological estimates for renal agenesis, age group 0–4 years, 1990.

Region	Incidence		Prevalence		Deaths		YLLs		YLDs		DALYs	
	Number ('000s)	Rate per100 000	Number ('000s)	Rate per100 000	Number ('000s)	Rate per100 000	Number ('000s)	Rate per100 000	Number ('000s)	Rate per100 000	Number ('000s)	Rate per100 000
						Males						
EME	1	3.59	0	0.04	1	3.60	32	120	0	0.00	32	120
FSE	0	1.60	0	0.02	0	1.60	7	54	0	0.00	7	54
IND	1	2.07	0	0.02	1	2.07	41	69	0	0.00	41	69
CHN	0	0.44	0	0.00	0	0.44	9	15	0	0.00	9	15
OAI	1	2.00	0	0.02	1	2.00	30	67	0	0.00	30	67
SSA	1	2.17	0	0.02	1	2.17	35	74	0	0.00	35	74
LAC	0	1.64	0	0.02	0	1.64	16	55	0	0.00	16	55
MEC	1	2.13	0	0.02	1	2.13	30	72	0	0.00	30	72
Developed	*1*	*2.91*	*0*	*0.03*	*1*	*2.91*	*39*	*97*	*0*	*0.00*	*39*	*97*
Developing	*5*	*1.89*	*0*	*0.02*	*5*	*1.89*	*160*	*64*	*0*	*0.00*	*160*	*64*
World	**6**	**1.84**	**0**	**0.02**	**6**	**1.84**	**199**	**62**	**0**	**0.00**	**199**	**62**
						Females						
EME	1	3.59	0	0.04	1	3.59	30	120	0	0.00	30	120
FSE	0	1.59	0	0.02	0	1.59	7	56	0	0.00	7	56
IND	1	2.08	0	0.02	1	2.08	40	71	0	0.00	40	71
CHN	0	0.45	0	0.00	0	0.45	9	15	0	0.00	9	15
OAI	1	2.00	0	0.02	1	2.00	29	68	0	0.00	29	68
SSA	1	2.17	0	0.02	1	2.17	35	74	0	0.00	35	74
LAC	0	1.63	0	0.02	0	1.63	15	55	0	0.00	15	55
MEC	1	2.14	0	0.02	1	2.14	29	73	0	0.00	29	73
Developed	*1*	*2.91*	*0*	*0.03*	*1*	*2.91*	*38*	*98*	*0*	*0.00*	*38*	*98*
Developing	*5*	*1.70*	*0*	*0.02*	*5*	*1.70*	*157*	*58*	*0*	*0.00*	*157*	*58*
World	**6**	**1.85**	**0**	**0.02**	**6**	**1.85**	**194**	**63**	**0**	**0.00**	**194**	**63**

Bower C, Stanley FJ (1989) Dietary folate as a risk factor for neural-tube defects: evidence from a case-control study in Western Australia. *Medical Journal of Australia*, 150:613–619.

Brewster MA, Heim MA (1985) Adverse pregnancy outcomes: information from the medical record. *Annals of Clinical and Laboratory Science*, 15:470–474.

Calzolari E, Cavazzuti GB, Cocchi G et al. (1987) Congenital malformations in 100,000 consecutive births in Emilia Romagna region, Northern Italy: comparison with the Eurocot data. *European Journal of Epidemiology*, 3:423–430.

Center for Disease Control. (1986) Premature mortality due to congenital anomalies. *Mortality and Morbidity Weekly Report*, 35:97–105.

Chaturvedi P, Banerjee KS (1989) Spectrum of congenital malformations in the newborns from rural Maharashtra. *Indian Journal of Pediatrics*, 56:501–507.

Chaturvedi P, Banerjee KS (1989) Spectrum of congenital malformations in the newborns from Rural Maharashtra. *Indian Journal of Pediatrics*, 56:501–507.

Chinara PK, Singh S (1982) East-west differentials in congenital malformations in India. *Indian Journal of Pediatrics*, 49:325–329.

Chinese Birth Defects Monitoring Program (1990) Central nervous system congenital malformations, especially neural tube defects in 29 provinces, metropolitan cities and autonomous regions of China. *International Journal of Epidemiology*, 19:987–982.

Choudhury AR, Mukherjee M, Sharma A, et al. (1989) Study of 126,266 consecutive births for major congenital defects. *Indian Journal of Pediatrics*, 56:493–499.

Chouhan GS, Rodrigues FM, Shaika BH, et al. (1985) Clinical and virological study of dengue fever outbreak in Jahore City, Rajasthan, 1985. *Indian Journal of Medical Research*, 91:414-418.

Cornell J, Nelson MM, Beighton P. (1983) Neural tube defects in the Cape Town area, 1975–1980. *South African Medical Journal*, 64:83–84.

Cuckle H, Wald N (1987) The impact of screening for open neural tube defects in England and Wales. *Prenatal Diagnosis*, 7:91–99.

Cuckle HS, Wald NJ,Cuckle PM (1989) Prenatal screening and diagnosis of neural tube defects in England and Wales in 1985. *Prenatal Diagnosis*, 9:393–400.

Czeizel A (1988) The activities of the Hungarian center for congenital anomaly control. *World Health Statistics Quarterly*, 41:219–227.

Czeizel AE (1993) Prevention of congenital abnormalities by periconceptional multivitamin supplementation. *British Medical Journal*, 306:1645–1648.

Czeizel AE, Dudas I (1992) Prevention of the first occurrence of neural-tube defects by periconceptional vitamin supplementation. *New England Journal of Medicine*, 327:1832–1835.

Czeizei A et al. (1972) Incidence of congenital heart defects in Budapest. *Acta Paediatrica Academiae Scientiarum Hungaricae* 13:191–202

Deaton JG (1973) The mortality rate and causes of death among institutionalized mongols in Texas. *Journal of Mental Deficiency Research*, 17:117–122.

Eckstein HB (1963) Exomphalos. A review of 100 cases. *British Journal of Surgery*, 50:405–410.

Ekanem AD, Chong H (1985) Easily identifiable congenital malformations. *British Journal of Obstetrics and Gynaecology*, 5:81–85 (suppl.).

Elixhauser A, Weschler JM, et al. (1993) Cost-benefit analysis of preconception care for women with established diabetes mellitus. *Diabetes Care*, 16:1146–1157.

Emanuel I, Culver BH, Erickson JD, et al. (1973) The further epidemiological differentiation of cleft lip and palate: a population study in King County, Washington, 1956–65. *Teratology*, 7:271–281.

Eskes T, Mooij P, Steegers-Theunissen, et al. (1992) Pregnancy care and prevention of birth defects. *Journal of Perinatal Medicine*, 20:253–265.

EUROCAT Working Group. (1991) *EUROCAT Report 4. Surveillance of congenital anomalies 1980–88*. Eurocat Central Registry, Department of Epidemiology, Catholic University of Leuven, Brussels.

Fauveau V, Wojtyniak B, Mostafa G, et al. (1990) Perinatal mortality in Matlab, Bangladesh: a community-based study. *International Journal of Epidemiology*, 19:606–612.

Ferencz C (1990) On the birth prevalence of congenital heart disease. *Journal of the American College of Cardiology*, 16:1701–1702

Fryers T (1986) Survival in Down syndrome. *Journal of Mental Deficiency Research*, 30:101–110.

Fulton MJ, Barer ML (1984) Screening for congenital dislocation of the hip: an economic appraisal. *Canadian Medical Association Journal*, 130:1149–1156.

Grosfeld JL, Weber TR (1982) Congenital abdominal wall defects: gastroschisis and omphalocele. *Current Problems in Surgery*, 19:159–213.

Grosfeld JL, Dawes L, Weber TR (1981) Congenital abdominal wall defects: current management and survival. *Surgical Clinics of North America*, 61:1037–1049.

Gross RH, Cox A, Tatyrek R, et al. (1983) Early management and decision making for the treatment of myelomeningocele. *Pediatrics*, 72:450–458.

Guvenc H, Ali Uslu M, Guvenc M, et al. (1993) Changing trend of neural tube defects in Eastern Turkey. *Journal of Epidemiology and Community Health*, 47:40–41.

Ho NK (1991) Congenital malformations in Toa Payoh Hospital-a 18 year experience (1972–1989). *Annals of the Academy of Medicine, Singapore*, 20:183–189.

Hoffman JIE, Christianson R (1978) Congenital heart disease in a cohort of 19,502 births with long-term follow up. *American Journal of Cardiology*, 42:641–647

Hoffman JIE (1990) Congenital heart disease: incidence and inheritance. *Paediatric Clinics of North America*, 37:25–43

Hoffman JIE (1968) Natural history of congenital heart disease. Problems in its assessment with special reference to ventricular septal defects. *Circulation*, 37:97–125.

Holmes LB (1978) Genetic counselling for the older pregnant women. *New England Journal of Medicine*, 298:1419–1421.

Holtxman NA (1990) Prenatal screening: when and for whom? *Journal of General Internal Medicine*, 5(suppl):s42–46.

Hunt GM, Lewin WS, Gleave J, et al. (1973) Predictive factors in open myelomenigocele, with special reference to sensory level. *British Medical Journal*, 4:197–201.

Hunt GM (1990) Open spina bifida: Outcome for a complete cohort treated unselectively and followed into adulthood. *Developmental Medicine and Child Neurology*, 32:108–118

Imaizumi Y, Yamamura H, Nishikawa M, et al. (1991) The prevalence at birth of congenital malformations at a maternity hospital in Osaka City, 1948–1990. *Japanese Journal of Human Genetics*, 36:275–287.

International Clearinghouse Birth Defects Monitoring Systems (ICBDMS). (1991) *Congenital malformations worldwide*. New York: Elsevier Science Publishers.

Iselius L, Lindsten J (1986) Changes in the incidence of Down syndrome in Sweden during 1968–82. *Human Genetics*, 72:133–139.

Jalil F, Lindblad BS, Hanson LA, et al. (1993) Early child health in Lahore, Pakistan: IX. Perinatal events. *Acta Paediatrica*, 82(suppl):95–107.

James WH (1986) Neural tube defects and sex ratios. *Lancet*, 2:573–574.

Jones MC (1988) Etiology of facial clefts: prospective evaluation of 428 patients. *Cleft Palate Journal*, 25:258–265.

Jones PG (1969) Exomphalos. A review of 45 cases. *Archives of Disease in Childhood*, 38:180–187.

Kalter H, Warkany J (1983) Congenital malformations: etiologic factors and their role in prevention. *New England Journal of Medicine*, 308:424–431 (Part 1) and 491–497 (Part 2).

Kalter H (1991) Five-decade international trends in the relation of perinatal mortality and congenital malformations: stillbirth and neonatal death compared. *International Journal of Epidemiology*, 20:173–179.

Khrouf N, Spang R, Podgorna T, et al. (1986) Malformations in 10,000 consecutive births in Tunis. *Acta Paediatrica Scandinavica*, 75:534–539.

Kishan J, Soni AL, Elzouki AY, et al. (1985) Neural tube defects. *Indian Pediatrics*, 22:545–546.

Kitzmiller JL, Gavin LA, Gin GD, et al. (1991) Preconception care of diabetes. Glycemic control prevents congenital anomalies. *JAMA*, 265:731–736.

Kock C (1989) Ultrachallscreening in der Scwangerachaft-eine kritische Literaturanalyse. *Wiener Klinische Wochenschrift*, 101:341–345.

Kohn MR, Shi EC (1990) Gastroschisis and exomphalos: recent trends and factors influencing survival. *New Zealand Journal of Surgery*, 60:199–202.

Kulkarni ML, Mathew MA, Ramchandran B (1987) High incidence of neural tube defects in South India. *Lancet*, 1:1260.

Kulkarni ML, Mathew MA, Reddy V (1989) The range of neural tube defects in southern India. *Archives of Disease in Childhood*, 645:201–204.

Laurence KM, James N, Miller M, et al. (1980) Increased risk of recurrence of pregnancies complicated by fetal neural tube defects in mothers receiving poor diets, and possible benefit of dietary counselling. *British Medical Journal*, 281:1592–1594.

Laurence KM (1974) Effects of early surgery for spina bifida cystica on survival and quality of life. *Lancet*, 1:301–304.

Laursen HB (1980) Some epidemiological aspects of congenital heart disease in Denmark. *Acta Pediatrica Scandinavia*, 69:619–624

Leck I (1969) Ethnic differences in the incidence of malformations following migration. *British Journal of Preventive and Social Medicine*, 23:166–173.

Leck I. (1983) Spina bifida and anencephaly: fewer patients, more problems. *British Medical Journal*, 286:1679–1680.

Leck I (1994) Structural Birth Defects. In: Pless IB ed. *The Epidemiology of Childhood Disorders*, New York: Oxford University Press, pp 66–117.

Lorber J (1971) Results of treatment of myelomenigeoele. An analysis of 524 unselected cases with special reference to possible selection for treatment. *Developmental Medicine and Child Neurology*, 13:279–303.

Lowry RB, Jones DC, Renwick DHG, et al. (1976) Down syndrome in British Columbia, 1952–73: Incidence and mean maternal age. *Teratology*, 14:29–34.

Mabogunje OA, Mahour GH (1984) Omphalocele and gastroschisis. Trends in survival across two decades. *American Journal of Surgery*, 148:679–686.

Mackeprang M, Hay S (1972) Cleft lip and palate mortality study. *Cleft Palate Journal*, 9:51–63.

MacMahon P, Sherins RS, Miller ML (1953) The incidence and life expectation of children with congenital heart disease. *British Heart Journal*, 15:121–129.

Mahour GH, Weitzman JJ, Rosenkrantz JG (1973) Omphalocele and gastroschisis. *Annals of Surgery*, 177:478–482.

Malone Q (1988) Mortality and survival of the Down syndrome population in Western Australia. *Journal of Mental Deficiency Research*, 32:59–65.

Manning PB, Weslwy JR, Behrendt DM, et al. (1986) Fifty year's experience with oesophageal atresia and tracheoesophageal fistula. Beginning with Cameron Haightís first operation in 1935. *Annals of Surgery*, 204:446–451.

Martinez-Frias ML, Frias JL, Salvador J (1989) Clinical/epidemiological analysis of malformations. *American Journal of Medical Genetics*, 35:121–125.

Masloman N, Mustadjab I, Munir M (1991) Congenital malformations at Gunung Wenang Hospital Manado: a five-year spectrum. *Paediatrica Indonesiana*, 31:294–302.

Mastroiacovo P, Bertollini R, Corchia C (1992) Survival of children with Down syndrome in Italy. *American Journal of Medical Genetics*, 42:208–212.

Mayer T, Black R, Matlak ME, et al. (1980) Gastroschisis and omphalocele: an eight-year review. *Annals of Surgery*, 192:783–787.

McLaughlin JF, Shurtleff DB, Lamers JY, et al. (1985) Influence of prognosis on decisions regarding the care of newborns with myelodysplasia. *New England Journal of Medicine*, 312:1589–1594.

Milunsky A, Alpert E (1978) Maternal serum AFP screening. *New England Journal of Medicine*, 298:738–739.

Milunsky A, Jick H, Jick SS, et al. (1989) Multivitamin/folic acid suuplementation in early pregnancy reduces the prevalence of neural tube defects. *Journal of the American Medical Association*, 262:2847–2852.

Modell B, Bulyzhenkov V (1988) Distribution and control of some genetic disorders. *World Health Statistics Quarterly*, 41:209–218.

Morgan SB (1979) Development and distribution of intellectual and adaptive skills in Down syndrome children: implications for early intervention. *Mental Retardation*, 247–249.

Morris CD, Menashe VD (1991) 25-year mortality after surgical repair of congenital heart defect in childhood. *JAMA*, 266:3447–3452.

MRC Vitamin Study Research Group (1991) Prevention of neural tube defects: results of the Medical Research Council Vitamin Study. *Lancet*, 338:131–137.

Mulcahy MT (1979) Down syndrome in Western Australia, mortality and survival. *Clinical Genetics*, 16:103–108.

Mulinare J, Cordero JF, Erickson JD, et al. (1988) Periconceptional use of multivitamins and the occurrence of anencephaly and spina bifida. *JAMA*, 260: 3141–3145.

Murray CJL and Lopez AD (1994) *Global comparative assessments in the health sector*. Geneva, World Health Organization.

Murray CJL and Lopez AD (1996) Estimating causes of death: new methods and global and regional applications for 1990. In: Murray CJL and Lopez AD, eds. *The global burden of disease: a comprehensive assessment of mortality and disability from diseases, injuries, and risk factors in 1990 and projected to 2020.* Cambridge, Harvard University Press.

Mustacchi P, Sherins BS, Miller MJ (1963) Congenital malformations of the heart and great vessels: prevalence, incidence and life expectancy in San Francisco. *JAMA*, 183:241–244.

Ncayiyana DJ (1986) Neural tube defects among rural blacks in a Transeki district. *South African Medical Journal*, 69:618–620.

Njoh J, Chellaram R, Ramas L (1991) Congenital abnormalities in Liberian neonates. *West African Journal of Medicine*, 10:439–442.

Oakley GP (1986) Frequency of human congenital malformations. *Clinics in Perinatology*, 13:545–554.

Pan American Health Organization. (1986) *Health conditions in the Americas*, 1990 edition. Washington, DC: PAHO (Scientific publication 524).

Pan American Health Organization. (1984) *Prevention and Control of Genetic Diseases and Congenital Defects*. Washington, DC: PAHO (Scientific Publication 460).

Parikh AP, Goyel NA (1990) Mental performance in Down syndrome. *Indian Journal of Pediatrics*, 57:261–263.

Pengsaa K, Taksaphan S (1987) Perinatal mortality at Srinagarind Hospital. *Journal of Medical Association of Thailand*, 70:667–672.

Pleydell MJ (1960) Anencephaly and other congenital abnormalities. Epidemiological study in Northamptonshire. *British Medical Journal*, 1:309–315.

Posaci C, Celiloglu M, Karabacak O (1992) The epidemiology of neural tube defects in Izmir, Turkey. *International Journal of Gynecology and Obstetrics*, 39:135–138.

Powell-Griner E, Woolbright A (1990) Trends in infant deaths from congenital anomalies: result from England and Wales, Scotland, Sweden and the United States. *International Journal of Epidemiology*, 19:391–398.

Roth MP, Dott B, Alembik Y, et al. (1987) Malformations congenitales dans une serie de 66,068 naissances consecutives. *Archives Francaises de Peditrie*, 44:173–176.

Samanek M (1994) Boy : girl ratio in children born with different forms of cardiac malformation: a population-based study. *Cardiology*, 15:53–57.

Sayed AR, Bourne DE, Nixon JM, et al. (1989) Birth defects surveillance. A pilot system in the Cape Peninsula. *South African Medical Journal*, 76:5–7.

Seller MJ. (1987) Neural tube defects and sex ratios. *American Journal of Medical Genetics*, 26:699–707.

Sever LE (1983) Incidence and prevalence as measures of the frequency of birth defects. *American Journal of Epidemiology*, 118:608–10.

Shapiro S, McCormick MC, Starfield BH, et al. (1983) Changes in infant morbidity associated with decreases in neonatal mortality. *Pediatrics*, 72:408–415.

Sharma AK, Shukla AK, Prabhakar G, et al. (1993)Oesophageal atresia: tragedies and triumphs over two decades in a developing country. *International Surgery*, 78:311–314.

Shinebourne EA et al. (1978) Coarctation of the aorta in infancy and childhood. *British Heart Journal* 38:375–385

Sharma JB, Gulati N (1992) Potential relationship between dengue fever and neural tube defects in a Northern District of India. *International Journal of Gynecology and Obstetrics*, 39:291–295.

Shyrock HS, Siegel JS (1976) *The Methods and Materials of Demography*. New York: Academic Press.

Sillen U, Hagberg S, Werkmaster K (1988) Management of oesophageal atresia: review of 16 year's experience. *Journal of Paediatric Surgery*, 23:805–809.

Simeonesson RJ (1991) Early prevention of childhood disability in developing countries. *International Journal of Rehabilitation Research*, 14:1–12.

Simpson JL (1991) Screening for fetal and genetic abnormalities. *Baillieres Clinical Obstetrics & Gynecology*, 5:675–696.

Singh M, Deorari AK, Paul VK, et al. (1990) Primary causes of neonatal deaths in a tertiary care hospital in Delhi: an autopsy study of 331 cases. *Annals of Tropical Paediatrics*, 10:151–157.

Smith WR, Leix F (1966) Omphalocele. *American Journal of Surgery*, 3:450–452.

Sood M, Agarwal N, Verma S, et al. (1991) Neural tube defects in an East Delhi Hospital. *Indian Journal of Pediatrics*, 58:363–365.

Staples AJ, Sutherland GR, Haan EA, et al. (1991) Epidemiology of Down syndrome in South Australia, 1960–89. *American Journal of Human Genetics*, 49:1014–1024.

Stoll C, Alembik Y, Dott B, et al. (1990) Epidemiology of Down syndrome in 118,265 consecutive births. *American Journal of Medical Genetics*, 7(suppl.):79–83.

Strodel WE, Coran AG, Kirsh MM, et al. (1979) Oesophageal atresia: A 41 year experience. *Archives of Surgery*, 114:523–527.

Taher AA (1992) Cleft lip and palate in Tehran. *Cleft Palate-Craniofacial Journal*, 29:15–16.

Tan KC, Ratnam SS, Kottegoda SR, et al. (1984) Anencephaly: a retrospective analysis in Singapore, 1976 to 1980. *Journal of Medical Genetics*, 21:350–354.

Thase ME (1982) Longevity and mortality in Down syndrome. *Journal of Mental Deficiency Research*, 26:177–192.

Thein MM, Koh D, Tan KL, et al. (1992) Descriptive profile of birth defects among livebirths in Singapore. *Teratology*, 46:277–284.

Thorburn MJ (1986) Early intervention for disabled children in the Caribbean. In: Marfo S, Walker S and Charles B eds. *Childhood Disability in Developing Countries*, New York: Praeger.

Tuohy PG, Counsell AM, Geddis DC (1993) The Plunket National Child Health Study: birth defects and sociodemographic factors. *New Zealand Medical Journal*, 106:489–492.

Tyan ML (1982) Differences in the reported frequencies of cleft lip plus cleft lip and palate in Asians born in Hawaii and the Continental United States. *Proceedings of the Society for Experimental Biology and Medicine*, 171:41–45.

Vanderas AP (1987) Incidence of cleft lip, cleft palate, and cleft lip and palate among races: a review. *Cleft Palate Journal*, 24:216–225.

Verma M, Chhatwal J, Singh D (1991) Congenital malformations-a retrospective study of 10,000 cases. *Indian Journal of Pediatrics*, 58:245–252.

Vesterby A et al. (1987) Congenital heart malformations in Jutland, Denmark: a three year necropsy study in children aged 0–14 years. *British Heart Journal* 58:653–658.

Weatherall JA (1982) A review of some effects of recent medical practices in reducing the numbers of children born with congenital abnormalities. *Health Trends*, 14:85–88.

Weatherall JAC, De Wals P, Lechat MF (1984) Evaluation of an information system for the surveillance of congenital malformations. *International Journal of Epidemiology*, 13:193–196.

World Bank (1993) *World Development Report 1993: investing in health*. New York, Oxford University Press for the World Bank.

Chapter 13

Unsafe Sex as a Risk Factor

Seth Berkley

Reproduction is one of the fundamental requirements of all forms of life. Without reproduction, life would cease. As such, there is a strong evolutionary biologic drive for reproduction and, for humans, this means sexual intercourse. Furthermore, sex is generally pleasurable and therefore desirable to most people. Yet, despite the universality and importance of sex, of all human behaviours, sexual behaviour may be the most complicated and most controversial. Standards of acceptable sexual behaviour vary by culture, economic and social status, gender and stage of life. These standards are part of the norms of the local culture. There are, however, often large differences between these norms and the practices that are followed. As a result, elaborate sexual rituals have been developed to rationalize these differences, and sexual activities are considered intensely private in most societies. Because of these values and the restrictions they place on discussing sexual behaviour, there are many gaps in our knowledge about this area.

Sexual intercourse also has another side. Pregnancy and childbirth can be hazardous for women. Gender relations around sexuality are complicated and can lead to violent behaviour. Furthermore, there are a number of infectious diseases that can be transmitted by sexual contact, many of which have severe sequelae. Thus, unsafe sexual activities can lead to a wide range of potentially harmful consequences ranging from social and/or physical discomfort and minor irritation, to life threatening illnesses or chronic psychological sequelae. Most of these consequences can be avoided by adherence to safe sexual practices, yet societies are often reluctant to openly discuss issues about sexuality or to teach safe sexual practices to their young adults; hence, the adoption of safe sexual practices has been less than ideal.

With the recent epidemic of sexually transmitted HIV and the renewed attention that has been placed on other sexually transmitted diseases, there has been an increasing effort to attempt to provide sexual education as a way to avoid the very severe complications of unsafe sex. Yet, there has

Table 1 Infections and complications of unsafe sex

Included in this chapter	*Excluded from this chapter*
Classical sexually transmitted infections: HIV, gonorrhoea, syphilis, chlamydia	Other STDs: chancroid, trichomoniasis, lymphogranuloma venereum, Herpes simplex virus, non-specific vaginitis, etc.
Sexually transmitted hepatitis B	Sexual transmission of Hepatitis C
Sexually transmitted HPV*	Infant infections from HSV
Complications of pregnancy in those wanting to use contraception but not having access	Post-traumatic stress disorder from rape
Complications of therapeutic abortions	Complications of pregnancy in those wanting to have children
	Pyelonephritis in women from ascending urinary tract infections.
	Homicide and violence related to sexual activity
	Complications of contraception methods
	Failure of contraceptives
	Poor maternal health from too many pregnancies.
	Poor child health from too closely spaced births
	Premature delivery from bacterial vaginosis

*Human papilloma virus

been no attempt to look at the overall burden that results from unsafe sexual practices. This chapter will attempt to quantify these effects using the information from the disease-specific Global Burden of Disease Study (GBD) and available data on risk practices. The fundamental question this chapter will attempt to answer is: what is the attributable risk of unsafe sexual behaviour for overall morbidity and mortality? A careful and extensive search has not revealed any such previous exercise. Yet, it appears that the disease burden is not trivial. As there is little information available on this topic, the estimates reported here must be interpreted cautiously since they are based on very limited data. In addition, this attempt has been carried out within the constraints of the GBD exercise and as a result, some consequences that might have made an important contribution to the burden of unsafe sex are not included in these calculations, as they were not separately enumerated in the GBD project.

As mentioned above, all sexual relations have some potential risk. As sex is required for the survival of the species, it is not meaningful to classify all sexual activity as hazardous. Rather, it is assumed that what is desirable is to eliminate unsafe sexual activities altogether. This requires an arbitrary definition of which behaviours are unsafe, and which are not.

Table 2 Estimated percentage of total HIV cases due to sexual transmission (heterosexual or homosexual), by region, 1990

Region	*% of total cases*
EME	60
FSE	60
IND	80
CHN	40
OAI	80
SSA	80
LAC	65
MEC	80

Source: Author's estimates

Table 1 lists the infections and complications that have been included and excluded from the assessment. The list of conditions included is necessarily rather limited. In fact, there are many other diseases that are the result of unsafe sex. This exercise has used a very narrow definition of safe sex: Safe sex is defined as consensual sexual contact with a partner who is not infected with any sexually transmitted pathogens and involving the use of appropriate contraceptives to prevent pregnancy unless the couple is intentionally attempting to have a child. Of the list of conditions not included in this review, some would legitimately be included if data were available (e.g. HSV, chancroid, violence related to sexual activity), while others should clearly not be included in the calculations (e.g. unavoidable complications from the appropriate use of modern contraceptives). Some of the exclusions relate to our inability to accurately define (with broad scientific consensus) what is unsafe behaviour (e.g. where to draw the cut-off for safe versus unsafe birth spacing).

HIV/AIDS

For the purposes of this review, all sexually transmitted (heterosexual and homosexual) HIV is considered to be from unsafe sex. Excluded from this analysis are infections arising from contact with infected blood including intravenous drug use. Table 2 presents the per cent of transmission that is estimated to be sexual in the different regions.

The GBD included secondary infections transmitted from mothers to infants as part of the overall burden of HIV. Some of these cases, however, were not due to infection of the mother through sexual contact. Including the full burden of maternal to child transmission would therefore overestimate the overall burden of unsafe sex and thus we have attempted to adjust the maternal transmission burden according to the estimated percentage of female transmission that is sexually acquired. As there are few data to reliably estimate this fraction for different regions,

Table 3 Estimated percentage of HIV transmission in females due to sexual contact, by region, 1990

Region	*% of total transmission*
EME	75
FSE	85
IND	95
CHN	85
OAI	95
SSA	95
LAC	85
MEC	95

Source: Author's estimates

conservative assumptions have been chosen and these must be considered very crude estimates (see Table 3).

Using the estimates from the Global Burden of Disease Study for HIV, including the adjustment for sexual transmission and maternal sexual transmission by region, the estimates of deaths and DALYs shown in Table 4 represent the burden from unsafe sex (including maternal transmission) attributed to HIV.

Classic bacterial sexually transmitted diseases (chlamydia, gonorrhoea and syphilis)

All of this transmission is considered to be sexual and all transmission is considered to be related to unsafe sex. The numbers involved (see Table 5) are the same as in Chapter 2 in this volume, except for the inclusion in these estimates of neonatal complications from sexually transmitted diseases (STDs), such as neonatal pneumonia, low birth weight and ectopic pregnancy, which in the GBD were listed under the burden of neonatal complications and maternal conditions respectively.

STDs are a major component of the burden. In 1990, there were over 412 000 deaths and almost 24 million DALYs lost. Most of the burden is seen in women and children (22.3 million or 90 per cent). Children account for a full 50 per cent of the burden (12.5 million DALYs). Of the adult burden, 96 per cent is in the most productive age group (15–44 years).

Human papilloma virus (HPV)

The means to diagnose HPV infection have only recently become available outside of the research setting. As a result, the incidence and prevalence of HPV are not reliably known, particularly in developing countries. Infection begins at an early age (at the onset of sexual activity) and in-

Table 4 Global burden of unsafe sex (heterosexual and homosexual) attributed to HIV infection, by region, 1990

Region	*DALYs (in '000s)*	*Deaths*
EME	760.4	24 877
FSE	24.6	592
IND	188.4	436
CHN	1.4	0
OAI	94.5	219
SSA	6 696.1	190 901
LAC	708.4	19 028
MEC	37.4	478
WORLD	8 511.2	236 531

Table 5 Global burden of unsafe sex (heterosexual and homosexual) attributed to classical bacterial STDs (chlamydia, gonorrhoea and syphilis), by region, 1990

Region	*DALYs (in '000s)*	*Deaths*
EME	423.9	1 024
FSE	449.0	2 277
IND	7 264.4	119 416
CHN	128.4	1 298
OAI	5 125.2	77 749
SSA	8 951.6	170 985
LAC	1 497.4	20 590
MEC	982.6	19 368
WORLD	24 822.6	412 728

creases to reach highest prevalence quickly. The few international studies that are available suggest very high numbers of infections. The type of diagnostic methods available in a clinical setting has a major impact on the prevalence observed. For example, a study in Denmark and Greenland reported HPV using ViraPap in 4.8 and 3.9 per cent respectively of random samples of 150 women aged 20–39 years (Schiffman et al. 1993). When type-specific Polymerase Chain Reaction (PCR) techniques were used, the total HPV detection rates in the same population 38.9 per cent and 43.4 per cent. As PCR is still a research technique and rarely used in clinical field settings, most studies will grossly underestimate the prevalence of HPV.

HPV infections can cause morbidity directly through clinical physical manifestation of warts. Warts can be localized and may only cause minor discomfort or can be widespread over the genital area, mouth and other parts of the body. Infants born to mothers with HPV infection can develop laryngeal warts and require costly and potentially hazardous surgery. It is, however, the association of HPV with cervical and penile cancer which is of most concern. Cervical cancer continues to be a problem in developed countries, despite the availability and use of PAP screening; more alarmingly, in developing countries, cervical cancer is a leading cause of cancer in women and leads to particularly high morbidity and mortality. Cervical cancer in 1990 was responsible for 5.4 million lost DALYs and over 200 000 deaths.

Only certain types of HPV are associated with an increased risk of cervical cancer. Because of problems with HPV diagnosis and the long time lag between infection and the onset of cancer, the attributable risk of HPV for cancer is difficult to estimate.

Most studies have shown the presence of HPV to be related to cervical dysplasia and most pathologists consider cervical dysplasia to be a precancerous condition (Nelson et al. 1989). Some cases of cervical dysplasia revert back to normal histology, but many progress. Progression is from dysplasia, to cervical intra-epithelial neoplasia (CIN) to invasive cancer. Further studies are needed to better understand the mechanisms and causes of progression.

In a study to assess risk factors for high-grade cervical dysplasia among southwestern Hispanic and non-Hispanic white women, the leading risk factor was cervical HPV infection detected by ELISA (odds ratio of 12.8) or PCR (odds ratio 20.8) (Becker et al. 1994). For the Hispanic women, the presence of HPV 16/18 was extremely strongly associated with cervical dysplasia (odds ratio 171).

Similar findings were seen in a study in Brazil. The adjusted odds ratio of cervical cancer associated with HPV 16, 18, 31 and 33 was 69.7 while for the unidentified types the odds ratio was 12 (Eluf-Neto et al. 1994).

In a large case-control study of HPV and cervical intra-epithelial neoplasia (CIN) carried out under the Kaiser Permanente health plan using PCR technology, 76 per cent of the cases were attributed to HPV infection. Review of cytopathologic material suggested that if the cytologic misclassification of condylomatous atypia were eliminated, the attributable risk would be even higher.

In fully developed squamous cancers of the cervix, HPV can be isolated from the cells of 95 per cent of the cases (Nelson et al. 1989). Presumed cervical squamous cell cancer precursors contain HPV in approximately 90 per cent of cases (Nelson et al. 1989). Recent studies using the most advanced microbiologic techniques for identifying HPV are reporting viral sequences in virtually all of the cases of cervical carcinoma. Most cases of CIN are likely to be caused by or require as a co-factor, HPV infection. The difficulty of diagnosis of both the HPV infection as well as CIN may account for a least some of the small percentage of CIN cases that are thought to have occurred without any exposure to HPV. On the contrary, not all cases of infection with HPV (even the strains which are closely associated with carcinogenesis) will lead to cancer. The other co-factors for oncogenesis are not well known but may include exposure to other sexually transmitted agents, smoking, increasing parity, diet, socio-economic status and race.

HPV and HIV are inter-related. Although HPV infection does not seem to increase the risk of HIV transmission, the presence of HIV infection in those co-infected with HPV increases the likelihood of HPV disease. Women infected with HIV have at least a ten fold increased risk of active HPV infection and a 12-fold increased risk of cervical dysplasia compared with uninfected women (Laga et al. 1992). HPV infection and cervical disease may also proceed more rapidly and be more refractory to treatment in women with HIV (Vernon et al. 1993). This modifier-effect has not been taken into account in this study, however, as heterosexual transmission of HIV continues to increase, the epidemic of cervical carcinoma is likely to accelerate and may contribute to higher rates of HPV transmission.

For the purposes of this study, it is estimated that 90 per cent of cases of cervical carcinoma are linked to acquired HPV infection which can be attributed to unsafe sexual practices. As the burden of penile cancer has not been estimated in the GBD and the link between HPV and penile cancer is much less clear and it is a relatively rare disease, penile cancer has been excluded the estimates.

Table 6 presents the estimates of DALYs and deaths from unsafe sex attributed to cervical carcinoma resulting from HPV infection, based on the estimates from the Global Burden of Disease for cervical carcinoma by region.

HEPATITIS B VIRUS

Hepatitis B virus (HBV) occurs throughout the world. Like HIV, transmission can occur via blood-borne exposure, sexual intercourse or from mother to child. Transmission of hepatitis B is much more efficient than

Table 6 Global burden of unsafe sex attributed to cervical carcinoma resulting from HPV infection, by region, 1990

Region	*DALYs (in '000s)*	*Deaths*
EME	173.2	14 077
FSE	167.3	13 827
IND	684.5	43 741
CHN	244.4	18 983
OAI	453.2	29 928
SSA	390.6	29 784
LAC	339.4	22 187
MEC	116.1	7 519
WORLD	2 568.8	180 045

HIV. Hepatitis B can cause both an acute infection and a chronic infection. Chronic infection is a major cause of chronic active hepatitis, cirrhosis and primary hepatocellular carcinoma and ultimately death. There are differences in how the immune system deals with infections acquired in childhood versus those acquired later in life. Infections which occur at birth will lead to the chronic carrier state 70–90 per cent of the time and infection during the first year of life has a high probability of leading to chronic infection. Conversely, infections acquired during adolescence and adulthood only lead to a chronic carrier state in about 5-10 per cent of cases (Kane et al. 1998). Most liver cancers associated with hepatitis B infection occur after a latent period of several decades. As a result, chronic infections acquired late in life may not have adequate time for progression to carcinoma. The incidence rate of primary hepatocellular carcinoma is quite low in those who acquire infections during adulthood probably as result of this latency as well as the different immunologic responses to the infection.

Transmission patterns vary by population. In countries where HBV is endemic, most transmission occurs from mother to child and only a small percentage occurs in adulthood. Due to the high prevalence of infection, however, the numbers of infections acquired in adulthood are not trivial. In countries with low rates of infection, infections are most often acquired in adulthood and sexual transmission is usually the most common route (Alter et al. 1986). Parenteral transmission is of concern in some populations although those at risk are usually less than those at risk through sexual contact. Because of the efficiency of transmission, hepatitis B is not only transmitted commonly through the reuse of shared injection equipment by intravenous drug users, but also in medical settings where nonsterile injection or skin piercing equipment is used. The ease of transmission means that health care personnel are also at high risk of iatrogenically-acquired infections.

Patterns of transmission are changing in those countries with low rates of infection. For example, in the United States, a study of hepatitis B in sentinel counties from 1981 to 1988 demonstrated a reduction in transmission through homosexual activity and health care employment and an increase in transmission through recreational parenteral drug use and heterosexual activity (80 per cent and 38 per cent respectively) (Alter et al. 1990). As Figure 1 shows, 26 per cent of transmission was from heterosexual contact, 7 per cent from homosexual contact and 37 per cent was transmission from unknown means. Thus sexual transmission accounted for almost half of the transmission. In areas without much recreational parenteral drug use, it is likely that the percentage attributed to sexual transmission would be much higher.

In populations where endemic transmission is common, but where vaccination of the population has already occurred, the pattern of hepatitis B transmission resembles that of less endemic areas. For example, in Taiwan, 15–20 per cent of the general population are HBV carriers. Before

Figure 1 Methods of transmission of hepatitis B in four U.S. counties, 1981–1988

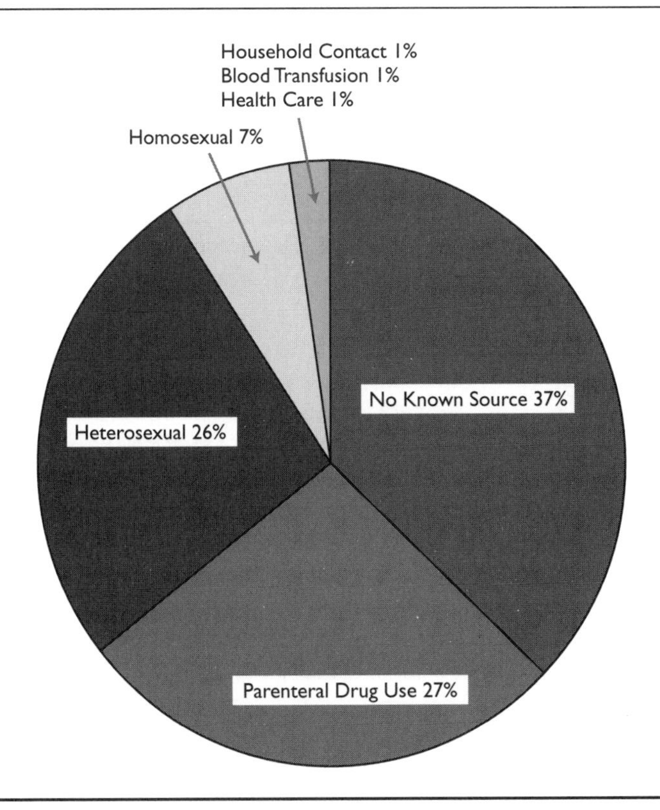

mass hepatitis B vaccination, most infections were acquired from birth. Now after vaccination, only about 20 per cent of the adult population are still susceptible to infection. In a study of risk factors for adults with acute infection, heterosexual contact was now the only factor in 83 per cent of the cases (Hou et al. 1993). However, global coverage with hepatitis B vaccine is probably not sufficient to yet affect transmission patterns substantially. For this chapter, we have ignored the effects of hepatitis B vaccination and have not stratified endemic countries according to the prevalence of hepatitis B vaccination. Rather, the attributable risks shown in Table 7 have been applied to the estimated percentage of hepatitis B cases associated with unsafe sex.

Using the estimates from the Global Burden of Disease for hepatitis B infections by region Table 8 presents DALYs and deaths from unsafe sex in 1990 that have been attributed to sexual transmission of hepatitis B infections.

Hepatitis C is becoming an increasingly common cause of hepatitis and a significant percentage of transmission is sexual. Unfortunately, as the etiologic agent has only recently been identified and the availability of test-

Table 7 Estimated percentage of cases of hepatitis B associated with unsafe sex, by endemicity

*Endemicity**	*Percentage associated with unsafe sex*
High (>5%)	5
Intermediate (2-5%)	20
Low (<2%)	60

* categories from Kane et al. 1998

Table 8 Global burden of unsafe sex attributed to sexual transmission of hepatitis B, by region, 1990

Region	*DALYs (in '000s)*	*Deaths*
EME	170.0	13 437
FSE	208.6	15 301
IND	368.2	19 458
CHN	286.3	18 974
OAI	129.6	7 870
SSA	60.8	3 470
LAC	71.7	3 581
MEC	144.4	7 948
WORLD	1 439.5	90 038

ing is limited, very little is known about the global incidence and prevalence of this infection. As a result, we have not attempted to include this agent in the calculations for unsafe sex.

Unintended Pregnancies

World-wide there are large numbers of women who become pregnant unintentionally. Some of these are caused by to contraceptive failure. Modern effective contraceptive methods (pill, IUD, foam, condom, Norplant and hormonal injectibles) have a low failure rate of 5–7/100 women when used correctly. As some failures are considered unavoidable due to the inherent limitations of these methods of contraception, complications of pregnancies resulting from use of these methods have not been considered in the burden of unsafe sex in this chapter.

Others pregnancies which we will count as unsafe sex, include those that occur from intentional non-use of contraception (being sexually active, but denying the personal risk of pregnancy) or from lack of knowledge about or access to contraception. Women who have these non-intended pregnancies tend to be poorer and more disadvantaged.

For example, in the United States, where the data are relatively good, it is estimated that fifty-five per cent of the six million pregnancies in 1980 were unwanted (World Health Organization Collaborating Center in

Perinatal Care and Health Service Research in Maternal and Child Care 1987). Of these, 27 per cent were in women who did not want another pregnancy and 73 per cent were in women who became pregnant before they wanted to become pregnant. More than 376 000 infants, 1 in 10 of all live births were born to women who did not want another child. The demographics of this are startling. Four of every 10 women became pregnant in their teens, 80 per cent of which were unintentional. These pregnancies are occurring disproportionately in poor households: black women are 2.5 times more likely to have an unintentional pregnancy than white women and poor women are twice as likely as other women. These are the groups least able to bear the cost and who will have the highest number of high risk (for mother and child) pregnancies. If all sexually active couples in the United States had used routinely one of the effective methods, the number of unintended pregnancies would have decreased from 2.4 million to 900 000; more than a 65 per cent reduction.

Unfortunately, good data are not widely available. Over the last two decades, however, a series of Demographic and Health Surveys (DHS) have been carried out in over 40 countries and serve as the primary source of data for fertility patterns, attitudes about pregnancy and use of contraceptives.

Of any group of women, there are some who at a given time, are sexually active, but are not using contraception and yet wish to control their fertility—either to postpone the next wanted birth or to prevent unwanted pregnancies after having the desired number of children. These women are defined as the fraction of the population with an "unmet need" for contraception (Westoff and Bankole 1995) and whose pregnancies contribute to unsafe sex. Unfortunately these studies are mostly carried out in women who are in union (either formal or informal) and some explicitly exclude unmarried women who are likely to have much higher levels of unmet need. Tables 9 and 10 summarize the data that are available from studies that have been carried oute in women 15–44 years old.

To adjust for unmet need in unmarried persons, we have assumed a large part of the primary demand for contraception would be in young and sexually active women and have added to these levels 15 per cent in Sub-Saharan Africa and Other Asia and Islands and 10 per cent in Latin America and the Caribbean, India, the Established Market Economies and the Formerly Socialist Economies of Europe and 5 per cent in the Middle Eastern Crescent and 2 per cent in China to account for this factor. It is still likely that this is an underestimate of the percentage of the unmarried population who are sexually active and not using modern methods of contraception and therefore are at risk of becoming, but do not wish to be pregnant. More data are needed globally to better understand the need for, and use of contraception in this group. We have also ignored the numbers of women below, 15 and above 44 years who are sexually active, fertile and have an unmet need for contraception.

Table 9 Estimated unmet contraceptive need in currently married women (in %), around 1990

Region	*Number of DHS studies*	*Range*	*Average*
EME		—	5*
FSE		—	5*
IND		—	15*
CHN		—	1*
OAI	3	11-16	14
SSA	9	21-40	32
MEC	3	20-25	23
LAC	10	13-36	20

* *Source:* Author's estimate based on DHS and other studies

Table 10 Total unmet need for contraception expressed as a percentage of women aged 15–44 years, by region

Region	*% unmet need*
EME	15
FSE	15
IND	25
CHN	3
OAI	29
SSA	47
LAC	30
MEC	28

Source: Author's estimates from unmet need data

Although complications of pregnancy will tend to cluster in those women of lower socio-economic status, we have assumed an equal distribution throughout the population for the purposes of estimating this burden. The effects of this assumption on the calculations are unknown but may well underestimate the burden as those who have an unmet need probably have less prenatal care, poorer nutrition and less access to health services and thus will have a higher pregnancy complication rate. We then used the GBD estimates for complications of pregnancy in women in each of these regions and adjusted them on the basis of these estimates. Table 11 summarizes the estimated DALYs and deaths from unsafe sex that can be attributed to complications of pregnancy in those women not wanting to be pregnant but not using an appropriate form of contraception.

Table 11 Global burden of unsafe sex attributed to complications of pregnancy in women with an unmet need for contraception, by region, 1990

Region	*DALYs (in '000s)*	*Deaths*
EME	47.3	91
FSE	59.8	133
IND	1 389.2	22 367
CHN	76.3	830
OAI	698.4	11 592
SSA	3 131.1	62 584
LAC	367.6	4 126
MEC	915.6	12 259
WORLD	6 885.3	113 983

ABORTIONS

This section only deals with disease burden due to therapeutic abortion, and does not consider any complications resulting from spontaneous abortions in women with desired pregnancies. Most of the morbidity and mortality from therapeutic abortions—whether medically or non-medically performed—probably occurs due to pregnancies resulting from unsafe sexual practices. Theoretically one should exclude the small number of abortions that result from inherent failure rates of properly used modern contraceptive methods. Unfortunately it is difficult to disaggregate the different reasons for seeking abortions and it probably can be safely assumed that the vast number of therapeutic abortions are not the result of inherent failure of properly used methods, but rather from non-use or improperl use. Even where data are available, however, abortion is difficult to study. Because of the stigma associated with abortion, reasons given for women seeking abortions may not accurately reflect the true situation.

Induced abortion on request is common in many countries of the world (40 per cent of the world's population live in countries where induced abortion is permitted on request), but almost all of these are developed countries (the exceptions being Cuba, China, Vietnam, Togo, and Tunisia) (Cleland and Benoit 1995). In other countries, menstrual regulation is permitted or abortion is permitted with only minimal social or medical justification. Fifty-three countries accounting for 25 per cent of the world's population restrict abortion to cases when it is necessary to save a women's life. In 1987, it was estimated that 26–31 million legal abortions were performed. In addition, there were between 10–22 million illegal abortions performed. These unsafe abortions are defined as those abortions not provided through approved facilities and/or persons. Mortality from legal abortion is generally low however, this partially relates to the quality of health services in the countries that permit abortion. In developed countries, mortality for legal abortion averages 0.6 deaths per 100 000 procedures (Henshaw and Morrow 1990). In developing countries, this figure might be 4–6 times higher. This compares to illegal abortion procedures where the death rate may be 50–500 times higher than that of an abortion performed professionally under safe conditions. The reasons for which women seek abortions vary by region. In most EME countries, about half of the abortions are obtained by young unmarried women seeking to delay a first birth, while in the FSE and many developing countries, abortion is most common among married women with two or more children.

Although information on the global number of abortions and abortion rates are incomplete, Table 12 lists what is known for a sub-sample of representative countries. Using the estimates from the Global Burden of Disease Study for complications from abortions by region results in the numbers of DALYs and deaths from unsafe sex shown in Table 13 that can be attributed to abortions.

Results

Globally, in 1990, unsafe sexual activity is estimated to have accounted for over one million deaths (2 per cent of all deaths worldwide) and close to 50 million lost disability adjusted life years (about 3.5 per cent of global DALYs lost in that year). The heaviest burdens occurs in females and infants and in the age group 15–44 years. Females account for 71 per cent of the overall disease burden from unsafe sex. If one includes females 15–44 and their infants, they account for 75 per cent of the burden. Overall, the age group 15–44 years accounts for 38 per cent of the deaths but 63 per cent of DALYs attributed to unsafe sex. This disparity between morbidity and mortality arises due to the rather large amount of mortality in newborns from the effects of sexually transmitted diseases and in those over 60 years from resulting carcinomas.

It is, within the 15–44 year old age group, a normally healthy and productive period of life, where the most severe effects of these unsafe sexual activities can be seen. In females in this age group, 12 per cent of the deaths and 15 per cent of the DALYs lost are due to conditions related to unsafe sex. In Sub-Saharan Africa, this proportion rises to 26 per cent of the deaths and 30 per cent of the DALY loss. This high burden is not only confined to Africa. In India, it is estimated that about 11 per cent of deaths and 20 per cent of DALYs at ages 15–44 can be attributed to unsafe sexual activity and even in Latin America and the Caribbean, the figures are 9 per cent and 14 per cent respectively. Tables 14 and 15 provide further detail on the burden of unsafe sex in those aged 15–44 years by region.

Many of the most severe sequelae (pelvic inflammatory disease, cervical carcinoma, infertility and abortions) occur in females. However, because of HIV infection and liver carcinoma from hepatitis B infection, the burden of unsafe sex for males is also comparatively high.

Table 12 Number and rate of legal abortions in selected countries

Country	*Number*	*Rate**
United States (1985)	1 588 600	28
United Kingdom (1987)	156 200	14.2
Germany (1984)	96 200	26.6
China (1987)	10 394 500	38.8
Tunisia (1988)	23 300	13.6
Vietnam (1980)	170 600	14.6
India (1987)#	588 400	3.0
France (1987)#	161 000	13.3
Poland (1987)#	122 600	14.9
Soviet Union (1982)^	11 000 000	181
Bangladesh (1986)^	241 400	12
Japan^	2 250 000	84

* per 1 000 women aged 15-44
# incomplete or poor statistics
^ by survey

Table 13 Global burden of unsafe sex attributed to therapeutic abortion (both medical and non-medical), by region, 1990

Region	*DALYs (in '000s)*	*Deaths*
EME	11.9	102
FSE	157.8	1 020
IND	1 600.4	17 037
CHN	76.5	2 539
OAI	775.2	6 959
SSA	1 674.5	25 179
LAC	445.3	4 344
MEC	355.9	3 998
WORLD	5 097.5	61 177

Table 14 Global burden of unsafe sex in those aged 15-44 years, 1990

Region	*DALYs (in '000s)*	*Deaths*
EME	1 592.4	21 813
FSE	1 048.5	5 189
IND	9 543.5	67 461
CHN	520.2	9 923
OAI	6 574.4	36 343
SSA	14 736.9	226 522
LAC	3 186.5	31 355
MEC	2 035.0	19 471
WORLD	39 237.4	418 077

Table 15 Estimated burden of disease attributable to unsafe sex in 15-44 year olds, by region, 1990

	Males				*Females*			
Region	**DALYs**	**% of Total**	**Deaths**	**% of Total**	**DALYs**	**% of Total**	**Deaths**	**% of Total**
EME	615.0	3	16 165	5	977.3	6	5 648	4
FSE	125.8	1	1 183	2	922.7	10	4 006	5
IND	1 767.6	5	3 914	1	7 776.0	20	63 547	11
CHN	120.7	<1	3 079	<1	399.5	1	6 844	1
OAI	1 221.8	4	1 517	<1	5 352.6	19	34 826	10
SSA	3 369.8	9	52 600	7	11 367.1	30	173 922	26
LAC	760.0	4	12 681	4	2 426.5	14	18 674	9
MEC	170.6	1	1 140	<1	1 864.4	10	18 331	7
WORLD	8 151.3	4	92 280	3	31 086.1	15	325 797	12

Table 16 Global burden of unsafe sex attributed to specific diseases, 1990

	Males		*Females*		*Total*	
Disease	**DALYs**	**Deaths**	**DALYs**	**Deaths**	**DALYs**	**Deaths**
HIV/AIDS	4 555.6	127 827	3 955.6	108 704	8 511.2	236 531
Classical bacterial STDs	8 915.0	182 803	15 907.6	229 925	24 822.6	412 728
Human papilloma virus infections	0*	0*	2 568.8	180 045	2 568.8	180 045
Hepatitis B infections	980.4	59 360	479.2	30 678	1 439.5	90 038
Complications of unintended pregnancies	0	0	6 885.2	113 983	6 885.2	113 983
Complications of therapeutic abortions	0	0	5 097.5	61 177	5 097.5	61 177
Total	12 004.3	369 990	36 698.0	724 512	48 702.3	1 094 502

* See discussion in HPV section, burden in males not included.

Figures 2 and 3 and Table 16 demonstrates the distribution of the burden and deaths by disease group.

Estimating the burden of unsafe sex

This chapter has attempted to provide an estimate of the burden of disease that can be attributed to unsafe sexual practices. The magnitude of the resultant disease burden from unsafe sex is substantial, with over 1 million deaths per year and almost 50 million DALYs. All of this is preventable. The significance of the burden of unsafe sex is not only due to its magnitude but also because its effects are largely felt in the most produc-

Figure 2 Estimated distribution of causes of death due to unsafe sex, 1990

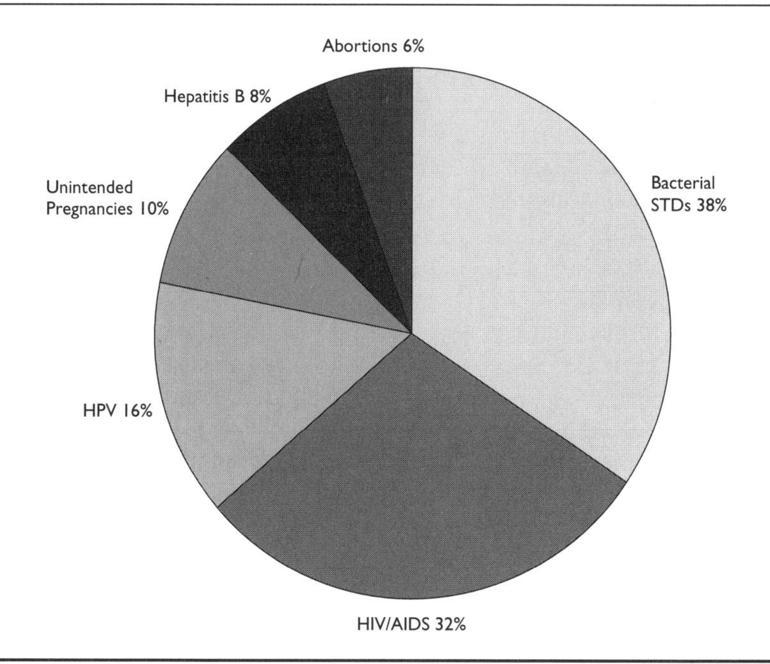

Figure 3 Estimated distribution of causes of DALYs due to unsafe sex, 1990

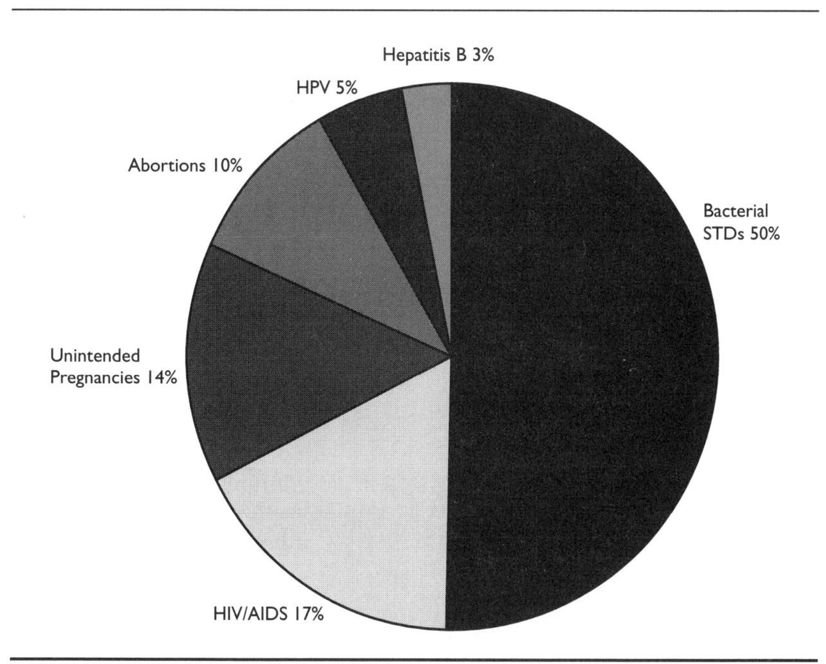

tive age groups of 15–44 years and in children. A dramatic difference in burden between the sexes is seen in reproductive health conditions. For males, unsafe sex accounts for only about one-quarter of the burden seen in females. Furthermore, in females 15–44 years, the disease burden from unsafe sex is not only extremely large, but until recently, relatively unrecognized.

The high burden of disease arising from unsafe sexual practices is not unexpected. Nonetheless, the estimates reported here are still subject to biases and confounding.

Obviously, if any of the diseases that are being considered as part of the burden of unsafe sex are themselves over reported, that alone would lead to an overestimate of the burden of unsafe sex. This is unlikely, however. We have attempted to be conservative in our calculations related to each of the individual diseases. In addition, external controls on the overall global burden of disease exercise assure at least internal consistency (for example, for deaths this means that the total of all deaths in each age group of all the diseases being studied as part of the global burden study must sum to the currently expected values).

It is possible that the percentages of these diseases attributed to sexual transmission or as risk factors are too high. For example, there will be controversy as to the attributable risk of HPV for cervical cancer. This field is changing, however, with the development of science. In the past, HPV was considered a minor factor. Now with better methods, pieces of the HPV genome can be identified in almost all cases of cervical cancer.

Finally, some percentage of the pregnancies that are terminated by unsafe abortion will be due to the failure of modern methods of contraception that are being correctly used. Given our framework, these should not be considered to be cases of unsafe sex. It is difficult to determine what this per cent is likely to be, but in any case, it is likely to be far less than the number of abortions that occur because of non-use or incorrect use of contraception.

The disease burden due to unsafe sex may also be under-reported here. Excluding the complications of desired pregnancies and of the unplanned failure of modern forms of contraception will omit a substantial burden of disease associated with sexual behaviour. In fact, some non-trivial percentage of these complications could also be classified as unsafe sexual behaviour. For example, pregnancy occurring too soon after the previous birth increases the risk of adverse complications for the mother, newborn and older children in the family. Having more than five children also dramatically increases the risk of maternal mortality and therefore having sexual relations without contraception, even if a pregnancy is wanted in those multiparous women, could be considered unsafe sex. One could also plausibly argue that the use of less reliable contraception (e.g. a diaphragm) could be considered less safe sex than using a more reliable method of contraception and we could, therefore, include the unwanted pregnancies and the complications that occur through the use of these less effective methods. As a result, the overall figures calculated in this chapter may well be an underestimation of the actual burden of unsafe sex.

Moreover, due to data availability, this chapter follows a rather strict definition of unsafe sex. If information were available on other diseases such as the proportion of sexually transmitted hepatitis C, the complications of non-specific bacterial vaginal infections, herpetic infections in newborns, and the psychiatric manifestations of unsafe sexual activities, there would undoubtedly be a further increase in the burden.

OTHER FACTORS THAT MIGHT INFLUENCE THE BURDEN OF UNSAFE SEX

Clearly there are other risk factors that influence unsafe sexual behaviour. These most notably include alcohol and the use of other drugs. There has been no attempt in this chapter to exclude the complications of unsafe sex in those who conduct unsafe sexual practices under the influence of these behaviour altering agents. It is likely, however, that in many societies a substantial percentage of unsafe sexual activities are conducted under the influence of these agents. But because we have estimated the burden by choosing attributable percentages from the diseases and their outcome rather than starting with modeling outcomes from their behaviours, we think this is unlikely to bias our estimates.

An interesting comparison would be to attempt to measure the burden of unsafe sex by starting with an analysis of known unsafe sexual behaviour in different parts of the world. From that, one could theoretically determine what proportion of sex is unsafe and then calculate number of contacts, transmission rates and ultimate disease cases and burden. Unfortunately, given current levels of knowledge this would be extremely difficult if not impossible to do. Knowledge about sexual behaviour in different parts of the world is rudimentary. Population-based studies are difficult to perform in many societies and as a result, there are serious reporting biases. At the beginning of the 1980s, the only broadly representative population based data available were the Kinsey data from the United States (already more than two decades old), and the World Fertility Survey. Since then, population based data on broad trends have been collected through the Demographic and Health Surveys. Unfortunately, these surveys target their questions primarily at married women and focus on fertility related behaviour (although questions on risk for HIV have been added recently). As a result, there are few comparable cross country data on sexuality, although some useful information has emerged dfrom a recent survey of behaviour in 13 countries coordinated by WHO/GPA (Cleland and Benoit 1995).

There are also a number of second-order consequences of unsafe sex that we have ignored. For example, the sexually transmitted epidemic of HIV sustains and increases the epidemic of tuberculosis. As a result of these infections, numbers of tuberculosis cases will rise. Furthermore, a number of sexually transmitted diseases such as syphilis and chancroid are more difficult to diagnose and treat in persons with HIV. As a result, these diseases are likely to increase.

Sexual Behaviour

Coexistent with the worldwide trend of globalization, there have been dramatic changes in sexual behaviour around the world. Some of these are global trends such as changes in the age of menarche, age at first intercourse, family size, use of contraception, and age at marriage. Others are highly variable and very culture specific. As a result there are important differences within countries and between countries. The age at menarche has been decreasing in both developed and developing countries. This has been attributed to changes in health and nutrition. This means that women are fertile at a younger age which may predispose them to early intercourse. This increases the period during which they are at risk of unsafe sex. There is also evidence that the age of first sexual intercourse has also been decreasing in many parts of the world, and this may not be linked to the changes in age at menarche (Sogolow et al. 1996). Despite this general trend, there remain enormous cultural differences in the age at the onset of sexual activity. For example, 10 per cent of never married males and females aged 15–19 years are sexually active in Burundi versus 69 per cent in Guinea Bissau (Cleland and Benoit 1995). In Asia, rates of early sexual activity tend to be lower but also vary dramatically from less than 5 per cent in Sri Lanka and Singapore where there exist enormous social sanctions against premarital intercourse to much higher rates (at least for males in Thailand) (Cleland and Benoit 1995). For example in Singapore, at age 20 years, 80 per cent of males and females report that they are sexually inexperienced and by age 25, 60 per cent remain so.

Concomitant with this trend towards early sexual activity, there have been dramatic global changes in family size—both desired and actual. The large and extended family characteristic of rural agricultural societies has been replaced by smaller families with less traditional values. This means that early childbearing may not always be desired. The wide availability and use of modern contraceptive methods has permitted the development of a new level of sexual freedom in many populations. This combined with a global trend towards an increasing age of marriage has meant that the opportunity for unsafe sex and the increased spread of sexually transmitted diseases particularly for adolescents has increased. Unfortunately, despite the onset of the AIDS epidemic and the resultant wave of studies of AIDS risk behaviours, there is still a sense of moral puritanism about discussing and studying sexuality, particularly in adolescents. As a result, there are few systematic studies of human sexuality or STDs in many developed and developing countries. This is unfortunate given the evidence of increasing STD transmission among adolescents in many parts of the world (Sanches et al. 1996).

Adolescents are especially at high risk of the complications of unsafe sex. Sexual norms vary widely among adolescents. Among unmarried individuals, available data suggest that age of sexual debut varies enormously, both within and across countries. Data from 14 surveys of sexual behaviour in developing countries carried out by the former WHO Global Programme on AIDS found that among males 15–19 years old, those reporting intercourse in the past 12 months varied from 1 to 69 per cent, and among females, from 0 to 56 per cent. The differences among the 9 sites in sub-Saharan Africa were very large, suggesting that the tendency to characterize this region as one of overall high sexual activity is misleading. These surveys also found that urban-rural patterns in sexual activity among 15–19 year olds were far more variable than the common expectation that urbanization encourages more relaxed sexual mores.

With respect to sexual orientation, the picture is also quite mixed. Tolerance for homosexuality and bi-sexuality is highly variable, although, in general, tolerance is generally lower in developing than in developed countries. The implications on the burden of unsafe sex from those practicing homosexuality is unclear. Male homosexuality appears to be associated with an increased risk of transmission of sexually transmitted agents, but will obviously not have the reproductive complications associated with infections in women. It is likely that homosexuality will increase the disease burden in males, but decrease it in females and so the effect on overall burden is unclear. The actual prevalence of the practices of homosexuality and bisexuality is only beginning to be documented in developing countries; research carried out since the onset of the HIV epidemic is revealing significant homosexual behaviour in many countries.

We have also not attempted to take into account here the burden arising from those practicing commercial sex. Clearly these persons are at higher risk for the sexually transmitted pathogens and their complications. They are also at higher risk of other complications such as sexually related violence that are not included in the burden estimates. These fators will have a multiplier effect on transmission. They serve effectively as a core group with enough frequency of contact to sustain high levels of sexually transmitted infections. In any population, however, the numbers of persons providing commercial sexual services will be small. In addition, in many countries, there has been active condom promotion in this group with the result that rates of disease transmission may be reduced.

Concluding Remarks

Interventions to reduce the burden of unsafe sex include the provision of sex education, and promoting the availability of condoms and other modern forms of contraception. The implications of providing these interventions varies. For example, the use of oral contraceptives results in a dramatic decrease in unsafe pregnancies, but has little impact on HIV and other sexually transmitted diseases. Condoms, as compared with oral contraceptives, will provide a slightly reduced level of protection against pregnancy and the resultant potential complications, but also has a mitigating effect on the other sexually transmitted infections. As a result, in areas of high risk in Africa, health policy makers have called for the use of both at the same time, although this is costly and difficult to maintain. Careful studies are required to determine the overall effect of varying these different interventions.

Proper sexual education is critical. It is particularly important for adolescents as they are at the highest risk of complications of unsafe sex and of adopting sexual practices which may increase risk for the rest of their lives. In addition, specific interventions for different diseases associated with unsafe sex would reduce the burden. All of the burden of unsafe sex (at least as we have defined it here) could be removed by primary prevention. From a disease standpoint, this is obviously preferable. Equally important, however, is that a substantial proportion, perhaps up to 50–60 per cent of the burden is probably preventable by secondary and tertiary prevention such as early treatment of sexually transmitted infections. Furthermore, a number of the diseases that result from unsafe sex have their own primary interventions; for example, early immunization for hepatitis B. For those that have an unwanted pregnancy, the availability of safe and legal abortion services rather than resorting to illicit services would also reduce the burden associated with their unsafe sexual behaviour.

In summary, although sexual relations may well be pleasurable, unsafe sex accounts for a very substantial part of the global burden of disease—particularly for those in the most productive age groups. Women carry the vast majority of this burden and much of it is unrecognized. If it were possible to include the full range of conditions contributing to the actual unsafe sex burden, the estimates reported here would be even higher and probably even more concentrated in women. Unsafe sexual activities can be addressed through many possible interventions at the primary, secondary and tertiary level. Many of these are extremely cost effective but require greater political will to ensure their widespread application.

Acknowledgements

I would like to acknowledge Dr Jane Rowley for her enormous help with the work reported in this book on the global burden of STDs and of unsafe sex, Chris Murray and Dean Jamison for pushing me to examine unsafe sex as a risk factor, Chris Murray and Alan Lopez for the incredible work they have done to put the overall Global Burden of Disease Study together.

REFERENCES

Alter MJ et al. (1986) Hepatitis B virus transmission between heterosexuals. *Journal of the American Medical Association*, 125:1307–10.

Alter MJ et al. (1990) The changing epidemiology of hepatitis B in the United States. *Journal of the American Medical Association*, 263:1218–1222.

Becker TM et al. (1994) Sexually transmitted diseases and other risk factors for cervical dysplasia among southwestern Hispanic and non-Hispanic white women. *Journal of the American Medical Association*, 271:1181–8.

Cleland J, Benoit F, eds. (1995) *Sexual Behaviour and AIDS in the Developing World.* Taylor and Francis, London.

Eluf-Neto J et al. (1994) Human papillomavirus and invasive cervical cancer in Brazil. *British Journal of Cancer,* 69:114–9.

Henshaw SK, Morrow E (1990) Induced Abortion: A world review, 1990. *Family Planning Perspectives,* 22:76–89.

Hou MC et al. (1993) Heterosexual transmission as the most common route of acute hepatitis B virus infection among adults in Taiwan—the importance of extending vaccination to susceptible adults. *Journal of Infectious Diseases,* 167:938–41.

Kane MA, Schatz GC, Hadler SC. (1998) The global burden of disease from hepatitis B. In: Murray CJL, Lopez AD, eds. *The global epidemiology of infectious diseases.* Cambridge, Harvard University Press.

Kjaer SK et al. (1993) Human papilloma virus, herpes simplex virus and other potential risk factors for cervical cancer in a high risk area (Greenland) and a low risk area (Denmark)—a second look. *British Journal of Cancer,* 67:830–7.

Laga M et al. (1992) Genital papillomavirus infection and cervical dysplasia—opportunistic complications of HIV infection. *International Journal of Cancer,* 50:45–8.

Nelson JH, Averette HE, Richart RM. (1989) Cervical Intraepithelial Neoplasia (dysplasia and carcinoma in situ) and early invasive cervical carcinoma. *Cancer,* 39:157–178.

Sanches K, Matida A, Pires D (1996) Trends in the AIDS epidemic among adolescents in Rio de Janeiro state-Brazil. Abstract Tu.C.2621 in the Program and Abstracts of the XI International Conference on AIDS, Vancouver, Canada.

Schiffman MH et al. (1993) Epidemiologic evidence showing that human papillomavirus infection causes most cervical intraepithelial neoplasia. *Journal of the National Cancer Institute,* 85:958–964.

Sogolow E et al. (1996) Initiation of sexual intercourse: ages and trends. Abstract Th.C. 4446 in the Program and Abstracts of the XI International Conference on AIDS, Vancouver, Canada.

United Nations (1988) Adolescent Reproductive Behaviour: Evidence from Developed Countries, Vol. I. Population Studies no. 109. United Nations, New York.

United Nations (1989) Adolescent Reproductive Behaviour: Evidence from Developing Countries, Vol. II. Population Studies no. 109. Ad. 1. United Nations, New York.

Vernon SD et al. (1993) Human papillomavirus, human immunodeficiency virus, and cervical cancer: newly recognized associations? *Infectious Agents and Disease,* 1:319–324.

Westoff CF, Bankole A (1995) *Unmet Need: 1990–1994.* DHS Comparative Studies #16, Macrointernational Inc. Calverton, Maryland.

World Health Organization Collaborating Center in Perinatal Care and Health Service Research in Maternal and Child Care (1987) Unintended Pregnancy and Infant Mortality/Morbidity. *American Journal of Preventive Medicine,* 3(5):130–142.

Index

R